PROSTATE CANCER: NEW HORIZONS IN RESEARCH AND TREATMENT

Prostate Cancer: New Horizons in Research and Treatment

Edited by

MICHAEL L. CHER
The Barbara Ann Karmanos
Cancer Institute, Detroit, MI,
USA

KENNETH V. HONN
Wayne State University School
of Medicine, Detroit, MI,
USA

AVRAHAM RAZ
Wayne State University School
of Medicine, Detroit, MI,
USA

Springer-Science+Business Media, B.V.

Electronic Services <http://www.wkap.nl>

Library of Congress Cataloging-in-Publication Data

A C.I.P Catalogue record for this book is available from the
library of Congress

ISBN 978-1-4757-8511-1   ISBN 978-0-306-48143-7 (eBook)
DOI 10.1007/978-0-306-48143-7

Printed on acid-free paper

Contents

vi

Preface

The incidence of prostate cancer has declined recently in the United States. Due to sustained efforts at early detection, however, a large number of men around the world continue to be diagnosed every year with early stage tumors. Fortunately, aggressive treatment approaches aimed at eradicating the primary tumor are capable of rendering most men free of tumor recurrence indefinitely. Without a doubt, technical refinements in surgery and radiation have led to quantifiable improvements in the quality of life of men choosing organ-ablative local treatment. Nonetheless many men continue to suffer recurrence and eventually develop metastatic disease. In addition, a significant number of men have metastatic disease when their prostate cancer is first diagnosed. Many of our patients continue to die of prostate cancer, and disease- and treatment-related morbidity continues to extract a heavy toll on the men with this disease, their families, and society in general.

In the last few years, the pace of research in prostate cancer has increased dramatically. New and emerging technologies have combined together with novel ideas from creative scientists leading to an explosion of new discovery. For example, genome- and transcriptome-wide analyses have led to a tremendous expansion of links between the fields of tumor genetics and tumor biology. Within the area of tumor biology, scientists are now focusing on the relationship between tumor cells and the surrounding microenvironment. These studies have increased our understanding of the processes of angiogenesis, apoptosis, androgen insensitivity, tumor cell dissemination, and growth at distant sites. These types of advances in prostate cancer research presage an era of new treatment approaches based on an understanding of the cellular and molecular mechanisms of disease. We look forward to an era of exciting and innovative investigations into the biological mechansims of cancer. We will soon see enhanced treatment efficacy together with reduced systemic and local effects of the disease and its treatment.

In this book, we are pleased to provide a series of reviews covering current basic, translational, and clinically-oriented research in prostate cancer. These articles appeared recently in three issues of *Cancer and Metastasis Reviews* devoted exclusively to prostate cancer. We chose topics and authors based on a desire to provide timely, interesting, and useful information to all readers of *Cancer and Metastasis Reviews*. Our aim was to cover a spectrum of research issues ranging from genetic, molecular, and cellular analyses all the way to epidemiological studies, refinements in local treatment strategies, and new biologically based non-hormonal treatments for systemic disease. We hope that these reviews will appeal to all with an interest in prostate cancer, including clinicians, clinician-scientists, basic scientists, and men with prostate cancer, their families and supporters.

Michael L. Cher, M.D.
Wayne State University and
The Barbara Ann Karmanos Cancer Institute
Detroit, Michigan, USA

M.L. Cher, K.V. Honn and A. Raz (eds): Prostate Cancer: New Horizons in Research and Treatment, 1.
© 2002 *Kluwer Academic Publishers.*

Pathology of prostate cancer

Mingxin Che[1] and David Grignon[2]
[1]Department of Pathology, Wayne State University School of Medicine, Karmanos Cancer Institute
and Detroit Medical Center, Detroit, MI, USA

Key words: prostate cancer, pathology, biopsy, radical prostatectomy, diagnostic criteria, Gleason score,
prognostic factors

I. Introduction

Prostate cancer poses a significant public health problem. Although a minority of men with newly diagnosed prostate carcinoma manifest metastatic disease,
a significant proportion of men will develop these
complications over the course of their lives. Pathological evaluation of prostate cancer in biopsy and radical
prostatectomy specimens has provided the most valuable factors in predicting cancer behavior and guiding
clinical management of prostate cancer patients.

II. Diagnosis

Over the past decade, the sextant biopsy technique has
emerged as the standard of care in the detection of
prostate cancer. However, limitations in cancer detection have been appreciated, particularly a false-negative
rate approaching 25%. Currently, recommendations to
reduce the false negative rate have included increasing
the biopsy number to a minimum of 10 cores, and sampling of the lateral peripheral and transition zones [1].

There are four major categories of diagnosis rendered on prostate needle biopsy, including (1) prostate
cancer, (2) high-grade prostatic intraepithelial neoplasia (HGPIN), (3) atypical small acinar proliferation
(ASAP), and (4) benign. Pathologists must not only
provide an accurate diagnosis but also prognostic
information to guide subsequent clinical management.

1. Diagnostic criteria of prostate cancer

The minimal criteria applied by Gleason for a diagnosis of a typical acinar type prostatic adenocarcinoma is
a proliferation of relatively uniform small glands lined

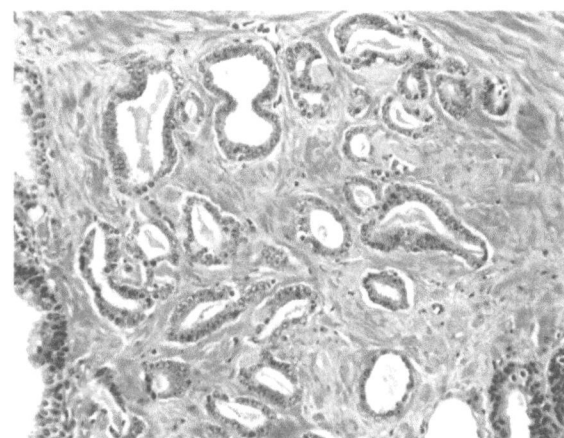

Figure 1. Prostatic adenocarcinoma with the minimal diagnostic
criteria present (uniform proliferation of small glands, single cell
layer and prominent nucleoli).

by a single layered epithelium with at least some cells
containing prominent nucleoli (Figure 1) [2]. These
criteria continue to be highlighted as the fundamental
basis for the diagnosis of cancer [3–5]. However, these
criteria have undergone revision in light of the nature of
the diagnostic tissue currently being submitted. While
the presence of prominent nucleoli remains one of the
cornerstones of a cancer diagnosis, it has become clear
that this is not an absolute. Kramer and Epstein [6] measured nucleolar size in 113 foci of Gleason grades 1 and
2 carcinoma and compared these with 18 examples of
adenosis. They concluded that while nucleoli remain
an important diagnostic feature, some cases of carcinoma (8%) contained no prominent nucleoli (defined
as being larger than 1.6 μm) and many examples of
adenosis (28%) had occasional or frequent prominent
nucleoli. It must be stressed that nucleoli by themselves

M.L. Cher, K.V. Honn and A. Raz (eds.), Prostate Cancer: New Horizons in Research and Treatment, 3–17.
© 2002 *Kluwer Academic Publishers.*

4

are not diagnostic of adenocarcinoma; nucleoli may be a feature of many benign mimics of cancer.

Thin needle biopsies sometimes contain only limited neoplastic glands. The most useful features in reaching a correct interpretation of adenocarcinoma in such cases are the enlarged nuclei, amphophilic cytoplasm, prominent nucleoli and absence of basal cells [7]. Ancillary features such as intraluminal secretions, crystalloids, collagenous micronodules and perineural invasion are also of considerable help (see below). Carcinomatous glands often contain granular eosinophilic luminal material sometimes with nuclear debris, a feature that is also helpful though not specific. The stroma in adenocarcinoma may be essentially normal giving the impression that the abnormal glands have been 'dropped onto the slide'. In contrast, many of the benign mimics of cancer will show stromal changes including fibrosis and associated inflammation. Perineural invasion when present is diagnostic of adenocarcinoma (Figure 2). Care must be taken not to overinterpret benign glands which may be located immediately adjacent to nerves and can appear to indent and distort the nerve fibers [8].

In summary, it is not possible to elaborate minimal absolute criteria for the diagnosis of prostatic adenocarcinoma. The diagnosis of cancer is based on a combination of architectural, cytological as well as ancillary features. The criteria established by Gleason remain the cornerstone for diagnosis but in many instances cannot and should not be rigidly adhered to. A similar conclusion was reached at an international consensus conference [9].

2. Ancillary features of prostate cancer

The presence of *acidic mucin* has been considered by many to be a marker of malignancy in the prostate gland (Figure 3) [10–12]. Several studies have shown that luminal acid mucin (wispy basophilic material on hematoxylin and eosin) is frequently present in adenocarcinoma and as such can aid in the diagnosis [13]. The presence of acidic mucin is however not specific for carcinoma but can also occur in potential cancer mimics such as atrophy, basal cell hyperplasia, atypical adenomatous hyperplasia and sclerosing adenosis [14–17].

Jensen et al. [18] first described the presence of so called *prostatic crystalloids* in association with well differentiated adenocarcinoma of the prostate. These crystalloids are intensely eosinophilic with a glassy appearance and sharp angulated edges giving an impression of birefringence (Figure 4). Several studies have since confirmed this association, but also demonstrated that these may be found in prostatic intraepithelial neoplasia and atypical adenomatous hyperplasia and even in normal glands [19–22]. The significance of the presence of crystalloids in benign glands in otherwise negative needle biopsies has been evaluated by Henneberry et al. [23] and Anton et al. [24]. Both studies revealed that the presence of crystalloids in otherwise benign biopsies was not associated with increased rate of prostate cancer in the subsequent biopsy although both studies were limited by small numbers of patients.

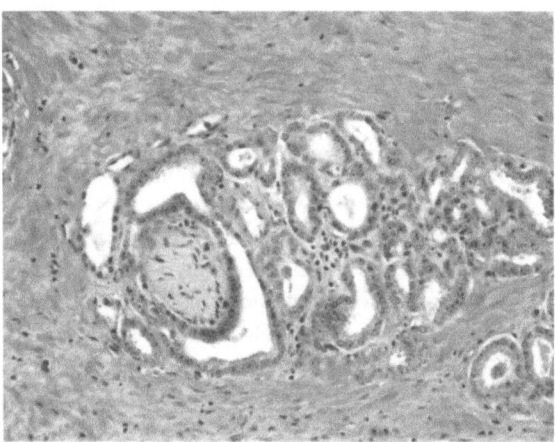

Figure 2. Prostatic adenocarcinoma with perineural invasion.

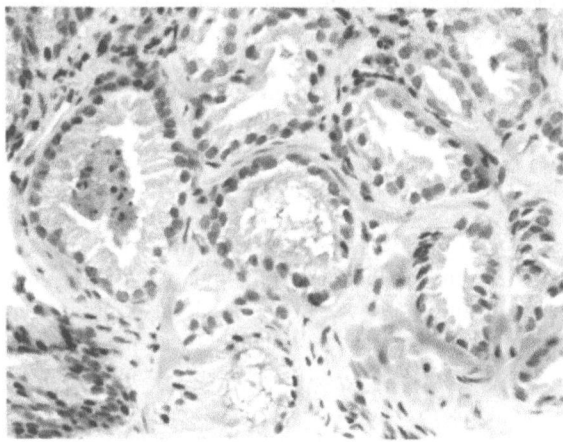

Figure 3. Prostatic adenocarcinoma with luminal acid mucin indicated by the flocculent material seen in the gland located in the center of the image.

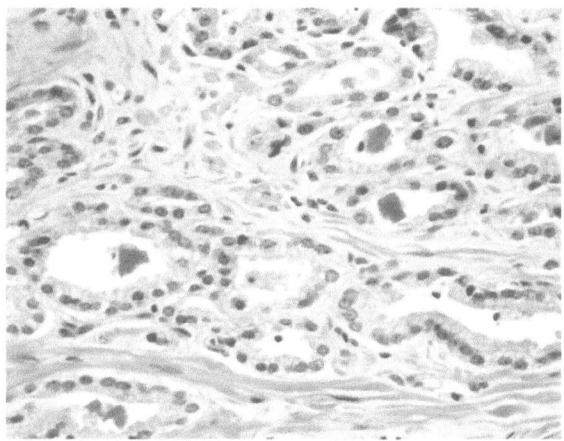

Figure 4. Prostatic adenocarcinoma with several acini containing prostatic crystalloids.

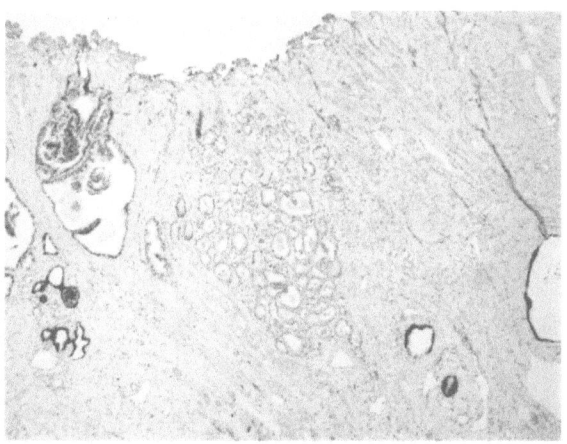

Figure 5. Prostatic tissue stained for high molecular weight cytokeratin by immunohistochemistry. Note the positive staining of the basal cell layer in benign glands around the periphery of the photomicrograph and absence of staining in the adenocarcinoma at the center.

It has been well established that the differential expression of intermediate cytokeratin filaments in the basal and secretory cells of the prostate gland, which was originally described by Nagle et al. [25], is diagnostically useful (Figure 5). Antibodies to *high molecular weight cytokeratin* can specifically label basal cells and not secretory cells. Benign mimics of adenocarcinoma are invariably positive with this antibody reflecting the presence of basal cells [26–27]. A positive stain for high molecular weight cytokeratin is especially valuable in excluding a diagnosis of cancer. Whereas it is dangerous to make a cancer diagnosis based on a negative immunoreaction alone. Although

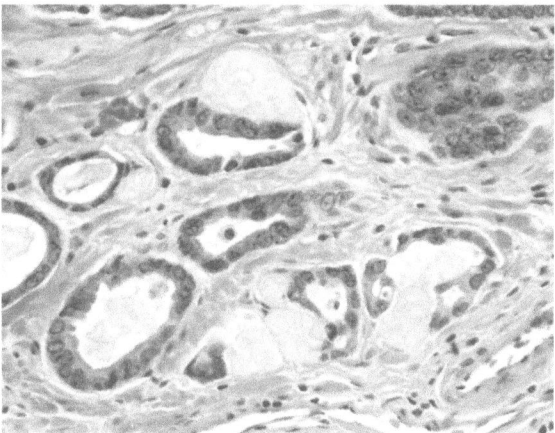

Figure 6. Prostatic adenocarcinoma with several fibrillar collagenous micro-nodules.

negative staining is a typical feature of adenocarcinoma, not all of benign glands exhibit visible positive stain. Therefore a diagnosis of carcinoma should still depend on histological criteria described above.

Collagenous micronodules has been recognized as another finding specific to adenocarcinoma [28]. These are eosinophilic fibrillar aggregates adjacent to neoplastic glands that are almost always associated with mucin producing carcinomas (Figure 6). This finding is rarely present in the small foci of well-formed glands that most often lead to significant diagnostic difficulty.

3. Histological variants of prostate cancer

The conventional acinar type of prostatic adenocarcinoma comprises over 90% of prostate cancer. Several uncommon variants are important because of their specific characteristics [29]. In general these rarely occur in a pure form and are generally seen in association with the conventional acinar type cancer. These tumors are almost all aggressive and in the Gleason system are considered to be grade 4 or grade 5. In the following sections, the more common variant types are briefly described.

A. Mucinous adenocarcinoma
The mucinous variant of prostate cancer is associated with elevated serum prostate specific antigen and exhibits similar metastasis pattern (including bone) and hormone sensitivity to conventional acinar type prostate cancer [30, 31]. Histologically, the tumor is characterized by mucin lakes containing suspended tumor cells arranged in cribriform or incomplete glands

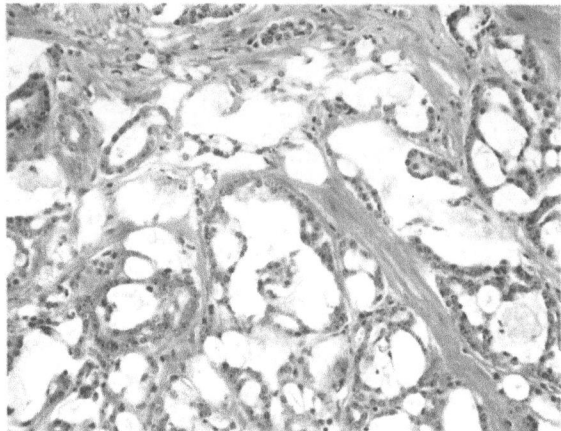

Figure 7. Prostatic adenocarcinoma with extensive mucin production both within the glandular lumens as well as involving the stroma.

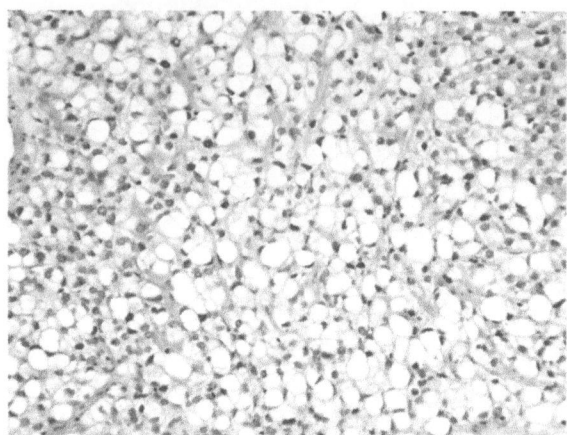

Figure 8. Prostatic adenocarcinoma with numerous signet ring cells.

(Figure 7). The diagnosis of mucinous adenocarcinoma is usually restricted to cases with at least 25% of the tumor volume made up of the extracellular mucin lakes. This pattern is considered to be Gleason grade 4. Pathologically these must be distinguished from mucinous carcinomas of bladder and rectum, which may directly invade the prostate gland. Positive immunohistochemical staining for prostate specific antigen (PSA) and prostatic acid phosphatase (PAP) are useful in confirming a prostatic origin.

B. Signet ring cell carcinoma

Signet ring cell carcinoma is a rare variant of prostate cancer and frequently presents at an advanced stage and is associated with an aggressive clinical course [32, 33]. The diagnosis has been restricted by most authors to cases with at least 25% signet ring cells. The tumor cells typically have a single large cytoplasmic vacuole displacing the nucleus resulting in the signet ring appearance and characteristically diffusely permeate the prostatic stroma (Figure 8). The cytoplasmic vacuoles generally represent intracytoplasmic lumens and are often mucin negative [32]. This pattern is almost always associated with other patterns of poorly differentiated adenocarcinoma. The tumor cells are however positive for PSA and PAP. As with mucinous carcinoma it is important to differentiate these carcinomas from signet ring cell carcinomas invading or metastasizing from other sites.

C. Ductal or endometrioid variant

This variant of prostatic adenocarcinoma generally presents in a similar manner to usual prostatic adenocarcinoma but the tumor can be exophytic into

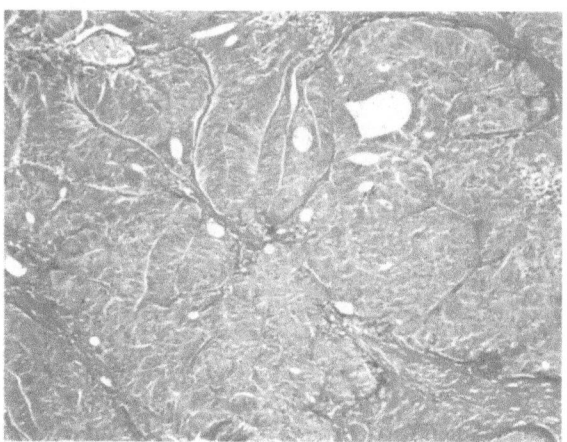

Figure 9. Prostatic adenocarcinoma of the ductal/endometrioid type with complex papillary cribriform architecture.

the urethra producing a papillary lesion visible cystoscopically [34–36]. These patients may present earlier with hematuria or obstruction and can be diagnosed on transurethral resection specimens. It has been reported that patients with this variant of prostate carcinoma have lower than expected levels of serum PSA on a stage for stage basis. Histologically these tumors are usually, though not always located in the larger prostatic ducts in the periurethral region. Architecturally they grow with a papillary or cribriform pattern and frequently there is a mixture of the two (Figure 9). The tumor cells are columnar with pseudostratification and show significant nuclear anaplasia with large vesicular nuclei having coarse chromatin, prominent nucleoli and frequent mitoses. In general these are graded as Gleason pattern 4 but comedonecrosis is common in this pattern and when present indicates a Gleason grade

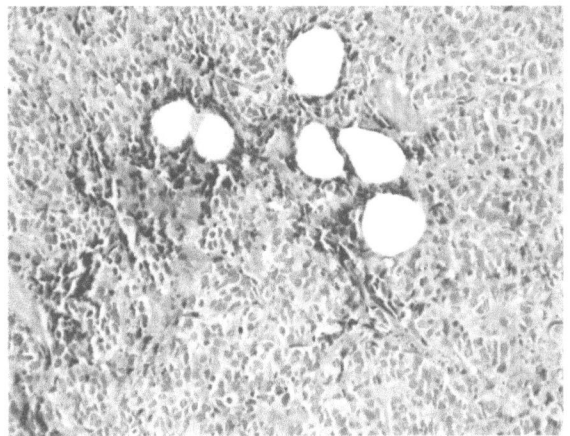

Figure 10. Small cell carcinoma of the prostate.

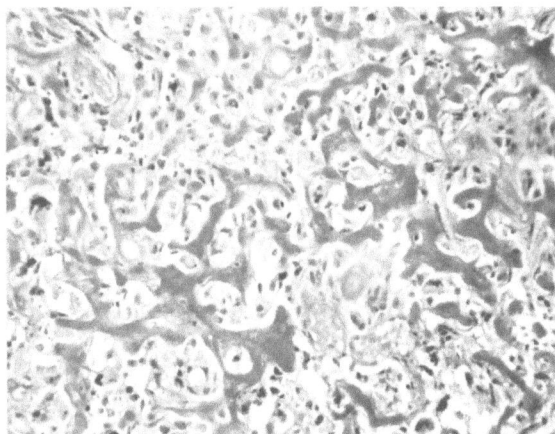

Figure 11. Sarcomatoid carcinoma of the prostate with the formation of osteoid in this area.

of 5 (pure ductal or endometrioid tumors almost always receive a Gleason score of 8 or 9). The tumors are PSA and PAP positive and this is helpful in differentiating them from transitional cell carcinoma and secondary involvement of the prostate by colon carcinoma

D. Small cell carcinoma

Small cell carcinoma is another rare variant of prostate carcinoma. It may occur *de novo* but more often presents with the development of rapid progression without the anticipated increase in PSA level in a patient being followed for known prostate cancer [37–39]. Patients usually have advanced disease, unusual metastatic patterns (e.g. liver involvement) and relatively mild increases in serum PSA. Rare cases with paraneoplastic syndromes are reported including Cushing's syndrome, Eaton-Lambert syndrome, hypercalcemia, SIADH and hyperglucagonemia. Histologically the diagnostic criteria are light microscopic and the same as for bronchogenic small cell carcinoma; the tumor is composed of cells with small to intermediate sized nuclei, finely distributed chromatin, inconspicuous nucleoli and scant cytoplasm (Figure 10). Nuclear molding is prominent and there are frequent mitoses and apoptotic bodies. In over 50% of cases a typical acinar pattern of adenocarcinoma is associated. Neuroendocrine markers (neuron specific enolase, chromogranin, serotonin, calcitonin, ACTH, bombesin, etc.) are positive in many but not all cases. PSA and PAP are only occasionally positive in the small cell component but are positive in acinar areas when present. These cases require clinical correlation to exclude metastatic spread from another site or more likely direct invasion from an adjacent organ, particularly the urinary bladder.

E. Sarcomatoid carcinoma

In rare cases, carcinomas of the prostate develop a malignant spindle cell component. These tumors are known by many terms including sarcomatoid carcinoma, carcinsarcoma, metaplastic carcinoma and spindle cell carcinoma [40–42]. These almost always develop in elderly patients in association with previous or concurrent high-grade prostate adenocarcinoma. There is a history of prior radiation therapy for prostate cancer in about 50% of cases. The serum PSA may be normal or only slightly elevated and there is a very poor prognosis. Histologically these are biphasic tumors with carcinomatous and sarcomatoid components (Figure 11). The spindle cells have marked nuclear pleomorphism and frequent mitotic figures with the most common patterns being malignant fibrous histiocytoma-like and high-grade sarcoma of no specific type. Heterologous elements such as osteosarcoma, chondrosarcoma and rhabdomyosarcoma can be present. Stains for cytokeratin, PSA and PAP are positive in the epithelial (carcinomatous) component but are only focally positive or absent in the sarcomatoid elements. These tumors must be distinguished from primary sarcomas, phyllodes tumor, postoperative spindle cell nodule and pseudosarcomatous fibromyxoid tumors.

4. High-grade prostatic intraepithelial neoplasia

HGPIN has a high predictive value as a marker for carcinoma, and its identification warrants repeat biopsy for concurrent or subsequent carcinoma. Its incidence ranges from 0.7% to 20% in all prostate biopsies and

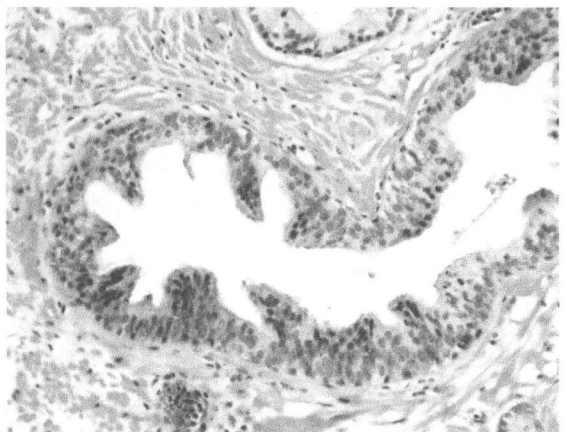

Figure 12. High-grade prostatic intraepithelial neoplasia.

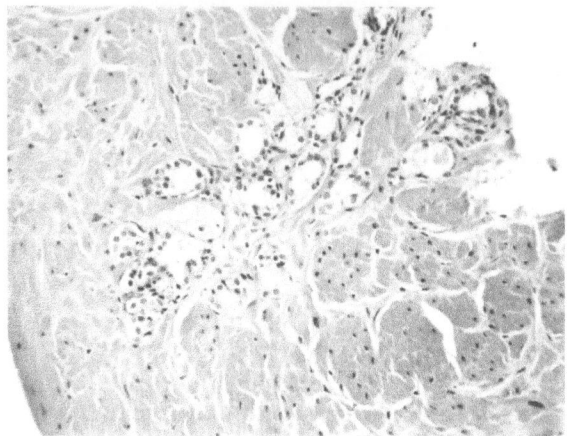

Figure 13. This focal collection of small glands is suspicious for adenocarcinoma but does not meet minimal diagnostic criteria. It would be reported as an ASAP.

carcinoma is identified in up to 50% of repeat biopsies [43–48]. In a recent study, Kronz et al. [49] analyzed 245 men in whom the only abnormal finding on the initial biopsy was HGPIN and who had at least one follow-up biopsy. Repeat biopsy identified cancer in 32.2% of men. The only independent histological predictor of a cancer diagnosis was the number of cores with HGPIN (risk of cancer: 30.2% with 1 or 2 cores, 40% with 3 cores, and 75% with >3 cores). They also demonstrated that if the first repeat biopsy were benign, high-grade PIN, or atypical, the eventual cancer rate was 10%, 25.9% and 57.1%, respectively.

Histologically, HGPIN is characterized by an intra-luminal proliferation of atypical secretory cells involving ducts and acini. Four histological patterns have been described including tufting, micropapillary, cribriform and flat [21]. However, the nuclear features including nuclear enlargement, hyperchromasia, especially the presence of prominent nucleoli are the hallmark of HGPIN (Figure 12). The basal cell layer is maintained, although it may be discontinuous. In difficult case, immunohistochemical stain for high molecular weight cytokeratin could be useful to reveal the presence of basal cells [50].

5. Atypical small acinar proliferation

In certain instances a biopsy contains a focus of small glands for which a specific diagnosis cannot be rendered (Figure 13). In these cases the focus does not show criteria sufficient for a diagnosis of cancer but at the same time does not show morphologic characteristics of a diagnosable benign entity. In a study in which a series of problematic small gland lesions was

reviewed by several urologic pathologists, the authors suggested the term ASAP for such situations [22]. It is accepted now that a diagnosis of ASAP suspicious for carcinoma is a reasonable diagnosis in cases where a minimal amount of atypical acini is present. Published experience with rebiopsy of patients having this type of finding indicates that in up to 45% a diagnosis of carcinoma will be rendered on repeat biopsy [51, 52]. In a study of 295 patients with ASAP, Iczkowski et al. [53] reported that adenocarcinoma was identified on follow-up biopsy in 42% of patients, with a median follow-up of 5.7 months (range 0.1–43). Gleason score varied from 4 to 9 (mean 6.2). Cumulative detection of 125 cancers was 90% after second biopsy and 99% after third biopsy. In 39% of patients, cancer was only contralateral to or in a different sextant site from the initial ASAP site.

It is currently recommended that the optimal repeat biopsy strategy in patients with ASAP or HGPIN should include bilateral biopsies of the standard sextant locations and transition zone sampling should also be considered [47].

III. Predicting outcome from the biopsy

There are numerous studies investigating pathologic prognostic factors of prostate cancer in needle biopsy specimen [54–56]. Multivariate models have shown that the combination of biopsy Gleason score, clinical stage and serum PSA provides reliable assessment of the risk for extraprostatic disease [57]. Other biopsy-derived parameters, especially quantitative histology, have demonstrated to contribute additional valuable prognostic information [57–60].

1. Gleason score

Histological grading of prostate cancer is among the most important predictors of biologic behavior. Although numerous systems have been described, currently the Gleason system is the most widely used and recommended [61]. The Gleason grading system, first described in 1966, is based on the architectural growth pattern of prostatic adenocarcinoma [2]. The multiple histological patterns, which can be seen in prostate cancer, are grouped into 5 broad grade categories, which are viewed as a continuum. Gleason grade 1 tumors consist of closely packed, uniform, round glands arranged in a nodule with pushing borders (Figure 14). This is a very uncommon pattern except in transition zone adenocarcinomas and is almost never seen in needle biopsy specimens. Gleason grade 2 tumors are similar to grade 1 except the glands show more variability in size and shape and are separated by more abundant stroma (Figure 15). The tumor nodules have a less circumscribed appearance although infiltration between benign glands is not seen. Gleason grade 3 includes three distinct architectural patterns, with the most common consisting of well formed, relatively uniform glands growing in an infiltrative manner; growth between benign glands is a useful clue to this grade (Figure 16). In the second pattern the glands are small with inconspicuous or even absent lumens and may have an angulated shape however they are still separate without fusion into cords or chains (a grade 4 pattern). Finally, grade 3 includes papillary and cribriform patterns with islands of tumor cells having smooth, rounded pushing type edges without stromal infiltration (Figure 17). Gleason grade 4 also includes multiple distinct architectures with the most common pattern consisting of small acinar structures, some with well-formed lumina, fusing into cords or chains; this pattern is frequently undergraded as 3 (Figure 18). Grade 4 also includes papillary-cribriform tumors where the edges are more irregular with an invasive appearance, many, though not all endometrioid carcinomas fall into this category. The hypernephroid pattern, characterized by nests of cells with abundant clear cytoplasm and small, hyperchromatic nuclei is considered to be grade 4. Gleason grade 5 includes 2 major patterns, first any carcinoma with little or no evidence of glandular differentiation falls into this

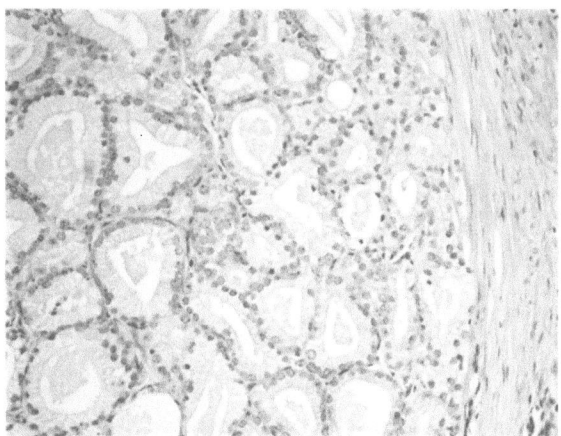

Figure 14. Prostatic adenocarcinoma, Gleason grade 1. The photomicrograph shows the edge of a well-circumscribed nodule of closely packed uniform glands.

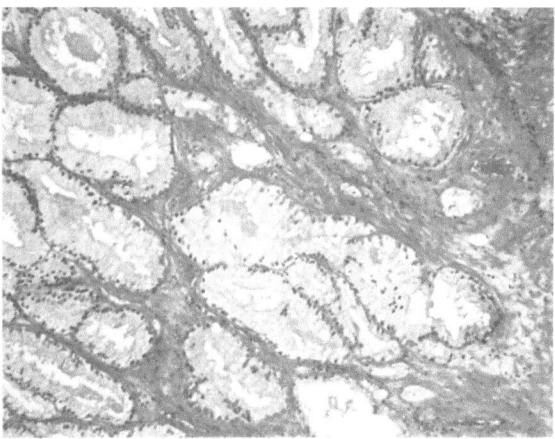

Figure 15. Prostatic adenocarcinoma, Gleason grade 2. This tumor also is forming relatively circumscribed nodules but the glands are more irregular in shape and are separated by increased amounts of stroma compared with Figure 14.

grade category; these can range from infiltrating single cells (including signet-ring cell carcinoma) to solid sheets of tumor cells (Figure 19). Grade 5 also includes papillary-cribriform carcinomas with central necrosis (comedocarcinoma pattern) (Figure 20).

Due to the nature of heterogeneity and multifocality of prostate cancer, several patterns can be seen in one tumor focus or different tumor foci of one prostate. The original Veterans Administration Cooperative Urologic Research Group studies found that tumors tended to behave more like the 'average' grade rather than the highest grade present. To account for this

10

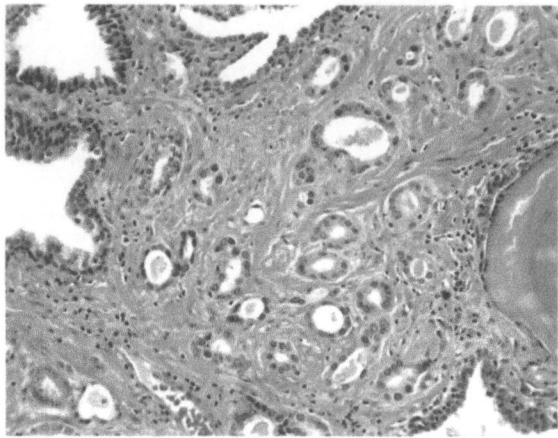

Figure 16. Prostatic adenocarcinoma, Gleason grade 3. This photomicrograph illustrates a collection of distinct well-formed glands infiltrating between benign glandular elements.

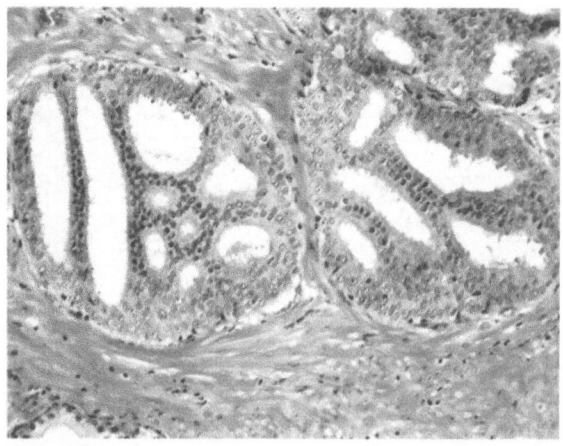

Figure 17. Prostatic adenocarcinoma, Gleason grade 3. In this focus the tumor is forming sharply circumscribed nests of glands with a cribriform architecture.

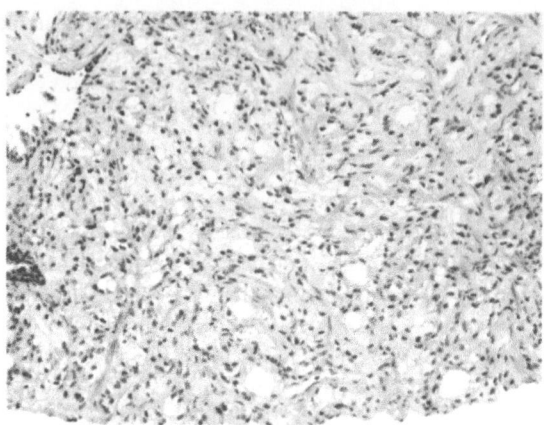

Figure 18. Prostatic adenocarcinoma, Gleason grade 4. This photomicrograph illustrates a tumor with variable gland formation and with many of the glands fused into poorly defined nests and cords.

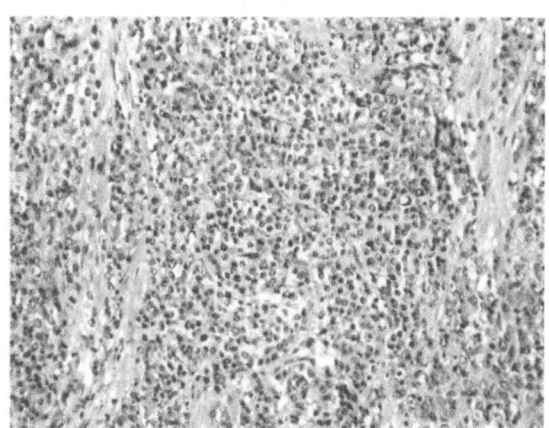

Figure 19. Prostatic adenocarcinoma, Gleason grade 5. The tumor is forming solid poorly defined masses with little evidence of gland formation.

Gleason developed a 'score' which sums the predominant grade with the second most prevalent grade (e.g. a tumor with a predominant grade of 4 and a secondary grade of 3 would be assigned a Gleason score of 7). Numerous clinical studies have repeatedly demonstrated the prognostic significance of Gleason score in patients managed by watchful waiting [62], radical prostatectomy [63], radiation therapy [64, 65, 113] or combined radiation and hormonal therapy [66, 67].

Gleason score 2–4 carcinomas are almost exclusively of transition zone origin and have a low malignant potential [68, 69]. Most now agree that Gleason score 7 cancers do not belong with the Gleason

score 5 and 6 tumors as an 'intermediate' category [70–72]. Currently, there has been a tendency to group Gleason scores into 4 broader categories. Gleason scores 2–4 as well differentiated, Gleason scores 5–6 as moderately well differentiated, Gleason score 7 as moderately poorly differentiated and Gleason scores 8–10 as poorly differentiated categories. More recent studies further demonstrated that in the category of Gleason score 7, there is significant prognostic difference in Gleason scores 4 + 3 and 3 + 4 subgroups [73–75]. In the updated prostate cancer staging nomograms (Partin table), the Gleason score 7 has

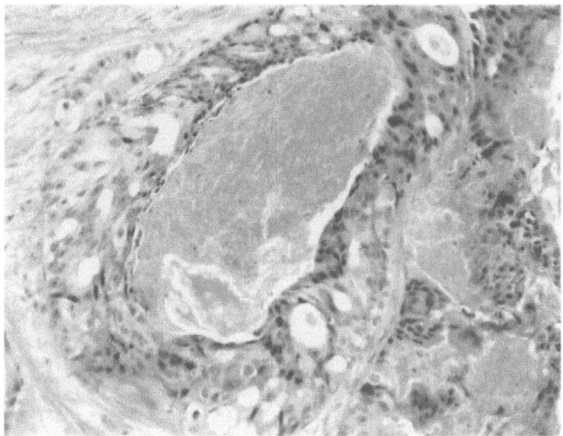

Figure 20. Prostatic adenocarcinoma, Gleason grade 5. The tumor is growing with a complex cribriform architecture having extensive central areas of comedonecrosis.

been divided into 2 subgroups according to the primary pattern being 3 or 4 [76].

2. Quantitative histology

Prostate biopsy quantitative histology is an area of great interest currently [60]. Several quantitation methods have been proposed and have been shown to have prognostic value in individual studies. Freedland et al. [77] and Grossklaus et al. [78] reported that the percentage of total biopsy tissue involved with cancer was the strongest independent predictor of PSA only recurrence after radical prostatectomy and also the predictor of pathological stage and tumor volume. Nelson et al. [56] showed that the greatest percentage of a biopsy core involved by cancer was highly predictive of PSA free-survival. Conrad et al. [59] found that the number of cores with predominant Gleason grade 4/5 is a predicting factor for pelvic lymph node metastasis. Grossfeld et al. [79] and D'Amico et al. [58] illustrated that the percentage of positive prostate biopsies was a significant predictor of disease recurrence. All these studies indicate that prostate biopsy quantitative histology may provide additional prognostic information in prostate cancer. Further studies will be needed to validate the reproducibility, reliability and feasibility of these quantitative histology approaches in prostate cancer diagnosis and prediction.

3. Perineural invasion

Considerable controversy exists as to the significance of perineural invasion. The growth of tumor cells along the nerve sheaths is defined as perineural invasion, which is a common finding in prostate cancer. Some studies indicate that perineural invasion is a significant preoperative predictor of progression [80, 112]. But other studies were not able to confirm the finding [26, 77].

Currently it is recommended that the pathological evaluation of prostate cancer in needle biopsy specimen should include the following parameters: (1) histological type, (2) Gleason score with primary and secondary grades, (3) quantitation of tumor (proportion [%] of prostatic tissue involved by neoplasm), (4) local invasion (periprostatic fat and seminal vesicle) and (5) perineural or vascular invasion.

IV. Pathologic evaluation of radical prostatectomy

It has been well recognized that the most important pathological parameters of radical prostatectomy specimen are tumor grade (Gleason score), pathological stage (Table 1) and surgical margins.

In a series of 925 consecutive men with clinical stage T1 or T2 prostate cancer underwent radical retropubic prostatectomy at Washington University, Catalona reported an overall 5-year progression rate of 22%. Biochemical disease free survival correlated with pathological tumor stage (91% for organ confined disease, 74% for positive margins or microscopic capsular perforation, 32% for seminal vesicle invasion and virtually nil for lymph node metastases) and tumor grade (89% for well, 78% for moderately and 51% for poorly differentiated tumors) [81]. Pound et al. [82] reported their

Table 1. Pathologic staging of prostate cancer (AJCC Cancer Staging Manual 2002)

pT2	Organ confined
pT2a	Unilateral, involving one-half of one lobe or less
pT2b	Unilateral, involving more than one-half of one lobe but not both lobes
pT2c	Bilateral disease
pT3	Extraprostatic extension
pT3a	Extraprostatic adipose tissue extension
pT3b	Seminal vesicle invasion
pT4	Invasion of bladder, rectum

12

experience on a series of 1623 men operated on at Johns Hopkins University. In this study, the likelihood of postoperative recurrence increased with increasing clinical stage, Gleason score, preoperative PSA level, and pathologic stage. They further demonstrated that the presence of a positive surgical margin was only important in high-grade tumors with capsular penetration. Tefilli et al. [72] evaluated pathologic characteristics and biochemical survival rate in a series of 652 patients underwent radical prostatectomy at the Detroit Medical Center and Wayne State University. The biochemical disease free survival was 34.5% for patients with Gleason score 8 or more, 75% for Gleason score 7, and 91.2% for Gleason score 6 or less prostate cancer. Mian et al. [83] demonstrated that in the patients with Gleason score 8 or higher prostate cancer, pathological status of radical prostatectomy specimen was the most significant independent predictor of disease recurrence. Age, ethnicity, clinical stage and preoperative PSA had no independent effect on disease recurrence.

Currently it is recommended that the pathological evaluation of prostate cancer in radical prostatectomy specimen should include the following parameters: (1) histological type, (2) Gleason score with primary and secondary grades, (3) location of tumor(s), (4) extent of local invasion including the status of extraprostatic extension and seminal vesicle involvement and (5) surgical margins (location and extent of margins involved with tumor. The Gleason score is assigned based on the apparent index tumor; in cases without an obvious major tumor nodule, the score is based on the complete gland [84].

V. Therapy effects

1. Hormonal therapy

Descriptions of the histological effects of hormonal therapy (usually total androgen blockade) on prostate cancer have been relatively consistent to date [85–87]. Total androgen blockade results in a significant decrease in the number (density) of cancer glands [86]. The residual neoplastic glands are usually small with compressed or absent lumens (Figure 21). We have noted the continued presence of acidic mucin and prostatic crystalloids within the lumens of some tumor glands. Occasionally there are only mucin lakes left behind in the prostatic stroma [114]. The secretory cells have cleared or vacuolated cytoplasms with

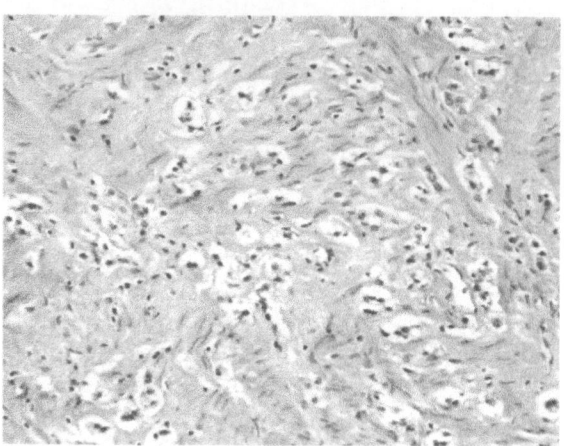

Figure 21. Prostatic adenocarcinoma after treatment with total androgen blockade. The malignant glands are shrunken with poorly defined lumens.

small, round, centrally located hyperchromatic nuclei and in many cells the nucleoli are inconspicuous. These vacuolated tumor cells can appear as single cells resulting in misinterpretation as histiocytes or in assigning a high Gleason grade [87]. This upward shift in grade parallels the degree of treatment effect noted [85]. This may result in a false impression of dedifferentiation and because of this, grading of tumors with the Gleason system following total androgen blockade may be an inaccurate assessment of biologic behavior [87]. This outcome has led to the recommendation that the Gleason scoring system should not be applied to prostate adenocarcinoma specimens after hormonal therapy [61]. However, a recent study suggested that despite the morphologic alterations induced by hormonal therapy, post-treatment Gleason score remained a significant prognostic measure [88]. Further studies are required to confirm this observation. The value of cytokeratin immunostaining for identifying residual tumor cells in those cases with severe treatment effects has been noted [87]. Immunohistochemical studies have demonstrated a significant decrease in the intensity of staining for PSA in most or some cases following treatment [85, 86].

2. Radiation therapy

The effect of radiation on prostate cancer is highly variable between different patients and heterogeneity can be seen within a single patient [89, 90]. The typical changes include: (1) decreased numbers of

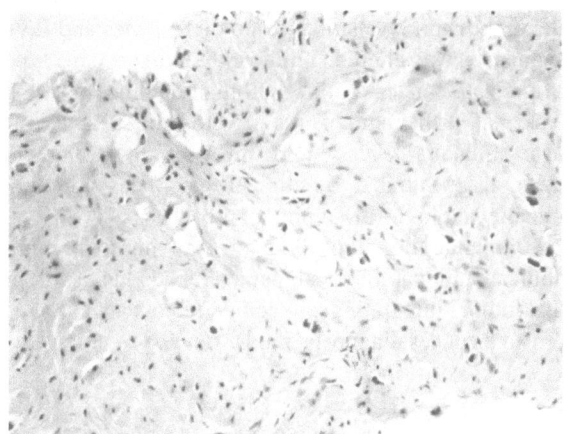

Figure 22. Prostatic adenocarcinoma after external beam radiotherapy. There are a few residual tumor glands and cells with atrophy and with cells having abundant cytoplasm.

cancer glands with those remaining being haphazardly arranged in the tissue, (2) irregularity in the shape and size of nuclei, hyperchromasia, nucleoli may or may not be prominent, (3) increased cytoplasmic volume with or without vacuolization. The increase in cytoplasm may be so great as to leave residual cancer cells appearing to have only cytoplasm without visible nuclei (Figure 22).

These morphologic alterations can impact on the interpretation of histological grade. For example, Bostwick et al. reported a change in the Gleason score of 2 or greater in 7 of 26 post radiation biopsies (27%) but did not specify the direction of change [91]. In the experience of Siders and Lee [92] the grade change following radiation therapy was usually a significant increase. Since the Gleason grading system is based on architecture, a tumor with the most severe treatment effects will consist of only scattered single cells, a Gleason grade 5 (score 10) pattern. It is seems unlikely that this reflects a dedifferentiation phenomenon related to the radiation *per se* [91]. Crook et al. [93] have suggested that grading may be of value only in those cases where the residual tumor shows minimal or no therapy effect. This is also our belief and at our institution post radiation therapy biopsies are not graded. We believe that the prognosis is best predicted by the pre-treatment Gleason score, although morphologic changes may be of significance in patients with positive post radiation biopsies [90, 93]. For cases with clinical local recurrence after radiation therapy (often several years following completion) the above may not hold true. In these cases the growing tumor may represent a new cancer. Such tumors have been reported to be of much higher grade than the initial, an observation which led Wheeler et al. [94] to conclude that this represented progression through clonal evolution.

3. Combined radiation and hormonal therapy

There is a very little published literature comparing the morphologic effects of radiation alone with radiation combined with total androgen blockade. In our experience, the frequency of positive biopsy following treatment is lower in the combined therapy group than the radiation only patients. Morphologically the residual tumor in the radiation only groups shows much more variability in terms of the degree of therapy effect. In contrast, residual tumor in the combined therapy groups exhibits significantly higher frequencies of moderate to marked treatment effect. It is not possible however to otherwise distinguish the two groups by the morphologic pattern alone. Crook et al. [93] had a similar experience; of the 89 patients with positive post-radiation therapy biopsies they studied, 32 had neoadjuvant hormonal therapy. They noted a 'consistently higher radiation effect score' in those patients receiving combined therapy, attributing the difference in score primarily to the more prominent cytoplasmic vacuolization in the combined treatment group.

VI. Metastatic prostate cancer

The prognosis of prostate cancer is mainly determined by the presence or absence of metastases. Well-differentiated lesions rarely metastasize and metastases are rarely well differentiated. Patients with moderately differentiated metastases have a statistically significant better survival than patients with poorly differentiated metastases [95]. Metastases typically disseminate as they dedifferentiate. Immunohistochemical studies for PSA and PAP and serum PSA levels may be helpful in determining whether a particular metastases is from the prostate.

In a recent study of 1589 autopsies with prostate cancer, hematogeneous metastases were present in 35% of patients, with most frequent involvement being bone (90%), lung (46%), liver (25%), pleura (21%) and adrenals (13%) [96]. Saitoh et al. [97] observed from their 1,885 autopsy study that the sites of metastasis were related to the number of organs involved. In the

14

cases of one organ involvement, bone was the most common site of metastasis. Whereas in the cases of multiple organ involvement, lymph nodes were slightly more common than bone to be involved.

VII. Molecular prognostic factors

Although Gleason Score, serum PSA and clinical stage are well established strong prognostic factors in prostate cancer, the most significant limitation of these parameters is the lack of ability to provide rationales for targeted individual treatment. With progress in cancer research, cancer biology will be better understood and therapeutic approaches targeted to specific molecules or pathways involved in cancer progression will be able to be developed. Molecular analysis at the time of diagnosis will be critical to the identification of the major molecules and main pathways involved in the cancer progression for an individual. Targeted therapy will only be possible if the tools to identify the target for individual patients are readily available. However, the lack of a reliable approach for molecular marker analysis using human specimens, especially routinely processed tissue, has been a major obstacle in translational research efforts. It has not been possible to convincingly validate the clinical relevance and utility of promising cancer – related molecules discovered from in vitro studies or animal models.

Various molecules including tumor suppressor genes, oncogenes, growth factors, as well as molecules involved in cell adhesion, signal transduction, apoptosis, angiogenesis and eicosanoid metabolism have been found to be abnormal in prostate cancer [98–106]. The potential prognostic values of molecular markers in prostate cancer have been comprehensively reviewed by several authors recently [104–107]. However, currently, none of the molecular markers can be recommended for routine use clinically for evaluation of prostate cancer [61, 108, 109]. Histopathological parameters remain the cornerstone for prostate cancer diagnosis and prediction. Nevertheless, histopathological features alone are insufficient in predicting biological behavior of prostate cancer and inadequate in guiding therapy strategy. Advances in human genome research and gene analysis technology have provided us the opportunity to investigate gene expression profile using high-throughout approaches. Recently, using gene-array technology, Luo et al. [110] have identified 84 largely novel genes and expressed sequence tag (EST) sequences whose expression levels were altered significantly in prostate cancer samples compared

with control normal tissues. They further found that the expression levels of a group of 12 genes and EST sequences was altered significantly in aggressive type of prostate cancers but not in organ-confined prostate cancers. Further study is required to validate and evaluate clinical relevance and utility of those markers using large number of clinical specimens applying reliable and high-throughout approaches.

Computational algorithms are evolving combining clinical and pathological parameters [111], and, in the future, integrating molecular factors to enhance prostate cancer diagnosis, prediction and treatment.

References

1. Cookson MS: Update on transrectal ultrasound-guided needle biopsy of the prostate. Mol Urol 4(3): 93–97, discussion 99, 2000
2. Gleason DF: Classification of prostatic carcinomas. Cancer Chemother Rep 50(3): 125–128, 1966
3. Kovi J: Microscopic differential diagnosis of small acinar adenocarcinoma of prostate. Pathol Annu 20(Pt 1): 157–196, 1985
4. Mostofi FK, Sesterhenn IA et al.: Prostatic carcinoma: Problems in the interpretation of prostatic biopsies. Hum Pathol 23(3): 223–241, 1992
5. Ro JY, Grignon DJ, Amin MB, Ayala A: Atlas of Surgical Pathology of the Male Reproductive Tract, W. B. Saunders Co., Philadelphia, 1997
6. Kramer CE, Epstein JI: Nucleoli in low-grade prostate adenocarcinoma and adenosis. Hum Pathol 24(6): 618–623, 1993
7. Epstein JI: Diagnostic criteria of limited adenocarcinoma of the prostate on needle biopsy. Hum Pathol 26(2): 223–229, 1995
8. Carstens PH: Perineural glands in normal and hyperplastic prostates. J Urol 123(5): 686–688, 1980
9. Algaba F, Epstein JI, et al.: Assessment of prostate carcinoma in core needle biopsy–definition of minimal criteria for the diagnosis of cancer in biopsy material. Cancer 78(2): 376–381, 1996
10. Taylor NS: Histochemistry in the diagnosis of early prostatic carcinoma. Hum Pathol 10(5): 513–520, 1979
11. Ro JY, Grignon DJ et al.: Mucin in prostatic adenocarcinoma. Semin Diagn Pathol 5(3): 273–283, 1988
12. Pinder SE, McMahon RF: Mucins in prostatic carcinoma. Histopathology 16(1): 43–46, 1990
13. Epstein JI, Fynheer J: Acidic mucin in the prostate: Can it differentiate adenosis from adenocarcinoma? Hum Pathol 23(12): 1321–1325, 1992
14. Grignon DJ, Ro JY, et al.: Basal cell hyperplasia, adenoid basal cell tumor, and adenoid cystic carcinoma of the prostate gland: An immunohistochemical study. Hum Pathol 19(12): 1425–1433, 1988
15. Grignon DJ, Ro JY, et al.: Sclerosing adenosis of the prostate gland. A lesion showing myoepithelial differentiation. Am J Surg Pathol 16(4): 383–391, 1992

16. Grignon DJ, O'Malley FP: Mucinous metaplasia in the prostate gland. Am J Surg Pathol 17(3): 287–290, 1993

17. Goldstein NS, Qian J, et al.: Mucin expression in atypical adenomatous hyperplasia of the prostate. Hum Pathol 26(8): 887–891, 1995

18. Jensen PE, Gardner WA Jr, et al.: Prostatic crystalloids: Association with adenocarcinoma. Prostate 1(1): 25–30, 1980

19. Ro JY, Ayala AG et al.: Intraluminal crystalloids in prostatic adenocarcinoma. Immunohistochemical, electron microscopic, and x-ray microanalytic studies. Cancer 57(12): 2397–2407, 1986

20. Ro JY, Grignon DJ et al.: Intraluminal crystalloids in whole-organ sections of prostate. Prostate 13(3): 233–239, 1988

21. Bostwick DG, Amin MB, et al.: Architectural patterns of high-grade prostatic intraepithelial neoplasia. Hum Pathol 24(3): 298–310, 1993

22. Bostwick DG, Srigley J, et al.: Atypical adenomatous hyperplasia of the prostate: Morphologic criteria for its distinction from well-differentiated carcinoma. Hum Pathol 24(8): 819–832, 1993

23. Henneberry JM, Kahane H, et al.: The significance of intraluminal crystalloids in benign prostatic glands on needle biopsy. Am J Surg Pathol 21(6): 725–728, 1997

24. Anton RC, Chakraborty S, et al.: The significance of intraluminal prostatic crystalloids in benign needle biopsies. Am J Surg Pathol 22(4): 446–449, 1998

25. Nagle RB, Ahmann FR et al.: Cytokeratin characterization of human prostatic carcinoma and its derived cell lines. Cancer Res 47(1): 281–286, 1987

26. O'Malley FP, Grignon DJ et al.: Usefulness of immunoperoxidase staining with high-molecular-weight cytokeratin in the differential diagnosis of small-acinar lesions of the prostate gland. Virchows Arch A Pathol Anat Histopathol 417(3): 191–196, 1990

27. Wojno KJ, Epstein JI: The utility of basal cell-specific anti-cytokeratin antibody (34 beta E12) in the diagnosis of prostate cancer. A review of 228 cases. Am J Surg Pathol 19(3): 251–260, 1995

28. Bostwick DG, Wollan P, et al.: Collagenous micronodules in prostate cancer. A specific but infrequent diagnostic finding. Arch Pathol Lab Med 119(5): 444–447, 1995

29. Randolph TL, Amin MB et al.: Histologic variants of adenocarcinoma and other carcinomas of prostate: Pathologic criteria and clinical significance. Mod Pathol 10(6): 612–629, 1997

30. Ro JY, Grignon DJ et al.: Mucinous adenocarcinoma of the prostate: Histochemical and immunohistochemical studies. Hum Pathol 21(6): 593–600, 1990

31. Teichman JM, Shabaik A et al.: Mucinous adenocarcinoma of the prostate and hormone sensitivity. J Urol 151(3): 701–702, 1994

32. Ro JY, el-Naggar A et al.: Signet-ring-cell carcinoma of the prostate. Electron-microscopic and immunohistochemical studies of eight cases. Am J Surg Pathol 12(6): 453–460, 1988

33. Guerin D, Hasan N, et al.: Signet ring cell differentiation in adenocarcinoma of the prostate: A study of five cases. Histopathology 22(4): 367–371, 1993

34. Christensen WN, Steinberg G, et al.: Prostatic duct adenocarcinoma. Findings at radical prostatectomy. Cancer 67(8): 2118–2124, 1991

35. Lee SS: Endometrioid adenocarcinoma of the prostate: A clinicopathologic and immunohistochemical study. J Surg Oncol 55(4): 235–238, 1994

36. Millar EK, Sharma NK et al.: Ductal (endometrioid) adenocarcinoma of the prostate: A clinicopathological study of 16 cases. Histopathology 29(1): 11–19, 1996

37. Tetu B, Ro JY et al.: Small cell carcinoma of the prostate. Part I. A clinicopathologic study of 20 cases. Cancer 59(10): 1803–1809, 1987

38. Oesterling JE, Hauzeur CG et al.: Small cell anaplastic carcinoma of the prostate: A clinical, pathological and immunohistological study of 27 patients. J Urol 147(3 Pt 2): 804–807, 1992

39. Rubenstein JH, Katin MJ et al.: Small cell anaplastic carcinoma of the prostate: Seven new cases, review of the literature, and discussion of a therapeutic strategy. Am J Clin Oncol 20(4): 376–380, 1997

40. Shannon RL, Ro JY et al.: Sarcomatoid carcinoma of the prostate. A clinicopathologic study of 12 patients. Cancer 69(11): 2676–2682, 1992

41. Lauwers GY, Schevchuk M, et al.: Carcinosarcoma of the prostate. Am J Surg Pathol 17(4): 342–349, 1993

42. Dundore PA, Cheville JC, et al.: Carcinosarcoma of the prostate. Report of 21 cases. Cancer 76(6): 1035–1042, 1995

43. Bostwick DG: Prospective origins of prostate carcinoma. Prostatic intraepithelial neoplasia and atypical adenomatous hyperplasia. Cancer 78(2): 330–336, 1996

44. Raviv G, Janssen T et al.: Prostatic intraepithelial neoplasia: Influence of clinical and pathological data on the detection of prostate cancer. J Urol 156(3): 1050–1054, discussion 1054–1055, 1996

45. Shepherd D, Keetch DW et al.: Repeat biopsy strategy in men with isolated prostatic intraepithelial neoplasia on prostate needle biopsy. J Urol 156(2 Pt 1): 460–462, discussion 462–463, 1996

46. Alsikafi NF, Brendler CB, et al.: High-grade prostatic intraepithelial neoplasia with adjacent atypia is associated with a higher incidence of cancer on subsequent needle biopsy than high-grade prostatic intraepithelial neoplasia alone. Urology 57(2): 296–300, 2001

47. Borboroglu PG, Sur RL, et al.: Repeat biopsy strategy in patients with atypical small acinar proliferation or high grade prostatic intraepithelial neoplasia on initial prostate needle biopsy. J Urol 166(3): 866–870, 2001

48. Park S, Shinohara K et al.: Prostate cancer detection in men with prior high grade prostatic intraepithelial neoplasia or atypical prostate biopsy. J Urol 165(5): 1409–1414, 2001

49. Kronz JD, Allan CH, et al.: Predicting cancer following a diagnosis of high-grade prostatic intraepithelial neoplasia on needle biopsy: Data on men with more than one follow-up biopsy. Am J Surg Pathol 25(8): 1079–1085, 2001

50. Amin MB, Ro JY, et al.: Prostatic intraepithelial neoplasia. Relationship to adenocarcinoma of prostate. Pathol Annu 29(Pt 2): 1–30, 1994

51. Iczkowski KA, MacLennan GT, et al.: Atypical small acinar proliferation suspicious for malignancy in prostate needle biopsies: Clinical significance in 33 cases. Am J Surg Pathol 21(12): 1489–1495, 1997

52. Ouyang RC, Kenwright DN et al.: The presence of atypical small acinar proliferation in prostate needle biopsy is predictive of carcinoma on subsequent biopsy. BJU Int 87(1): 70–74, 2001

53. Iczkowski KA, Bassler TJ, et al.: Diagnosis of suspicious for malignancy in prostate biopsies: Predictive value for cancer. Urology 51(5): 749–757, discussion 757–758, 1998

54. Sebo TJ, Cheville JC et al.: Predicting prostate carcinoma volume and stage at radical prostatectomy by assessing needle biopsy specimens for percent surface area and cores positive for carcinoma, perineural invasion, Gleason score, DNA ploidy and proliferation, and preoperative serum prostate specific antigen: A report of 454 cases. Cancer 91(11): 2196–2204, 2001

55. Egevad L, Granfors T, et al.: Prognostic value of the Gleason score in prostate cancer. BJU Int 89(6): 538–542, 2002

56. Nelson CP, Rubin MA et al.: Preoperative parameters for predicting early prostate cancer recurrence after radical prostatectomy. Urology 59(5): 740–745, 2002

57. Feneley MR, Partin AW: Indicators of pathologic stage of prostate cancer and their use in clinical practice. Urol Clin North Am 28(3): 443–458, 2001

58. D'Amico AV, Whittington R, et al.: Clinical utility of the percentage of positive prostate biopsies in defining biochemical outcome after radical prostatectomy for patients with clinically localized prostate cancer. J Clin Oncol 18(6): 1164–1172, 2000

59. Conrad S, Graefen M, et al.: Prospective validation of an algorithm with systematic sextant biopsy to predict pelvic lymph node metastasis in patients with clinically localized prostatic carcinoma. J Urol 167(2 Pt 1): 521–525, 2002

60. Moul JW: Prostate biopsy quantitative histology as a staging and prognostic factor. J Urol 167(2 Pt 1): 526–527, 2002

61. Grignon DJ, Hammond EH: College of American Pathologists Conference XXVI on clinical relevance of prognostic markers in solid tumors. Report of the Prostate Cancer Working Group. Arch Pathol Lab Med 119(12): 1122–1126, 1995

62. Chodak GW, Thisted RA, et al.: Results of conservative management of clinically localized prostate cancer. N Engl J Med 330(4): 242–248, 1994

63. Epstein JI, Pizov G, et al.: Correlation of pathologic findings with progression after radical retropubic prostatectomy. Cancer 71(11): 3582–3593, 1993

64. Zagars GK, Pollack A et al.: Prognostic factors for clinically localized prostate carcinoma: Analysis of 938 patients irradiated in the prostate specific antigen era. Cancer 79(7): 1370–1380, 1997

65. Roach M 3rd, Lu J et al.: Long-term survival after radiotherapy alone: Radiation therapy oncology group prostate cancer trials. J Urol 161(3): 864–868, 1999

66. Pilepich MV, Krall JM et al.: Androgen deprivation with radiation therapy compared with radiation therapy alone for locally advanced prostatic carcinoma: A randomized comparative trial of the Radiation Therapy Oncology Group. Urology 45(4): 616–623, 1995

67. Pilepich MV, Winter K et al.: Phase III radiation therapy oncology group (RTOG) trial 86-10 of androgen deprivation adjuvant to definitive radiotherapy in locally advanced carcinoma of the prostate. Int J Radiat Oncol Biol Phys 50(5): 1243–1252, 2001

68. McNeal JE, Redwine EA, et al.: Zonal distribution of prostatic adenocarcinoma. Correlation with histologic pattern and direction of spread. Am J Surg Pathol 12(12): 897–906, 1988

69. Lee F, Siders DB, et al.: Prostate cancer: transrectal ultrasound and pathology comparison. A preliminary study of outer gland (peripheral and central zones) and inner gland (transition zone) cancer. Cancer 67(4 Suppl): 1132–1142, 1991

70. Epstein JI, Pound CR, et al.: Disease progression following radical prostatectomy in men with Gleason score 7 tumor. J Urol 160(1): 97–100, discussion 101, 1998

71. Tefilli MV, Gheiler EL et al.: Prognostic indicators in patients with seminal vesicle involvement following radical prostatectomy for clinically localized prostate cancer. J Urol 160(3 Pt 1): 802–806, 1998

72. Tefilli MV, Gheiler EL et al.: Should Gleason score 7 prostate cancer be considered a unique grade category? Urology 53(2): 372–377, 1999

73. Sakr WA, Tefilli MV et al.: Gleason score 7 prostate cancer: A heterogeneous entity? Correlation with pathologic parameters and disease-free survival. Urology 56(5): 730–734, 2000

74. Han M, Partin AW, et al.: Long-term biochemical disease-free and cancer-specific survival following anatomic radical retropubic prostatectomy. The 15-year Johns Hopkins experience. Urol Clin North Am 28(3): 555–565, 2001

75. Makarov DV, Sanderson H, et al.: Gleason Score 7 Prostate Cancer on Needle Biopsy: Is the Prognostic Difference in Gleason Scores 4 3 and 3 4 Independent of the Number of Involved Cores? J Urol 167(6): 2440–2442, 2002

76. Partin AW, Mangold LA et al.: Contemporary update of prostate cancer staging nomograms (Partin Tables) for the new millennium. Urology 58(6): 843–848, 2001

77. Freedland SJ, Csathy GS, et al.: Percent prostate needle biopsy tissue with cancer is more predictive of biochemical failure or adverse pathology after radical prostatectomy than prostate specific antigen or Gleason score. J Urol 167(2 Pt 1): 516–520, 2002

78. Grossklaus DJ, Coffey CS, et al.: Percent of cancer in the biopsy set predicts pathological findings after prostatectomy. J Urol 167(5): 2032–2035, discussion 2036, 2002

79. Grossfeld GD, Latini DM, et al.: Predicting disease recurrence in intermediate and high-risk patients undergoing radical prostatectomy using percent positive biopsies: Results from CaPSURE. Urology 59(4): 560–565, 2002

80. Bonin SR, Hanlon AL, et al.: Evidence of increased failure in the treatment of prostate carcinoma patients who have perineural invasion treated with three-dimensional conformal radiation therapy. Cancer 79(1): 75–80, 1997

81. Catalona WJ, Smith DS: 5-year tumor recurrence rates after anatomical radical retropubic prostatectomy for prostate cancer. J Urol 152(5 Pt 2): 1837–1842, 1994

82. Pound CR, Partin AW et al.: Prostate-specific antigen after anatomic radical retropubic prostatectomy. Patterns of recurrence and cancer control. Urol Clin North Am 24(2): 395–406, 1997

83. Mian BM, Troncoso P et al.: Outcome of patients with Gleason score 8 or higher prostate cancer following radical prostatectomy alone. J Urol 167(4): 1675–1680, 2002

84. Sakr WA, Grignon DJ: Prostate. Practice parameters, pathologic staging, and handling radical prostatectomy specimens. Urol Clin North Am 26(3): 453–463, 1999

85. Murphy WM, Soloway MS et al.: Pathologic changes associated with androgen deprivation therapy for prostate cancer. Cancer 68(4): 821–828, 1991

86. Tetu B, Srigley JR et al.: Effect of combination endocrine therapy (LHRH agonist and flutamide) on normal prostate and prostatic adenocarcinoma. A histopathologic and immunohistochemical study. Am J Surg Pathol 15(2): 111–120, 1991

87. Armas OA, Aprikian AG, et al.: Clinical and pathobiological effects of neoadjuvant total androgen ablation therapy on clinically localized prostatic adenocarcinoma. Am J Surg Pathol 18(10): 979–991, 1994

88. Bentley G, Dey J, et al.: Significance of the Gleason scoring system after neoadjuvant hormonal therapy. Mol Urol 4(3): 125, discussion 131, 2000

89. Dhom G, Degro S: Therapy of prostatic cancer and histopathologic follow-up. Prostate 3(6): 531–542, 1982

90. Rakozy C, FJ, Tekyi-Mensah S et al.: Post-radiation prostate needle bipsies in 121 patients with and without neoadjuvant hormonal therapy: Histologic grading and clinical outcome (abstract). Mod Pathol 13: 111A, 2000

91. Bostwick DG, Egbert BM, et al.: Radiation injury of the normal and neoplastic prostate. Am J Surg Pathol 6(6): 541–551, 1982

92. Siders DB, Lee F: Histologic changes of irradiated prostatic carcinoma diagnosed by transrectal ultrasound. Hum Pathol 23(4): 344–351, 1992

93. Crook JM, Bahadur YA, et al.: Evaluation of radiation effect, tumor differentiation, and prostate specific antigen staining in sequential prostate biopsies after external beam radiotherapy for patients with prostate carcinoma. Cancer 79(1): 81–89, 1997

94. Wheeler JA, Zagars GK et al.: Dedifferentiation of locally recurrent prostate cancer after radiation therapy. Evidence for tumor progression. Cancer 71(11): 3783–3787, 1993

95. Brawn P: Histologic features of metastatic prostate cancer. Hum Pathol 23(3): 267–272, 1992

96. Bubendorf L, Schopfer A, et al.: Metastatic patterns of prostate cancer: An autopsy study of 1,589 patients. Hum Pathol 31(5): 578–583, 2000

97. Saitoh H, Hida M et al.: Metastatic patterns of prostatic cancer. Correlation between sites and number of organs involved. Cancer 54(12): 3078–3084, 1984

98. Turkeri LN, Sakr WA et al.: Comparative analysis of epidermal growth factor receptor gene expression and protein product in benign, premalignant, and malignant prostate tissue. Prostate 25(4): 199–205, 1994

99. Gao X, Chen YQ, et al.: Somatic mutations of the WAF1/CIP1 gene in primary prostate cancer. Oncogene 11(7): 1395–1398, 1995

100. Gao X, Grignon DJ, et al.: Elevated 12-lipoxygenase mRNA expression correlates with advanced stage and poor differentiation of human prostate cancer. Urology 46(2): 227–237, 1995

101. Macoska JA, Trybus TM, et al.: Evidence for three tumor suppressor gene loci on chromosome 8p in human prostate cancer. Cancer Res 55(22): 5390–5395, 1995

102. Sakr WA, Grignon DJ: Prostate cancer: Indicators of aggressiveness. Eur Urol 32(Suppl 3): 15–23, 1997

103. Sarkar FH, Li Y et al.: Relationship of p21(WAF1) expression with disease-free survival and biochemical recurrence in prostate adenocarcinomas (PCa). Prostate 40(4): 256–260, 1999

104. Dunsmuir WD, Gillett CE, et al.: Molecular markers for predicting prostate cancer stage and survival. BJU Int 86(7): 869–878, 2000

105. Gopalkrishnan RV, Kang DC, et al.: Molecular markers and determinants of prostate cancer metastasis. J Cell Physiol 189(3): 245–256, 2001

106. Mora LB, Buettner R et al.: Prostate adenocarcinoma: Cellular and molecular abnormalities. Cancer Control 8(6): 551–561, 2001

107. Hamdy FC: Prognostic and predictive factors in prostate cancer. Cancer Treat Rev 27(3): 143–151, 2001

108. Bostwick DG, Grignon DJ, et al.: Prognostic factors in prostate cancer. College of American Pathologists Consensus Statement 1999. Arch Pathol Lab Med 124(7): 995–1000, 2000

109. Hammond ME, Fitzgibbons PL, et al.: College of American Pathologists Conference XXXV: Solid tumor prognostic factors-which, how and so what? Summary document and recommendations for implementation. Cancer Committee and Conference Participants. Arch Pathol Lab Med 124(7): 958–965, 2000

110. Luo JH, Yu YP, et al.: Gene expression analysis of prostate cancers. Mol Carcinog 33(1): 25–35, 2002

111. Veltri RW, Miller MC et al.: Prediction of prostate carcinoma stage by quantitative biopsy pathology. Cancer 91(12): 2322–2328, 2001

112. Sebo TJ, Cheville JC et al.: Perineural invasion and MIB-1 positivity in addition to Gleason score are significant preoperative predictors of progression after radical retropubic prostatectomy for prostate cancer. Am J Surg Pathol 26(4): 431–439, 2002

113. Roach M, Lu J et al.: Four prognostic groups predict long-term survival from prostate cancer following radiotherapy alone on Radiation Therapy Oncology Group clinical trials. Int J Radiat Oncol Biol Phys 47(3): 609–615, 2000

114. Tran TA, Jennings TA et al.: Pseudomyxoma ovariilike posttherapeutic alteration in prostatic adenocarcinoma: A distinctive pattern in patients receiving neoadjuvant androgen ablation therapy. Am J Surg Pathol 22(3): 347–354, 1998

Address for offprints: Mingxin Che, Department of Pathology, Harper University Hospital, 3990 John R, Detroit MI 48202, USA; *Tel:* +1 313 745 8555; *e-mail:* mche@dmc.org

Prostate cancer susceptibility genes: Many studies, many results, no answers

Nina N. Nupponen and John D. Carpten
Cancer Genetics Branch, National Human Genome Research Institute, National Institutes of Health, Bethesda, MD, USA

Key words: hereditary, prostate cancer, predisposition, mutation

Abstract

Since the first report of a genome-wide scan for hereditary prostate cancer (HPCA hereinafter) in 1996, several publications have presented data implicating various chromosomal regions by linkage analysis without any consequential identifications of the target genes. The most intensive attention has been focused on chromosome 1, and it has been proposed to contain at least three sub-chromosomal regions (HPC1, PCAP, CAPB) harboring putative prostate cancer susceptibility genes. Nevertheless, one susceptibility gene, ELAC2/HPC2 at chromosome 17, has now been identified. Yet it seems to have a questionable role in prostate cancer predisposition. HPCA susceptibility loci have become undeniable archenemies of prostate cancer investigators, as the results of candidate gene analyses have been bewilderingly inconclusive. Predisposition to prostate cancer is most likely to be caused by several genes, different models of Mendelian inheritance, incomplete penetrance and varying population ethnicity frequencies. We will review the current state of the HPCA field and discuss the difficulties associated with identifying prostate cancer susceptibility genes.

Introduction

Prostate cancer is the most common non-cutaneous cancer in men in the US with approximately 198 100 cases diagnosed per year [1]. It has been estimated that one out of eight males will be diagnosed with prostate cancer in their lifetime [2]. The risk for prostate cancer increases with age, with the mean age at diagnosis in the US currently being 71 years for Caucasian Americans and 69 years for African Americans [3]. Risk factors associated with prostate cancer are not well understood. The relative risk of prostate cancer is higher for those men with a family history of prostate cancer when compared to men without an affected relative [4,5]. Family history is the most significant risk factor known for developing prostate cancer.

Results from segregation analyses suggest that familial clustering of prostate cancer can best be explained by transmission of a rare hereditary factor accounting for 5–10% of total prostate cancer cases [6]. These findings support the identification of prostate cancer susceptibility genes by positional cloning methods. Twenty hereditary cancer genes have been successfully identified by positional cloning strategies. Traditionally, the chromosomal location of the gene in a hereditary disease is detected using linkage analysis. The power of linkage analysis is tremendous when it is associated with disease phenotypes adhering strongly to the rules of Mendelian inheritance. Parametric linkage analysis is based on the presumption that a single locus is causative for an indistinguishable disease phenotype with a known model of inheritance. A major dilemma in prostate cancer genetics is the assignment of the correct mode of inheritance for familial prostate cancer, as several studies have suggested different modes of inheritance for prostate cancer, e.g. dominant, recessive or X-linked inheritance [7–10]. Non-parametric linkage analyses can be used because they do not require knowledge of a precise genetic model, and chromosomal locations are identified from affected family individuals sharing a common set of genetic marker alleles surrounding the disease locus. In other words, all affected individuals within a family will share a similar pattern of adjacent

M.L. Cher, K.V. Honn and A. Raz (eds.), Prostate Cancer: New Horizons in Research and Treatment, 19–28.
© 2002 *Kluwer Academic Publishers.*

20

genetic markers that is not shared by the unaffected members of the family. Both methods have been used in prostate cancer genetic studies.

Several issues have hampered prostate cancer genetics including the high prevalence of sporadic prostate cancers, the late age of disease onset and heterogeneity. The first issue is that of phenocopies, or affected individuals in the family that are purely sporadic cases. Linkage results are substantially diminished in these families, as the sporadic cases are analyzed as affected individuals, but they do not share the disease locus with the hereditary cases in the family. The second issue involves ascertainment, as prostate cancer is a late age disease. Therefore, in many instances parents are deceased, so obtaining genetic information on the parents is usually not possible. Even in the case of affected siblings, several may have died of diseases other than prostate cancer, so obtaining genetic information on these individuals is not possible. This limits the number of samples ascertained, which decreases the amount of genetic information, ultimately reducing the linkage results. Finally, there is the issue of heterogeneity, where more than one locus may be responsible for the same phenotype. Therefore, within any collection of high-risk prostate cancer families, only a fraction of the families will be genetically linked to the same susceptibility locus. Heterogeneity is evident in several hereditary cancer types and is quite evident in prostate cancer as will be discussed later in this article.

Altogether, it is evident that hereditary prostate cancer (HPCA) is a more complex disease than expected a decade ago in the dawn of identifying the first tumor suppressor genes in familial cancers. HPCA undoubtedly involves more loci than, for instance, breast or colorectal cancers. However, efforts to identify susceptibility genes will yield insights into mechanisms of prostate cancer development. Table 1 summarizes the published genetic linkage studies for prostate cancer susceptibility genes, which will be discussed in detail below.

What lies beneath chromosome 1?

The first evidence of a HPCA predisposition locus was published in 1996 [11]. The data set consisted of 91 high-risk prostate cancer families from Northern-America (including two African-American) and Sweden. The family inclusion criteria for this study were: prostate cancer present in three generations (maternal or paternal lineage but not both); three first-degree relatives with a prostate cancer diagnosis, or two relatives affected before age 55 [6,12]. Assuming heterogeneity, a multipoint LOD of 5.43 was observed for markers mapping to chromosome 1, 1q24–q31, with the estimation that 34% of families used in the analysis were linked to this chromosomal region. The LOD score is the log 10 of an odds ratio for a genetic marker being linked to a disease versus being unlinked. A LOD of 3 is equivalent to 1000 : 1 odds that the marker is linked to the disease locus. Therefore, the higher the LOD score the more likely the marker is linked. For simple Mendelian disorders, a LOD of 3 or higher is generally accepted as true linkage. However, due to heterogeneity and other factors, lower LOD scores are accepted for complex diseases such as prostate cancer. The locus, designated at HPC1, has been either confirmed or excluded by several publications

Table 1. Hereditary prostate cancer genome-wide scans in chronological order by publication

Chromosomal region	HLOD	Number of families	Reference
1q24–q25 (HPC1)	Multipoint 5.43	91	Smith et al. (1996)
Xq27–q28 (HPCX)	Two-point 2.57	360	Xu et al. (1998)
1q42–q43 (PCAP)	Multipoint 2.2	47	Berethon et al. (1998)
1p35–p36 (CAPB)	Two-point 3.65	12	Gibbs et al. (1999)
20q13	Multipoint 3.02	162	Berry et al. (2000)
17p13 (HPC2/ELAC2)	Two-point 4.5	33	Tavtigian et al. (2001)
5q31–q33, 7q32–q36, 19q12	P-values 0.0002, 0.0007, 0.0004	513 sibpairs	Witte et al. (2001)
2q37–q38, 12p13–p12, 15q26, 16p13, 16q23–q24	Multipoint 2.92, 2.0, 1.71, 2,81, 3.15	564 sibpairs	Suarez et al. (2001)
5p13–q13, 12p13–p12, 19p13	Multipoint 2.03, 2.78, 2.87	98	Hsieh et al. (2001)
8p22–p23	Multipoint 1.84	159	Xu et al. (2001)

Table 2. Confirmatory reports of original HPCA linkage studies

Chromosomal region	HLOD	Number of families	Reference
1q24–q25 (HPC1)	NPL 1.72	59	Cooney et al. (1997)
1q24–q25 (HPC1)	Single-point 1.93	92	Hsieh et al. (1997)
1q24–q25 (HPC1)	Three-point 2.82	41	Neuhausen et al. (1999)
1q24–q25 (HPC1)	NPL 1.64	40	Gronberg et al. (1999)
1q24–q25 (HPC1)	NPL 1.99	144	Berry et al. (2000)
1q24–q25 (HPC1)	Multipoint 2.56	772	Xu et al. (2000)
1q24–q25 (HPC1)	NPL 3.47	150	Goode et al. (2000)
1q24–q25 (HPC1)	Single-point 1.93	98	Hsieh et al. (2001)
1q24–q25 (HPC1)	Multipoint 2.54	159	Xu et al. (2001)
1q24–q25 (HPC1)	NPL 2.61	149	Goode et al. (2001)
Xq27–q28 (HPCX)	NPL 1.89	153	Lange et al. (1999)
Xq27–q28 (HPCX)	Two-point 2.05	57	Schleutker et al. (2000)
Xq27–q28 (HPCX)	Single-point 1.62	42	Hsieh et al. (2001)
1q42–q43 (PCAP)	Two-point 1.99	152	Gibbs et al. (2000)
1q42–q43 (PCAP)	Multipoint 2.10	230	Suarez et al. (2000)
1q42–q43 (PCAP)	Multipoint 1.90	254	Goddard et al. (2001)
1q42–q43 (PCAP)	Multipoint 2.65	64	Cancel-Tassin et al. (2001)
1p35–p36 (CAPB)	NPL 2.28	152	Gibbs et al. (2000)
1p35–p36 (CAPB)	Single-point 3.78	13	Suarez et al. (2000)
1p35–p36 (CAPB)	NPL 1.02	207	Badzioch et al. (2000)
1p35–p36 (CAPB)	NPL 1.50	149	Goode et al. (2001)

producing an apparent lack of agreement for the HPC1 putative prostate cancer predisposition gene [13–22] (Table 2). The most comprehensive analysis of HPC1 linkage was recently reported by the International Consortium for Prostate Cancer Genetics. In this study, 772 families were analyzed for six genetic markers surrounding the original HPC1 locus [18]. The results showed positive linkage. However, the estimated frequency of linked families was reduced to 6% as compared to 34% in the original HPC1 linkage study. Also, HPC1 linkage was strongest in families with male-to-male transmission and an early age of diagnosis.

Following chromosomal location of HPC1 by linkage analysis, a detailed physical map of the region was constructed [23,24]. Physical mapping aims at constructing clone 'contigs' by obtaining overlapping, large-insert genomic clones (e.g. YACs, BACs, PACs, P1s) that cover the region of interest. These maps also play an important role in candidate gene mapping and in the mapping of genetic markers for refining the critical genetic interval. Currently, the existence of the HPC1 gene remains a mystery, as no mutations have been reported in families linked to the HPC1 locus.

The predisposing for cancer of prostate (PCAP) putative susceptibility locus at 1q42–q43 was the second HPCA predisposition locus reported, which mapped to chromosome 1 [25]. The PCAP locus was detected using 47 German and French families. Linkage analysis was performed assuming heterogeneity and a multipoint HLOD value of 2.2 was achieved. Non-parametric analysis yielded an NPL value of 3.1. This locus appears to be the main predisposing locus of HPCA originating from western and southern parts of Europe [26–29] (Table 2).

The third chromosome 1 putative prostate cancer susceptibility locus is known as Cancer of prostate and brain (CAPB) and was mapped to 1p36 by linkage analysis [30]. The linked prostate cancer families also had several cases of primary brain tumors (12 out of 141 families, LOD 3.22), in which allelic imbalance at 1p36 is a frequent phenomenon [31–33]. One candidate gene at 1p36, designated as TP73, is a TP53 family member [34]. However, mutation and expression analyses of the TP73 gene in prostate cancer have revealed that it is not frequently mutated in familial prostate–brain or sporadic prostate cancer patients [35–37].

The indication of X-linked inheritance in prostate cancer

An X-linked mode of inheritance of prostate cancer had been suggested earlier based on a hypothesis that an individual's risk for acquiring prostate cancer is higher if his brother rather than father has a diagnosis of prostate cancer [8,9]. This suggestion is now supported by linkage implicating a chromosome X prostate cancer susceptibility locus, designated HPCX, at Xq27–q28 [38]. This study used a combined set of 360 families from North America, Finland and Sweden that were further stratified into two categories based on the presence/absence of male-to-male transmission. A notable two-point LOD score of 4.6 was obtained for markers at Xq27–q28 within families showing no male-to-male transmission and it was predicted to account for 16% of prostate cancers in this set. The HPCX linkage has been confirmed independently by others [39–42] (Table 2).

The newly identified gene, ELAC2, involvement in HPCA predisposition

A genome-wide scan of a large number of high-risk prostate cancer families from the Mormon population suggested linkage at 17p11 [43]. The original set of families ($n = 127$) gave a significant two-point LOD score of 4.3. Genetic refinement led to the subsequent mapping and mutational analysis of a gene known as HPC2/ELAC. The function of the ELAC2 protein serves as a metal-dependent hydrolase in orthologs of *S. cerevisiae*, *C. elegans*, *D. melanogaster*, etc., and displays amino acid sequence similarity with DNA interstrand crosslink repair proteins [43]. Mutational analysis revealed one germline frameshift mutation in one 17p-linked family that led to the premature truncation of the protein. However, the segregation of this mutation in this family was inconsistent. Furthermore, two missense mutations (ALA541THR and SER217LEU) were reported to segregate within two high-risk families and these missense mutations seemed to be associated with early-onset disease.

Prior to the report of the identification of HPC2/ELAC, an association study was performed to assess the Ala541Thr carrier rate in prostate cancer cases versus controls [44]. The Ala541Thr carrier rate was 7.5% among individuals with clinically diagnosed prostate cancer compared to 5.7% among the controls suggesting a statistically significant difference in cases versus controls. Thus far, four independent analysis of the ELAC2 gene involvement in HPCA have been published [45–48]. Only one of these publications demonstrated a novel nonsense mutation appearing in

exon 7 of the ELAC2 gene (Glu216Stop), but showing an incomplete segregation pattern [48]. The missense mutations mentioned above were not found to indicate a statistically increased risk for HPCA in any of the replication reports. In addition, a study regarding the role of these two polymorphisms detected in individuals with an elevated serum PSA level could not observe any statistical difference between persons with high PSA levels and healthy females [49].

Chromosome 17 contains two famous tumor suppressor genes, TP53 (17p13.1) and BRCA1 (17q12). It has been shown that there seems to be an increased relative risk for developing prostate cancer in males carrying mutations in the BRCA1 gene [50–52]. In sporadic prostate cancers, loss of chromosome 17 has been found in up to 50% of advanced prostate cancer by loss of heterogeneity (LOH) and comparative genomic hybridization (CGH) studies [53–58]. In addition, a microcell-mediated transfer of human chromosome 17 suppresses growth in highly metastatic prostate cancer cells, thus presenting additional evidence for the presence of a prostate cancer susceptibility gene on chromosome 17 [59]. Nevertheless, the role of ELAC/HPC2 in HPCA remains inconclusive.

Other HPCA loci discovered by genome-wide linkages

In addition to the above-mentioned HPCA loci identified through linkage efforts, several other loci have been reported to confer susceptibility to prostate cancer. One such chromosomal locus maps to the long arm of chromosome 20 (20q11–q13) and has been designated as HPC20 [60]. Positive LOD scores were achieved using both parametric and non-parametric analyses with a non-parametric LOD score of 3.69 in families with no male-to-male transmission, <5 affected individuals and an age at diagnosis >65 years of age. These findings have been confirmed by three other studies strongly suggesting the presence of a prostate cancer predisposition gene at 20q13 [61,62] (Table 1).

Using tumor aggressiveness as a quantitative trait, non-parametric analysis was performed on 513 brothers to identify prostate cancer aggressiveness loci [63]. Statistically significant signals were detected at three distinct genomic regions, 5q31–q33, 7q32 and 19q12. Another study using multiplex sibships that resulted in several chromosomal loci is listed in Table 1.

Classical chromosomal loci in sporadic prostate cancer correlate to novel HPCA loci

A number of regions commonly associated with allelic imbalance in prostate cancer have also recently been implicated in prostate cancer susceptibility. A recent analysis using 504 brothers representing 230 multiplex sibships with prostate cancer revealed positive linkage results at 16p13 (HLOD 2.81) and 16q23–q24 (HLOD 3.15) [27]. The latter is a chromosomal region commonly lost in sporadic prostate carcinomas [64–66]. The E-cadherin (CDH1) is located at 16q22.1 and its dysfunction has been associated with an invasive tumor phenotype in sporadic prostate cancer [67–69]. Nevertheless, no mutations in prostate cancer have been detected within the coding sequence of this gene. Furthermore, E-cadherin is a known susceptibility gene for hereditary diffuse gastric cancer characterized by several different nonsense mutations displaying an autosomal dominant pattern of inheritance [70]. Interestingly, an elevated risk for both prostate and gastric carcinoma was seen among relatives of prostate cancer patients in a population based study in Finland [71].

Loss of heterozygosity at 8p is the most common genetic rearrangement detected in each and every phase of prostate cancer development, emerging from prostatic intraepithelial neoplasia (PIN) to metastatic lesions. Several reports indicate multiple homozygous deletions and at least two minimal common regions of loss, 8p12–p21 and 8p22, suggesting the presence of several candidate tumor suppressor genes [72,73]. Further intriguing evidence has recently been obtained from genome-wide scans of HPCA revealing linkage to genetic markers at 8p, thus increasing the evidence for the importance of this chromosomal region in prostate cancer development [11,74,75]. A putative prostate cancer susceptibility gene known as PG1, which is localized to 8p22, was evaluated for the association of variants in this gene to prostate cancer [75]. Although there was evidence of over-transmission of a specific PG1 allele in prostate cancer patients in this study, no obvious functionally relevant changes have been identified. Further investigation is warranted.

Both CGH and LOH studies have shown that the most frequently lost chromosome arms in prostate cancer are 8p, 10q, 13q, 16q and 17p implicating important putative tumor suppressor genes in prostate cancer development and progression (reviewed in [76–80]). Information gathered from both hereditary and sporadic prostate cancer studies point intriguingly to the same chromosomal regions, forming a riddle whether coincidence means multiplied probability.

Polymorphisms detected in genes involved in the androgen pathway

Regulation of prostate cells involves a network of hormonal control including an age-related decrease of dihydrosterone (DHT) as well as elevated androgen receptor gene (AR) expression in prostate basal cells. The most extensively studied genes in steroid hormone metabolism include AR, steroid 5α-reductase gene (SRD5A2), hydroxysteroid dehydrogenases (HSDs), enzymes that promote steroid hormone biotransformation such as glutathione S-transferase (GST), N-acetyltransferase (NAT), cytochrome P450C17α (CYP17) and vitamin D receptor (VDR). The nucleotide differences in DNA sequence among individuals or populations are referred to as polymorphisms. All studies including these genes have been performed using association analysis in order to test whether a particular polymorphism detected in an individual's blood DNA is enriched in a disease when compared with unaffected controls. This analysis might then produce a statistically significant association between that allele and the disease. For that reason, these studies fall into the category of genes implicated in susceptibility to cancer.

The transactivation domain of the AR is encoded by the first exon, which features polymorphic CAG and GGC trinucleotide repeats [81]. The length of the CAG-repeat (40 or more) has been associated with androgen insensitivity syndromes (AIS) and the reduction of this repeat length (<15 repeats) may lead to elevated transactivation potentials [82]. The shorter form of the CAG-repeat is believed to be associated with increased prostate cancer risk, especially in African-American males, as the frequency of the (<15 repeat) allele is higher in African Americans when compared to men of other ethnic groups [82,83].

The AIS mutation repertoire of the AR gene contains all known classical types of mutations (missense, nonsense, frame-shift, splice-site) (reviewed extensively in [84]). In the Finnish population, a polymorphism (Asp726Leu) has been suggested to increase the risk for prostate cancer up to 6-fold [85–87]. AR gene rearrangements are highly correlated with sporadic prostate cancer progression as well. About 30% of hormone-refractory tumors show amplification and/or over-expression of the AR [55,88,89]. The tumors that develop during anti-androgen treatment may acquire a specific mutation (Thr877Ala) that may explain response failures by utilizing hormones other than DHT [90,91].

The 3'-UTR of the SRD5A2 gene contains dinucleotide TA-repeats (the most common form has 87 bp) and only African-American males are represented in the category of long TA-repeat alleles not found in other populations [92,93]. The functional relevance of this polymorphism is unknown. In addition, two other polymorphisms in the SRD5A2 gene have been identified, Val89Leu and Ala89Thr [94,95] of which the former confers a 30% reduction in steroid 5α reductase activity in Asian males if the allele is in a homozygous state, e.g. leucine–leucine [94]. This genotype is more common in Asian males (28%) than in African Americans (2.5%) suggesting an association for extremely high prostate cancer risk based on testosterone hormonal regulatory mechanisms behind the disease [96]. Other genes involved in the testosterone pathway (VDR, CYP17, HSDs, GSTs and NAT) have been recently reviewed comprehensively [97,98].

Conclusions

Several susceptibility genes implicated by positional cloning in familial cancers have been identified, however, the molecular genetics behind prostate cancer predisposition remain unknown. The increasing number of publications, novel linkages on various chromosomes and the lack of confirmatory studies are among the many issues confounding the field of prostate cancer susceptibility. Heterogeneity, likelihood of reduced penetrance and the existence of numerous sporadic cases are all obstacles that can only be overcome by enormous combined efforts from numerous prostate cancer investigation groups. The ICPCG represents such a consortium and should continue to prove extremely useful in the overall evaluation of prostate cancer susceptibility genes. Furthermore, although men of African descent have higher incidence rates and mortality rates when compared to men of other ethnicities, there has been very little targeted recruitment to assess the role of HPCA factors in men of African descent. A consortium of investigators, clinicians and health professionals known as the African American Hereditary Prostate Cancer Study Network has been established to address the issue of HPCA in African Americans. Although no linkage data has yet been published from this group, information on the recruitment strategy and experience has been reported and should help other groups tailor their recruitment strategies to increase the representation of men of African descent, namely African Americans, in prostate cancer genetic studies [99]. It is our hope that large meta-analyses of thousands of high-risk prostate cancer families will be performed to help us gain a true understanding of HPCA. Likewise, the analysis of thousands of prostate cancer cases and controls must be accumulated and analyzed concurrently to allow researchers to gain insights into the role of low penetrant alleles in the genetics of prostate cancer. The last decade has seen breakthroughs in the sequencing of the human genome and the development of novel methods in molecular genetics such as microarrays. These tools should aid researchers to get a better grasp of the biology and genetics behind prostate cancer susceptibility, development and progression. As prostate cancer has become a major health issue in the US and other countries alike, continued funding for research in these areas must be supported. As early diagnosis is the best way of combating this disease, the research discussed above will provide insights into the pathways involved in prostate cancer, which will ultimately allow for the identification of novel diagnostic and therapeutic tools to give men diagnosed with this disease a better overall quality of life.

Acknowledgements

Nina N. Nupponen has been supported by The Helsingin Sanomat Foundation, the Ella and Georg Ehrnrooth Foundation, the Maud Kuistila Foundation, the Paulo Foundation and the Finnish Cultural Foundation.

References

1. Ries L, Kosary CL, Hankey BA, Miller B, Clegg L, Edwards BK: SEER cancer statistics review, 1973–97. National Cancer Institute, Bethesda, MD, 2000
2. Ries L, Esner M, Kosary CL, Hankey B, Miller B, Clegg L, Edwards B: SEER cancer statistics review, 1973–96. National Cancer Institute, Bethesda, MD, 1999
3. Stanford JL, Stephenson RA, Coyle LM, Cerhan J, Correa R, Eley JW, Gilliland F, Hankey B, Kolonel LN, Kosary CL, Ross R, Severson R, West D: Prostate cancer trends 1973–1995, SEER program. National Cancer Institute, Bethesda, MD, 1999
4. Steinberg GD, Carter BS, Beaty TH, Childs B, Walsh PC: Family history and the risk of prostate cancer. Prostate 17: 337–347, 1990

5. Isaacs SD, Kiemeney LA, Baffoe-Bonnie A, Beaty TH, Walsh PC: Risk of cancer in relatives of prostate cancer probands. J Natl Cancer Inst 87: 991–996, 1995

6. Carter BS, Bova GS, Beaty TH, Steinberg GD, Childs B, Isaacs WB, Walsh PC: Hereditary prostate cancer: epidemiologic and clinical features. J Urol 150: 797–802, 1993

7. Carter BS, Beaty TH, Steinberg GD, Childs B, Walsh PC: Mendelian inheritance of familial prostate cancer. Proc Natl Acad Sci USA 89: 3367–3371, 1992

8. Monroe KR, Yu MC, Kolonel LN, Coetzee GA, Wilkens LR, Ross RK, Henderson BE: Evidence of an X-linked or recessive genetic component to prostate cancer risk. Nat Med 1: 827–829, 1995

9. Narod SA, Dupont A, Cusan L, Diamond P, Gomez JL, Suburu R, Labrie F: The impact of family history on early detection of prostate cancer. Nat Med 1: 99–101, 1995

10. Schaid DJ, McDonnell SK, Blute ML, Thibodeau SN: Evidence for autosomal dominant inheritance of prostate cancer. Am J Hum Genet 62: 1425–1438, 1998

11. Smith JR, Freije D, Carpten JD, Gronberg H, Xu J, Isaacs SD, Brownstein MJ, Bova GS, Guo H, Bujnovszky P, Nusskern DR, Damber JE, Bergh A, Emanuelsson M, Kallioniemi OP, Walker-Daniels J, Bailey-Wilson JE, Beaty TH, Meyers DA, Walsh PC, Collins FS, Trent JM, Isaacs WB: Major susceptibility locus for prostate cancer on chromosome 1 suggested by a genome-wide search. Science 274: 1371–1374, 1996

12. Walsh PC, Partin AW: Family history facilitates the early diagnosis of prostate carcinoma. Cancer 80: 1871–1874, 1997

13. Cooney KA, McCarthy JD, Lange E, Huang L, Miesfeldt S, Montie JE, Oesterling JE, Sandler HM, Lange K: Prostate cancer susceptibility locus on chromosome 1q: a confirmatory study. J Natl Cancer Inst 89: 955–959, 1997

14. Hsieh CL, Oakley-Girvan I, Gallagher RP, Wu AH, Kolonel LN, Teh CZ, Halpern J, West DW, Paffenbarger RS Jr. Whittemore AS: Re: prostate cancer susceptibility locus on chromosome 1q: a confirmatory study. J Natl Cancer Inst 89: 1893–1894, 1997

15. Eeles RA, Durocher F, Edwards S, Teare D, Badzioch M, Hamoudi R, Gill S, Biggs P, Dearnaley D, Ardern-Jones A, Dowe A, Shearer R, McLennan DL, Norman RL, Ghadirian P, Aprikian A, Ford D, Amos C, King TM, Labrie F, Simard J, Narod SA, Easton D, Foulkes WD: Linkage analysis of chromosome 1q markers in 136 prostate cancer families. The Cancer Research Campaign/British Prostate Group U.K. Familial Prostate Cancer Study Collaborators. Am J Hum Genet 62: 653–658, 1998

16. Neuhausen SL, Skolnick MH, Cannon-Albright L: Familial prostate cancer studies in Utah. Br J Urol 79(Suppl 1): 15–20, 1997

17. Gronberg H, Smith J, Emanuelsson M, Jonsson BA, Bergh A, Carpten J, Isaacs W, Xu J, Meyers D, Trent J, Damber JE: In Swedish families with hereditary prostate cancer, linkage to the HPC1 locus on chromosome 1q24–25 is restricted to families with early-onset prostate cancer. Am J Hum Genet 65: 134–140, 1999

18. Xu J: Combined analysis of hereditary prostate cancer linkage to 1q24–25: results from 772 hereditary prostate cancer families from the International Consortium for Prostate Cancer Genetics. Am J Hum Genet 66: 945–957, 2000

19. Berry R, Schaid DJ, Smith JR, French AJ, Schroeder JJ, McDonnell SK, Peterson BJ, Wang ZY, Carpten JD, Roberts SG, Tester DJ, Blute ML, Trent JM, Thibodeau SN: Linkage analyses at the chromosome 1 loci 1q24–25 (HPC1), 1q42.2–43 (PCAP), and 1p36 (CAPB) in families with hereditary prostate cancer. Am J Hum Genet 66: 539–546, 2000

20. Goode EL, Stanford JL, Chakrabarti L, Gibbs M, Kolb S, McIndoe RA, Buckley VA, Schuster EF, Neal CL, Miller EL, Brandzel S, Hood L, Ostrander EA, Jarvik GP: Linkage analysis of 150 high-risk prostate cancer families at 1q24–25. Genet Epidemiol 18: 251–275, 2000

21. Xu J, Zheng SL, Chang B, Smith JR, Carpten JD, Stine OC, Isaacs SD, Wiley KE, Henning L, Ewing C, Bujnovszky P, Bleeker ER, Walsh PC, Trent JM, Meyers DA, Isaacs WB: Linkage of prostate cancer susceptibility loci to chromosome 1. Hum Genet 108: 335–345, 2001

22. Goode EL, Stanford JL, Peters MA, Janer M, Gibbs M, Kolb S, Badzioch MD, Hood L, Ostrander EA, Jarvik GP: Clinical characteristics of prostate cancer in an analysis of linkage to four putative susceptibility loci. Clin Cancer Res 7: 2739–2749, 2001

23. Carpten JD, Makalowska I, Robbins CM, Scott N, Sood R, Connors TD, Bonner TI, Smith JR, Faruque MU, Stephan DA, Pinkett H, Morgenbesser SD, Su K, Graham C, Gregory SG, Williams H, McDonald L, Baxevanis AD, Klingler KW, Landes GM, Trent JM: A 6-Mb high-resolution physical and transcription map encompassing the hereditary prostate cancer 1 (HPC1) region. Genomics 64: 1–14, 2000

24. Sood R, Bonner TI, Makalowska I, Stephan DA, Robbins CM, Connors TD, Morgenbesser SD, Su K, Faruque MU, Pinkett H, Graham C, Baxevanis AD, Klinger KW, Landes GM, Trent JM, Carpten JD: Cloning and characterization of 13 novel transcripts and the human rgs8 gene from the 1q25 region encompassing the hereditary prostate cancer (hpc1) locus. Genomics 73: 211–222, 2001

25. Berthon P, Valeri A, Cohen-Akenine A, Drelon E, Paiss T, Wohr G, Latil A, Millasseau P, Mellah I, Cohen N, Blanche H, Bellane-Chantelot C, Demenais F, Teillac P, Le Duc A, de Petriconi R, Hautmann R, Chumakov I, Bachner L, Maitland NJ, Lidereau R, Vogel W, Fournier G, Mangin P, Cussenot O: Predisposing gene for early-onset prostate cancer, localized on chromosome 1q42.2–43. Am J Hum Genet 62: 1416–1424, 1998

26. Gibbs M, Chakrabarti L, Stanford JL, Goode EL, Kolb S, Schuster EF, Buckley VA, Shook M, Hood L, Jarvik GP, Ostrander EA: Analysis of chromosome 1q42.2–43 in 152 families with high risk of prostate cancer. Am J Hum Genet 64: 1087–1095, 1999

27. Suarez BK, Lin J, Burmester JK, Broman KW, Weber JL, Banerjee TK, Goddard KA, Witte JS, Elston RC, Catalona WJ: A genome screen of multiplex sibships with prostate cancer. Am J Hum Genet 66: 933–944, 2000

28. Cancel-Tassin G, Latil A, Valeri A, Mangin P, Fournier G, Berthon P, Cussenot O: PCAP is the major known prostate

26

cancer predisposing locus in families from south and west Europe. Eur J Hum Genet 9: 135–142, 2001

29. Goddard KA, Witte JS, Suarez BK, Catalona WJ, Olson JM: Model-free linkage analysis with covariates confirms linkage of prostate cancer to chromosomes 1 and 4. Am J Hum Genet 68: 1197–1206, 2001

30. Gibbs M, Stanford JL, McIndoe RA, Jarvik GP, Kolb S, Goode EL, Chakrabarti L, Schuster EF, Buckley VA, Miller EL, Brandzel S, Li S, Hood L, Ostrander EA: Evidence for a rare prostate cancer-susceptibility locus at chromosome 1p36. Am J Hum Genet 64: 776–787, 1999

31. Cairncross JG, Ueki K, Zlatescu MC, Lisle DK, Finkelstein DM, Hammond RR, Silver JS, Stark PC, MacDonald DR, Ino Y, Ramsay DA, Louis DN: Specific genetic predictors of chemotherapeutic response and survival in patients with anaplastic oligodendrogliomas. J Natl Cancer Inst 90: 1473–1479, 1998

32. Smith JS, Alderete B, Minn Y, Borell TJ, Perry A, Mohapatra G, Hosek SM, Kimmel D, O'Fallon J, Yates A, Feuerstein BG, Burger PC, Scheithauer BW, Jenkins RB: Localization of common deletion regions on 1p and 19q in human gliomas and their association with histological subtype. Oncogene 18: 4144–4152, 1999

33. Bigner SH, Matthews MR, Rasheed BK, Wiltshire RN, Friedman HS, Friedman AH, Stenzel TT, Dawes DM, McLendon RE, Bigner DD: Molecular genetic aspects of oligodendrogliomas including analysis by comparative genomic hybridization. Am J Pathol 155: 375–386, 1999

34. Kaghad M, Bonnet H, Yang A, Creancier L, Biscan JC, Valent A, Minty A, Chalon P, Lelias JM, Dumont X, Ferrara P, McKeon F, Caput D: Monoallelically expressed gene related to p53 at 1p36, a region frequently deleted in neuroblastoma and other human cancers. Cell 90: 809–819, 1997

35. Takahashi H, Ichimiya S, Nimura Y, Watanabe M, Furusato M, Wakui S, Yatani R, Aizawa S, Nakagawara A: Mutation, allelotyping, and transcription analyses of the p73 gene in prostatic carcinoma. Cancer Res 58: 2076–2077, 1998

36. Yokomizo A, Mai M, Bostwick DG, Tindall DJ, Qian J, Cheng L, Jenkins RB, Smith DI, Liu W: Mutation and expression analysis of the p73 gene in prostate cancer. Prostate 39: 94–100, 1999

37. Peters MA, Janer M, Kolb S, Jarvik GP, Ostrander EA, Stanford JL: Germline mutations in the p73 gene do not predispose to familial prostate-brain cancer. Prostate 48: 292–296, 2001

38. Xu J, Meyers D, Freije D, Isaacs S, Wiley K, Nusskern D, Ewing C, Wilkens E, Bujnovszky P, Bova GS, Walsh P, Isaacs W, Schleutker J, Matikainen M, Tammela T, Visakorpi T, Kallioniemi OP, Berry R, Schaid D, French A, McDonnell S, Schroeder J, Blute M, Thibodeau S, Grönberg H, Emanuelsson M, Damber J, Bergh A, Jonsson B, Smith J, Bailey-Wilson J, Carpten J, Stephan D, Gillanders E, Amundson I, Kainu T, Freas-Lutz D, Baffoe-Bonnie A, Van Aucken A, Raman Sood S, Collins F, Brownstein M, Trent J: Evidence for a prostate cancer susceptibility locus on the X chromosome. Nat Genet 20: 175–179, 1998

39. Lange EM, Chen H, Brierley K, Perrone EE, Bock CH, Gillanders E, Ray ME, Cooney KA: Linkage analysis of 153 prostate cancer families over a 30-cM region containing the putative susceptibility locus HPCX. Clin Cancer Res 5: 4013–4020, 1999

40. Schleutker J, Matikainen M, Smith J, Koivisto P, Baffoe-Bonnie A, Kainu T, Gillanders E, Sankila R, Pukkala E, Carpten J, Stephan D, Tammela T, Brownstein M, Bailey-Wilson J, Trent J, Kallioniemi OP: A genetic epidemiological study of hereditary prostate cancer (HPC) in Finland: frequent HPCX linkage in families with late-onset disease. Clin Cancer Res 6: 4810–4815, 2000

41. Peters MA, Jarvik GP, Janer M, Chakrabarti L, Kolb S, Goode EL, Gibbs M, DuBois CC, Schuster EF, Hood L, Ostrander EA, Stanford JL: Genetic linkage analysis of prostate cancer families to Xq27–28. Hum Hered 51: 107–113, 2001

42. Hsieh CL, Oakley-Girvan I, Balise RR, Halpern J, Gallagher RP, Wu AH, Kolonel LN, O'Brien LE, Lin IG, Van Den Berg DJ, Teh CZ, West DW, Whittemore AS: A genome screen of families with multiple cases of prostate cancer: evidence of genetic heterogeneity. Am J Hum Genet 69: 148–158, 2001

43. Tavtigian SV, Simard J, Teng DH, Abtin V, Baumgard M, Beck A, Camp NJ, Carillo AR, Chen Y, Dayananth P, Desrochers M, Dumont M, Farnham JM, Frank D, Frye C, Ghaffari S, Gupte JS, Hu R, Iliev D, Janecki T, Kort EN, Laity KE, Leavitt A, Leblanc G, McArthur-Morrison J, Pederson A, Penn B, Peterson KT, Reid JE, Richards S, Schroeder M, Smith R, Snyder SC, Swedlund B, Swensen J, Thomas A, Tranchant M, Woodland AM, Labrie F, Skolnick MH, Neuhausen S, Rommens J, Cannon-Albright LA: A candidate prostate cancer susceptibility gene at chromosome 17p. Nat Genet 27: 172–180, 2001

44. Rebbeck TR, Walker AH, Zeigler-Johnson C, Weisburg S, Martin AM, Nathanson KL, Wein AJ, Malkowicz SB: Association of HPC2/ELAC2 genotypes and prostate cancer. Am J Hum Genet 67: 1014–1019, 2000

45. Xu J, Zheng SL, Carpten JD, Nupponen NN, Robbins CM, Mestre J, Moses TY, Faith DA, Kelly BD, Isaacs SD, Wiley KE, Ewing CM, Bujnovszky P, Chang B, Bailey-Wilson J, Bleecker ER, Walsh PC, Trent JM, Meyers DA, Isaacs WB: Evaluation of linkage and association of HPC2/ELAC2 in patients with familial or sporadic prostate cancer. Am J Hum Genet 68: 901–911, 2001

46. Suarez BK, Gerhard DS, Lin J, Haberer B, Nguyen L, Kesterson NK, Catalona WJ: Polymorphisms in the prostate cancer susceptibility gene HPC2/ELAC2 in multiplex families and health controls. Cancer Res 61: 4982–4984, 2001

47. Rokman A, Ikonen T, Mononen N, Autio V, Matikainen MP, Koivisto PA, Tammela TL, Kallioniemi OP, Schleutker J: ELAC2/HPC2 involvement in hereditary and sporadic prostate cancer. Cancer Res 61: 6038–6041, 2001

48. Wang L, McDonnell SK, Elkins DA, Slager SL, ChristensenE, Marks AF, Cunningham JM, Peterson BJ, Jacobsen SJ, Cerhan JR, Blute ML, Schaid DJ, Thibodeau SN: Role of HPC2/ELAC2 in hereditary prostate cancer. Cancer Res 61: 6494–6499, 2001

49. Vesprini D, Nam RK, Trachtenberg J, Jewett MA, Tavtigian SV, Emami M, Ho M, Toi A, Narod SA: HPC2 variants and screen-detected prostate cancer. Am J Hum Genet 68: 912–917, 2001

50. Langston AA, Stanford JL, Wicklund KG, Thompson JD, Blazej RG, Ostrander EA: Germ-line BRCA1 mutations in selected men with prostate cancer. Am J Hum Genet 58: 881–884, 1996

51. Struewing JP, Hartge P, Wacholder S, Baker SM, Berlin M, McAdams M, Timmerman MM, Brody LC, Tucker MA: The risk of cancer associated with specific mutations of BRCA1 and BRCA2 among Ashkenazi Jews. N Engl J Med 336: 1401–1408, 1997

52. Gayther SA, de Foy KA, Harrington P, Pharoah P, Dunsmuir WD, Edwards SM, Gillett C, Ardern-Jones A, Dearnaley DP, Easton DF, Ford D, Shearer RJ, Kirby RS, Dowe AL, Kelly J, Stratton MR, Ponder BA, Barnes D, Eeles RA: The frequency of germ-line mutations in the breast cancer predisposition genes BRCA1 and BRCA2 in familial prostate cancer. The cancer research campaign/British prostate group United Kingdom familial prostate cancer study collaborators. Cancer Res 60: 4513–4518, 2000

53. Gao X, Wu N, Grignon D, Zacharek A, Liu H, Salkowski A, Li G, Sakr W, Sarkar F, Porter AT, et al.: High frequency of mutator phenotype in human prostatic adenocarcinoma. Oncogene 9: 2999–3003, 1994

54. Gao X, Zacharek A, Grignon DJ, Sakr W, Powell IJ, Porter AT, Honn KV: Localization of potential tumor suppressor loci to a <2 Mb region on chromosome 17q in human prostate cancer. Oncogene 11: 1241–1247, 1995

55. Visakorpi T, Kallioniemi AH, Syvanen AC, Hyytinen ER, Karhu R, Tammela T, Isola JJ, Kallioniemi OP: Genetic changes in primary and recurrent prostate cancer by comparative genomic hybridization. Cancer Res 55: 342–347, 1995

56. Cher ML, Bova GS, Moore DH, Small EJ, Carroll PR, Pin SS, Epstein JI, Isaacs WB, Jensen RH: Genetic alterations in untreated metastases and androgen-independent prostate cancer detected by comparative genomic hybridization and allelotyping. Cancer Res 56: 3091–3102, 1996

57. Cunningham JM, Shan A, Wick MJ, McDonnell SK, Schaid DJ, Tester DJ, Qian J, Takahashi S, Jenkins RB, Bostwick DG, Thibodeau SN: Allelic imbalance and microsatellite instability in prostatic adenocarcinoma. Cancer Res 56: 4475–4482, 1996

58. Nupponen NN, Kakkola L, Koivisto P, Visakorpi T: Genetic alterations in hormone-refractory recurrent prostate carcinomas. Am J Pathol 153: 141–148, 1998

59. Chekmareva MA, Kadkhodaian MM, Hollowell CM, Kim H, Yoshida BA, Luu HH, Stadler WM, Rinker-Schaeffer CW: Chromosome 17-mediated dormancy of AT6.1 prostate cancer micrometastases. Cancer Res 58: 4963–4969, 1998

60. Berry R, Schroeder JJ, French AJ, McDonnell SK, Peterson BJ, Cunningham JM, Thibodeau SN, Schaid DJ: Evidence for a prostate cancer-susceptibility locus on chromosome 20. Am J Hum Genet 67: 82–91, 2000

61. Bock CH, Cunningham JM, McDonnell SK, Schaid DJ, Peterson BJ, Pavlic RJ, Schroeder JJ, Klein J, French AJ, Marks A, Thibodeau SN, Lange EM, Cooney KA: Analysis of the prostate cancer-susceptibility locus HPC20 in 172 families affected by prostate cancer. Am J Hum Genet 68: 795–801, 2001

62. Zheng SL, Xu J, Isaacs SD, Wiley K, Chang B, Bleecker ER, Walsh PC, Trent JM, Meyers DA, Isaacs WB: Evidence for a prostate cancer linkage to chromosome 20 in 159 hereditary prostate cancer families. Hum Genet 108: 430–435, 2001

63. Witte JS, Goddard KA, Conti DV, Elston RC, Lin J, Suarez BK, Broman KW, Burmester JK, Weber JL, Catalona WJ: Genome-wide scan for prostate cancer-aggressiveness loci. Am J Hum Genet 67: 92–99, 2000

64. Suzuki H, Komiya A, Emi M, Kuramochi H, Shiraishi T, Yatani R, Shimazaki J: Three distinct commonly deleted regions of chromosome arm 16q in human primary and metastatic prostate cancers. Genes Chromosomes Cancer 17: 225–233, 1996

65. Latil A, Cussenot O, Fournier G, Driouch K, Lidereau R: Loss of heterozygosity at chromosome 16q in prostate adenocarcinoma: identification of three independent regions. Cancer Res 57: 1058–1062, 1997

66. Elo JP, Harkonen P, Kyllonen AP, Lukkarinen O, Poutanen M, Vihko R, Vihko P: Loss of heterozygosity at 16q24.1–q24.2 is significantly associated with metastatic and aggressive behavior of prostate cancer. Cancer Res 57: 3356–3359, 1997

67. Umbas R, Schalken JA, Aalders TW, Carter BS, Karthaus HF, Schaafsma HE, Debruyne FM, Isaacs WB: Expression of the cellular adhesion molecule E-cadherin is reduced or absent in high-grade prostate cancer. Cancer Res 52: 5104–5109, 1992

68. Umbas R, Isaacs WB, Bringuier PP, Schaafsma HE, Karthaus HF, Oosterhof GO, Debruyne FM, Schalken JA: Decreased E-cadherin expression is associated with poor prognosis in patients with prostate cancer. Cancer Res 54: 3929–3933, 1994

69. Tomita K, van Bokhoven A, van Leenders GJ, Ruijter ET, Jansen CF, Bussemakers MJ, Schalken JA: Cadherin switching in human prostate cancer progression. Cancer Res 60: 3650–3654, 2000

70. Guilford P, Hopkins J, Harraway J, McLeod M, McLeod N, Harawira P, Taite H, Scoular R, Miller A, Reeve AE: E-cadherin germline mutations in familial gastric cancer. Nature 392: 402–405, 1998

71. Matikaine MP, Pukkala E, Schleutker J, Tammela TL, Koivisto P, Sankila R, Kallioniemi OP: Relatives of prostate cancer patients have an increased risk of prostate and stomach cancers: a population-based, cancer registry study in Finland. Cancer Causes Control 12: 223–230, 2001

72. Kagan J, Stein J, Babaian RJ, Joe YS, Pisters LL, Glassman AB, von Eschenbach AC, Troncoso P: Homozygous deletions at 8p22 and 8p21 in prostate cancer implicate these regions as the sites for candidate tumor suppressor genes. Oncogene 11: 2121–2126, 1995

73. Vocke CD, Pozzatti RO, Bostwick DG, Florence CD, Jennings SB, Strup SE, Duray PH, Liotta LA,

Emmert-Buck MR, Linehan WM: Analysis of 99 microdissected prostate carcinomas reveals a high frequency of allelic loss on chromosome 8p12–21. Cancer Res 56: 2411–2416, 1996

74. Gibbs M, Stanford JL, Jarvik GP, Janer M, Badzioch M, Peters MA, Goode EL, Kolb S, Chakrabarti L, Shook M, Basom R, Ostrander EA, Hood L: A genomic scan of families with prostate cancer identifies multiple regions of interest. Am J Hum Genet 67: 100–109, 2000

75. Xu J, Zheng SL, Hawkins GA, Faith DA, Kelly B, Isaacs SD, Wiley KE, Chang B, Ewing CM, Bujnovszky P, Carpten JD, Bleecker ER, Walsh PC, Trent JM, Meyers DA, Isaacs WB: Linkage and association studies of prostate cancer susceptibility: evidence for linkage at 8p22–23. Am J Hum Genet 69: 341–35, 2001

76. Kallioniemi OP, Visakorpi T: Genetic basis and clonal evolution of human prostate cancer. Adv Cancer Res 68: 225–255, 1996

77. Bookstein R, Bova GS, MacGrogan D, Levy A, Isaacs WB: Tumour-suppressor genes in prostatic oncogenesis: a positional approach. Br J Urol 79 (Suppl 1) 28–36, 1997

78. Verma RS, Manikal M, Conte RA, Godec CJ: Chromosomal basis of adenocarcinoma of the prostate. Cancer Invest 17: 441–447, 1999

79. Nupponen N, Visakorpi T: Molecular biology of progression of prostate cancer. Eur Urol 35: 351–354, 1999

80. Brothman AR, Maxwell TM, Cui J, Deubler DA, Zhu XL: Chromosomal clues to the development of prostate tumors. Prostate 38: 303–312, 1999

81. Hakimi JM, Rondinelli RH, Schoenberg MP, Barrack ER: Androgen-receptor gene structure and function in prostate cancer. World J Urol 14: 329–337, 1996

82. Chamberlain NL, Driver ED, Miesfeld RL: The length and location of CAG trinucleotide repeats in the androgen receptor N-terminal domain affect transactivation function. Nucleic Acids Res 22: 3181–3186, 1994

83. Irvine RA, Yu MC, Ross RK, Coetzee GA: The CAG and GGC microsatellites of the androgen receptor gene are in linkage disequilibrium in men with prostate cancer. Cancer Res 55: 1937–1940, 1995

84. Brinkmann AO: Molecular basis of androgen insensitivity. Mol Cell Endocrinol 179: 105–109, 2001

85. Elo JP, Kvist L, Leinonen K, Isomaa V, Henttu P, Lukkarinen O, Vihko P: Mutated human androgen receptor gene detected in a prostatic cancer patient is also activated by estradiol. J Clin Endocrinol Metab 80: 3494–3500, 1995

86. Koivisto PA, Schleutker J, Helin H, Ehren-van Eekelen C, Kallioniemi OP, Trapman J: Androgen receptor gene alterations and chromosomal gains and losses in prostate carcinomas appearing during finasteride treatment for benign prostatic hyperplasia. Clin Cancer Res 5: 3578–3582, 1999

87. Mononen N, Syrjakoski K, Matikainen M, Tammela TL, Schleutker J, Kallioniemi OP, Trapman J, Koivisto PA: Two percent of Finnish prostate cancer patients have a germ-line mutation in the hormone-binding domain of the androgen receptor gene. Cancer Res 60: 6479–6481, 2000

88. Visakorpi T, Hyytinen E, Koivisto P, Tanner M, Keinanen R, Palmberg C, Palotie A, Tammela T, Isola J, Kallioniemi OP: In vivo amplification of the androgen receptor gene and progression of human prostate cancer. Nat Genet 9: 401–406, 1995

89. Koivisto P, Kononen J, Palmberg C, Tammela T, Hyytinen E, Isola J, Trapman J, Cleutjens K, Noordzij A, Visakorpi T, Kallioniemi OP: Androgen receptor gene amplification: a possible molecular mechanism for androgen deprivation therapy failure in prostate cancer. Cancer Res 57: 314–319, 1997

90. Taplin ME, Bubley GJ, Ko YJ, Small EJ, Upton M, Rajeshkumar B, Balk SP: Selection for androgen receptor mutations in prostate cancers treated with androgen antagonist. Cancer Res 59: 2511–2515, 1999

91. Sack JS, Kish KF, Wang C, Attar RM, Kiefer SE, An Y, Wu GY, Scheffler JE, Salvati ME, Krystek SR Jr. Weinmann R, Einspahr HM: Crystallographic structures of the ligand-binding domains of the androgen receptor and its T877A mutant complexed with the natural agonist dihydrotestosterone. Proc Natl Acad Sci USA 98: 4904–4909, 2001

92. Davis DL, Russell DW: Unusual length polymorphism in human steroid 5 alpha-reductase type 2 gene (SRD5A2). Hum Mol Genet 2: 820, 1993

93. Reichardt JK, Makridakis N, Henderson BE, Yu MC, Pike MC, Ross RK: Genetic variability of the human SRD5A2 gene: implications for prostate cancer risk. Cancer Res 55: 3973–3975, 1995

94. Makridakis N, Ross RK, Pike MC, Chang L, Stanczyk FZ, Kolonel LN, Shi CY, Yu MC, Henderson BE, Reichardt JK: A prevalent missense substitution that modulates activity of prostatic steroid 5alpha-reductase. Cancer Res 57: 1020–1022, 1997

95. Makridakis NM, Ross RK, Pike MC, Crocitto LE, Kolonel LN, Pearce CL, Henderson BE, Reichardt JK: Association of missense substitution in SRD5A2 gene with prostate cancer in African-American and Hispanic men in Los Angeles, USA. Lancet 354: 975–978, 1999

96. Lunn RM, Bell DA, Mohler JL, Taylor JA: Prostate cancer risk and polymorphism in 17 hydroxylase (CYP17) and steroid reductase (SRD5A2). Carcinogenesis 20: 1727–1731, 1999

97. Bosland MC: The role of steroid hormones in prostate carcinogenesis. J Natl Cancer Inst Monogr 27: 39–66, 2000

98. Henderson BE, Feigelson HS: Hormonal carcinogenesis. Carcinogenesis 21: 427–433, 2000

99. Royal C, Baffoe-Bonnie A, Kittles R, Powell I, Bennett J, Hoke G, Pettaway C, Weinrich S, Vijayakumar S, Ahaghotu C, Mason T, Johnson E, Obeikwe M, Simpson C, Mejia R, Boykin W, Roberson P, Frost J, Faison-Smith L, Meegan C, Foster N, Furbert-Harris P, Carpten J, Bailey-Wilson J, Trent J, Berg K, Dunston G, Collins F: Recruitment experience in the first phase of the African American Hereditary Prostate Cancer (AAHPC) study. Ann Epidemiol 10(Suppl 8): S68–S77, 2000

Address for offprints: Cancer Genetics Branch, National Human Genome Research Institute, National Institutes of Health, 50 South Drive, Bethesda, MD-20892; Tel: 301-435-5626; Fax: 301-480-4866; e-mail: jdc@nhgri.nih.gov

Molecular profiling in prostate cancer

F. Feroze-Merzoug[1], M.S. Schober[1] and Y.Q. Chen[1,2]
[1]*Department of Pathology,* [2]*Center for Molecular Medicine and Genetics, Wayne State University, Detroit, MI, USA*

Key words: prostate, androgen receptor, androgen regulation, differential expression, microarray, expressed sequence tags, serial analysis of gene expression, proteomics

Abstract

Prostate cancer is the most diagnosed cancer and the second leading cause of cancer death among men in the United States. Ability to detect this cancer early and availability of better prognostic markers are critical in order to decrease morbidity and mortality of prostate cancer. With the recent development in gene expression analysis methodology, expression profiles of thousands of genes can be generated in tissue samples and cell lines. Comparison of the global gene expression patterns between normal prostate and tumors at different stages may allow us to understand better the molecular mechanism of prostate tumorigenesis and progression. Different cancer cell lines and tissues appear to have different gene expression patterns that provide a new tool to classify tumors. Molecular classification of prostate cancer holds great promise for early detection and prognosis of this disease in the future. In this review, we summarize some of the recent mRNA and protein expression profiling studies performed in prostate cancer. Further, we discuss the potential benefits and limitations of current profiling technology.

Introduction

Prostate cancer is the most frequently diagnosed cancer and the second leading cause of cancer death among men in the United States. Considerable progress has been made in the early detection and treatment of prostate cancer over the last two decades. Nonetheless, mortality from prostate cancer remains a significant health care problem. Two critical issues for reduction of mortality and morbidity from this disease are early detection and improved prognostic markers. Interestingly, a majority of men will develop histological prostate carcinoma by their fifth decade [1], however, many will never progress to clinically relevant disease. Some clinical cancers are more aggressive, and many are slow-growing. Early detection of aggressive prostate cancer is important, especially in the organ-confined stage, as treatment at this phase will likely cure the cancer. However, even if the prostate cancer is left untreated, many men with clinically-diagnosed, less aggressive prostate cancers will not die of this disease rather other causes. With an increasing number of men with clinically-diagnosed prostate cancer, this

problem leads to an enormous cost to the health care system as well as the emotional trauma and potential physiological side effects to the individual. Therefore, development of better prognostic markers is critical to the effort to identify and treat patients with unfavorable prognosis.

Prostate is a hormone-regulated organ. Androgens affect prostatic epithelial cell proliferation and differentiation, and play a critical role in tumorigenesis. A common treatment of prostate cancer involves the deprivation of androgen, clinically known as androgen ablation. Despite the initial response of patients to hormonal therapy, the vast majority of patients eventually relapse. Molecular mechanisms involved in the development of hormone-refractory prostate cancer are unknown. However, several biological processes may contribute to this development. Mutations on the androgen receptor (AR) can cause a ligand-independent activation, or promiscuity of the receptor, i.e. alteration in the ligand binding specificity such that it binds hormones such as progesterone and estradiol [2,3]. Another phenomenon observed in 28–30% of recurrent hormone-refractory prostate cancer tumors

M.L. Cher, K.V. Honn and A. Raz (eds.), Prostate Cancer: New Horizons in Research and Treatment, 29–35.
© 2002 *Kluwer Academic Publishers.*

30

is AR amplification [4–6]. Increased levels of AR may allow tumor cells to survive and thrive in low androgen environments. Specific growth factors and cytokines, such as insulin-like growth factor-I (IGF-I) [7] and interleukin-6 (IL-6) [8] may also activate the AR in a ligand-independent manner. Coregulators can affect receptor transactivation depending upon the delicate balance between coactivator and corepressor expression levels [9,10]. Regardless of the mechanism leading to androgen independence, downstream genes in the androgen pathway play a critical role in the development of hormone-refractory prostate cancer.

Identification of differentially expressed genes

One of the keys to understanding prostate growth and tumorigenesis is the identification of differentially expressed genes between normal and tumor prostate cells, and genes regulated by androgens. Much effort has been directed to identify such genes over the years. Prostate-specific antigen (PSA) is probably the best characterized androgen-regulated gene and a common diagnostic marker. Many other genes related to growth, adhesion, cell cycle and apoptosis have been studied.

Several lines of evidence suggest that insulin-like growth factors (IGFs) may play an important role in prostate cancer. IGF-I is a potent serum maker for prostate cancer risk [11]. Increased expression of IGF-I and its receptor may be associated with tumor progression [12]. In addition, the AR can be activated by IGF-I in a ligand-independent manner [7]. A reduction in the cell adhesion molecule E-cadherin and its interacting molecule catenin may play a role in prostate cancer metastasis [13,14] and is associated with poor prognosis and survival [15,16]. Over the last decade, it has become apparent that AR requires accessory factors for optimal activation of target genes. Numerous coregulators have been identified with diverse structures and potential mechanisms of coregulation. Expression level of some AR coregulators may correlate with the grade of prostate cancer [17]. Many genes involved in cell cycle regulation such as P53, RB, P21, P27 and P16, and in apoptosis such as BCL-2 and BAX have been evaluated in prostate cancer. Recently, the tumor suppressor PTEN has also been assessed. Progresses have been made in understanding the molecular mechanism of prostate cancer development. However, critical issues remain, i.e. early detection of aggressive

tumors and markers for better prognosis of clinical disease.

Comprehensive gene expression analyses

With the recent development in gene expression analysis methodology, expression profiles of thousands of genes can be generated in cancer cells. Different cancer cell lines and tissues appear to have different gene expression patterns [18,19], and such differences allow for molecular classifications of cancer [20,21].

Using the well established Expressed Sequence Tag (EST) method, prostate specific cDNA libraries were constructed [22], individual cDNA clones were sequenced [22,23], and a web-based prostate expression database (PEDB) was constructed [24]. ESTs and full-length cDNA sequences derived from more than 40 human prostate cDNA libraries are maintained and represent a wide spectrum of normal and pathological conditions. Prostate ESTs were assembled into distinct species groups using the multiple alignment program CAP2 and were annotated with information from the GenBank, dbEST and UniGene databases. Differential expression of each EST species can be viewed across all libraries using a Virtual Expression Analysis Tool. The PEDB is a useful addition to the public EST project originated and organized by the National Institutes of Health (http://www.ncbi.nlm.nih.gov/). Prostate tumor tissues are highly heterogeneous. A given tissue often contains benign, PIN lesions and carcinoma cells of various grades as well as stromal cells. With the development of laser capture microdissection method, cells of specific types and from specific areas can be precisely dissected. Prostate cDNA libraries have also been successfully constructed from microdissected tissues [25].

Although thousands of genes can be determined, the EST method is relatively slow and expensive. Using the Serial Analysis of Gene Expression (SAGE) method, a large number of genes can be quantified more efficiently [26]. An expression profile of androgen-regulated genes from LNCaP cells has been generated by SAGE [26]. Among 123,371 transcripts analyzed, a total of 28,844 distinct SAGE tags were identified representing 16,570 genes. Some 351 genes were significantly affected by dihydrotestosterone (DHT) treatment at the RNA level ($p < 0.05$), of which 147 were induced and 204 repressed by DHT treatment [27]. In another study, also conducted using LNCaP cells, a total of 83,489 SAGE tags representing 23,448 known genes or ESTs and 1,655 potentially novel genes were identified [28]. Comparison of transcripts between control and R1881-treated LNCaP cells revealed the induction of 136 genes and repression of 215 genes in response to the synthetic androgen ($p < 0.05$). These identified genes are most likely comprised of two groups; namely those regulated directly by androgen and those targeted by androgen-regulated gene products. Interestingly, both studies suggested that there were approximately 300 genes regulated by androgen and, somewhat surprisingly, there were more genes repressed than stimulated by androgen treatment in LNCaP cells. It is noteworthy that the androgen-regulated genes ($\approx$300 per study) identified by these two studies are different with some overlaps. Such discrepancy may be contributed to the use of DHT [27] versus a more stable synthetic androgen analog R1881 [28] and dosage of 10^{-9} M [27] versus 10^{-8} M [28]. Induction or repression of androgen-regulated genes is also time-dependent. Indeed, PSA was found to be induced at 4–6 h, peaked between 6 and 20 h, and gradually declined after 20 h post-treatment of DHT [27].

Differentially expressed genes between normal and prostate tumor tissues have also been determined by SAGE. In one study, a total of 133,217 transcripts were analyzed, with 35,185 distinct SAGE tags identified representing 19,287 genes. Comparison of the transcripts in normal and tumor tissue revealed 156 differentially expressed genes ($p < 0.05$), of which 88 genes were up-regulated and 68 genes were down-regulated in the tumor tissue [29]. Based on SAGE data, the transcriptome for human prostate was estimated to be approximately 37,000 distinct transcripts [29]. SAGE data for another study (Library PR317 normal versus Library PR317 tumor) is available at the Cancer Genome Anatomy Project (CGAP) web site and a third independent SAGE experiment (Library PrCA-1 versus Library Normal prostate) is ongoing (http://www.ncbi.nlm.nih.gov/SAGE/sagexpsetup.cgi).

A comprehensive SAGE database for many human cancers, including the prostate, is accessible through the CGAP web site. The levels of gene expression can be determined virtually by searching this database using either a SAGE tag or a UniGene number. More importantly, differential expression of genes between tissues or cell lines can be explored by the xProfiler algorithm (http://www.ncbi.nlm.nih.gov/SAGE/sagexpsetup.cgi).

The use of DNA microarray for expression profiling has steadily gained popularity during the past five years. Gene expression was measured in normal and organ-confined prostate cancer by 588-gene arrays [30]. Levels of the GSTM1, MCP-1, TNFR-1, TGF-β3 and ID-1 genes were found to be significantly reduced in tumor cells. In another study, expression profiling was performed in primary human prostate cancer and benign prostatic hyperplasia (BPH) using 6500-gene arrays. Gene expression in each of the 16 prostate cancer and 9 BPH specimens was compared with a common reference to generate normalized measures for each gene across all of the samples. Using an analysis of complete pairwise comparisons of all expression profiles, discernable patterns of overall gene expression that differentiate prostate cancer from BPH were clearly observed [31]. Further analysis of the data identified 210 genes with statistically significant differences in expression between prostate cancer and BPH [31]. Microarray analysis conducted by a different group identified IGFBP2 as one of the genes highly expressed in CWR22R hormone-refractory prostate tumor xenograft and hormone-refractory clinical tumors [32]. Protein levels of IGFBP2 were analyzed by immunohistochemistry on tissue arrays. High expression of the protein was observed in 100% of the hormone-refractory clinical tumors, and 36% of the primary tumors, but not in the benign prostatic specimens [32]. Another gene of interest, hepsin, a transmembrane serine protease, was identified by four independent studies [31,33–35]. Expression of hepsin was significantly correlated with measures of clinical outcome. Two independent SAGE analyses and a cDNA microarray study, however, did not identify hepsin as a differentially expressed gene [29,36] (http://www.ncbi.nlm.nih.gov/SAGE/sagexpsetup.cgi; Library PR317 normal versus Library PR317 tumor). The failure in detecting differential expression of hepsin by SAGE may be due to the difference in tissue samples.

EST, SAGE and cDNA microarray studies reveal significant and widespread differences in gene expression patterns between normal adjacent prostate, BPH, localized, metastatic and hormone-refractory prostate cancer. Gene expression analysis of prostate tissues should help to delineate the molecular mechanisms underlying prostate malignant growth and identify molecular markers for diagnostic, prognostic and therapeutic use. Indeed, many novel genes have been cloned as the result of gene expression profiling [37–42]. Gene expression patterns will undoubtedly be used for molecular classification of prostate cancer in the future.

32

Proteomics

Much effort in gene expression profiling has been at the transcript level. However, it is clear that mRNA expression data alone are insufficient to predict cellular functional outcomes. For instance, mRNA expression data provide very little information about activation state, post-translational modification or localization of corresponding proteins. Moreover, there is evidence highlighting the disparity between mRNA transcript and protein expression levels. In a study of androgen-regulated genes by SAGE and proteomics, some 351 genes out of a total of 16,570 genes measured were found to be significantly affected by DHT treatment at the RNA level. Proteomic analysis demonstrated that 44 protein spots were affected at least two-fold in response to androgen, out of a total of 1,031 protein spots analyzed. The change in intensity for most of the affected proteins identified could not be predicted based on the level of their corresponding RNA [27]. It is believed that there is a tight coupling between transcription and translation in prokaryotes and disparity between the levels of mRNA and protein increases from prokaryotes to low eukaryotes in mammals. The lack of correlation between mRNA and corresponding protein is evident even in low eukaryotic cells such as yeast [43]. Therefore, it will be necessary to profile both mRNA and protein for a complete picture of how cells are altered during malignant transformation.

Compared to mRNA profiling, classical quantitative analysis of protein expression levels is much more time-consuming because proteins are analyzed one at a time. Another limitation is the fact that only proteins expressed at relatively high levels can be determined. Nevertheless, progress has been made in proteomic analysis of prostate cancer. A study, involving the collection of cells from prostate hyperplasia and prostate carcinoma, subsequently subjected to two-dimensional gel electrophoresis (2-DE) and computer assisted analysis, demonstrated considerable differences in expressed protein patterns [44]. Malignant tumors showed significant increases in the expression level of proliferating cell nuclear antigen (PCNA), calreticulin, HSP 90 and pHSP 60, oncoprotein 18(v), elongation factor 2, glutathione-S-transferase pi (GST-pi), superoxide dismutase and triose phosphate isomerase. In addition, decreases in the levels of tropomyosin-1 and -2, and cytokeratin 18 were observed in prostate carcinomas compared to prostate hyperplasias [44]. In a subsequent study, the decrease in tropomyosin

expression was confirmed in malignant tissues [45]. These studies were done with grossly dissected prostate tissues. It has been shown that 2-DE analysis can also be performed with laser capture microdissected samples [46].

The effects of androgen on protein expression have also been studied. Protein expression profiles of androgen-stimulated prostate cancer cells were generated by 2-DE. Mass spectrometric (MS) analysis of androgen-regulated proteins in these cells identified the metastasis-suppressor gene NDKA/nm23; a finding that may explain a marked reduction in metastatic potential when these cells express a functional androgen receptor pathway [47]. Using surface-enhanced laser desorption/ionization (SELDI) MS analysis, reproducible and discriminatory protein biomarker profiles can be obtained from as few as 25 cells in less than 5 min, from the time of dissection to the generation of the protein fingerprint. Furthermore, these protein pattern profiles are discriminatory for different tumor types, and reveal reproducible changes in expression as cells undergo malignant transformation. Consistent protein changes were identified in microdissected cells from patient-matched tumor and normal epithelium in three out of three malignant prostate tissue sets [48]. A reverse-phase protein microarray study, in which cell lysates from matched normal prostate epithelium, PIN and invasive prostate cancer were spotted onto slides, showed that cancer progression was associated with increased phosphorylation of Akt, a suppressor of apoptosis pathways, as well as decreased phosphorylation of ERK [49]. At the transition from histologically normal epithelium to PIN, a statistically significant surge was observed in phosphorylated Akt and a concomitant suppression of downstream apoptosis pathways which proceed the transition into invasive carcinoma [49].

Conclusion and future directions

Functional genomics is an exciting and rapidly changing field. Array technology has significantly improved and proteomic techniques are swiftly evolving. Still, molecular profiling of prostate cancer is in its infancy. The massive amounts of data generated by mRNA and protein profiling require efficient, capable bioinformatics to extract biologically meaningful conclusions. Preliminary studies in prostate and other cancers suggest that different cancer cell lines and tissues have different gene expression patterns (see previous section)

[18,19], and such differences allow for molecular classification of cancer [20,21].

Like any emerging technology, many limitations must be overcome before it can be applied to clinical practice. Although microarrays show great promise, this methodology has not matured to the point of consistently generating robust and reliable data when used in the average laboratory [50]. It will also require the integration of other sources of biological information, such as gene identity, biochemical pathway for a given gene and pathology of tissues, to understand the cellular program of gene expression and molecular basis of cell transformation [51]. The industrialization of proteomics demands reproducible and high-throughput profiling technologies that current 2-DE cannot achieve. New technologies in protein arrays, either on chips or with self-encoded elements in solution, hold much promise for deciphering the diverse and immense proteome [52–54]. Imaging mass spectrometry is an interesting new technology that allows direct mapping of proteins present in tissue sections [55]. Protein–protein interaction mapping [56–58] and protein subcellular localization [59,60] should provide useful complementary information. In molecular profiling of cancer tissues, perhaps the most important of all, is the preparation of tissue samples. Profiling results are only as good as the tissues isolated for the experiment. Accordingly, laser capture microdissection may be the standard for tissue procurement in the future [61]. With the advances of profiling technology, expression patterning holds great promise for prognosis, early detection and molecular classification of prostate cancer.

References

1. Sakr WA, Grignon DJ, Crissman JD, Heilbrun LK, Cassin BJ, Pontes JJ, Haas GP: High grade prostatic intraepithelial neoplasia (HGPIN) and prostatic adenocarcinoma between the ages of 20–69: An autopsy study of 249 cases. *In Vivo* 8: 439–443, 1994
2. Taplin ME, Bubley GJ, Ko YJ, Small EJ, Upton M, Rajeshkumar B, Balk SP: Selection for androgen receptor mutations in prostate cancers treated with androgen antagonist. Cancer Res 59: 2511–2515, 1999
3. Marcelli M, Ittmann M, Mariani S, Sutherland R, Nigam R, Murthy L, Zhao Y, DiConcini D, Puxeddu E, Esen A, Eastham J, Weigel NL, Lamb DJ: Androgen receptor mutations in prostate cancer. Cancer Res 60: 944–949, 2000
4. Visakorpi T, Hyytinen E, Koivisto P, Tanner M, Keinanen R, Palmberg C, Palotie A, Tammela T, Isola J, Kallioniemi OP: *In vivo* amplification of the androgen receptor gene and progression of human prostate cancer. Nat Genet 9: 401–406, 1995
5. Koivisto P, Kononen J, Palmberg C, Tammela T, Hyytinen E, Isola J, Trapman J, Cleutjens K, Noordzij A, Visakorpi T, Kallioniemi OP: Androgen receptor gene amplification: A possible molecular mechanism for androgen deprivation therapy failure in prostate cancer. Cancer Res 57: 314–319, 1997
6. Wallen MJ, Linja M, Kaartinen K, Schleutker J, Visakorpi T: Androgen receptor gene mutations in hormone-refractory prostate cancer. J Pathol 189: 559–563, 1999
7. Culig Z, Hobisch A, Cronauer MV, Radmayr C, Trapman J, Hittmair A, Bartsch G, Klocker H: Androgen receptor activation in prostatic tumor cell lines by insulin-like growth factor-I, keratinocyte growth factor, and epidermal growth factor. Cancer Res 54: 5474–5478, 1994
8. Hobisch A, Eder IE, Putz T, Horninger W, Bartsch G, Klocker H, Culig Z: Interleukin-6 regulates prostate-specific protein expression in prostate carcinoma cells by activation of the androgen receptor. Cancer Res 58: 4640–4645, 1998
9. Bautista S, Valles H, Walker RL, Anzick S, Zeillinger R, Meltzer P, Theillet C: In breast cancer, amplification of the steroid receptor coactivator gene AIB1 is correlated with estrogen and progesterone receptor positivity. Clin Cancer Res 4: 2925–2929, 1998
10. Smith CL, Nawaz Z, O'Malley BW: Coactivator and corepressor regulation of the agonist/antagonist activity of the mixed antiestrogen, 4-hydroxytamoxifen. Mol Endocrinol 11: 657–666, 1997
11. Chan JM, Stampfer MJ, Giovannucci E, Gann PH, Ma J, Wilkinson P, Hennekens CH, Pollak M: Plasma insulin-like growth factor-I and prostate cancer risk: A prospective study. Science 279: 563–566, 1998
12. Nickerson T, Chang F, Lorimer D, Smeekens SP, Sawyers CL, Pollak M: *In vivo* progression of LAPC-9 and LNCaP prostate cancer models to androgen independence is associated with increased expression of insulin-like growth factor I (IGF-I) and IGF-I receptor (IGF-IR). Cancer Res 61: 6276–6280, 2001
13. Morton RA, Ewing CM, Nagafuchi A, Tsukita S, Isaacs WB: Reduction of E-cadherin levels and deletion of the alpha-catenin gene in human prostate cancer cells. Cancer Res 53: 3585–3590, 1993
14. Umbas R, Schalken JA, Aalders TW, Carter BS, Karthaus HF, Schaafsma HE, Debruyne FM, Isaacs WB: Expression of the cellular adhesion molecule E-cadherin is reduced or absent in high-grade prostate cancer. Cancer Res 52: 5104–5109, 1992
15. Umbas R, Isaacs WB, Bringuier PP, Schaafsma HE, Karthaus HF, Oosterhof GO, Debruyne FM, Schalken JA: Decreased E-cadherin expression is associated with poor prognosis in patients with prostate cancer. Cancer Res 54: 3929–3933, 1994
16. Richmond PJ, Karayiannakis AJ, Nagafuchi A, Kaisary AV, Pignatelli M: Aberrant E-cadherin and alpha-catenin expression in prostate cancer: Correlation with patient survival. Cancer Res 57: 3189–3193, 1997
17. Fujimoto N, Mizokami A, Harada S, Matsumoto T: Different expression of androgen receptor coactivators in human prostate. Urology 58: 289–294, 2001

34

18. Ross DT, Scherf U, Eisen MB, Perou CM, Rees C, Spellman P, Iyer V, Jeffrey SS, Van de Rijn M, Waltham M, Pergamenschikov A, Lee JC, Lashkari D, Shalon D, Myers TG, Weinstein JN, Botstein D, Brown PO: Systematic variation in gene expression patterns in human cancer cell lines. Nat Genet 24: 227–235, 2000

19. Perou CM, Sorlie T, Eisen MB, van de Rijn M, Jeffrey SS, Rees CA, Pollack JR, Ross DT, Johnsen H, Akslen LA, Fluge O, Pergamenschikov A, Williams C, Zhu SX, Lonning PE, Borresen-Dale AL, Brown PO, Botstein D: Molecular portraits of human breast tumours. Nature 406: 747–752, 2000

20. Sorlie T, Perou CM, Tibshirani R, Aas T, Geisler S, Johnsen H, Hastie T, Eisen MB, van de Rijn M, Jeffrey SS, Thorsen T, Quist H, Matese JC, Brown PO, Botstein D, Eystein Lonning P, Borresen-Dale AL: Gene expression patterns of breast carcinomas distinguish tumor subclasses with clinical implications. Proc Natl Acad Sci USA 98: 10869–10874, 2001

21. Golub TR, Slonim DK, Tamayo P, Huard C, Gaasenbeek M, Mesirov JP, Coller H, Loh ML, Downing JR, Caligiuri MA, Bloomfield CD, Lander ES: Molecular classification of cancer: Class discovery and class prediction by gene expression monitoring. Science 286: 531–537, 1999

22. Nelson PS, Ng WL, Schummer M, True LD, Liu AY, Bumgarner RE, Ferguson C, Dimak A, Hood L: An expressed-sequence-tag database of the human prostate: Sequence analysis of 1168 cDNA clones. Genomics 47: 12–25, 1998

23. Huang GM, Ng WL, Farkas J, He L, Liang HA, Gordon D, Yu J, Hood L: Prostate cancer expression profiling by cDNA sequencing analysis. Genomics 59: 178–186, 1999

24. Hawkins V, Doll D, Bumgarner R, Smith T, Abajian C, Hood L, Nelson PS: PEDB: The prostate expression Database. Nucleic Acids Res 27: 204–208, 1999

25. Krizman DB, Chuaqui RF, Meltzer PS, Trent JM, Duray PH, Linehan WM, Liotta LA, Emmert-Buck MR: Construction of a representative cDNA library from prostatic intraepithelial neoplasia. Cancer Res 56: 5380–5383, 1996

26. Velculescu VE, Zhang L, Vogelstein B, Kinzler KW: Serial analysis of gene expression. Science 270: 484–487, 1995

27. Waghray A, Feroze F, Schober M, Yao F, Wood C, Puravs E, Krause M, Hanash S, Chen YQ: Identification of androgen-regulated genes in the prostate cancer cell line LNCaP by serial analysis of gene expression and proteomics analysis. Proteomics 1: 1327–1338, 2001

28. Xu LL, Su YP, Labiche R, Segawa T, Shanmugam N, McLeod DG, Moul JW, Srivastava S: Quantitative expression profile of androgen-regulated genes in prostate cancer cells and identification of prostate-specific genes. Int J Cancer 92: 322–328, 2001

29. Waghray A, Schober M, Feroze F, Yao F, Virgin J, Chen YQ: Identification of differentially expressed genes by serial analysis of gene expression in human prostate cancer. Cancer Res 61: 4283–4286, 2001

30. Chetcuti A, Margan S, Mann S, Russell P, Handelsman D, Rogers J, Dong Q: Identification of differentially expressed genes in organ-confined prostate cancer by gene expression array. Prostate 47: 132–140, 2001

31. Luo J, Duggan DJ, Chen Y, Sauvageot J, Ewing CM, Bittner ML, Trent JM, Isaacs WB: Human prostate cancer and benign prostatic hyperplasia: Molecular dissection by gene expression profiling. Cancer Res 61: 4683–4688, 2001

32. Bubendorf L, Kolmer M, Kononen J, Koivisto P, Mousses S, Chen Y, Mahlamaki E, Schraml P, Moch H, Willi N, Elkahloun AG, Pretlow TG, Gasser TC, Mihatsch MJ, Sauter G, Kallioniemi OP: Hormone therapy failure in human prostate cancer: Analysis by complementary DNA and tissue microarrays. J Natl Cancer Inst 91: 1758–1764, 1999

33. Magee JA, Araki T, Patil S, Ehrig T, True L, Humphrey PA, Catalona WJ, Watson MA, Milbrandt J: Expression profiling reveals hepsin overexpression in prostate cancer. Cancer Res 61: 5692–5696, 2001

34. Dhanasekaran SM, Barrette TR, Ghosh D, Shah R, Varambally S, Kurachi K, Pienta KJ, Rubin MA, Chinnaiyan AM: Delineation of prognostic biomarkers in prostate cancer. Nature 412: 822–826, 2001

35. Welsh JB, Sapinoso LM, Su AI, Kern SG, Wang-Rodriguez J, Moskaluk CA, Frierson HF Jr, Hampton GM: Analysis of gene expression identifies candidate markers and pharmacological targets in prostate cancer. Cancer Res 61: 5974–5978, 2001

36. Chaib H, Cockrell EK, Rubin MA, Macoska JA: Profiling and verification of gene expression patterns in normal and malignant human prostate tissues by cDNA microarray analysis. Neoplasia 3: 43–52, 2001

37. Vasmatzis G, Essand M, Brinkmann U, Lee B, Pastan I: Discovery of three genes specifically expressed in human prostate by expressed sequence tag database analysis. Proc Natl Acad Sci USA 95: 300–304, 1998

38. Cole KA, Chuaqui RF, Katz K, Pack S, Zhuang Z, Cole CE, Lyne JC, Linehan WM, Liotta LA, Emmert-Buck MR: cDNA sequencing and analysis of POV1 (PB39): A novel gene up-regulated in prostate cancer. Genomics 51: 282–287, 1998

39. Nelson PS, Gan L, Ferguson C, Moss P, Gelinas R, Hood L, Wang K: Molecular cloning and characterization of prostase, an androgen-regulated serine protease with prostate-restricted expression. Proc Natl Acad Sci USA 96: 3114–3119, 1999

40. Xu LL, Shanmugam N, Segawa T, Sesterhenn IA, McLeod DG, Moul JW, Srivastava S: A novel androgen-regulated gene, PMEPA1, located on chromosome 20q13 exhibits high level expression in prostate. Genomics 66: 257–263, 2000

41. Xu J, Stolk JA, Zhang X, Silva SJ, Houghton RL, Matsumura M, Vedvick TS, Leslie KB, Badaro R, Reed SG: Identification of differentially expressed genes in human prostate cancer using subtraction and microarray. Cancer Res 60: 1677–1682, 2000

42. Lin B, White JT, Ferguson C, Bumgarner R, Friedman C, Trask B, Ellis W, Lange P, Hood L, Nelson PS: Part-1: A novel human prostate-specific, androgen-regulated gene that maps to chromosome 5q12. Cancer Res 60: 858–863, 2000

43. Gygi SP, Rochon Y, Franza BR, Aebersold R: Correlation between protein and mRNA abundance in yeast. Mol Cell Biol 19: 1720–1730, 1999

44. Alaiya A, Roblick U, Egevad L, Carlsson A, Franzen B, Volz D, Huwendiek S, Linder S, Auer G: Polypeptide expression in prostate hyperplasia and prostate adenocarcinoma. Anal Cell Pathol 21: 1–9, 2000

45. Alaiya AA, Oppermann M, Langridge J, Roblick U, Egevad L, Brindstedt S, Hellstrom M, Linder S, Bergman T, Jornvall H, Auer G: Identification of proteins in human prostate tumor material by two-dimensional gel electrophoresis and mass spectrometry. Cell Mol Life Sci 58: 307–311, 2001

46. Ornstein DK, Gillespie JW, Paweletz CP, Duray PH, Herring J, Vocke CD, Topalian SL, Bostwick DG, Linehan WM, Petricoin EF 3rd, Emmert-Buck MR: Proteomic analysis of laser capture microdissected human prostate cancer and in vitro prostate cell lines. Electrophoresis 21: 2235–2242, 2000

47. Nelson PS, Han D, Rochon Y, Corthals GL, Lin B, Monson A, Nguyen V, Franza BR, Plymate SR, Aebersold R, Hood L: Comprehensive analyses of prostate gene expression: Convergence of expressed sequence tag databases, transcript profiling and proteomics. Electrophoresis 21: 1823–1831, 2000

48. Paweletz CP, Gillespie JW, Ornstein DK, Simone NL, Brown MR, Cole KA, Wang QH, Huang J, Hu N, Yip TT, Rich WE, Kohn EC, Linehan WM, Weber T, Taylor P, Emmert-Buck MR, Liotta LA, Petricoin IEF: Rapid protein display profiling of cancer progression directly from human tissue using a protein biochip. Drug Dev Res 49: 34–42, 2000

49. Paweletz CP, Charboneau L, Bichsel VE, Simone NL, Chen T, Gillespie JW, Emmert-Buck MR, Roth MJ, Petricoin IE, Liotta LA: Reverse-phase protein microarrays which capture disease progression show activation of prosurvival pathways at the cancer invasion front. Oncogene 20: 1981–1989, 2001

50. Hess KR, Zhang W, Baggerly KA, Stivers DN, Coombes KR: Microarrays: Handling the deluge of data and extracting reliable information. Trends Biotechnol 19: 463–468, 2001

51. Noordewier MO, Warren PV: Gene expression microarrays and the integration of biological knowledge. Trends Biotechnol 19: 412–415, 2001

52. Zhu H, Bilgin M, Bangham R, Hall D, Casamayor A, Bertone P, Lan N, Jansen R, Bidlingmaier S, Houfek T, Mitchell T, Miller P, Dean RA, Gerstein M, Snyder M: Global analysis of protein activities using proteome chips. Science 293: 2101–2105, 2001

53. Haab BB, Dunham MJ, Brown PO: Protein microarrays for highly parallel detection and quantitation of specific proteins and antibodies in complex solutions. Genome Biol 2: 4.1–4.13, 2001

54. Zhou H, Roy S, Schulman H, Natan MJ: Solution and chip arrays in protein profiling. Trends Biotechnol 19: S34–S39, 2001

55. Stoeckli M, Chaurand P, Hallahan DE, Caprioli RM: Imaging mass spectrometry: A new technology for the analysis of protein expression in mammalian tissues. Nat Med 7: 493–496, 2001

56. Uetz P, Giot L, Cagney G, Mansfield TA, Judson RS, Knight JR, Lockshon D, Narayan V, Srinivasan M, Pochart P, Qureshi-Emili A, Li Y, Godwin B, Conover D, Kalbfleisch T, Vijayadamodar G, Yang M, Johnston M, Fields S, Rothberg JMA: A comprehensive analysis of protein–protein interactions in Saccharomyces cerevisiae. Nature 403: 623–627, 2000

57. Walhout AJ, Sordella R, Lu X, Hartley JL, Temple GF, Brasch MA, Thierry-Mieg N, Vidal M: Protein interaction mapping in C. elegans using proteins involved in vulval development. Science 287: 116–122, 2000

58. Stanyon CA, Finley RL Jr: Progress and potential of Drosophila protein interaction maps. Pharmacogenomics 1: 417–431, 2000

59. Simpson JC, Wellenreuther R, Poustka A, Pepperkok R, Wiemann S: Systematic subcellular localization of novel proteins identified by large-scale cDNA sequencing. EMBO Rep 1: 287–292, 2000

60. Remy I, Michnick SW: Visualization of biochemical networks in living cells. Proc Natl Acad Sci USA 98: 7678–7683, 2001

61. Craven RA, Banks RE: Laser capture microdissection and proteomics: Possibilities and limitation. Proteomics 1: 1200–1204, 2001

Address for offprints: Y.Q. Chen, Department of Cancer Biology, Wake Forest University, Medical Center Blvd., Winston-Salem, NC 27157; Tel: 336-7137655; Fax: 336-7137660; e-mail: yq-chen@WFUBMC.edu

Chromosomal deletions and tumor suppressor genes in prostate cancer

Jin-Tang Dong
Department of Pathology, Department of Biochemistry and Molecular Genetics,
University of Virginia Health System, Charlottesville, VA, USA

Key words: prostate cancer, chromosomal deletion, tumor suppressor gene, CGH, LOH, FISH

Abstract

Chromosomal deletion appears to be the earliest as well as the most frequent somatic genetic alteration during carcinogenesis. It inactivates a tumor suppressor gene in three ways, that is, revealing a gene mutation through loss of heterozygosity as proposed in the two-hit theory, inducing haploinsufficiency through quantitative hemizygous deletion and associated loss of expression, and truncating a genome by homozygous deletion. Whereas the two-hit theory has guided the isolation of many tumor suppressor genes, the haploinsufficiency hypothesis seems to be also useful in identifying target genes of chromosomal deletions, especially for the deletions detected by comparative genomic hybridization (CGH). At present, a number of chromosomal regions have been identified for their frequent deletions in prostate cancer, including 2q13–q33, 5q14–q23, 6q16–q22, 7q22–q32, 8p21–p22, 9p21–p22, 10q23–q24, 12p12–13, 13q14–q21, 16q22–24, and 18q21–q24. Strong candidate genes have been identified for some of these regions, including NKX3.1 from 8p21, PTEN from 10q23, p27/Kip1 from 12p13, and KLF5 from 13q21. In addition to their location in a region with frequent deletion, there are functional and/or genetic evidence supporting the candidacy of these genes. Thus far PTEN is the most frequently mutated gene in prostate cancer, and KLF5 showed the most frequent hemizygous deletion and loss of expression. A tumor suppressor role has been demonstrated for NKX3.1, PTEN, and p27/Kip1 in knockout mice models. Such genes are important targets of investigation for the development of biomarkers and therapeutic regimens.

Introduction

It is well established that cancer is a genetic disease resulting from the malfunction of a set of genes [1]. Such malfunction can be inherited as in hereditary cancer, can be induced by carcinogenic factors as in most sporadic cancers, or can result from epigenetic mechanisms such as DNA methylation and imprinting. According to their roles in a cell, genes related to cancer can be categorized into two groups, that is, tumor suppressor genes and oncogenes.

Tumor suppressor genes refer to the genes whose function is to restrain cells from uncontroled growth and migration. The concept of tumor suppressor gene was developed from cell fusion studies by Harris et al. [2], in which the hybrids between two tumor cell lines became nontumorigenic if both genomes were retained and the hybrids became tumorigenic if specific chromosomes were lost. By studying both hereditary and sporadic retinoblastoma, Knudson [3,4] discovered that inactivation of the RB1 tumor suppressor gene followed two genetic 'hits', that is, mutation in one allele and deletion or mutation in the other. As the 'hit' revealing a mutation, chromosomal deletion has been widely used to localize tumor suppressor genes in human cancer [5], and many tumor suppressor genes have been discovered.

Chromosomal loss is one of the most frequent genetic alterations detected in a cancer cell [6]. It can also occur in early stages of carcinogenesis, as deletion has been detected in normal cells [7]. Such loss can involve a region of a chromosome or an entire chromosome. Regional chromosomal loss, which is widely used to detect tumor suppressor loci, can occur in three forms with different consequences (Figure 1). First, the deletion occurs in one chromosome but it was patched using its counterpart as a template. In this situation, loss of heterozygosity (LOH) occurred but no quantitative loss occurred. This type of loss could either reveal a recessive mutation at a locus in the retained allele as

M.L. Cher, K.V. Honn and A. Raz (eds.), Prostate Cancer: New Horizons in Research and Treatment, 37–57.
© 2002 *Kluwer Academic Publishers.*

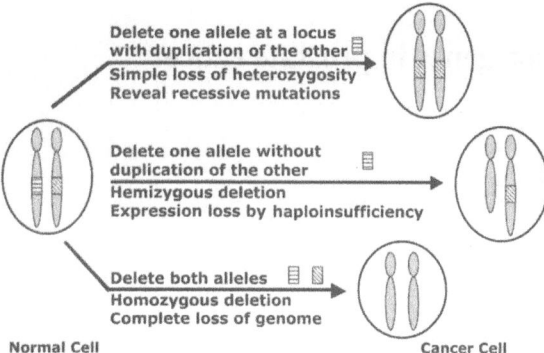

Figure 1. Type and consequence of a chromosomal deletion during the development of cancer. One pair of chromosomes are shown, and the two alleles at a locus are indicated by boxes with horizontal and hatched lines respectively.

Table 1. Chromosomal deletions detected by cytogenetic analysis

Break points	Number of cases with interstitial deletion	Number of cases	Number of studies	References
10q23–q25	0	12	8	[19,28,44, 62–65,125]
6q13–q23	1, q15q23	7	3	[28,45,55]
7q22	0	7	4	[62–65]
1q11–q12	0	6	3	[19–21]
1p11–p34	1, p11p31	5	4	[19,28,62,64]
8p12–p22	0	5	4	[28,44,64,65]
3p12–p23	2, p12p14, p22p23	4	4	[42–45]
3q13–q25	1, q13q24	4	3	[29,43,125]
10p13	0	4	2	[45,216]
17p11–p12	0	4	3	[45,159,207]
12q12–q22	2, q12q13, q14q21	3	3	[28,216,217]
2q13–q33	1, q13q23	2	2	[28,29]
14q13–q24	1, q21q24	2	2	[28,45]
15q24–q25	0	2	2	[19,28]
16q22	0	2	2	[28,55]

Note: Data were primarily collected from the Mitelman Database of Chromosome Aberrations in Cancer [6]. Only the chromosomes with at least two cases showing deletions and reported in at least two studies are listed.

proposed in the two-hit theory [4,5], or have no effect on a cell's phenotype if the retained allele has no mutations. The second type of regional deletion is hemizygous deletion, in which one chromosome is deleted but is not repaired, resulting in the loss of half genome for a locus. In addition to revealing a mutation, such hemizygous deletion can induce haploinsufficiency, in which loss of half genome results in insufficient gene product. Therefore, when haploinsufficiency occurs, a hemizygous deletion still has significant consequence even if the other allele is not mutated. The third type of deletion is homozygous deletion, in which both chromosomes are deleted for a locus, thus the gene product is either absent if its entire genome is deleted or truncated if the deletion involves a part of its genome. In either case, a gene's function is most likely abolished.

LOH analysis has been widely used to localize tumor suppressor loci, and a large number of chromosomal regions have been identified as tumor suppressor loci. In addition, CGH studies also demonstrated a number of chromosomal regions that are lost in cancer cells [8]. The number of tumor suppressor genes identified to fit the two-hit theory, however, has been quite small. One explanation for this discrepancy is that many chromosomal deletions may inactivate a tumor suppressor gene by hemizygous deletion-induced loss of expression, that is, haploinsufficiency, which most likely does not involve gene mutations. Haploinsufficiency is one mechanism underlying human genetic diseases [9,10]. A role for tumor suppressor haploinsufficiency in hereditary cancer has been suggested [11]. Using knockout

mice, haploinsufficiency-induced tumor formation has been demonstrated for several tumor suppressor genes including *PTEN* in multiple cancers [12], *SMAD4/DPC4* in gastric cancer [13], and *p27Kip1* in multiple tumors [14]. Frequent haploinsufficiency at the *KLF5* gene has been detected in prostate cancer [15]. Therefore, searching for genes with haploinsufficiency in addition to point mutations would facilitate the identification of target genes of chromosomal regions deleted in human cancer.

In prostate cancer, a number of chromosomal regions have been identified for their frequent deletions, as detected by conventional cytogenetic analysis (Table 1), by comparative genomic hybridization (CGH) (Table 2), by fluorescence *in situ* hybridization (FISH), and by LOH analysis. At present, however, only a few genes from the common regions of deletion, that is, NKX3.1 from 8p21, PTEN from 10q23, p27/Kip1 from 12p13, and KLF5 from 13q21, have been implicated significantly in prostate cancer. Many more target genes of the deletion regions remain to be identified. The goal of this review is to summarize the current status of common regions of deletion and identification of target genes, and thus to facilitate our understanding of genetic basis of prostate cancer.

Table 2. Regional chromosomal deletions detected by comparative genomic hybridization analysis

Band	Number of cases with loss	Total cases analyzed	%	References
8p11–p22	175	417	42	[16–18,31–33,36, 37,49–51,57,58]
13q14–q22	160	411	39	[16–18,31–37, 50,51,57,58]
19q13	26	73	36	[16,17,35]
16q13–23	105	339	31	[16–18,33,35,36, 49,51,57]
1p34–ptel	31	109	28	[16–18]
5q14–q23	112	396	28	[18,31–33,36, 37,49–51]
6q15–q22	126	443	28	[16,18,31–34,36, 37,49–51,57,58]
17p	25	89	28	[16,31–33]
22q	26	93	28	[16,17,32]
10q22–25	77	289	27	[16–18,33, 35–37,49]
4q21–31	32	141	23	[18,33,34,36,37]
15q22–q23	33	160	21	[16,17,31–33,36]
2q21–32	47	230	20	[18,31–37]
18q21	57	305	19	[16,18,32,34,36, 37,50,51,57]
20q	17	102	17	[17,31,32]
Y	30	174	17	[18,31,36,37,51]
9p21–pter	14	96	15	[18,32]
12q21–q24	9	64	14	[17,36,37]
16p	7	49	14	[31,32]
11q22–q23	4	37	11	[17,58]
12p11–p13	13	114	11	[18,34,51]

Note: The frequency of losses for a region is based on all the studies that showed loss for that region in >10% of the cases examined. Only the regions with loss in at least two studies were included. The majority of the studies were included in a previous review article [8].

Chromosome 1

In three CGH studies, deletion of 1p34–pter was detected in 31 of 109 (28%) prostate cancers examined [16–18]. Deletions also occur at 1q. Based on cytogenetic analyses, deletion of 1q involves several break points. Deletion at 1q11–q12 appears to be more frequent, being detected in 6 cases from 3 studies thus far (Table 1) [19–21]. At present, however, no frequent deletion at 1q has been detected by either CGH or LOH analysis.

Three prostate cancer susceptibility genes have been linked to different regions on chromosome 1, that is, HPC1 at 1q24–25 [22], PCAP at 1q42–43 [23], and CAPB at 1p36 [24]. These loci have been confirmed

in additional studies [25]. Microsatellite markers from the linked regions at 1q24–q25 and 1p36 have been analyzed for LOH in familial prostate cancers [26,27]. LOH was infrequent in both studies, occurring in 3 of 27 (11%) for both 1q24–25 and 1p36 in one study [26] and in 7.5% of 35 cases in another study [27]. Forty sporadic tumors were also analyzed for 1q24–25, and similar frequency of LOH was found [27].

Chromosome 2q

In cytogenetic analyses, deletion of chromosome 2 with break points at 2q13–q33, including one interstitial deletion of del(2)(q13q23), has been detected in 2 cases [28,29]. The CWR22 prostate cancer xenograft also has an interstitial deletion, which is at 2q13–q33 [30]. By CGH analyses, loss of chromosome 2, with 2q21–32 commonly involved, has been detected in 9 studies at a frequency of 20% (47 of 230 cases) [18,31–37]. No comprehensive LOH analysis has been reported for 2q deletion.

One gene, named Bin1, has been tested as the target gene of deletion at 2q. This gene is within the deletion region at 2q14. It is an ubiquitous adaptor protein that can suppress malignant transformation by c-Myc [38] and it has been linked to cell death and differentiation decisions [39]. In prostate cancer, LOH at Bin1 was detected in 40% of informative cases and aberrant splicing of the gene frequently occurred in metastatic tumors and androgen-independent tumor cell lines [40]. Ectopic expression of Bin1 suppressed the growth of prostate cancer lines *in vitro*. These findings suggest that Bin1 is a candidate gene for the 2q deletion.

Chromosome 3p

Deletion at 3p is frequent in many other cancers including that of the lung and the breast, and a region of homozygous deletion has been identified [41]. In prostate cancer, 4 cases with deletions at 3p12–p23 have been reported in 4 cytogenetic studies [42–45]. Two of the 4 cases showed interstitial deletions, one involved p12p14 and the other p22p23. CGH studies, however, have not detected deletions at 3p (Table 2). In one molecular study [46], in which 38 microdissected prostate cancers were examined for 6 polymorphic markers from 3p, LOH was identified in 34 of 38 cases (89%) with at least one marker, and 2 clusters of LOH were suggested, one at 3p24–p26 and the other at 3p22–p12.

Chromosome 4q

Although not detected by cytogenetic studies, deletions of chromosome 4 occur at a noticeable frequency in 5 CGH analyses of prostate cancer [18,33,34,36,37]. Thirty-two of 141 (23%) tumors analyzed had deletions, and the common region of deletion involves 4q21–q31. The same region appears to be affected in other cancers including esophageal adenocarcinoma. In CGH analysis of prostate cancer cell lines TSU-Pr1, NCI-H660, PC-3, DU145, and LNCaP, deletion at 4q was one of the most frequent losses [47].

Chromosome 5q

Deletion at 5q is a frequent event in prostate cancer. Although not reported in primary tumor specimens, deletion of 5q11 has been detected by cytogenetic analysis in 5 cell lines, that is, TSU-Pr1, NCI-H660, PC-3, DU145, and LNCaP [47]. FISH analyses of 5 additional prostate cancer cell lines demonstrated deletions of 5q in 2 of them, one was del(5)(q23q35) in the SP2964 (i.e. ARCaP) cell line, and the other was del(5)(q23q33) in the SP3316 line [48].

In 9 CGH analyses, deletion at 5q was detected in 112 of 396 (28%) prostate cancers, and the common region of deletion was in 5q14–q23 [18,31–33,36,37,49–51]. Whereas deletion at 5q has been detected in prostatic intraepithelial neoplasia (PIN) lesions by CGH [37], more advanced tumors appear to have more frequent deletions [51].

Using the restriction fragment length polymorphism (RFLP) technique, LOH at the APC locus of 5q21–q22 was detected in 3 of 7 informative prostate cancers [52]. In a genome wide screening for LOH in prostate cancer [53], LOH at 5q was also frequent, and such LOH was associated with higher tumor stage. Frequent LOH was also detected for 5q (D5S806, 20%) in PIN lesions [54]. At present, no detailed deletion mapping studies are available.

Chromosome 6q

Deletion of the long arm of chromosome 6, with the common region at 6q15–q22, is a frequent genetic alteration in prostate cancer. In cytogenetic studies, deletion at 6q13–q23 has been detected in 7 cases in 3 studies [28,45,55], and 6q is the second most frequently deleted chromosome (after 10q, which has 10 cases

and harbors the *PTEN* gene). One cancer showed an interstitial deletion of 6q15–q23. Cytogenetic deletion of chromosome 6 has also been detected in a human prostate cancer xenograft [56]. CGH analyses provide even stronger evidence for a region of deletion at 6q, as deletion involving 6q15–q22 has been detected in 126 of 443 (28%) cases analyzed in 13 reports [16,18,31–34,36,37,49–51,57,58]. The common region of deletion appears to be the same as detected in cytogenetic studies. Metastases and recurrent tumors have more frequent deletions at 6q than do primary tumors [16,32,33]. These studies indicate that one or more suppressor genes are located on 6q15–q22 in prostate cancer.

LOH analyses also showed frequent deletions at 6q in prostate cancer. In a genome wide screening for LOH in prostate cancer [53], 6q was one of the frequently deleted chromosomal regions (24%). Another study of one 6q marker showed that LOH was more frequent in metastases than in PIN lesions as well as primary tumors of prostate cancer [54]. Cooney et al. [59] analyzed 52 tumors with 9 polymorphic markers from 6q and mapped a common LOH region to a DNA segment of 19 cM between markers D6S251 and D6S283 at 6q14–q21. They also found a separate region of deletion centering around marker D6S404. In another analysis of 38 primary prostate cancers for LOH using 13 microsatellite loci on 6q, the most frequent LOH was also found at markers located within the region identified in Cooney's study [60].

In a recent analysis of 44 primary tumors and 23 cell lines/xenografts of prostate cancer with 46 microsatellite markers [61], LOH at 6q16–q22 was detected in 21 of 44 (48%) primary tumors and in 12 of 23 (52%) cell lines/xenografts. Two regions of LOH were defined. One was 7.5 cM at 6q16–q21 between markers D6S1716 and D6S1580, and the other was 4.3 cM at 6q22 between D6S261 and D6S1702. The two regions overlapped with that defined in Cooney's study respectively [59]. Whereas no correlation was found between LOH at 6q16–q22 and patient age at diagnosis or Gleason score, tumors at higher stage appear to have more frequent LOH.

Chromosome 7q

Deletion of 7q is a frequent event in cytogenetic analyses of prostate cancer (Table 1) [62–65]. The common breakpoint is in 7q22–q32. In the CGH analyses of prostate cancer so far, however, deletion of 7q has not been detected [8], which could be due to the occurrence of trisomy 7, one of the most frequent genetic alterations in prostate cancer [66,67].

Analysis of microsatellite markers, on the other hand, showed frequent LOH at 7q [53,68]. High frequency of LOH at 7q has been confirmed in different studies including one using both RFLP and microsatellite analyses [69]. Examination of 16 primary prostate carcinomas with 14 polymorphic microsatellite markers spanning 7q21–qter revealed that 5 of 6 informative cases lost marker D7S522 at 7q31, and the percentage of LOH was normally distributed around this marker [70]. Similarly, a study of 43 samples using both RFLP and microsatellite procedures demonstrated that the most frequently deleted region was at 7q31.1, with the percentage of LOH normally distributed around marker D7S480 [71]. Marker D7S480 is only 1.9 cM telomeric to D7S522. In a third deletion mapping study with 54 prostate cancers and 21 microsatellite markers, LOH was detected in 15 tumors (28%) and the most common site of deletion involved markers D7S523 and D7S486 at 7q31.1; both are less than 1.1 cM centromeric to D7S522 [72]. Therefore, the common region of deletion could be in a 2.9 cM interval between D7S523 and D7S480. A correlation between LOH at 7q31 and higher tumor grade or lymph node metastasis was reported [72]. These studies clearly identify a LOH region at 7q31 in prostate cancer.

In addition to frequent LOH at 7q31, trisomy 7 is also frequent in prostate cancer [66,67], and this abnormality is correlated with aggressiveness of prostate cancer [73]. In understanding both trisomy 7 and deletion at 7q31 in the same tumors, Cui et al. [74] conducted a dual-color FISH analysis on isolated nuclei from 28 primary prostate cancers. Nine of them were trisomy 7 and 2 other cases, both high grade tumors, showed deletions at 7q31.1. It was suggested that deletions at 7q31.1 precede reduplications of chromosome 7. Similarly, in a FISH analysis of 25 prostate cancers with chromosome 7 probes, 9 tumors showed apparent simple gain of a whole chromosome 7, 1 had apparent simple loss of a whole chromosome 7, and 3 had gain of the chromosome 7 centromere and loss of the 7q31 region [75]. Mutation screening and DNA sequencing of the MET gene, which is mapped to 7q31, revealed only the presence of simple sequence polymorphisms but no apparent disease-associated mutations. One of the DNA probes showing deletions, that is, the one for marker D7S522, spans the common fragile site FRA7G at 7q31, raising the question whether the second most common aphidicolin-

inducible fragile site in the human genome may be responsible for 7q31 deletions.

Functionally, microcell-mediated chromosome transfer studies have shown that introduction of an intact chromosome 7 can restore senescence to human fibroblasts known to have LOH within 7q31–q32 [76]. In addition, introduction of chromosome 7 inhibits the tumorigenicity of a mouse squamous carcinoma cell line [77]. In the human prostate cancer cell line PC-3, introduction of chromosome 7 induced longer tumor latency [78], and the common region of deletion was approximately 1.5 Mb between markers D7S486 and D7S655 at 7q31. To facilitate the cloning of the putative tumor suppressor gene, Zenklusen et al. [79] have constructed a high-resolution physical map of yeast artificial chromosome (YAC), bacterial artificial chromosome (BAC), and expressed sequence tags (ESTs) spanning markers D7S522 and D7S677 in approximately a 1-Mb region of human chromosome 7q31.1–q31.2.

More recently, a candidate tumor suppressor gene, ST7, has been identified from 7q31 using a positional cloning strategy [80]. The ST7 gene is ubiquitously expressed in human tissues including prostate and showed mutations in cell lines derived from breast tumors and primary colon carcinomas. Introduction of the ST7 cDNA into the PC-3 prostate cancer cell line had no effect on the in vitro proliferation of the cells, but abrogated their in vivo tumorigenicity [80]. The role of ST7 in prostate cancer needs further investigations.

Chromosome 8p

Deletion at the short arm of chromosome 8 is one of the most frequent genetic alterations in prostate cancer. Although cytogenetic studies only detected 5 cases with deletion of 8p12–p22 in 4 reports [28,44,64,65], deletion of this region is the most frequent in CGH studies, occurring in 175 of 417 (42%) cancers examined [16–18,31–33,36,37,49–51,57,58]. In a group of prostate cancer metastases from 20 patients, which were highly enriched for tumor cells, loss of 8p occurred in 80% of them [33]. CGH analysis of prostate cancer cell lines also showed loss of 8p as one of the most frequent losses [47].

Using the method of FISH, frequent aneosomy of chromosome 8 with simultaneous p arm deletion and q arm gain was detected [31,81]. Using probes from 2 deletion regions, that is, lipoprotein lipase (LPL) from 8p22 and D8S7 from 8p23, FISH analyses revealed 8p deletion in 32 of 42 (71%) specimens. Most cases lost both regions. Dual-color FISH, using a control probe from the centromere of chromosome 8, confirmed frequent deletion of 8p in prostate cancer [82,83].

A large number of studies have been published on 8p LOH in prostate cancer. Using the RFLP method, LOH of 8p was detected in 3 of 6 informative cases [84]. Bova et al. [85] analyzed prostate cancer specimens from 52 patients for allelic loss using 8 polymorphic probes from 8p. The common region of deletion was at 8p22–8p21.2, and loss of the D8S220 marker at 8p21.3–8p21.2 was the most frequent, occurring in 16 of 27 (59%) tumors. The smallest region of overlap (SRO) for deletion was defined to a 14-cM interval at 8p22 between the D8S163 and LPL loci. A large number of LOH studies using microsatellite markers have been performed, and frequent LOH at 8p22 has been repeatedly detected [53,54,68,69,86–91]. In one analysis of 32 primary tumors with 16 markers, the most frequent LOH occurred at the LPL locus (46%) on 8p22 and at the D8S360 (45%) and NEFL (43%) loci on 8p21 [92]. The minimal region of deletion was around the LPL locus within a 9 cM region between loci MSR and D8S258. Additional LOH studies using microdissected tumors have identified additional regions of deletion within 8p12–p21 [53,86,89,93–96]. In addition to 8p22, a different region was at 8p21 in a segment of 12 cM between markers D8S1128 and D8S131 [92]. In another analysis of 46 prostate cancers with 12 RFLP markers from 8p [94], the 2 regions of LOH were defined as one in a 1.2 Mb interval at 8p22–p21.3 between markers cMSR-32 and C18-1051 and the other at 8p21–8p11.22 between C18-1312 and C18-494. In Macoska et al.'s [89] study of 135 tumors with 9 markers from 8p, another 2 regions in addition to the one at 8p22 were identified, which encompass the NEFL locus and D8S87-ANK1 loci respectively. In a high-resolution mapping study, Vocke et al. [95] investigated 99 microdissected tumors with 25 microsatellite markers from 8p, and very frequent LOH was detected at markers D8S133, D8S136, NEFL, and D8S137, which are located at 8p12–21. In one study [96], even 4 regions appear to be involved, that is, D8S262 at 8p23, D8S259 at 8p22, D8S255 and D8S285 at 8p12, and D8S260 and D8S528 at 8q12–13. Multiple regions of deletion at 8p have also been demonstrated by FISH analysis [83].

After Bova et al.'s [85] report of an interstitial homozygous deletion in a metastatic prostate cancer, which removed the candidate tumor suppressor gene N33, homozygous deletion involving the loci of LPL, NEFL, and D8S87 has been detected in other studies [92,97]. The homozygous deletion could be as frequent as 16% in some tumors [98]. Using sequence tagged site (STS) markers, a homozygous deletion of 730–1,320 kb was found in one prostate cancer xenograft, that is, PC133, among 14 cell lines/xenografts analyzed [99]. The deletion was confirmed and extended by FISH analysis of PC133 chromosome spreads.

LOH at 8p21 appears to be an early event in prostatic carcinogenesis, as it has been detected in PIN lesions by the analyses of LOH, FISH, and CGH [37,93,100]. Using microdissected samples from 30 patients with concomitant cancer and PIN, LOH at 8p12–21 was detected in 34 of 54 (63%) PIN foci and 29 of 32 (91%) tumors. Whereas multiple foci of PIN from the same patient often show different patterns of LOH at 8p, the same pattern of LOH was detected in both tumor and its adjacent PIN for 16 of 29 (55%) cases [93]. Similar findings were reported in another study [101]. Detection of common genetic events shared by primary tumors and adjacent PIN lesions supports the hypothesis that PIN is the precursor of prostate carcinoma.

Although loss of 8p appears to be an early event in prostatic carcinogenesis, an association between such loss and various clinicopathologic parameters has been reported. For example, LOH at 8p was associated with higher tumor grade [53,86]. FISH analysis also showed that the degree of 8p deletion was correlated with tumor grade and tumor stage [31]. Based on the defined LOH regions, a detailed FISH analysis of 42 primary tumors showed that deletions of 8p22 and 8p21.3 were correlated with tumor grade, and deletion at 8p21.1–p21.2 occurred more frequently in tumors which were positive for lymph node metastases [83]. No clinicopathologic parameters had significant relation to deletions at 8p12. Using the FISH technique [102], 8p22 deletions were detected in 58 of 97 (60%) prostate cancer specimens, and the frequency of 8p22 deletion was statistically higher in patients with pT3 or pT4 tumors than in those with pT2. In this study, 8p22 deletion is also a strong parameter to predict disease progression.

Target genes. In order to clone the target gene for 8p deletion, Bova et al. [103] has constructed a physical map for about 2 Mb DNA at 8p22. Using this map, the region of 8p22 homozygous deletion in a metastasis has been narrowed to a segment of 730–970 kb, which contains microsatellite markers D8S549, D8S1991, and D8S1992. From this region of homozygous deletion, a gene named N33 has been identified [104,105], which has 11 coding exons spanning 205–220 kb of the 730–970 kb deletion. The N33 gene is expressed as an 1.5-kb mRNA in most tissues including prostate, but neither mutation nor loss of expression has been detected in prostate cancer cells [105], suggesting a minor role for N33 in prostate cancer.

Another candidate for the target gene of 8p deletion is FEZ1/LZTS1 [106], which was isolated from 8p22 and contains a leucine-zipper region with similarity to the DNA-binding domain of the cAMP-responsive activating-transcription factor 5. Northern blot hybridization revealed that expression of FEZ1 was not detectable in more than 60% of epithelial tumors. One mutation was found in the PC-3 cell line. Transcript analysis from several FEZ1-expressing tumors revealed truncated mRNAs, including a frameshift change, and one aberrant transcript was also detected in the DU145 cell line. Alteration and inactivation of the FEZ1 gene in prostate cancer support its candidacy for the target gene of 8p22 deletion. In functional studies, overexpression of FEZ1 in cancer cells appeared to inhibit colony-forming efficiencies, suppressed tumorigenicity, and reduced cell growth with the accumulation of cells at late S-G(2)/M stage of the cell cycle [107,108], suggesting that FEZ1 inhibits cancer cell growth through regulation of mitosis, and that its alterations result in abnormal cell growth.

The third candidate gene for 8p21 deletion region is dematin, a cytoskeletal protein that bundles actin filaments in a phosphorylation-dependent manner [109]. This gene is between two frequently deleted markers D8S258 and D8S137, and its LOH occurred in the majority of 8p21-linked prostate tumors. In addition, overexpression of wild-type dematin in PC-3 cells resulted in the restoration of a more polarized, epithelial-like phenotype.

The strongest candidate for the target gene of 8p deletion so far, however, is the NKX3.1 gene, which was isolated from 8p21 as a prostate-specific gene in humans with homology to the Drosophila NK homeobox gene family [110]. Northern blot analyses indicate that this gene is expressed at a high level in adult prostate and at a much lower level in testis, and little or not at all in most other tissues. In the LNCaP androgen-dependent prostate cancer line, NKX3.1 mRNA is expressed at a basal level that was increased upon androgen stimulation. The NKX3.1 mRNA was undetectable in two androgen-independent prostate carcinoma lines.

The function of NKX3.1 has been examined in mice using a gene targeting technique [111,112]. Homozygous mutant mice for NKX3.1 were viable and fertile, and the phenotype was confined to the prostate and palatine glands. The homozygous mutant mice exhibited defective branching morphogenesis of these glands. Moreover, epithelial cells of the mutant prostate showed significant hyperplasia, similar to PIN lesions in human prostate. Interestingly, heterozygous mice also developed PIN-like hyperplasia in prostate, indicating that haploinsufficiency of NKX3.1 induces preneoplastic lesions in the prostate [111]. Taken together with the fact that deletion of 8p is also frequent in PIN lesions of human prostate, it is likely that loss of NKX3.1 makes prostate epithelial cells proliferate more rapidly; thus additional genetic events could occur to fully transform a cell.

On the other hand, mutations of the NKX3.1 coding sequence have not been detected in several studies of over 100 prostate cancer specimens using different methods [113–115]. Protein expression of NKX3.1 was found to be in nuclei of normal prostate epithelial cells [116]. In 507 samples of neoplastic prostate epithelium on a tissue microarray, loss of NKX3.1 expression was found in 20% of high grade PIN lesions, 28% of primary tumors, 34% of hormone-refractory cancers, and 78% of metastases, suggesting an association between loss of NKX3.1 expression with hormone-refractory disease and advanced tumor stage in prostate cancer. In another two studies in which NKX3.1 RNA was analyzed for expression change, however, no consistent changes were noticed [114,115]. Considering that haploinsufficiency may be a major mechanism for the loss of NKX3.1 function, that is, NKX3.1 may be subject to partial instead of complete loss of expression, the techniques used in these studies may not have been sensitive enough to detect quantitative reduction of NKX3.1 expression.

Chromosome 9p

Although deletion of the short arm of chromosome 9 has not been detected in cytogenetic studies, CGH analyses of 96 prostate cancer specimens have showed deletion of 9p21–pter in 14 (15%) cases [18,32]. In cell lines, in particular, deletion of 9p is one of the most frequent detected by CGH [47]. These studies suggest a role for 9p deletion in prostate cancer.

Analysis of two microsatellite markers from 9p21–p22 showed that LOH at 9p22 is frequent in metastases but not in high grade PIN lesions and primary tumors [54]. In a more detailed LOH mapping study, in which 40 samples were analyzed for 15 microsatellite markers on 9p, frequent deletion was detected at 9p21, involving markers D9S1748 (50%) and D9S171 (51.4%) [117]. Cairns et al. [118] found that a small region of homozygous deletion at 9p21 identified from bladder cancer is also deleted in prostate cancer.

The p16/MTS1 tumor suppressor gene is located within the small region of homozygous deletion identified by Cairns et al. [118]. This gene encodes a 16 kDa inhibitor of cyclin-dependent kinases, and its inactivation by homozygous deletion, point mutation, and aberrant methylation in the 5' promoter region may enhance progression through the cell cycle in other types of tumors. Examination of p16/MTS1 in 20 primary prostate tumors and 4 established cell lines by PCR-SSCP revealed no homozygous deletions but 2 mutations, one at codon 76 in the DU145 cell line and the other at codon 55 in a primary tumor [119]. Another analysis of 18 cancers using the same approach detected no homozygous deletion and one sequence alteration at codon 140, but this change was present in both tumor cells and matched nonneoplastic cells and thus may represent a polymorphism [120]. No mutations were detected in 3 additional primary tumors and 7 lymph node metastases examined [121]. In Jarrard et al.'s [121] study, LOH at loci close to p16 was detected in 12 of 60 (20%) primary tumors and in 13 of 28 (46%) metastases, and promoter methylation was detected in 5 of 40 prostate cancer samples. These results indicate that homozygous deletion and point mutations in the p16/MTS1 gene are rare but promoter methylation may inactivate p16 in a subset of tumors.

Chromosome 10p

Cytogenetic study by Teixeira et al. [45] showed a recurrent deletion, del(10)(p13), in 3 of 12 tumors analyzed. In one of the tumors, the terminal nature of the deletion was confirmed by two-color FISH. Using the RFLP approach, deletion at 10p was detected in 4 of 19 informative cases [52]. Examination of 35 prostate tumors with 24 polymorphic microsatellite loci spanning chromosome 10 showed frequent deletions at 10p, including loci D10S211, D10S89, and D10S111, which were mapped to 10p11.2 by FISH analysis [122]. Presence of a region of deletion at 10p was also demonstrated in other LOH analyses, in which a total of 131 tumors were examined, and D10S111 was one of the most frequently deleted markers [123,124]. Therefore, deletion at 10p11–13 may play a role in prostate cancer.

Chromosome 10q

Deletion of the long arm of chromosome 10 is the most frequent chromosomal deletion detected by cytogenetic analyses in prostate cancer. In 8 studies, deletion of 10q23–q25 was detected in 12 cases [19,28,44,62–65,125].

In CGH studies, deletion of 10q22–q25 occurred in 77 of 289 (27%) tumors analyzed [16–18,33, 35–37,49]. CGH analyses of five prostate cancer cell lines showed a recurrent breakpoint at 10q22 in each of them [47]. FISH analysis also demonstrated frequent loss of 10q in prostate cancer and PIN lesions [100].

A number of LOH studies have showed frequent deletion of 10q in prostate cancer. Using the RFLP method, Carter et al. [126] first reported LOH of 10q in 30% of tumors. Using the same technique, a higher frequency of LOH (42%) was reported in another study [52]. Frequent LOH of 10q has also been detected by PCR based microsatellite analyses [54,68,69]. Using high density microsatellite markers, even more frequent LOH (62%) was detected, and the region of deletion was localized to the q23–q25 bands of chromosome 10, centering on the 10q23–q24 boundary, as markers at the boundary were deleted in the overwhelming majority (22 of 23) of tumors [127]. The same small region of LOH was also mapped in another analysis [128], as the D10S221 locus at 10q23–q24 presented the highest rate of LOH. D10S185 is also among the most frequently deleted markers [123]. The region of deletion was further defined to a 7 cM interval in an study of 48 tumors [124]. LOH at this locus appeared to be more frequent in tumors from fatal cases (stage D tumor) than in localized tumors (stage B and/or C) [124]. From this region, the PTEN tumor suppressor gene has been identified [129,130]. In addition to the 1023–24 locus, another locus at distant 10q, probably at 10q26, has been suggested, and the region was mapped to a DNA segment of 17 cM [123,124].

There are several genes that have been considered as the target genes of deletion at 10q. One is the ANX7 gene from 10q21 [131], to which deletions at 10q23 often extend. This gene suppressed cell proliferation and colony formation when transfected into LNCaP and DU145 cells. Using a tissue microarray of 301 prostate specimens, loss of protein expression for ANX7 is more frequent in metastases and recurrent hormone-refractory tumors of prostate cancer as compared with primary tumors. Analysis of 4 microsatellite markers at or near the ANX7 locus in microdissected tumor cells showed allelic loss of ANX7 in 35% of tumors, with the microsatellite marker closest to the ANX7 locus showing the highest rate of LOH [131].

Another candidate gene for the 10q deletion is MXI1 at 10q24–q25, a member of the helix-loop-helix gene family which negatively regulates the Myc oncogene. Mutations of MXI1 were detected in 4 primary tumors that had LOH at 10q24–q25 [132], which fits the two-hit theory of tumor suppressor inactivation and suggests a suppressive role of MXI1 in prostate cancer. In addition, mice deficient for MXI1 exhibit significant prostate hyperplasia, and introduction of MXI1 into the DU145 prostate carcinoma cells resulted in reduced cell proliferation and soft agar colony formation and a higher proportion of cells in the G(2)/M phase of the cell cycle [133]. This G(2)/M growth arrest was associated with reduced levels of c-Myc, supporting a role for MXI1 loss in the pathogenesis of a subset of human prostate cancers. In other studies, however, loss of the MXI1 locus is rare (1 in 23 tumors) and no mutation of MXI1 could be detected in a total of 65 tumors of different stages [127,134], questioning a substantial role of MXI1 in prostate cancer. In 38 families with either 3 cases of prostate cancer or 2 affected siblings both diagnosed below the age of 67 years, no mutations were found in 2 coding regions of MXI1 [135].

The strongest candidate for the target gene of 10q deletion is the *PTEN* gene at 10q23.3, which was designated *PTEN*, *MMAC1*, or *TEP-1* in different studies [129,130,136]. The *PTEN* gene has 9 exons that encode a 403-amino acid protein of a dual-specific phosphatase with putative actin-binding and tyrosine phosphatase domains. Introduction of PTEN into cancer cells that lack *PTEN* function negatively regulates cell migration and survival, inducing cell cycle arrest and apoptosis via negative regulation of the phosphatidylinositol 3'-kinase/protein kinase B/Akt signaling pathway [137–139]. Mutation and down-regulation of the *PTEN* gene have been detected in various human cancers [140–142]. In addition, germline mutations in *PTEN* are associated with Cowden disease [143], in which patients are at increased risk for certain cancers.

Thus far, *PTEN* is the most frequently mutated gene in metastases of prostate cancer, occurring in at least 1 metastatic site in 12 of 19 (63%) patients who had multiple metastases [144] and in 9 of 15 (60%) cell lines and xenografts primarily derived from metastases of prostate cancer [145]. These results indicate a role for *PTEN* in the progression of prostate cancer. Mutations of *PTEN* in localized prostate cancers have been found at lower frequencies including 1/28 (4%) [146], 1/25 (4%) [147], 1/40 (2.5%) [148], 0/45 [149], and 1/22 (5%) [150]. Somewhat higher rates of mutations were observed in some other studies including 10/80 (12.5%) (10/23 43%) in cases with LOH at *PTEN* [151], 5/37 (13.5%) [152], 8/60 (13%) [153], and 1/10 (10%) [140]. In familial prostate cancer, *PTEN*'s role was not detected [154,155].

The difference in mutation frequency of *PTEN* in primary prostate cancer among different studies appear to be largely due to differences in tumor grade and stage in the study populations. Summarizing 5 studies in which both tumor grade and PTEN mutations were available [147–149,152], 9 of 67 (13.4%) high grade tumors showed PTEN mutations, while only 3 of 117 (2.6%) lower grade cases showed mutations. In a study of PTEN in prostate cancer from Chinese patients, who were diagnosed with clinical symptoms but without the aid of the serum PSA screening test and the majority of tumors were high grade, *PTEN* mutations occurred in 5 of 32 (16%) cases [156], which is more frequent than 1 of 40 (2.5%) frequency in American patients studied by the same group [148]. Consistent with mutation studies, loss of PTEN expression has also been shown to correlate with higher grade of primary tumors [140,142]. Mutational spectrum of PTEN in human tumors and the molecular pathways through which PTEN acts to suppress tumor growth have been reviewed in different articles [141,157].

Chromosome 11p

A deletion at 11p14 was reported in a cytogenetic study [44]. Allelic loss at 11p has also been detected in prostate cancer, and multiple regions on both p and q arms were suggested [54,158]. In CGH studies, however, no obvious deletion has been observed [8]. At present no detailed deletion mapping studies are available.

Chromosome 12p12–13

Deletion of 12p with a breakpoint at 12p11 was reported in 1 case in a cytogenetic study [159]. In

CGH studies, deletion of 12p11–p13 was a noticeable event in prostate cancer, occurring in 13 of 114 (11%) cases [18,34,51]. In a FISH analysis, 11 of 20 (55%) prostate cancers showed significant loss of chromosome 12 [160].

Using the representational difference analysis (RDA) procedure, Kibel et al. [161] found that HSU59962, a genomic sequence in 12p12–p13, was homozygously deleted in a prostate cancer xenograft. The region of deletion was mapped to a 1–5 cM region using STS markers. LOH at markers from this region was demonstrated in 9 of 19 (47%) patients [161]. In a subsequent study, the same group constructed a physical map for the deletion region and further defined it to a 1–2-Mb DNA segment between markers WI-664 and D12S358 [162]. LOH at markers from this region of homozygous deletion was identified in 14 of 60 (23%) primary tumors, 6 of 20 (30%) lymph node metastasis, and 9 of 19 (47%) distant metastases [163]. A higher rate of LOH at these markers was detected in 27 sporadic prostate tumors in another study [164]. Among the genes/ESTs mapped to the region of homozygous deletion are the p27/Kip1 and ETV6 genes, suggesting their candidacy as the target gene of deletion in prostate cancer.

Whereas loss of RNA expression for ETV6 was detected in 7 of 27 (26%) tumors, which suggests a role of this gene in prostate cancer [164], the p27/Kip1 gene is more interesting, because it is able to inhibit cyclin-dependent kinases and block cell proliferation. Low p27/Kip1 expression predicts recurrence and poor disease-free survival in prostate cancer [165,166] and correlated with a number of prognostic morphologic features including higher Gleason scores/tumor grade, positive surgical margins, seminal vesicle involvement, and lymph node metastasis [167–169]. Most interestingly, both p27/Kip1 nullizygous and heterozygous mice develop hyperplasia in prostate and are predisposed to tumors in multiple tissues when challenged with gamma-irradiation or a chemical carcinogen [14]. Molecular analyses of tumors in p27/Kip1 heterozygous mice show that the remaining wild-type allele is neither mutated nor silenced, indicating that haploinsufficiency of p27/Kip1 may play a role in tumorigenesis. Concomitant inactivation of one PTEN allele and one or both p27/Kip1 alleles accelerates spontaneous neoplastic transformation and incidence of tumors of various histological origins in mice [170].

Mutation analyses of 44 samples including some metastatic tumors showed no mutations except for homozygous deletions [171]. Even the rate of homozygous deletion is low and is not responsible for the frequent loss of expression for p27/Kip1. Methylation analysis of 4 cell lines and 9 xenografts did not detect promoter methylation that could silence gene transcription [171]. Therefore, haploinsufficiency rather than two-hit mechanism appears to be the major mechanism for the inactivation of p27/Kip1 in prostate cancer.

Chromosome 13q

Deletion of the long arm of human chromosome 13 (13q) is a frequent event in prostate cancer. In addition to cytogenetically visible deletions [56,172], CGH studies have indicated that chromosome 13 is the second most commonly deleted chromosome (after chromosome 8) in prostate cancer, showing loss of 13q14–q22 in 160 of 411 (39%) tumors studied [16–18, 31–37,50,51,57,58]. Moreover, each of the cell lines derived from prostate cancers, that is, LNCaP, DU-145, PC-3, and NCI-H660, showed loss of 13q sequence with the minimal common region of deletion at 13q21 [47,173].

Whereas deletion at 13q has been detected in PIN lesions by CGH [37], many studies have showed that deletion at 13q is related to clinical aggressiveness of prostate cancer [174,175]. For example, deletion at 13q14 is correlated with prostate cancers of advanced stage or grade [176,177], is more frequent in recurrent as compared to those localized prostate cancer [32], is extremely frequent in metastases of prostate cancer [178], and is associated with younger patient age at diagnosis in localized prostate neoplasms [178]. Frequent loss at 13q has also been detected in tumors from patients with familial prostate cancer [58].

13q14 region. At least 2 distinct regions of deletion occur on chromosome 13 in prostate cancer. One is at 13q14, the other at 13q21 [175,177,178]. Two known tumor suppressor genes important in some types of carcinoma are located on the q arm of chromosome 13, that is, *BRCA2* at 13q12 and *RB1* at 13q14. Although *BRCA2* appears not to be involved in the development of prostate cancer [174,179–181], allelic loss and somatic mutations of the *RB1* gene have been detected in some prostate tumors [182–184]. No correlation between LOH and mutation or absence of expression of the *RB1* gene has been observed, however [179–181]. LOH at loci encompassing the *RB1* gene has been examined in several studies in prostate cancer, and frequent LOH at 13q has been detected [52,53,69,174,178,179,181,185–187]. Using 7 microsatellite markers, Latil et al. [181] found that the region with the most frequent LOH on 13q was located in a 7 cM interval between *D13S263* and *RB1* (*D13S153*). Li et al. [185], using 8 markers, found that the most frequently deleted region was between *D13S218* and *D13S153*, which includes the area defined in the study of Latil et al. [181]. Cooney et al. [179] studied 9 markers and identified a region between *D13S153* and *D13S133*, which spans the *RB1* but not the *BRCA2* gene and overlaps with the regions identified in Li and Latil's studies. Consistent with these findings, Hyytinen et al. [178] also found that the region of deletion at 13q14 is located between *RB1* and *BRCA2*. Different from most studies, the region of deletion was defined by markers close to but telomeric to the RB1 locus in two other studies [186,187].

Detailed mapping of the region of deletion at 13q14 has been performed [188]. Analysis of 134 prostate cancers for hemizygous/homozygous deletion using markers from the LOH region detected homozygous deletion in 13 of 134 tumors (10%). Based on the high-resolution YAC/BAC/STS/EST physical map, homozygous/hemizygous deletion analyses of 61 cell lines/xenografts derived from human cancers of the prostate, breast, ovary, endometrium, cervix, and bladder defined the region of deletion between markers A005X38 and WI-7773 [188]. LOH analysis of the 61 cell lines/xenografts, using the homozygosity-mapping-of-deletion (HOMOD) approach and 26 microsatellite markers, defined the region of deletion between markers M1 and M5. Combination of homozygous/hemizygous deletion and LOH results defined the SRO for deletion to an 800 kb DNA interval between markers A005X38 and M5 [188]. This region of deletion is at least 2 Mb centromeric to the *RB1* tumor suppressor gene and the leukemia-associated genes 1 and 2, each of which is located at 13q14. At this time, however, no strong candidate gene has been identified for the deletion region at 13q14 [188]. The C13 gene at 13q12–14, identified by differential display, showed epithelial expression, allelic imbalance, and down-regulation in advanced cancer [189], but it is outside the deletion region [188].

13q21 region. In Hyytinen's LOH assay, a distinct region of LOH in a 7-cM DNA segment involving markers D13S269 and D13S162 at 13q21 was identified [178]. The deletion region defined by a large number of CGH analyses also centers at 13q21 [8].

Consistent with CGH findings, hemizygous deletion of 13q21 was detected in 9% of 147 tumor specimens analyzed by duplex PCR assay, and the common region of deletion was defined to a 3.3 Mb interval between D13S152 and D13S162 in the prostate cancer cell line/xenograft LNCaP and PC-82 [175]. Based on a physical map of YAC/BAC/STS/EST, the minimal region of deletion was further defined to about 700 Kb between markers D13S791 and D13S166 by LOH analysis of 42 primary prostate cancers, 8 prostate cancer cell lines/xenografts, and 49 cell lines from cancers of the breast, ovary, endometrium, and cervix, using 18 microsatellite markers encompassing the deletion region [190]. A gene that is homologous to the *WT1* tumor suppressor gene, *AP-2rep (KLF12)*, was mapped in this region but it was expressed at low levels in both normal and neoplastic cells of the prostate, and did not have any mutations in a group of aggressive prostate cancers and cell lines/xenografts. In another study, the region of deletion was further narrowed to 200 kb, and the transcription factor KLF5 was identified as the only complete gene in the minimal region of deletion [15]. Both duplex PCR assay and real time PCR assay demonstrated frequent hemizygous deletion and loss of expression for KLF5 in prostate cancer, suggesting a tumor suppressive role of KLF5 in prostate cancer. No mutations of the gene were detected and promoter methylation is not responsible for the loss of KLF5 expression, suggesting that haploinsufficiency is the primary mechanism of KLF5 inactivation [15].

Chromosome 15q

There are 6 CGH studies showing deletion of 15q22–q23 in 33 of 160 (21%) tumors analyzed [16,17,31–33,36], but no detailed deletion mapping studies have been reported.

Chromosome 16q

Whereas deletion of 16q22 was detected in 2 cases so far by cytogenetic analysis of prostate cancer [28,55], it has been frequent in CGH studies, occurring in 105 of 339 (31%) cases examined [16–18,33,35,36,49,51,57]. Most cases involved 16q13–23 in the regions of deletion. In a group of 20 metastases, deletion of 16q occurred in 11 (55%) of them [33].

Using the RFLP technique, 16q was one of the two chromosomal regions showing frequent LOH (30%)

[126]. Additional studies with the same method confirmed this finding [52,84], and the rate of LOH was up to 60% in one study [84]. Frequent LOH at 16q has also been detected by PCR-based microsatellite analyses [53].

LOH at 16q was associated with aneuploidy and higher Gleason score [53,191]. Allelic losses on 16q were observed more frequently in the cancer-death cases than in early-stage tumor cases [191–195] as well as in higher stage tumors than in lower stage ones [196].

Analysis of 48 prostate cancer specimens suggested 3 distinct commonly deleted regions, that is, 16q22.1–q22.3, 16q23.2-q24.1, and 16q24.3–qter [192]. The estimated sizes of deletions were 4.7 cM (16q22.1–q22.3), 17.2 cM (16q23.2–q24.1), and 8.4 cM (16q24.3–qter). Three similar regions of LOH were detected in another analysis of 59 tumors with 14 microsatellite markers [194], in which the region at 16q22 is close to the E-cadherin gene. In this study, the regions were limited by markers D16S347 and D16S318 at 16q22.1, D16S518 and D16S507 at 16q23.2, and D16S520 and D16S413 at 16q24.3. Two common regions of LOH at 16q were defined in another study [197], one at 16q21–22 (50%) and another at 16q24.2–qter (56%). Based on these studies, the common LOH region appears to be at 16q23–q24, between loci D16S504 and D16S422 [191,193,195,198]. Furthermore, linkage analysis identified a prostate cancer susceptibility locus at 16q23 in an interval of 12.4 cM between markers D16S515 and D16S3040 [199]. In a follow-up study, 51 prostate cancers were investigated for LOH using the markers showing linkage. Interestingly, the minimal region of deletion was located between markers D16S3096 and D16S516 at 16q23.2, which flank 1 cM DNA within the linked region [200]. A positive association between LOH at this locus and family history was noticed.

The FISH method has also been used to determine the location of 16q deletion [201]. Hybridization of region-specific cosmid contig probes to interphase prostatic carcinoma nuclei detected physical deletion of 16q23.1–q24 in 15 of 30 tumors (50%), which is consistent with LOH data. In some FISH studies, deletion at 16q was also detected in PIN lesions, and metastases showed more frequent deletion than primary tumors [100,202]. LOH at 16q in PIN lesions has also been detected by microsatellite analysis [54,196]. Consistent with LOH at 16q in the PIN lesions, deletion of 16q was detected in an E1A-immortalized nonneoplastic prostatic epithelial cell line by both cytogenetic and FISH analyses [203].

Homozygous deletion at 16q has been found in multiple cancers including prostate cancer, and a 700 kb physical map spanning the region has been constructed [204], which spans the common fragile site FRA16D. Based on another physical map spanning markers D16S518 and D16S516 [205], a gene named *WWOX* was identified. Although located in the region of homozygous deletion, this gene did not show mutation or expression loss in cancer cells.

The E-cadherin gene is located at 16q22, and LOH at this locus has been detected in some prostate cancers. Reduced E-cadherin expression also occurs in prostate cancer [191]. However, the LOH at 16q22 does not center at this locus [191,206], and no mutations for this gene were detected in two studies [191,192], suggesting that E-cadherin is not the target gene of deletion at 16q. No other strong candidate genes for 16q deletion have been reported.

Chromosome 17p

Deletion of 17p is a relatively frequent event in cytogenetic studies, as 4 cases with deletions at 17p11–p12 have been reported in 3 studies [45,159,207]. In CGH studies, deletion of 17p is also frequent, occurring in 25 of 89 cases (28%) [16,31–33]. One LOH study demonstrated LOH at 17p in prostate cancer [54], but no detailed deletion mapping studies are available. Chromosomal banding study also detected a deletion at 17p11 in a PIN lesion [45].

Chromosome 17q21

Deletion of 17q has been detected in one cytogenetic study [45] but not in any of the CGH studies. Examination of aneusomies in 20 prostate cancers by FISH showed frequent loss of chromosome 17 [160]. LOH analysis also showed frequent deletion of 17q in prostate cancer (34% of 42 cases) [69], and the LOH involves the proximal long arm of chromosome 17 [208]. Using several markers spanning 17q12–q21, including one marker from BRCA1, frequent LOH was detected at the BRCA1 locus and the D17S856 locus [209]. Further analysis of this region identified a frequent region of deletion between markers D17S776 and D17S855, which is centromeric to BRCA1 at 17q21 [210]. A FISH analysis of 23 prostate cancers, on the other hand, suggested a deletion region distal to the BRCA1 locus [211].

Chromosome 18q

Deletion of 18q, with the common region of deletion at 18q21, is relatively frequent in prostate cancer, as 57 of 305 cases (19%) examined by CGH showed losses [16,18,32,34,36,37,50,51,57]. FISH analysis also detected frequent deletion of 18q in prostate cancer [100], and the region of deletion involves 18q21–qter. Loss of 18q was more frequent in higher stage tumors [50,212], and was associated with ane-uploidy [53]. Loss of 18q in PIN lesions has also been detected by both FISH analysis [100] and a CGH study [37].

Using the RFLP method, LOH at 18q was detected in 3 of 7 informative cases (43%) [84]. Microsatellite analysis also detected frequent LOH at 18q [53,54,68,69], and the region of deletion was suggested to be between the centromere and the D18S19 locus [68]. Detailed deletion mapping using 46 prostate cancers and 32 microsatellite markers identified a distinct commonly deleted region within a 5-cM interval in 18q21.1 [212]. Another analysis of 32 tumors with 17 markers suggested two regions of LOH, one between markers D18S1119 and D18S64, and the other between D18S848 and D18S58 at a more distal locus [213]. The most frequent deletion involves markers D18S51 and D18S858 at 18q21, likely in an interval of 0.58 cM flanked by D18S41 and D18S381 [214]. The Smad2 gene resides within this region at 18q21, but it was not mutated in 6 prostate cell lines examined. In addition, both the DCC and DPC4/Smad4 tumor suppressor genes are centromeric to this region of deletion, and no mutations were detected for these genes in prostate cancer [212], suggesting other gene(s) as the target gene of 18q deletion in prostate cancer. Introduction of chromosome 18 into the DU145 and TSU-Pr1 prostate cancer cell lines led to a longer population doubling time, retarded growth in soft agar, and slowed tumor growth in nude mice, providing functional evidence for a tumor suppressor gene on 18q in prostate cancer [215].

Chromosomes 19q, 20q, 21q, and Y

Based on CGH studies, loss of several other chromosomes is relatively frequent in prostate cancer, including 19q13 (26/73 or 36%) [16,17,35], 22q (26/93 or 28%) [16,17,32], 20q (17/102 or 17%) [17,31,32], and Y (30/174 or 17%) [18,31,36,37,51]. Except for 21q whose LOH was frequent in one study [54], no other deletion mapping studies are available for these chromosomal regions.

Conclusions

(1) Chromosomal deletion appears to be the earliest as well as the most common genetic alteration in prostate cancer. (2) The pattern of chromosomal deletions is similar between sporadic tumors and tumors from familial prostate cancer. (3) In addition to the two-hit theory of tumor suppressor inactivation, hemizygous deletion-induced expression loss, that is, haploinsufficiency, may be a more common mechanism for the loss of tumor suppressor function. (4) Strong candidates have been identified for the target genes of deletion for several chromosomal regions, including NKX3.1 at 8p21, PTEN at 10q23.3, p27/Kip1 at 12p13, and KLF5 at 13q21.

Key unanswered questions

The role of tumor suppressor haploinsufficiency in human prostatic carcinogenesis needs to be determined. The application of gene targeting technique in mice has demonstrated roles of haploinsufficiency at NKX3.1, PTEN, and p27/Kip1 in prostate cancer. Such techniques, including gene knockout in nonneoplastic human epithelial cells, appear to provide the most convincing evidence in defining a tumor suppressor gene.

Second, the target genes remain to be identified for the majority of the chromosomal regions deleted in prostate cancer. Among more than a dozen frequently deleted chromosomal regions, strong candidate genes are available for only four of them. The emerging haploinsufficiency hypothesis of tumor suppressor inactivation should facilitate the identification of target genes for the deleted chromosomal regions in prostate cancer.

For some of the strong candidate genes identified thus far, especially NKX3.1 and KLF5, studies need to be carried out to examine how these genes act in a cell and what molecular pathways are involved.

References

1. Vogelstein B, Kinzler KW: The genetic basis of human cancer. McGraw-Hill, New York, 1998, p 731
2. Harris H, Miller OJ, Klein G, Worst P, Tachibana T: Suppression of malignancy by cell fusion. Nature 223: 363–368, 1969

3. Knudson AG, Jr: Mutation and cancer: Statistical study of retinoblastoma. Proc Natl Acad Sci USA 68: 820–823, 1971

4. Knudson AG, Jr: Genetics and etiology of human cancer. Adv Hum Genet 8: 1–66, 1977

5. Cavenee WK, Dryja TP, Phillips RA, Benedict WF, Godbout R, Gallie BL, Murphree AL, Strong LC, White RL: Expression of recessive alleles by chromosomal mechanisms in retinoblastoma. Nature 305: 779–784, 1983

6. Mitelman F, Johansson B, Mertens F: Mitelman database of chromosome aberrations in cancer. http://cgap.nci.nih.gov/Chromosomes/Mitelman2001

7. Deng GR, Lu Y, Zlotnikov G, Thor AD, Smith HS: Loss of heterozygosity in normal tissue adjacent to breast carcinomas. Science 274: 2057–2059, 1996

8. Knuutila S, Aalto Y, Autio K, Bjorkqvist AM, El-Rifai W, Hemmer S, Huhta T, Kettunen E, Kiuru-Kuhlefelt S, Larramendy ML, Lushnikova T, Monni O, Pere H, Tapper J, Tarkkanen M, Varis A, Wasenius VM, Wolf M, Zhu Y: DNA copy number losses in human neoplasms. Am J Pathol 155: 683–694, 1999

9. Song WJ, Sullivan MG, Legare RD, Hutchings S, Tan X, Kufrin D, Ratajczak J, Resende IC, Haworth C, Hock R, Loh M, Felix C, Roy DC, Busque L, Kurnit D, Willman C, Gewirtz AM, Speck NA, Bushweller JH, Li FP, Gardiner K, Poncz M, Maris JM, Gilliland DG: Haploinsufficiency of CBFA2 causes familial thrombocytopenia with propensity to develop acute myelogenous leukaemia. Nat Genet 23: 166–175, 1999

10. Sisodiya SM, Free SL, Williamson KA, Mitchell TN, Willis C, Stevens JM, Kendall BE, Shorvon SD, Hanson IM, Moore AT, van Heyningen V: PAX6 haploinsufficiency causes cerebral malformation and olfactory dysfunction in humans. Nat Genet 28: 214–216, 2001

11. Bay JO, Uhrhammer N, Pernin D, Presneau N, Tchirkov A, Vuillaume M, Laplace V, Grancho M, Verrelle P, Hall J, Bignon YJ: High incidence of cancer in a family segregating a mutation of the ATM gene: Possible role of ATM heterozygosity in cancer. Hum Mutat 14: 485–492, 1999

12. Di Cristofano A, Pesce B, Cordon-Cardo C, Pandolfi PP: Pten is essential for embryonic development and tumour suppression. Nat Genet 19: 348–355, 1998

13. Xu X, Brodie SG, Yang X, Im YH, Parks WT, Chen L, Zhou YX, Weinstein M, Kim SJ, Deng CX: Haploid loss of the tumor suppressor Smad4/Dpc4 initiates gastric polyposis and cancer in mice. Oncogene 19: 1868–1874, 2000

14. Fero ML, Randel E, Gurley KE, Roberts JM, Kemp CJ: The murine gene p27Kip1 is haplo-insufficient for tumour suppression. Nature 396: 177–180, 1998

15. Chen C, Vessella RL, Dong JT: Defining KLF5 as a tumor suppressor gene at 13q21 in human prostate cancer. Cancer Res submitted: 2002

16. Nupponen NN, Kakkola L, Koivisto P, Visakorpi T: Genetic alterations in hormone-refractory recurrent prostate carcinomas. Am J Pathol 153: 141–148, 1998

17. Sattler HP, Rohde V, Bonkhoff H, Zwergel T, Wullich B: Comparative genomic hybridization reveals DNA copy number gains to frequently occur in human prostate cancer. Prostate 39: 79–86, 1999

18. Alers JC, Rochat J, Krijtenburg PJ, Hop WC, Kranse R, Rosenberg C, Tanke HJ, Schroder FH, van Dekken H: Identification of genetic markers for prostatic cancer progression. Lab Invest 80: 931–942, 2000

19. Arps S, Rodewald A, Schmalenberger B, Carl P, Bressel M, Kastendieck H: Cytogenetic survey of 32 cancers of the prostate. Cancer Genet Cytogenet 66: 93–99, 1993

20. Qi H, Dal Cin P, Van de Voorde W, Elgamal AA, Van Poppel H, Baert L, Van Den Berghe H: del(1)(q12) in adenocarcinomas of the prostate. Cancer Genet Cytogenet 87: 79–81, 1996

21. Carvalho-Salles AB, Mesquita JC, Tajara EH: Deletion (1)(q12) and double minutes in a metastatic adenocarcinoma of the prostate. Cancer Genet Cytogenet 116: 50–53, 2000

22. Smith JR, Freije D, Carpten JD, Gronberg H, Xu J, Isaacs SD, Brownstein MJ, Bova GS, Guo H, Bujnovszky P, Nusskern DR, Damber JE, Bergh A, Emanuelsson M, Kallioniemi OP, Walker-Daniels J, Bailey-Wilson JE, Beaty TH, Meyers DA, Walsh PC, Collins FS, Trent JM, Isaacs WB: Major susceptibility locus for prostate cancer on chromosome 1 suggested by a genome-wide search. Science 274: 1371–1374, 1996

23. Berthon P, Valeri A, Cohen-Akenine A, Drelon E, Paiss T, Wohr G, Latil A, Millasseau P, Mellah I, Cohen N, Blanche H, Bellane-Chantelot C, Demenais F, Teillac P, Le Duc A, de Petriconi R, Hautmann R, Chumakov I, Bachner L, Maitland NJ, Lidereau R, Vogel W, Fournier G, Mangin P, Cohen D, Cussenot O: Predisposing gene for early-onset prostate cancer, localized on chromosome 1q42.2–43. Am J Hum Genet 62: 1416–1424, 1998

24. Gibbs M, Stanford JL, McIndoe RA, Jarvik GP, Kolb S, Goode EL, Chakrabarti L, Schuster EF, Buckley VA, Miller EL, Brandzel S, Li S, Hood L, Ostrander EA: Evidence for a rare prostate cancer-susceptibility locus at chromosome 1p36. Am J Hum Genet 64: 776–787, 1999

25. Xu J, Zheng SL, Chang B, Smith JR, Carpten JD, Stine OC, Isaacs SD, Wiley KE, Henning L, Ewing C, Bujnovszky P, Bleeker ER, Walsh PC, Trent JM, Meyers DA, Isaacs WB: Linkage of prostate cancer susceptibility loci to chromosome 1. Hum Genet 108: 335–345, 2001

26. Ahman AK, Jonsson BA, Damber JE, Bergh A, Emanuelsson M, Gronberg H: Low frequency of allelic imbalance at the prostate cancer susceptibility loci HPC1 and 1p36 in Swedish men with hereditary prostate cancer. Genes Chromosomes Cancer 29: 292–296, 2000

27. Dunsmuir WD, Edwards SM, Lakhani SR, Young M, Corbishley C, Kirby RS, Dearnaley DP, Dowe A, Ardern-Jones A, Kelly J, Eeles RA: Allelic imbalance in familial and sporadic prostate cancer at the putative human prostate cancer susceptibility locus, HPC1. CRC/BPG UK Familial Prostate Cancer Study Collaborators. Cancer Research Campaign/British Prostate Group. Br J Cancer 78: 1430–1433, 1998

28. Webb HD, Hawkins AL, Griffin CA: Cytogenetic abnormalities are frequent in uncultured prostate cancer cells. Cancer Genet Cytogenet 88: 126–132, 1996

29. Azar GM, DiPillo F, Gogineni SK, Godec CJ, Verma RS: Highly complex chromosomal aberrations in bone marrow of a patient with metastatic prostate neoplasm. Cancer Genet Cytogenet 99: 116–120, 1997

30. Kochera M, Depinet TW, Pretlow TP, Giaconia JM, Edgehouse NL, Pretlow TG, Schwartz S: Molecular cytogenetic studies of a serially transplanted primary prostatic carcinoma xenograft (CWR22) and four relapsed tumors. Prostate 41: 7–11, 1999

31. Cher ML, MacGrogan D, Bookstein R, Brown JA, Jenkins RB, Jensen RH: Comparative genomic hybridization, allelic imbalance, and fluorescence in situ hybridization on chromosome 8 in prostate cancer. Genes Chromosomes Cancer 11: 153–162, 1994

32. Visakorpi T, Kallioniemi AH, Syvanen AC, Hyytinen ER, Karhu R, Tammela T, Isola JJ, Kallioniemi OP: Genetic changes in primary and recurrent prostate cancer by comparative genomic hybridization. Cancer Res 55: 342–347, 1995

33. Cher ML, Bova GS, Moore DH, Small EJ, Carroll PR, Pin SS, Epstein JI, Isaacs WB, Jensen RH: Genetic alterations in untreated metastases and androgen-independent prostate cancer detected by comparative genomic hybridization and allelotyping. Cancer Res 56: 3091–3102, 1996

34. Koivisto PA, Schleutker J, Helin H, Ehren-van Eekelen C, Kallioniemi OP, Trapman J: Androgen receptor gene alterations and chromosomal gains and losses in prostate carcinomas appearing during finasteride treatment for benign prostatic hyperplasia. Clin Cancer Res 5: 3578–3582, 1999

35. Verhagen PC, Zhu XL, Rohr LR, Cannon-Albright LA, Tavtigian SV, Skolnick MH, Brothman AR: Microdissection, DOP-PCR, and comparative genomic hybridization of paraffin-embedded familial prostate cancers. Cancer Genet Cytogenet 122: 43–48, 2000

36. El Gedaily A, Bubendorf L, Willi N, Fu W, Richter J, Moch H, Mihatsch MJ, Sauter G, Gasser TC: Discovery of new DNA amplification loci in prostate cancer by comparative genomic hybridization. Prostate 46: 184–190, 2001

37. Zitzelsberger H, Engert D, Walch A, Kulka U, Aubele M, Hofler H, Bauchinger M, Werner M: Chromosomal changes during development and progression of prostate adenocarcinomas. Br J Cancer 84: 202–208, 2001

38. Elliott K, Sakamuro D, Basu A, Du W, Wunner W, Staller P, Gaubatz S, Zhang H, Prochownik E, Eilers M, Prendergast GC: Bin1 functionally interacts with Myc and inhibits cell proliferation via multiple mechanisms. Oncogene 18: 3564–3573, 1999

39. Sakamuro D, Prendergast GC: New Myc-interacting proteins: A second Myc network emerges. Oncogene 18: 2942–2954, 1999

40. Ge K, Minhas F, Duhadaway J, Mao NC, Wilson D, Buccafusca R, Sakamuro D, Nelson P, Malkowicz SB, Tomaszewski J, Prendergast GC: Loss of heterozygosity and tumor suppressor activity of Bin1 in prostate carcinoma. Int J Cancer 86: 155–161, 2000

41. Lerman MI, Minna JD: The 630-kb lung cancer homozygous deletion region on human chromosome 3p21.3: Identification and evaluation of the resident candidate tumor suppressor genes. The International Lung Cancer Chromosome 3p21.3 Tumor Suppressor Gene Consortium. Cancer Res 60: 6116–6133, 2000

42. Gibas Z, Pontes JE, Sandberg AA: Chromosome rearrangements in a metastatic adenocarcinoma of the prostate. Cancer Genet Cytogenet 16: 301–304, 1985

43. Johnson BE, Whang-Peng J, Naylor SL, Zbar B, Brauch H, Lee E, Simmons A, Russell E, Nam MH, Gazdar AF: Retention of chromosome 3 in extrapulmonary small cell cancer shown by molecular and cytogenetic studies. J Natl Cancer Inst 81: 1223–1228, 1989

44. Jones E, Zhu XL, Rohr LR, Stephenson RA, Brothman AR: Aneusomy of chromosomes 7 and 17 detected by FISH in prostate cancer and the effects of selection in vitro. Genes Chromosomes Cancer 11: 163–170, 1994

45. Teixeira MR, Waehre H, Lothe RA, Stenwig AE, Pandis N, Giercksky KE, Heim S: High frequency of clonal chromosome abnormalities in prostatic neoplasms sampled by prostatectomy or ultrasound-guided needle biopsy. Genes Chromosomes Cancer 28: 211–219, 2000

46. Dahiya R, McCarville J, Hu W, Lee C, Chui RM, Kaur G, Deng G: Chromosome 3p24–26 and 3p22–12 loss in human prostatic adenocarcinoma. Int J Cancer 71: 20–25, 1997

47. Pan Y, Lui WO, Nupponen N, Larsson C, Ji, Visakorpi T, Bergerheim US, Kytola S: 5q11, 8p11, and 10q22 are recurrent chromosomal breakpoints in prostate cancer cell lines. Genes Chromosomes Cancer 30: 187–195, 2001

48. Ozen M, Navone NM, Multani AS, Troncoso P, Logothetis CJ, Chung LW, von Eschenbach AC, Pathak S: Structural alterations of chromosome 5 in twelve human prostate cancer cell lines. Cancer Genet Cytogenet 106: 105–109, 1998

49. Cher ML, Lewis PE, Banerjee M, Hurley PM, Sakr W, Grignon DJ, Powell IJ: A similar pattern of chromosomal alterations in prostate cancers from African-Americans and Caucasian Americans. Clin Cancer Res 4: 1273–1278, 1998

50. Fu W, Bubendorf L, Willi N, Moch H, Mihatsch MJ, Sauter G, Gasser TC: Genetic changes in clinically organ-confined prostate cancer by comparative genomic hybridization. Urology 56: 880–885, 2000

51. Alers JC, Krijtenburg PJ, Vis AN, Hoedemaeker RF, Wildhagen MF, Hop WC, van Der Kwast TT, Schroder FH, Tanke HJ, van Dekken H: Molecular cytogenetic analysis of prostatic adenocarcinomas from screening studies: Early cancers may contain aggressive genetic features. Am J Pathol 158: 399–406, 2001

52. Phillips SM, Morton DG, Lee SJ, Wallace DM, Neoptolemos JP: Loss of heterozygosity of the retinoblastoma and adenomatous polyposis susceptibility gene loci and in chromosomes 10p, 10q and 16q in human prostate cancer. Br J Urol 73: 390–395, 1994

53. Cunningham JM, Shan A, Wick MJ, McDonnell SK, Schaid DJ, Tester DJ, Qian J, Takahashi S, Jenkins RB, Bostwick DG, Thibodeau SN: Allelic imbalance and microsatellite instability in prostatic adenocarcinoma. Cancer Res 56: 4475–4482, 1996

54. Saric T, Brkanac Z, Troyer DA, Padalecki SS, Sarosdy M, Williams K, Abadesco L, Leach RJ, O'Connell P: Genetic pattern of prostate cancer progression. Int J Cancer 81: 219–224, 1999

55. Zitzelsberger H, Szucs S, Robens E, Weier HU, Hofler H, Bauchinger M: Combined cytogenetic and molecular genetic analyses of fifty-nine untreated human prostate carcinomas. Cancer Genet Cytogenet 90: 37–44, 1996

56. Pittman S, Russell PJ, Jelbart ME, Wass J, Raghavan D: Flow cytometric and karyotypic analysis of a primary small cell carcinoma of the prostate: A xenografted cell line. Cancer Genet Cytogenet 26: 165–169, 1987

57. Joos S, Bergerheim USR, Pan Y, Matsuyama H, Bentz M, Dumanoir S, Lichter P: Mapping of chromosomal gains and losses in prostate cancer by comparative genomic hybridization. Genes Chromosomes Cancer 14: 267–276, 1995

58. Rokman A, Koivisto PA, Matikainen MP, Kuukasjarvi T, Poutiainen M, Helin HJ, Karhu R, Kallioniemi OP, Schleutker J: Genetic changes in familial prostate cancer by comparative genomic hybridization. Prostate 46: 233–239, 2001

59. Cooney KA, Wetzel JC, Consolino CM, Wojno KJ: Identification and characterization of proximal 6q deletions in prostate cancer. Cancer Res 56: 4150–4153, 1996

60. Srikantan V, Sesterhenn IA, Davis L, Hankins GR, Avallone FA, Livezey JR, Connelly R, Mostofi FK, McLeod DG, Moul JW, Chandrasekharappa SC, Srivastava S: Allelic loss on chromosome 6Q in primary prostate cancer. Int J Cancer 84: 331–335, 1999

61. Hyytinen ER, Saduut R, Chen C, Paull L, Koivisto PA, Vessella RL, Frierson HF, Dong JT: Defining the region(s) of deletion at 6q16–q22 in human prostate cancer. Genes Chromosomes Cancer in press: 2002

62. Atkin NB, Baker MC: Chromosome study of five cancers of the prostate. Hum Genet 70: 359–364, 1985

63. Lundgren R, Kristoffersson U, Heim S, Mandahl N, Mitelman F: Multiple structural chromosome rearrangements, including del(7q) and del(10q), in an adenocarcinoma of the prostate. Cancer Genet Cytogenet 35: 103–108, 1988

64. Lundgren R, Mandahl N, Heim S, Limon J, Henrikson H, Mitelman F: Cytogenetic analysis of 57 primary prostatic adenocarcinomas. Genes Chromosomes Cancer 4: 16–24, 1992

65. Milasin J, Micic S: Double minute chromosomes in an invasive adenocarcinoma of the prostate. Cancer Genet Cytogenet 72: 157–159, 1994

66. Bandyk MG, Zhao L, Troncoso P, Pisters LL, Palmer JL, von Eschenbach AC, Chung LW, Liang JC: Trisomy 7: A potential cytogenetic marker of human prostate cancer progression. Genes Chromosomes Cancer 9: 19–27, 1994

67. Wang R-Y, Troncoso P, Palmer JL, El-Naggar AK, Liang JC: Trisomy 7 by dual-color fluorescence *in situ* hybridization: A potential biological marker for prostate cancer progression. Clin Cancer Res 2: 1553–1558, 1996

68. Latil A, Baron JC, Cussenot O, Fournier G, Soussi T, Boccon-Gibod L, Le Duc A, Rouesse J, Lidereau R: Genetic alterations in localized prostate cancer: Identification of a common region of deletion on chromosome arm 18q. Genes Chromosomes Cancer 11: 119–125, 1994

69. Latil A, Fournier G, Cussenot O, Lidereau R: Differential chromosome allelic imbalance in the progression of human prostate cancer. J Urol 156: 2079–2083, 1996

70. Zenklusen JC, Thompson JC, Troncoso P, Kagan J, Conti CJ: Loss of heterozygosity in human primary prostate carcinomas: A possible tumor suppressor gene at 7q31.1. Cancer Res 54: 6370–6373, 1994

71. Latil A, Cussenot O, Fournier G, Baron JC, Lidereau R: Loss of heterozygosity at 7q31 is a frequent and early event in prostate cancer. Clin Cancer Res 1: 1385–1389, 1995

72. Takahashi S, Shan AL, Ritland SR, Delacey KA, Bostwick DG, Lieber MM, Thibodeau SN, Jenkins RB: Frequent loss of heterozygosity at 7q31.1 in primary prostate cancer is associated with tumor aggressiveness and progression. Cancer Res 55: 4114–4119, 1995

73. Matturri L, Biondo B, Cazzullo A, Montanari E, Radice F, Timossi R, Turconi P, Lavezzi AM: Detection of trisomy 7 with fluorescence *in situ* hybridization and its correlation with DNA content and proliferating cell nuclear antigen-positivity in prostate cancer. Am J Clin Oncol 21: 253–257, 1998

74. Cui J, Deubler DA, Rohr LR, Zhu XL, Maxwell TM, Changus JE, Brothman AR: Chromosome 7 abnormalities in prostate cancer detected by dual-color fluorescence *in situ* hybridization. Cancer Genet Cytogenet 107: 51–60, 1998

75. Jenkins RB, Qian J, Lee HK, Huang H, Hirasawa K, Bostwick DG, Proffitt J, Wilber K, Lieber MM, Liu W, Smith DI: A molecular cytogenetic analysis of 7q31 in prostate cancer. Cancer Res 58: 759–766, 1998

76. Ogata T, Ayusawa D, Namba M, Takahashi E, Oshimura M, Oishi M: Chromosome 7 suppresses indefinite division of nontumorigenic immortalized human fibroblast cell lines KMST-6 and SUSM-1. Mol Cell Biol 13: 6036–6043, 1993

77. Zenklusen JC, Oshimura M, Barrett JC, Conti CJ: Inhibition of tumorigenicity of a murine squamous cell carcinoma (SCC) cell line by a putative tumor suppressor gene on human chromosome 7. Oncogene 9: 2817–2825, 1994

78. Zenklusen JC, Hodges LC, LaCava M, Green ED, Conti CJ: Definitive functional evidence for a tumor suppressor gene on human chromosome 7q31.1 neighboring the Fra7G site. Oncogene 19: 1729–1733, 2000

79. Zenklusen JC, Weintraub LA, Green ED: Construction of a high-resolution physical map of the ~1-Mb region of human chromosome 7q31.1–31.2 harboring a putative tumor suppressor gene. Neoplasia 1: 16–22, 1999

80. Zenklusen JC, Conti CJ, Green ED: Mutational and functional analyses reveal that ST7 is a highly conserved tumor-suppressor gene on human chromosome 7q31. Nat Genet 27: 392–398, 2001

81. Macoska JA, Trybus TM, Sakr WA, Wolf MC, Benson PD, Powell IJ, Pontes JE: Fluorescence *in situ* hybridization analysis of 8p allelic loss and chromosome 8 instability in human prostate cancer. Cancer Res 54: 3824–3830, 1994

82. Huang SF, Xiao S, Renshaw AA, Loughlin KR, Hudson TJ, Fletcher JA: Fluorescence *in situ* hybridization evaluation

of chromosome deletion patterns in prostate cancer. Am J Pathol 149: 1565–1573, 1996

83. Oba K, Matsuyama H, Yoshihiro S, Kishi F, Takahashi M, Tsukamoto M, Kinjo M, Sagiyama K, Naito K: Two putative tumor suppressor genes on chromosome arm 8p may play different roles in prostate cancer. Cancer Genet Cytogenet 124: 20–26, 2001

84. Kunimi K, Bergerheim US, Larsson IL, Ekman P, Collins VP: Allelotyping of human prostatic adenocarcinoma. Genomics 11: 530–536, 1991

85. Bova GS, Carter BS, Bussemakers MJ, Emi M, Fujiwara Y, Kyprianou N, Jacobs SC, Robinson JC, Epstein JI, Walsh PC, Isaacs WB: Homozygous deletion and frequent allelic loss of chromosome 8p22 loci in human prostate cancer. Cancer Res 53: 3869–3873, 1993

86. MacGrogan D, Levy A, Bostwick D, Wagner M, Wells D, Bookstein R: Loss of chromosome arm 8p loci in prostate cancer: Mapping by quantitative allelic imbalance. Genes Chromosomes Cancer 10: 151–159, 1994

87. Sakr WA, Macoska JA, Benson P, Grignon DJ, Wolman SR, Pontes JE, Crissman JD: Allelic loss in locally metastatic, multisampled prostate cancer. Cancer Res 54: 3273–3277, 1994

88. Trapman J, Sleddens HF, van der Weiden MM, Dinjens WN, Konig JJ, Schroder FH, Faber PW, Bosman FT: Loss of heterozygosity of chromosome 8 microsatellite loci implicates a candidate tumor suppressor gene between the loci D8S87 and D8S133 in human prostate cancer. Cancer Res 54: 6061–6064, 1994

89. Macoska JA, Trybus TM, Benson PD, Sakr WA, Grignon DJ, Wojno KD, Pietruk T, Powell IJ: Evidence for three tumor suppressor gene loci on chromosome 8p in human prostate cancer. Cancer Res 55: 5390–5395, 1995

90. Crundwell MC, Chughtai S, Knowles M, Takle L, Luscombe M, Neoptolemos JP, Morton DG, Phillips SM: Allelic loss on chromosomes 8p, 22q and 18q (DCC) in human prostate cancer. Int J Cancer 69: 295–300, 1996

91. Washburn JG, Wojno KJ, Dey J, Powell IJ, Macoska JA: 8pter-p23 deletion is associated with racial differences in prostate cancer outcome. Clin Cancer Res 6: 4647–4652, 2000

92. Kagan J, Stein J, Babaian RJ, Joe YS, Pisters LL, Glassman AB, von Eschenbach AC, Troncoso P: Homozygous deletions at 8p22 and 8p21 in prostate cancer implicate these regions as the sites for candidate tumor suppressor genes. Oncogene 11: 2121–2126, 1995

93. Emmert-Buck MR, Vocke CD, Pozzatti RO, Duray PH, Jennings SB, Florence CD, Zhuang Z, Bostwick DG, Liotta LA, Linehan WM: Allelic loss on chromosome 8p12-21 in microdissected prostatic intraepithelial neoplasia. Cancer Res 55: 2959–2962, 1995

94. Suzuki H, Emi M, Komiya A, Fujiwara Y, Yatani R, Nakamura Y, Shimazaki J: Localization of a tumor suppressor gene associated with progression of human prostate cancer within a 1.2 Mb region of 8p22-p21.3. Genes Chromosomes Cancer 13: 168–174, 1995

95. Vocke CD, Pozzatti RO, Bostwick DG, Florence CD, Jennings SB, Strup SE, Duray PH, Liotta LA, Emmert-Buck MR, Linehan WM: Analysis of 99 microdissected prostate carcinomas reveals a high frequency of allelic loss on chromosome 8p12-21. Cancer Res 56: 2411–2416, 1996

96. Perinchery G, Bukurov N, Nakajima K, Chang J, Hooda M, Oh BR, Dahiya R: Loss of two new loci on chromosome 8 (8p23 and 8q12-13) in human prostate cancer. Int J Oncol 14: 495–500, 1999

97. Prasad MA, Trybus TM, Wojno KJ, Macoska JA: Homozygous and frequent deletion of proximal 8p sequences in human prostate cancers: Identification of a potential tumor suppressor gene site. Genes Chromosomes Cancer 23: 255–262, 1998

98. Kalapurakal JA, Jacob AN, Kim PY, Najjar DD, Hsieh YC, Ginsberg P, Daskal I, Asbell SO, Kandpal RP: Racial differences in prostate cancer related to loss of heterozygosity on chromosome 8p12-23. Int J Radiat Oncol Biol Phys 45: 835–840, 1999

99. Van Alewijk DC, Van der Weiden MM, Eussen BJ, Van Den Andel-Thijssen LD, Ehren-van Eekelen CC, Konig JJ, van Steenbrugge GJ, Dinjens WN, Trapman J: Identification of a homozygous deletion at 8p12–21 in a human prostate cancer xenograft. Genes Chromosomes Cancer 24: 119–126, 1999

100. Qian J, Jenkins RB, Bostwick DG: Genetic and chromosomal alterations in prostatic intraepithelial neoplasia and carcinoma detected by fluorescence *in situ* hybridization. Eur Urol 35: 479–483, 1999

101. Haggman MJ, Wojno KJ, Pearsall CP, Macoska JA: Allelic loss of 8p sequences in prostatic intraepithelial neoplasia and carcinoma. Urology 50: 643–647, 1997

102. Matsuyama H, Pan Y, Oba K, Yoshihiro S, Matsuda K, Hagarth L, Kudren D, Naito K, Bergerheim US, Ekman P: Deletions on chromosome 8p22 may predict disease progression as well as pathological staging in prostate cancer. Clin Cancer Res 7: 3139–3143, 2001

103. Bova GS, MacGrogan D, Levy A, Pin SS, Bookstein R, Isaacs WB: Physical mapping of chromosome 8p22 markers and their homozygous deletion in a metastatic prostate cancer. Genomics 35: 46–54, 1996

104. MacGrogan D, Levy A, Bova GS, Isaacs WB, Bookstein R: Structure and methylation-associated silencing of a gene within a homozygously deleted region of human chromosome band 8p22. Genomics 35: 55–65, 1996

105. Bookstein R, Bova GS, MacGrogan D, Levy A, Isaacs WB: Tumour-suppressor genes in prostatic oncogenesis: a positional approach. British J Urol 79: 28–36, 1997

106. Ishii H, Baffa R, Numata SI, Murakumo Y, Rattan S, Inoue H, Mori M, Fidanza V, Alder H, Croce CM: The FEZ1 gene at chromosome 8p22 encodes a leucine-zipper protein, and its expression is altered in multiple human tumors. Proc Natl Acad Sci USA 96: 3928–3933, 1999

107. Cabeza-Arvelaiz Y, Sepulveda JL, Lebovitz RM, Thompson TC, Chinault AC: Functional identification of LZTS1 as a candidate prostate tumor suppressor gene on human chromosome 8p22. Oncogene 20: 4169–4179, 2001

108. Ishii H, Vecchione A, Murakumo Y, Baldassarre G, Numata S, Trapasso F, Alder H, Baffa R,

54

Croce CM: FEZ1/LZTS1 gene at 8p22 suppresses cancer cell growth and regulates mitosis. Proc Natl Acad Sci USA 14: early edition, 2001

109. Lutchman M, Pack S, Kim AC, Azim A, Emmert-Buck M, van Huffel C, Zhuang Z, Chishti AH: Loss of heterozygosity on 8p in prostate cancer implicates a role for dematin in tumor progression. Cancer Genet Cytogenet 115: 65–69, 1999

110. He WW, Sciavolino PJ, Wing J, Augustus M, Hudson P, Meissner PS, Curtis RT, Shell BK, Bostwick DG, Tindall DJ, Gelmann EP, Abate-Shen C, Carter KC: A novel human prostate-specific, androgen-regulated homeobox gene (NKX3.1) that maps to 8p21, a region frequently deleted in prostate cancer. Genomics 43: 69–77, 1997

111. Bhatia-Gaur R, Donjacour AA, Sciavolino PJ, Kim M, Desai N, Young P, Norton CR, Gridley T, Cardiff RD, Cunha GR, Abate-Shen C, Shen MM: Roles for Nkx3.1 in prostate development and cancer. Genes Dev 13: 966–977, 1999

112. Tanaka M, Komuro I, Inagaki H, Jenkins NA, Copeland NG, Izumo S: Nkx3.1, a murine homolog of Ddrosophila bagpipe, regulates epithelial ductal branching and proliferation of the prostate and palatine glands. Dev Dyn 219: 248–260, 2000

113. Voeller HJ, Augustus M, Madike V, Bova GS, Carter KC, Gelmann EP: Coding region of NKX3.1, a prostate-specific homeobox gene on 8p21, is not mutated in human prostate cancers. Cancer Res 57: 4455–4459, 1997

114. Xu LL, Srikantan V, Sesterhenn IA, Augustus M, Dean R, Moul JW, Carter KC, Srivastava S: Expression profile of an androgen regulated prostate specific homeobox gene NKX3.1 in primary prostate cancer. J Urol 163: 972–979, 2000

115. Ornstein DK, Cinquanta M, Weiler S, Duray PH, Emmert-Buck MR, Vocke CD, Linehan WM, Ferretti JA: Expression studies and mutational analysis of the androgen regulated homeobox gene NKX3.1 in benign and malignant prostate epithelium. J Urol 165: 1329–1334, 2001

116. Bowen C, Bubendorf L, Voeller HJ, Slack R, Willi N, Sauter G, Gasser TC, Koivisto P, Lack EE, Kononen J, Kallioniemi OP, Gelmann EP: Loss of NKX3.1 expression in human prostate cancers correlates with tumor progression. Cancer Res 60: 6111–6115, 2000

117. Perinchery G, Bukurov N, Nakajima K, Chang J, Li LC, Dahiya R: High frequency of deletion on chromosome 9p21 may harbor several tumor-suppressor genes in human prostate cancer. Int J Cancer 83: 610–614, 1999

118. Cairns P, Polascik TJ, Eby Y, Tokino K, Califano J, Merlo A, Mao L, Herath J, Jenkins R, Westra W, et al.: Frequency of homozygous deletion at p16/CDKN2 in primary human tumours. Nat Genet 11: 210–212, 1995

119. Tamimi Y, Bringuier PP, Smit F, Vanbokhoven A, Debruyne F, Schalken JA: p16 mutations/deletions are not frequent events in prostate cancer. Brit J Cancer 74: 120–122, 1996

120. Chen W, Weghorst CM, Sabourin CL, Wang Y, Wang D, Bostwick DG, Stoner GD: Absence of p16/MTS1 gene mutations in human prostate cancer. Carcinogenesis 17: 2603–2607, 1996

121. Jarrard DF, Bova GS, Ewing CM, Pin SS, Nguyen SH, Baylin SB, Cairns P, Sidransky D, Herman JG, Isaacs WB: Deletional, mutational, and methylation analyses of CDKN2 (p16/MTS1) in primary and metastatic prostate cancer. Genes Chromosomes Cancer 19: 90–96, 1997

122. Trybus TM, Burgess AC, Wojno KJ, Glover TW, Macoska JA: Distinct areas of allelic loss on chromosomal regions 10p and 10q in human prostate cancer. Cancer Res 56: 2263–2267, 1996

123. Ittmann M: Allelic loss on chromosome 10 in prostate adenocarcinoma. Cancer Res 56: 2143–2147, 1996

124. Komiya A, Suzuki H, Ueda T, Yatani R, Emi M, Shimazaki J: Allelic losses at loci on chromosome 10 are associated with metastasis and progression of human prostate cancer. Genes Chromosomes Cancer 17: 245–253, 1996

125. Brothman AR, Lesho LJ, Somers KD, Schellhammer PF, Ladaga LE, Merchant DJ: Cytogenetic analysis of four primary prostatic cultures. Cancer Genet Cytogenet 37: 241–248, 1989

126. Carter BS, Ewing CM, Ward WS, Treiger BF, Aalders TW, Schalken JA, Epstein JI, Isaacs WB: Allelic loss of chromosomes 16q and 10q in human prostate cancer. Proc Natl Acad Sci USA 87: 8751–8755, 1990

127. Gray IC, Phillips SM, Lee SJ, Neoptolemos JP, Weissenbach J, Spurr NK: Loss of the chromosomal region 10q23–25 in prostate cancer. Cancer Res 55: 4800–4803, 1995

128. Lacombe L, Orlow I, Reuter VE, Fair WR, Dalbagni G, Zhang ZF, Cordoncardo C: Microsatellite instability and deletion analysis of chromosome 10 in human prostate cancer. Int J Cancer 69: 110–113, 1996

129. Li J, Yen C, Liaw D, Podsypanina K, Bose S, Wang SI, Puc J, Miliaresis C, Rodgers L, McCombie R, Bigner SH, Giovanella BC, Ittmann M, Tycko B, Hibshoosh H, Wigler MH, Parsons R: PTEN, a putative protein tyrosine phosphatase gene mutated in human brain, breast, and prostate cancer. Science 275: 1943–1947, 1997

130. Steck PA, Pershouse MA, Jasser SA, Yung WKA, Lin H, Ligon AH, Langford LA, Baumgard ML, Hattier T, Davis T, Frye C, Hu R, Swedlund B, Teng DHF, Tavtigian SV: Identification of a candidate tumour suppressor gene, MMAC1, at chromosome 10q23.3 that is mutated in multiple advanced cancers. Nat Genet 15: 356–362, 1997

131. Srivastava M, Bubendorf L, Srikantan V, Fossom L, Nolan L, Glasman M, Leighton X, Fehrle W, Pittaluga S, Raffeld M, Koivisto P, Willi N, Gasser TC, Kononen J, Sauter G, Kallioniemi OP, Srivastava S, Pollard HB: ANX7, a candidate tumor suppressor gene for prostate cancer. Proc Natl Acad Sci USA 98: 4575–4580, 2001

132. Eagle LR, Yin X, Brothman AR, Williams BJ, Atkin NB, Prochownik EV: Mutation of the MXI1 gene in prostate cancer. Nat Genet 9: 249–252, 1995

133. Taj MM, Tawil RJ, Engstrom LD, Zeng Z, Hwang C, Sanda MG, Wechsler DS: MXI1, a Myc antagonist, suppresses proliferation of DU145 human prostate cells. Prostate 47: 194–204, 2001

134. Kuczyk MA, Serth J, Bokemeyer C, Schwede J, Herrmann R, Machtens S, Grunewald V, Hofner K,

Jonas U: The MXI1 tumor suppressor gene is not mutated in primary prostate cancer. Oncol Rep 5: 213–216, 1998

135. Edwards SM, Dearnaley DP, Ardern-Jones A, Hamoudi RA, Easton DF, Ford D, Shearer R, Dowe A, Eeles RA: No germline mutations in the dimerization domain of MXI1 in prostate cancer clusters. The CRC/BPG UK Familial Prostate Cancer Study Collaborators. Cancer Research Campaign/British Prostate Group. Br J Cancer 76: 992–1000, 1997

136. Li DM, Sun H: TEP1, encoded by a candidate tumor suppressor locus, is a novel protein tyrosine phosphatase regulated by transforming growth factor beta. Cancer Res 57: 2124–2129, 1997

137. Wu X, Senechal K, Neshat MS, Whang YE, Sawyers CL: The PTEN/MMAC1 tumor suppressor phosphatase functions as a negative regulator of the phosphoinositide 3-kinase/Akt pathway. Proc Natl Acad Sci USA 95: 15587–15591, 1998

138. Davies MA, Koul D, Dhesi H, Berman R, McDonnell TJ, McConkey D, Yung WK, Steck PA: Regulation of Akt/PKB activity, cellular growth, and apoptosis in prostate carcinoma cells by MMAC/PTEN. Cancer Res 59: 2551–2556, 1999

139. Persad S, Attwell S, Gray V, Delcommenne M, Troussard A, Sanghera J, Dedhar S: Inhibition of integrin-linked kinase (ILK) suppresses activation of protein kinase B/Akt and induces cell cycle arrest and apoptosis of PTEN-mutant prostate cancer cells. Proc Natl Acad Sci USA 97: 3207–3212, 2000

140. Whang YE, Wu X, Suzuki H, Reiter RE, Tran C, Vessella RL, Said JW, Isaacs WB, Sawyers CL: Inactivation of the tumor suppressor PTEN/MMAC1 in advanced human prostate cancer through loss of expression. Proc Natl Acad Sci USA 95: 5246–5250, 1998

141. Ali IU, Schriml LM, Dean M: Mutational spectra of PTEN/MMAC1 gene: A tumor suppressor with lipid phosphatase activity. J Natl Cancer Inst 91: 1922–1932, 1999

142. McMenamin ME, Soung P, Perera S, Kaplan I, Loda M, Sellers WR: Loss of PTEN expression in paraffin-embedded primary prostate cancer correlates with high Gleason score and advanced stage. Cancer Res 59: 4291–4296, 1999

143. Liaw D, Marsh DJ, Li J, Dahia PLM, Wang SI, Zheng ZM, Bose S, Call KM, Tsou HC, Peacocke M, Eng C, Parsons R: Germline mutations of the PTEN gene in Cowden-disease, an inherited breast and thyroid cancer syndrome. Nat Genet 16: 64–67, 1997

144. Suzuki H, Freije D, Nusskern DR, Okami K, Cairns P, Sidransky D, Isaacs WB, Bova GS: Interfocal heterogeneity of PTEN/MMAC1 gene alterations in multiple metastatic prostate cancer tissues. Cancer Res 58: 204–209, 1998

145. Vlietstra RJ, van Alewijk DC, Hermans KG, van Steenbrugge GJ, Trapman J: Frequent inactivation of PTEN in prostate cancer cell lines and xenografts. Cancer Res 58: 2720–2723, 1998

146. Facher EA, Law JC: PTEN and prostate cancer. J Med Genet 35: 790, 1998

147. Feilotter HE, Nagai MA, Boag AH, Eng C, Mulligan LM: Analysis of PTEN and the 10q23 region in primary prostate carcinomas. Oncogene 16: 1743–1748, 1998

148. Dong JT, Sipe TW, Hyytinen ER, Li CL, Heise C, McClintock DE, Grant CD, Chung LW, Frierson HF, Jr: PTEN/MMAC1 is infrequently mutated in pT2 and pT3 carcinomas of the prostate. Oncogene 17: 1979–1982, 1998

149. Orikasa K, Fukushige S, Hoshi S, Orikasa S, Kondo K, Miyoshi Y, Kubota Y, Horii A: Infrequent genetic alterations of the PTEN gene in Japanese patients with sporadic prostate cancer. J Hum Genet 43: 228–230, 1998

150. Pesche S, Latil A, Muzeau F, Cussenot O, Fournier G, Longy M, Eng C, Lidereau R: PTEN/MMAC1/TEP1 involvement in primary prostate cancers. Oncogene 16: 2879–2883, 1998

151. Cairns P, Okami K, Halachmi S, Halachmi N, Esteller M, Herman JG, Isaacs WB, Bova GS, Sidransky D: Frequent inactivation of PTEN/MMAC1 in primary prostate cancer. Cancer Res 57: 4997–5000, 1997

152. Gray IC, Stewart LM, Phillips SM, Hamilton JA, Gray NE, Watson GJ, Spurr NK, Snary D: Mutation and expression analysis of the putative prostate tumour-suppressor gene PTEN. Br J Cancer 78: 1296–1300, 1998

153. Wang SI, Parsons R, Ittmann M: Homozygous deletion of the PTEN tumor suppressor gene in a subset of prostate adenocarcinomas. Clin Cancer Res 4: 811–815, 1998

154. Cooney KA, Tsou HC, Petty EM, Miesfeldt S, Ping XL, Gruener AC, Peacocke M: Absence of PTEN germ-line mutations in men with a potential inherited predisposition to prostate cancer. Clin Cancer Res 5: 1387–1391, 1999

155. Forrest MS, Edwards SM, Hamoudi RA, Dearnaley DP, Arden-Jones A, Dowe A, Murkin A, Kelly J, Teare MD, Easton DF, Knowles MA, Bishop DT, Eeles RA: No evidence of germline PTEN mutations in familial prostate cancer. J Med Genet 37: 210–212, 2000

156. Dong JT, Li CL, Sipe TW, Frierson HFJ: Mutations of PTEN/MMAC1 in primary prostate cancers from Chinese patients. Clin Cancer Res 7: 304–308, 2001

157. Simpson L, Parsons R: PTEN: Life as a tumor suppressor. Exp Cell Res 264: 29–41, 2001

158. Dahiya R, McCarville J, Lee C, Hu W, Kaur G, Carroll P, Deng G: Deletion of chromosome 11p15, p12, q22, q23-24 loci in human prostate cancer. Int J Cancer 72: 283–288, 1997

159. Molenaar WM, Stoepker ME, de Ruiter AJ, Hoekstra HJ, van den Berg E: Cytogenetic support for primary prostatic cancer in a patient presenting with a soft tissue mass in the leg. Cancer Genet Cytogenet 86: 147–149, 1996

160. Brothman AR, Watson MJ, Zhu XL, Williams BJ, Rohr LR: Evaluation of 20 archival prostate tumor specimens by fluorescence in situ hybridization (FISH). Cancer Genet Cytogenet 75: 40–44, 1994

161. Kibel AS, Schutte M, Kern SE, Isaacs WB, Bova GS: Identification of 12p as a region of frequent deletion in advanced prostate cancer. Cancer Res 58: 5652–5655, 1998

162. Kibel AS, Freije D, Isaacs WB, Bova GS: Deletion mapping at 12p12-13 in metastatic prostate cancer. Genes Chromosomes Cancer 25: 270–276, 1999

163. Kibel AS, Faith DA, Bova GS, Isaacs WB: Loss of heterozygosity at 12p12–13 in primary and metastatic prostate adenocarcinoma. J Urol 164: 192–196, 2000

164. Latil A, Guerard M, Berthon P, Cussenot O: 12p12–13 deletion in prostate tumors and quantitative expression of CDKN1B and ETV6 candidate genes. Genes Chromosomes Cancer 31: 199–200, 2001

165. Cote RJ, Shi Y, Groshen S, Feng AC, Cordon-Cardo C, Skinner D, Lieskovosky G: Association of p27Kip1 levels with recurrence and survival in patients with stage C prostate carcinoma. J Natl Cancer Inst 90: 916–920, 1998

166. Yang RM, Naitoh J, Murphy M, Wang HJ, Phillipson J, deKernion JB, Loda M, Reiter RE: Low p27 expression predicts poor disease-free survival in patients with prostate cancer. J Urol 159: 941–945, 1998

167. Guo Y, Sklar GN, Borkowski A, Kyprianou N: Loss of the cyclin-dependent kinase inhibitor p27(Kip1) protein in human prostate cancer correlates with tumor grade. Clin Cancer Res 3: 2269–2274, 1997

168. Cheville JC, Lloyd RV, Sebo TJ, Cheng L, Erickson L, Bostwick DG, Lohse CM, Wollan P: Expression of p27kip1 in prostatic adenocarcinoma. Mod Pathol 11: 324–328, 1998

169. Macri E, Loda M: Role of p27 in prostate carcinogenesis. Cancer Metastasis Rev 17: 337–344, 1998

170. Di Cristofano A, De Acetis M, Koff A, Cordon-Cardo C, Pandolfi PP: Pten and p27KIP1 cooperate in prostate cancer tumor suppression in the mouse. Nat Genet 27: 222–224, 2001

171. Kibel AS, Christopher M, Faith DA, Bova GS, Goodfellow PJ, Isaacs WB: Methylation and mutational analysis of p27(kip1) in prostate carcinoma. Prostate 48: 248–253, 2001

172. Gibas Z, Becher R, Kawinski E, Horoszewicz J, Sandberg AA: A high-resolution study of chromosome changes in a human prostatic carcinoma cell line (LNCaP). Cancer Genet Cytogenet 11: 399–404, 1984

173. Nupponen NN, Hyytinen ER, Kallioniemi AH, Visakorpi T: Genetic alterations in prostate cancer cell lines detected by comparative genomic hybridization. Cancer Genet Cytogenet 101: 53–57, 1998

174. Melamed J, Einhorn JM, Ittmann MM: Allelic loss on chromosome 13q in human prostate carcinoma. Clin Cancer Res 3: 1867–1872, 1997

175. Dong JT, Chen C, Stultz BG, Isaacs JT, Frierson HF, Jr: Deletion at 13q21 is associated with aggressive prostate cancers. Cancer Res 60: 3880–3883, 2000

176. Afonso A, Emmert-Buck MR, Duray PH, Bostwick DG, Linehan WM, Vocke CD: Loss of heterozygosity on chromosome 13 is associated with advanced stage prostate cancer. J Urol 162: 922–926, 1999

177. Dong JT, Boyd JC, Frierson HF, Jr: Loss of heterozygosity at 13q14 and 13q21 in high grade, high stage prostate cancer. Prostate 49: 166–171, 2001

178. Hyytinen ER, Frierson HF, Boyd JC, Chung LWK, Dong JT: Three distinct regions of allelic loss at 13q14, 13q21–22, and 13q33 in prostate cancer. Genes Chromosomes Cancer 25: 108–114, 1999

179. Cooney KA, Wetzel JC, Merajver SD, Macoska JA, Singleton TP, Wojno KJ: Distinct regions of allelic loss on 13q in prostate cancer. Cancer Res 56: 1142–1145, 1996

180. Ittmann MM, Wieczorek R: Alterations of the retinoblastoma gene in clinically localized, stage B prostate adenocarcinomas. Hum Pathol 27: 28–34, 1996

181. Latil A, Cussenot O, Fournier G, Lidereau R: The BRCA2 gene is not relevant to sporadic prostate tumours. Int J Cancer 66: 282–283, 1996

182. Bookstein R, Rio P, Madreperla SA, Hong F, Allred C, Grizzle WE, Lee WH: Promoter deletion and loss of retinoblastoma gene expression in human prostate carcinoma. Proc Natl Acad Sci USA 87: 7762–7766, 1990

183. Brooks JD, Bova GS, Isaacs WB: Allelic loss of the retinoblastoma gene in primary human prostatic adenocarcinomas. Prostate 26: 35–39, 1995

184. Kubota Y, Fujinami K, Uemura H, Dobashi Y, Miyamoto H, Iwasaki Y, Kitamura H, Shuin T: Retinoblastoma gene mutations in primary human prostate cancer. Prostate 27: 314–320, 1995

185. Li CD, Larsson C, Futreal A, Lancaster J, Phelan C, Aspenblad U, Sundelin B, Liu Y, Ekman P, Auer G, Bergerheim USR: Identification of two distinct deleted regions on chromosome 13 in prostate cancer. Oncogene 16: 481–487, 1998

186. Ueda T, Emi M, Suzuki H, Komiya A, Akakura K, Ichikawa T, Watanabe M, Shiraishi T, Masai M, Igarashi T, Ito H: Identification of a 1-cM region of common deletion on 13q14 associated with human prostate cancer. Genes Chromosomes Cancer 24: 183–190, 1999

187. Yin Z, Spitz MR, Babaian RJ, Strom SS, Troncoso P, Kagan J: Limiting the location of a putative human prostate cancer tumor suppressor gene at chromosome 13q14.3. Oncogene 18: 7576–7583, 1999

188. Chen C, Frierson HF, Jr, Haggerty PF, Theodorescu D, Gregory CW, Dong JT: An 800 kb region of deletion at 13q14 in human prostate and other carcinomas. Genomics 77: 135–144, 2001

189. Schmidt U, Fiedler U, Pilarsky CP, Ehlers W, Fussel S, Haase M, Faller G, Sauter G, Wirth MP: Identification of a novel gene on chromosome 13 between BRCA-2 and RB-1. Prostate 47: 91–101, 2001

190. Chen C, Brabham WW, Stultz BG, Frierson HFJ, Barrett JC, Sawyers CL, Isaacs JT, Dong JT: Defining a common region of deletion at 13q21 in human cancers. Genes Chromosomes Cancer 31: 333–344, 2001

191. Li C, Berx G, Larsson C, Auer G, Aspenblad U, Pan Y, Sundelin B, Ekman P, Nordenskjold M, van Roy F, Bergerheim US: Distinct deleted regions on chromosome segment 16q23–24 associated with metastases in prostate cancer. Genes Chromosomes Cancer 24: 175–182, 1999

192. Suzuki H, Komiya A, Emi M, Kuramochi H, Shiraishi T, Yatani R, Shimazaki J: Three distinct commonly deleted regions of chromosome arm 16q in human primary and metastatic prostate cancers. Genes Chromosomes Cancer 17: 225–233, 1996

193. Elo JP, Harkonen P, Kyllonen AP, Lukkarinen O, Poutanen M, Vihko R, Vihko P: Loss of heterozygosity at 16q24.1–q24.2 is significantly associated with metastatic

and aggressive behavior of prostate cancer. Cancer Res 57: 3356–3359, 1997

194. Latil A, Cussenot O, Fournier G, Driouch K, Lidereau R: Loss of heterozygosity at chromosome 16q in prostate adenocarcinoma: Identification of three independent regions. Cancer Res 57: 1058–1062, 1997

195. Elo JP, Harkonen P, Kyllonen AP, Lukkarinen O, Vihko P: Three independently deleted regions at chromosome arm 16q in human prostate cancer: Allelic loss at 16q24.1–q24.2 is associated with aggressive behaviour of the disease, recurrent growth, poor differentiation of the tumour and poor prognosis for the patient. Br J Cancer 79: 156–160, 1999

196. Strup SE, Pozzatti RO, Florence CD, Emmert-Buck MR, Duray PH, Liotta LA, Bostwick DG, Linehan WM, Vocke CD: Chromosome 16 allelic loss analysis of a large set of microdissected prostate carcinomas. J Urol 162: 590–594, 1999

197. Godfrey TE, Cher ML, Chhabra V, Jensen RH: Allelic imbalance mapping of chromosome 16 shows two regions of common deletion in prostate adenocarcinoma. Cancer Genet Cytogenet 98: 36–42, 1997

198. Osman I, Scher H, Dalbagni G, Reuter V, Zhang ZF, Cordon-Cardo C: Chromosome 16 in primary prostate cancer: A microsatellite analysis. Int J Cancer 71: 580–584, 1997

199. Suarez BK, Lin J, Burmester JK, Broman KW, Weber JL, Banerjee TK, Goddard KA, Witte JS, Elston RC, Catalona WJ: A genome screen of multiplex sibships with prostate cancer. Am J Hum Genet 66: 933–944, 2000

200. Paris PL, Witte JS, Kupelian PA, Levin H, Klein EA, Catalona WJ, Casey G: Identification and fine mapping of a region showing a high frequency of allelic imbalance on chromosome 16q23.2 that corresponds to a prostate cancer susceptibility locus. Cancer Res 60: 3645–3649, 2000

201. Cher ML, Ito T, Weidner N, Carroll PR, Jensen RH: Mapping of regions of physical deletion on chromosome 16q in prostate cancer cells by fluorescence *in situ* hybridization (FISH). J Urol 153: 249–254, 1995

202. Pan Y, Matsuyama H, Wang N, Yoshihiro S, Haggarth L, Li C, Tribukait B, Ekman P, Bergerheim US: Chromosome 16q24 deletion and decreased E-cadherin expression: Possible association with metastatic potential in prostate cancer. Prostate 36: 31–38, 1998

203. Chin RK, Hawkins AL, Isaacs WB, Griffin CA: E1A transformed normal human prostate epithelial cells contain a 16q deletion. Cancer Genet Cytogenet 103: 155–163, 1998

204. Paige AJ, Taylor KJ, Stewart A, Sgouros JG, Gabra H, Sellar GC, Smyth JF, Porteous DJ, Watson JE: A 700-kb physical map of a region of 16q23.2 homozygously deleted in multiple cancers and spanning the common fragile site FRA16D. Cancer Res 60: 1690–1697, 2000

205. Bednarek AK, Laflin KJ, Daniel RL, Liao Q, Hawkins KA, Aldaz CM: WWOX, a novel WW domain-containing protein mapping to human chromosome 16q23.3–24.1, a region frequently affected in breast cancer. Cancer Res 60: 2140–2145, 2000

206. Murant SJ, Rolley N, Phillips SM, Stower M, Maitland NJ: Allelic imbalance within the E-cadherin gene is an infrequent event in prostate carcinogenesis. Genes Chromosomes Cancer 27: 104–109, 2000

207. Konig JJ, Teubel W, Kamst E, Romijn JC, Schroder FH, Hagemeijer A: Cytogenetic analysis of 39 prostate carcinomas and evaluation of short-term tissue culture techniques. Cancer Genet Cytogenet 101: 116–122, 1998

208. Brothman AR, Steele MR, Williams BJ, Jones E, Odelberg S, Albertsen HM, Jorde LB, Rohr LR, Stephenson RA: Loss of chromosome 17 loci in prostate cancer detected by polymerase chain reaction quantitation of allelic markers. Genes Chromosomes Cancer 13: 278–284, 1995

209. Gao X, Zacharek A, Salkowski A, Grignon DJ, Sakr W, Porter AT, Honn KV: Loss of heterozygosity of the BRCA1 and other loci on chromosome 17q in human prostate cancer. Cancer Res 55: 1002–1005, 1995

210. Gao X, Zacharek A, Grignon DJ, Sakr W, Powell IJ, Porter AT, Honn KV: Localization of potential tumor suppressor loci to a <2 Mb region on chromosome 17q in human prostate cancer. Oncogene 11: 1241–1247, 1995

211. Williams BJ, Jones E, Zhu XL, Steele MR, Stephenson RA, Rohr LR, Brothman AR: Evidence for a tumor suppressor gene distal to BRCA1 in prostate cancer. J Urol 155: 720–725, 1996

212. Ueda T, Komiya A, Emi M, Suzuki H, Shiraishi T, Yatani R, Masai M, Yasuda K, Ito H: Allelic losses on 18q21 are associated with progression and metastasis in human prostate cancer. Genes Chromosomes Cancer 20: 140–147, 1997

213. Padalecki SS, Troyer DA, Hansen MF, Saric T, Schneider BG, O'Connell P, Leach RJ: Identification of two distinct regions of allelic imbalance on chromosome 18Q in metastatic prostate cancer. Int J Cancer 85: 654–658, 2000

214. Yin Z, Babaian RJ, Troncoso P, Strom SS, Spitz MR, Caudell JJ, Stein JD, Kagan J: Limiting the location of putative human prostate cancer tumor suppressor genes on chromosome 18q. Oncogene 20: 2273–2280, 2001

215. Padalecki SS, Johnson-Pais TL, Killary AM, Leach RJ: Chromosome 18 suppresses the tumorigenicity of prostate cancer cells. Genes Chromosomes Cancer 30: 221–229, 2001

216. Brothman AR, Peehl DM, Patel AM, McNeal JE: Frequency and pattern of karyotypic abnormalities in human prostate cancer. Cancer Res 50: 3795–3803, 1990

217. Limon J, Lundgren R, Elfving P, Heim S, Kristoffersson U, Mandahl N, Mitelman F: Double minutes in two primary adenocarcinomas of the prostate. Cancer Genet Cytogenet 39: 191–194, 1989

Address for offprints: Jin-Tang Dong, Department of Pathology, University of Virginia Health System, Box 800214, Charlottesville, Virginia 22908, USA; *Fax:* 434-924 9206; *e-mail:* jdong@virginia.edu

Role of eicosanoids in prostate cancer progression

Daotai Nie[1], Mingxin Che[2], David Grignon[2], Keqin Tang[1] and Kenneth V. Honn[1,2]
[1]*Department of Radiation Oncology*, [2]*Department of Pathology Wayne State University School of Medicine and Karmanos Cancer Institute, Detroit, MI, USA*

Key words: eicosanoid, cyclooxygenase, lipoxygenase, tumor metastasis, apoptosis

Abstract

Metabolism of arachidonic acid through cyclooxygenase, lipoxygenase, or P450 epoxygenase pathways leads to the formation of various bioactive eicosanoids. In this review, we discuss alterations in expression pattern of eicosanoid-generating enzymes found during prostate tumor progression and expound upon their involvement in tumor cell proliferation, apoptosis, motility, and tumor angiogenesis. The expression of cyclooxygenase-2, 12-lipoxygenase, and 15-lipoxygenase-l are up-regulated during prostate cancer progression. It has been demonstrated that inhibitors of cyclooxygenase-2, 5-lipoxygenase and 12-lipoxygenase cause tumor cell apoptosis, reduce tumor cell motility and invasiveness, or decrease tumor angiogenesis and growth. The eicosanoid product of 12-lipoxygenase, 12(S)-hydroeicosatetraenoic acid, is found to activate Erkl/2 kinases in LNCaP cells and PKCα in rat prostate AT2.1 tumor cells. Overexpression of 12-lipoxygenase and 15-lipoxygenase-l in prostate cancer cells stimulate prostate tumor angiogenesis and growth, suggesting a facilitative role for 12-lipoxygenase and 15-lipoxygenase-l in prostate tumor progression. The expression of 15-lipoxygenase-2 is found frequently to be lost during the initiation and progression of prostate tumors. 15(S)-hydroxyeicosatetraenoic acid, the product of 15-lipoxygenase-2, inhibits proliferation and causes apoptosis in human prostate cancer cells, suggesting an inhibitory role for 15-lipoxygenase-2 in prostate tumor progression. The regulation of prostate cancer progression by eicosanoids, in either positive or negative ways, provides an exciting possibility for management of this disease.

I. Introduction

Cancer of prostate (CaP) is one of most common cancers in US males. With an aging population and more sophisticated screening, new cases of CaP have steadily risen in the past two decades. Progression of prostate cancer to a more invasive and metastatic stage contributes to deterioration of life quality and mortality. It remains unknown what genetic, physiologic, or environmental factors lead to the invasion and metastasis of prostate tumor cells to distant organs such as bone. A number of epidemiologic studies suggest that high consumption of fat, especially red meat, is a risk factor for prostate cancer [1]. Arachidonic acid and its precursor, linoleic acid, are major ingredients in animal fats and many vegetable oils. At the cellular level, mobilization and subsequent metabolism of arachidonic acid by enzymes such as cyclooxygenase (COX) and lipoxygenase (LOX) generate a group of lipids, termed as eicosanoids, which have potent and diverse biological activities. Eicosanoids have been implicated in a variety of human diseases such as inflammation, fever, arthritis, and cancer. For example, eicosanoids have been shown to play important roles in regulating tumor initiation, progression, and metastasis. In this review, we attempt to provide an overview of eicosanoids and discuss their biologic activities in the context of prostate cancer progression and metastasis.

II. Arachidonic acid metabolism: an overview of eicosanoids

Arachidonic acid is mobilized by phospholipase A_2 (PLA_2) from cellular membrane glycerolipid pools in response to many stimuli such as cytokines, growth

M.L. Cher, K.V. Honn and A. Raz (eds.), Prostate Cancer: New Horizons in Research and Treatment, 59–70.
© 2002 *Kluwer Academic Publishers.*

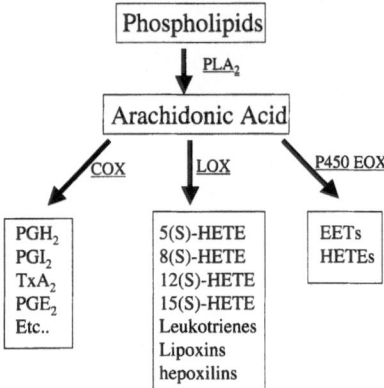

Figure 1. Arachidonic acid metabolism and eicosanoid biosynthesis. Arachidonic acid is mobilized from cellular membrane phospholipids by PLA_2. Arachidonic acid released can be oxidized by COX-1 and COX-2 to form various prostanglandins, prostacyclin, or thromboxane; by various LOXs to form 5(S)-, 8(S)-, 12(S)-, and 15(S)-HETE, leukotrienes, lipoxins, and hepoxilins; or by p450 EOX to form EETs and HETEs.

factors, and hormones. Arachidonic acid released can be oxidized by COX, LOX, or P450 epoxygenase (EOX) to form a variety of eicosanoids as shown in Figure 1. The COX enzymes catalyze a key step in the conversion of arachidonate to an endoperoxide precursor, PGH_2, for formation of prostanglandins, prostacyclin, or thromboxane. Prostaglandins play critical roles in numerous biologic processes, including the regulation of immune function, kidney development, reproductive biology, and gastrointestinal integrity.

Another important arm of arachidonic acid metabolism to form bioactive eicosanoids is the LOX pathway. Arachidonate metabolism by LOXs leads to the formation of regioisomeric *cis/trans* conjugated hydroxyeicosatetraenoic acids (HETEs), leukotrienes, lipoxins, and hepoxilins. There are a number of members in the lipoxygenase family including 5-, 8-, 12-, and 15-lipoxygenases whose main products are 5(S)-, 8(S)-, 12(S)-, and 15(S)-HETE, respectively. Among them, 12(S)-HETE, has a plethora of biological activities including stimulating tumor cell adhesion, invasion, and metastasis.

In the P450 epoxygenase pathway, arachidonic acid is converted into EETs and HETEs. There are few studies regarding the potential role of eicosanoids generated from P450 epoxygenase pathway in tumor biology. Therefore, this review focuses on COX and LOX arms of arachdonic acid metabolism in the context of prostate tumor biology.

III. Role of COX in prostate cancer progression

A. *Up-regulation of COX-2 expression in human prostate cancer*

Cyclooxygenase has two isoforms which differ mainly in their pattern of expression. COX-1 is widely expressed in most tissues, whereas COX-2 expression is usually absent but readily inducible by numerous stimuli such as TNFα, phorbol ester, and many oncogenes. Aberrant or increased expression of COX-2 has been implicated in the pathogenesis of many diseases. In cancer, COX-2 has been found up-regulated in pancreatic cancer, lung, colon, and head and neck cancer.

In prostate cancer, there are several reports describing an increase in COX-2 expression in tumor tissues when compared to normal epithelial tissues or cells. Using reverse transcription-PCR (RT-PCR), Gupta et al. [2] assessed COX-2 expression in 12 samples of pair-matched benign and cancer tissues obtained from the same prostate cancer patient and found that the mean levels of COX-2 mRNA were 3.4-fold higher in prostate cancer tissue compared with the paired benign tissue. The increased COX-2 expression in prostate tumor tissues is further confirmed by immunoblot analysis in 10 of 12 samples examined [2]. The increased expression of COX-2 in prostate cancer was also reported by Lee et al. [3], in which they found an increase in COX-2 expression in 15 out of 18 (83%) prostate cancer samples whereas it was detected in only 22% (4 of 18) of paired benign tissues. Yoshimura et al. [4] examined the expression of both COX-1 and COX-2 in 28 prostate carcinoma (CaP) patients, 8 benign prostatic hyperplasia (BPH) patients, 1 prostatic intraepithelial neoplasia (PIN) patient, and 8 specimens of normal prostate tissue. They found a very weak expression of COX-1 and marked expression of immunoreactive COX-2 in tumor cells, in comparison to a very weak expression of both isoforms in all cases of BPH and in the NP tissues. The extent and intensity of immunoreactive COX-2 polypeptides in tumor cells was statistically much greater than those of cells from BPH. By RT-PCR analysis, enhanced expression of COX-2, but not COX-1, was observed in CaP tissue [4].

Kirschenbaum et al. [5] also examined the expression of both COX-1 and COX-2 in 31 specimens of CaP and 10 specimens of BPH. They found that COX-1 was predominantly expressed in the basal epithelium of non-cancerous prostatic tissue (90% positive staining), but not in non-cancerous luminal epithelial cells

(0–10%). Interestingly, the expression of COX-1 in luminal epithelial cells was up-regulated in CaP (63% of CaP specimens). COX-2 was strongly expressed in prostate smooth muscle cells of the prostate. COX-2 was also expressed in the basal epithelial cells (60% BPH, 94% peripheral zone, 75% PIN). Luminal epithelial cells derived from BPH did not express COX-2 whereas those from PIN expressed COX-2 in 86% of samples. In CaP, COX-2 expression was intense and uniform, with 87% of samples demonstrating immunoreactivity [5]. The study suggests that in addition to COX-2, COX-1 expression is up-regulated in prostate cancer.

Uotila et al. [6] examined the expression of COX-1 and COX-2 in 12 cases of prostate cancer specimens, in comparison to 13 cases of normal control prostates. They found that the intensity of COX-2 immunostaining was significantly stronger in prostate cancer cells than in the non-malignant glandular epithelium of the control prostates. COX-2 also was expressed in PIN lesions in control prostates. They did not find significant difference in COX-1 expression between control and cancer prostates [6].

From the above-described studies, it is in consensus that the expression of COX-2 is elevated during initiation of prostate cancer and its subsequent progression to more advanced stages. In contrast, there is no clear consensus regarding the expression of COX-1 in prostate cancer. It is interesting to explore the molecular mechanism by which COX-2 expression is increased in prostate cancer. Clinically, the elevation of COX-2 expression in prostate cancer, if functionally important for tumor progression, may raise an exciting possibility of using selective COX-2 inhibitors as chemotherapeutic agents in those patients who have COX-2 positive tumors.

Subbarayan et al. [7] found normal and malignant prostate cancer cells responded differently to TNFα treatment regarding COX-2 expression. They found different patterns and kinetics of expression for COX-1 and COX-2 among normal cells and tumor cells in response to TNFα. In particular, COX-2 protein levels increased, and the subcellular distribution formed a distinct perinuclear ring in the normal cells at 4 h after TNFα exposure. In cancer cells, the COX-2 protein levels also increased in response to TNFα treatment, but the subcellular distribution was less organized; COX-2 protein appeared diffuse in some cells and accumulated as focal deposits in the cytoplasm of other cells [7]. In addition to TNFα, prostaglandin E_2 (PGE_2) also stimulated COX-2 expression in PC-3 and LNCaP cells [8].

Although TNFα and PGE_2 are found to be part of the regulatory circuit controling the expression of COX-2 in prostate cancer cells, its relevance with the observed up-regulation of COX-2 in prostate cancer is unknown. With various reports finding an increased expression of COX-2 in prostate tumor tissues, there is certainly need to further study the molecular mechanism by which COX-2 expression is increased in human prostate cancer cells.

B. Induction of apoptosis by COX inhibitors

Under some extracellular cues, cells may commit themselves to programmed cell death, termed apoptosis. Some cells become tumorigenic when they become resistant to apoptosis. Induction of apoptosis in tumor cells, therefore, is a promising approach for inhibition of tumor growth. Liu et al. [9] found that NS398, a specific inhibitor of COX-2, could induce apoptosis in LNCaP cells at concentration of $100\,\mu M$ in a time- and dose-dependent fashion. The induction of apoptosis was associated with a down-regulation in bcl-2 protein expression and with many apoptotic morphologic features such as chromatin condensation and chromosomal DNA fragmentation. In contrast, NS398 treatment had no effect on either cell viability or nuclear function and morphology in human fetal prostate fibroblasts [9]. The study suggests a possible functional role of COX-2 in tumor cell resistance to apoptosis. However, caution should be exercised in correlating inhibition of COX-2 with the induction of apoptosis by NS398. Since NS398 inhibits COX-2 with IC_{50} of $1\,\mu M$, the induction of apoptosis by NS398 at $100\,\mu M$ may not be pharmacologically or physiologically relevant.

Hsu et al. [10] found another COX-2 inhibitor, celecoxib, also induced apoptosis in prostate carcinoma cells by reducing Akt phosphorylation. Interestingly, celecoxib is more potent in apoptosis induction than other COX-2 inhibitors they examined, despite the observation that these inhibitors exhibit similar IC_{50} in COX-2 inhibition. The lack of correlation between induction of apoptosis and COX-2 inhibition suggests that additional factors are involved in induction of apoptosis by COX-2 inhibitors [10]. Lim et al. [11] examined the activities of two metabolites of sulindac (a non-steroidal anti-inflammatory drug), sulindac sulfide and sulindac sulfone (exisulind, Prevatec), and exisulind (CP248) on a series of human prostate epithelial cell lines. They found marked growth inhibition in BPH-1, LNCaP, and PC-3 cell lines with IC_{50} values of about $66\,\mu M$ for sulindac sulfide, $137\,\mu M$ for exisulind, and $64\,nM$ for CP248. The growth inhibition in the presence of these three compounds is accompanied by induction of apoptosis in all of these cell lines. Interestingly, they found that CP248 and exisulind, which do not inhibit COX-1 or COX-2 activities even at concentrations up to $10\,mM$, were very potent in inhibition of tumor cell growth and induction of apoptosis. The results suggest a COX-independent mechanism in apoptosis induction by CP248 and exisulid. They also found that three benign and malignant prostate cell lines, which have various levels of COX-1 and COX-2 expression, showed similar sensitivity to growth inhibition and induction of apoptosis by these three compounds. The results further suggest a COX-independent mechanism in growth inhibition and apoptosis induction in human prostate cancer cells by sulindac derivatives [11].

C. Regulation of tumor angiogenesis and growth by COX

The elaboration of capillary blood vessel ingrowth in tumors is a critical stage during tumor progression. Without angiogenesis, the expansion of tumors is limited to several millimeters duo to the limitation of oxygen and nutrient supply. Tumor cells can produce a number of growth factors and cytokines such as vascular endothelial growth factor (VEGF) and basic fibroblast growth factor (bFGF) to stimulate angiogenesis. It has been shown that COX-2 plays a role in tumor angiogenesis and also in regulation of VEGF expression. Liu et al. [12] examined the relationship between COX-2 expression and VEGF induction in response to cobalt chloride ($CoCl_2$)-simulated hypoxia in three human prostate cancer cell lines. They found, in a human metastatic prostate cancer cell line, that VEGF induction by $CoCl_2$-simulated hypoxia is maintained by a concomitant, persistent induction of COX-2 expression and sustained elevation of PGE_2 synthesis. Their results suggest that COX-2 activity, reflected by PGE_2 production, is involved in hypoxia-induced VEGF expression, and thus, modulates prostatic tumor angiogenesis [12].

Liu et al. [13] further evaluated the *in vivo* efficacy of a COX-2 inhibitor, NS398, in inhibition of the growth of tumors from PC-3 cells in mice. They found that NS398 induced a sustained inhibition of PC-3 tumor cell growth and a regression of existing tumors. Immunohistochemical analysis revealed that NS398 had no effect on proliferation (PCNA), but induced apoptosis (TUNEL) and

decreased MVD (angiogenesis). VEGF expression was also significantly down-regulated in the NS398-treated tumors. The results demonstrate that a selective COX-2 inhibitor suppresses PC-3 cell tumor growth *in vivo* by induction of tumor cell apoptosis and down-regulation of tumor VEGF with decreased angiogenesis [13].

D. Regulation of tumor cell invasion and metastasis by COX products

Eicosanoids modulate the interaction of tumor cells with various host components in cancer metastasis. It has been shown that COX-2 enhanced the metastatic potential of colon cancer cells [14]. Limited study has been conducted on the potential role of COX in regulating the metastatic phenotypes of prostate cancer. Attiga et al. [15] tested the effect of inhibitors of PLA_2, COX, or LOX on the invasion of prostate tumor cells through Matrigel *in vitro* using the Boyden chamber assay and fibroblast-conditioned medium as the chemoattractant. They found that invasion through Matrigel was inhibited by the PLA_2 inhibitor 4-bromophenacyl bromide (4-BPB), the general COX inhibitor ibuprofen (IB), and the highly selective COX-2 inhibitor NS398. Inhibition of cell invasiveness by 4-BPB ($1.0\,\mu M$), IB ($10.0\,\mu M$), and NS398 ($10.0\,\mu M$) was reversed by the addition of PGE_2. PGE_2 alone, however, did not stimulate invasiveness, which suggests that its production is necessary for rendering the cells invasive–permissive but not sufficient for inducing invasiveness [15].

To summarize, it has been shown in many studies that COX-2 expression is up-regulated in prostate cancer. Inhibitors of COX-2 have been found to inhibit proliferation, invasion, and expression of VEGF in various prostate tumor cells. Several COX-2 inhibitors also induce tumor cell apoptosis, although its relevance with the inhibition of COX-2 activities remains to be established. Further studies are needed to confirm the functional role of COX-2 in tumor cell proliferation, survival, expression of VEGF, and invasiveness.

IV. Role of 5-LOX in prostate cancer progression

A. Expression of 5-LOX in human prostate cancer

Gupta et al. [16] studied the expression and activities of 5-LOX in 22 pair-matched benign and malignant tissue samples that were obtained from the same patients with CaP. Using RT-PCR, they found a six-fold increase in the mean level of 5-LOX mRNA in malignant tissue as compared with benign tissue. Westen blot analysis demonstrated that, compared with benign tissue, 5-LOX protein was overexpressed in 16 of 22 samples examined and was 2.6-fold greater ($P < 0.001$) in malignant tissue. Immunohistochemical studies further verified 5-LOX up-regulation in malignant tissue that was not present in benign tissue. The level of 5-HETE, which is a metabolic product of arachidonic acid, was found to be 2.2-fold greater ($P < 0.001$) in malignant tumor tissue compared with benign tissue. The study suggests an increase in 5-LOX expression and activity in human prostate tumors [16]. However, caution should be exercised during interpretation of the data. Foremost, the PCR products were not sequenced to confirm that the bands shown are *bona fide* segments of 5-LOX cDNA. This is especially important in light of a discrepancy between the size of the PCR product shown in the paper (561 bp) and the expected size of PCR product based on the primers used in this study. If a BLAST search is conducted using the sequences of forward and reverse primers provided in the article, a PCR product with a size of 415 bp, rather than 561 bp, is expected from 5-LOX cDNA. The pitfalls in the validity of RT-PCR measurement of 5-LOX mRNA levels compromise the observations. As a final note, Shappell et al. [17] did not observe any 5-LOX activity in prostate tumor tissues, as indicated by the absence of any detectable 5-HETE. Therefore, further studies are needed to confirm the expression of 5-LOX in prostate tumor cells *in vivo* and *in vitro* [17].

B. Induction of apoptosis by 5-LOX inhibitors

In addition to COX inhibitors, inhibitors of 5-LOX or its activating protein (FLAP) have been reported to induce apoptosis in prostate cancer cells. Anderson et al. [18] found that SC41661A and MK886, two selective inhibitors of 5-LOX cellular enzyme activity, reduced PC-3 prostate cell proliferation and with continued culture, induced apoptosis. Interestingly, they observed a difference in the mode of cell death between SC41661A-treated groups and those treated with MK886. SC41661A-treated cells exhibited 'foamy,' vacuolated cytoplasm and mitochondria with disrupted cristae and limiting membranes, while some cells contained numerous polysomes and extended hypertrophic

Golgi and secretory cisternal networks. A proportion of the treated cells detached and the nuclei of these cells were characteristic of type 1 'apoptotic' programmed cell death. MK886, which inhibits 5-LOX activity by inhibiting the 5-LOX activating protein, induced non-necrotic changes largely confined to the cytoplasm, most consistent with type 2 'autophagic' programmed cell death [18].

Ghosh and Meyers [19] further confirmed the ability of MK886 to induce cell apoptosis in prostate cancer cells. They found inhibition of 5-LOX by MK886 completely blocked the biosynthesis of 5-HETE and induced massive and rapid apoptosis in LNCaP and PC-3 cells. Cells treated with MK886 demonstrated mitochondrial permeability transition between 30 and 60 min, externalization of phosphatidylserine within 2 h, and degradation of DNA to nucleosomal subunits beginning within 2–4 h. Exogenous 5-HETE protects these cells from apoptosis induced by 5-LOX inhibitors. Interestingly, they did not observe cell death when cells were treated with inhibitors of 12-LOX, COX, or cytochrome P450 pathways of arachidonic acid metabolism, in contrast to the observations from other research groups [9,19].

While the induction of apoptosis by MK886 is a valid observation, controversy exists as to whether or not the observed apoptosis is due to the inhibition of 5-LOX enzymatic activities. First, the concentration of MK886 required to induce apoptosis is approximately $10 \mu M$, a concentration $4000\times$ greater than the IC_{50} for inhibition of leukotriene biosynthesis in intact leukocytes [20] and $100\times$ higher than that required to affect 5-LOX enzymatic activity [21]. Second, MK886 induces apoptosis in cells that do not express 5-LOX [22] and by a mechanism independent of FLAP inhibition [23]. Third, in addition to inhibition of FLAP, MK886 has been found to inhibit peroxisome-proliferator-activated receptor (PPAR) alpha [24]. Finally, if 5-LOX is the convergent point for apoptosis induction by MK886 and other 5-LOX inhibitors, one would expect cells to die by a similar mechanism. Yet, as described above, two different inhibitors induce apoptosis by morphologically distinct pathways [18]. The fact that two types of 5-LOX inhibitors induce cell death in a drastically different manner argues against the contention that apoptosis is initiated as a result of 5-LOX inhibition. Clearly, more work is needed to further ascertain the functional role of 5-LOX and its eicosanoid products in prostate cancer.

64

V. Role of 12-LOX in human prostate cancer progression

A. Up-regulation of 12-LOX expression during prostate cancer progression

12-LOX was found to be expressed in a variety of tumor cells. The mRNA of 12-LOX has been detected in erythroleukemia, colon carcinoma, epidermoid carcinoma A431 cells, human glioma, and breast cancer cells [25]. Rat and murine tumor cell lines also express 12-LOX [26,27]. The sequence of RT-PCR 12-LOX products from human epidermoid A431 cells was found identical to platelet-type 12-LOX [26]. The product of 12-LOX activity in tumor cells has been identified as predominantly the S enantiomer by chiral HPLC and its structure confirmed by GC-MS spectral analysis [28]. In addition, 12-LOX mRNA has been found to be up-regulated in some cancer cell lines by cytokines such as epidermal growth factor and autocrine motility factor [29].

Gao et al. [30] investigated the expression pattern of 12-LOX at the mRNA level in 122 matching prostate normal and cancerous tissues by quantitative RT-PCR and analyzed for a possible association between 12-LOX expression and histologic grade, pathologic and clinical stage, margin positivity, age, and race [30]. When compared with the matching normal tissues, 46 (38%) of 122 evaluable patients showed elevated levels of 12-LOX mRNA in prostate cancer tissues. A statistically significantly greater number of cases were found to have an elevated level of 12-LOX among T3, high grade, and surgical margin-positive than T2, intermediate, and low grade, and surgical margin-negative prostatic adenocarcinomas. The study suggests that an elevation of 12-LOX mRNA expression occurs more frequently in advanced stage, high-grade prostate cancer [30].

It should be noted that Shappell et al. [17] did not find detectable 12-LOX activity in prostate tumor tissues, as indicated by the absence of 12-HETE. We conducted immunohistochemical analysis of 12-LOX at the protein level in frozen human prostate tumor tissues. (The antibody utilized does not work well with paraffin-embedded tissue, unpublished observations.) As shown in the figure, 12-LOX immunoreactivity appears correlated with tumor grade. Neoplastic glands are weakly, moderately or strongly positive for 12-LOX in low-grade tumor (Figure 2A), intermediate-grade tumor (Figure 2B,C), or in high-grade tumor (Figure 2D) correspondingly.

B. Stimulation of prostate tumor angiogenesis and growth by overexpression of 12-LOX

To study the role of 12-LOX in CaP progression, we generated stable 12-LOX-transfected PC-3 cells. These transfectants constitutively expressed high levels of 12-LOX at both mRNA and protein levels and synthesized larger amount of 12(S)-HETE. In contrast, PC-3 parental cell lines and vector control cells had minimal levels of endogenous 12-LOX expression and activity. In vitro, 12-LOX-transfected PC-3 cells demonstrated a proliferation rate similar to neo controls in the presence of fetal bovine serum. In serum-limited conditions, however, 12-LOX-transfected PC-3 cells had a higher proliferation rate than neo-vector controls or PC-3 parental cells (Nie and Honn, unpublished observations). Following s.c. injection into athymic nude mice, 12-LOX-transfected PC-3 cells formed larger tumors than did the controls. Decreased necrosis and increased vascularization were observed in the tumors from 12-LOX-transfected PC-3 cells. Both endothelial cell migration and Matrigel implantation assays indicate that 12-LOX-transfected PC-3 cells were more angiogenic than their neo controls. These data indicate that 12-LOX stimulates human CaP tumor growth by increasing the angiogenecity of prostate tumor cells [31]. It should be noted that a similar observation regarding the role of 12-LOX in tumor growth and angiogenesis also was observed independently by Connoly and Rose [32] in breast cancer.

C. Regulation of tumor cell invasion and metastasis by 12(S)-HETE

Extensive works have reported that 12(S)-HETE augments tumor cell metastatic potential. 12(S)-HETE is found to modulate several parameters related to the metastatic potential of tumor cells, such as motility [33], secretion of lysosomal proteinases cathepsin B and L [34], expression of integrin receptor αIIbβ3 [35], tumor cell adhesion to endothelium and spreading on subendothelial matrix [36], and lung colonizing ability in vivo [28]. The plethora of activities of 12(S)-HETE is related to its ability to activate multiple cellular signaling events in various tumor cells. Early experiments demonstrated that 12(S)-HETE mimicked the phorbol ester PMA in enhancing tumor cell integrin expression and adhesion [35]. It was also shown that 12(S)-HETE induced a 100% increase in membrane associated PKC activity [37]. It was further demonstrated that the

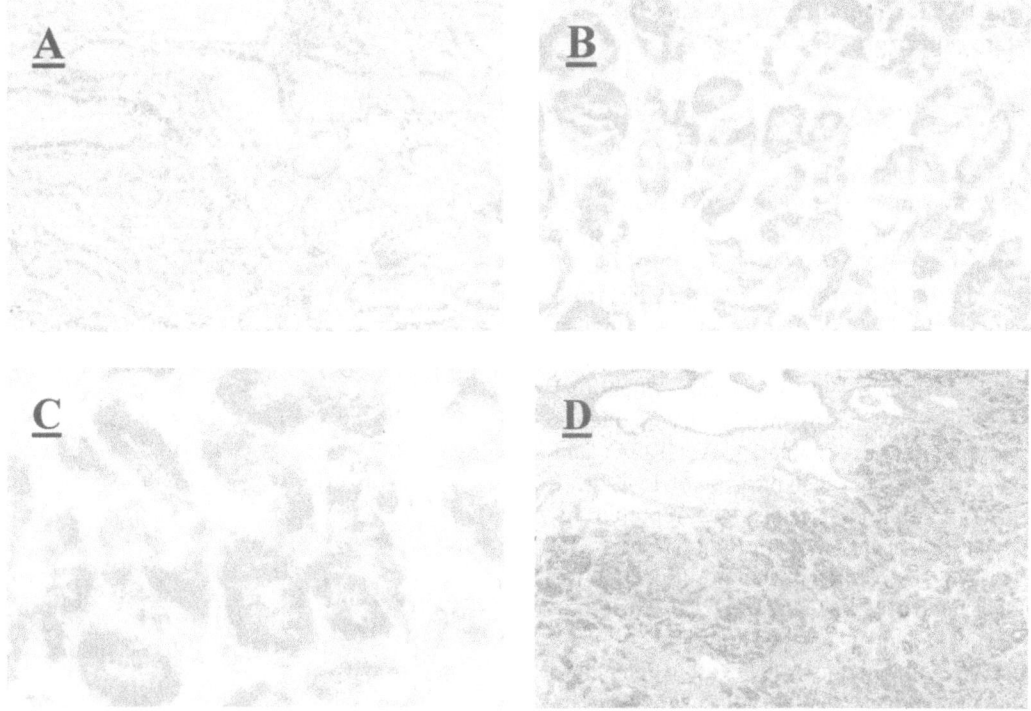

Figure 2. Immunohistochemical staining for 12-LOX in frozen prostate tumor tissues. Sections of frozen specimens were probed with a 12-LOX polyclonal antibody (Oxford Biomedical Research Inc, Oxford, MI). Positive immunoreactivity is indicated by staining with brownish color. A, A low-grade tumor; B,C, intermediate-grade tumor; D, a high-grade tumor.

stimulation of tumor cells with 12(S)-HETE was followed by a rapid accumulation of DAG and IP3 via activating an upstream G protein and PLC [37]. In addition to its activation of the PKC pathway, 12(S)-HETE was shown to activate p42/44 MAP kinase [38] and PI3 kinase [39] in A431 cells.

Liu et al. [40] investigated the effect of 12(S)-HETE on the motility and invasion of low-metastatic rat prostate AT2.1 tumor cells and the effect of 12(S)-HETE activation of specific PKC isoform(s) in these processes. They found that 12(S)-HETE increased the motility and invasion of AT2.1 cells, and this 12(S)-HETE-increased motility and invasion were inhibited by a PKC inhibitor, calphostin C, as well as a Ca^{2+} chelator, bis-(*o*-aminophenoxy)ethane-N,N,N′,N′-tetraacetic acid/tetra(acetoxy-methyl)ester. AT2.1 cells expressed the PKC isoforms alpha and delta, and 12(S)-HETE increased the membrane association of PKC alpha but not delta. Further, the motility and invasion of AT2.1 cells were increased by thymelea toxin, a selective activator of PKC alpha over PKC delta. The study suggests 12(S)-HETE augments the invasiveness of AT2.1 cells via selective activation of PKC alpha [40].

D. Expression of 12-LOX in LNCaP cells and its role in cell survival

It has been shown that arachidonate 12-LOX regulates cell proliferation and apoptosis [41]. In hormone-sensitive LNCaP cells, we found 12-LOX expressed at the protein level (Figure 3A). Baicalein and BHPP, two selective inhibitors of 12-LOX [42], induced apoptosis in LNCaP cells (Figure 3B), suggesting that 12-LOX also participates in the regulatory circuit controling cell proliferation and death, in contrast to the results reported by Ghosh and Meyers [19]. The arachidonate product of 12-LOX, 12(S)-HETE, induced a significant activation of p42/44 MAP kinase in LNCaP cells (Figure 3C). Considering the putative role of p42/44 MAP kinase in cell growth and apoptosis, it is not surprising to observe a regulatory role of 12-LOX and 12(S)-HETE in prostate tumor cell growth and survival.

VI. Role of 15-LOX and their metabolites in prostate cancer progression

A. Expression of 15-LOX in human prostate cancer

The major arachidonate product of 15-LOX is 15(S)-HETE. So far, two isoforms of 15-LOX have been identified, that is, 15-LOX-1 and 15-LOX-2. In addition to the formation of 15(S)-HETE from arachidonic acid, 15-LOX-1 can utilize linoleic acid to form 13-(S)-hydroxyoctadecadienoic acid (13-HODE). 15-LOX-2 is a recently identified lipoxygenase that has approximately 40% sequence identity to the known human 5S-, 12S-, and 15S-lipoxygenases [43]. The expression of 15-LOX-1 in both LNCaP and PC-3 cells was reported by Spindler et al. [44] using Western blot and RT-PCR. They developed a polyclonal antibody specific for 13(S)-HODE and used the antibody to detect this bioactive lipid in human prostate tumor specimens. They observed immunohistochemically detectable 13-HODE in human CaP, whereas adjacent normal tissue showed no immunoreactivity [44].

The expression of 15-LOX-1 was found to be regulated by tumor suppressor p53 [45]. Kelavkar et al. [46] examined the expression of 15-LOX-1 and mutant p53 (mtp53) in human prostatic tissues in 48 prostatectomy specimens of different Gleason grades ($n = 48$) using immunostaining with antibodies specific for 15-LOX-1 and mtp53. They found robust staining in cancer foci for both 15-LOX-1 (36 of 48, 75%) and mtp53 (19 of 48, 39%). Furthermore, the intensities of expression of 15-LOX-1 and mtp53 were correlated positively with each other ($P < 0.001$) and with the degree of malignancy, as assessed by Gleason grading ($P < 0.01$). By immunohistochemistry, 15-LOX-1 was located in secretory cells of peripheral zone glands, prostatic ducts, and seminal vesicles, but not in the basal cell layer or stroma. The study suggests a possible role for 15-LOX-1 expression in influencing the malignant potential and pathobiological behavior of adenocarcinomas [46].

Shappell et al. [17] found a loss of 15-LOX-2 during prostate cancer progression. By immunohistochemistry, they found that 15-LOX-2 is located in secretory cells of peripheral zone glands and large prostatic ducts and somewhat less uniformly in apical cells of transition and central zone glands. 15-LOX-2 was not detected in the basal cell layer, stroma, ejaculatory ducts, seminal vesicles, or transitional epithelium.

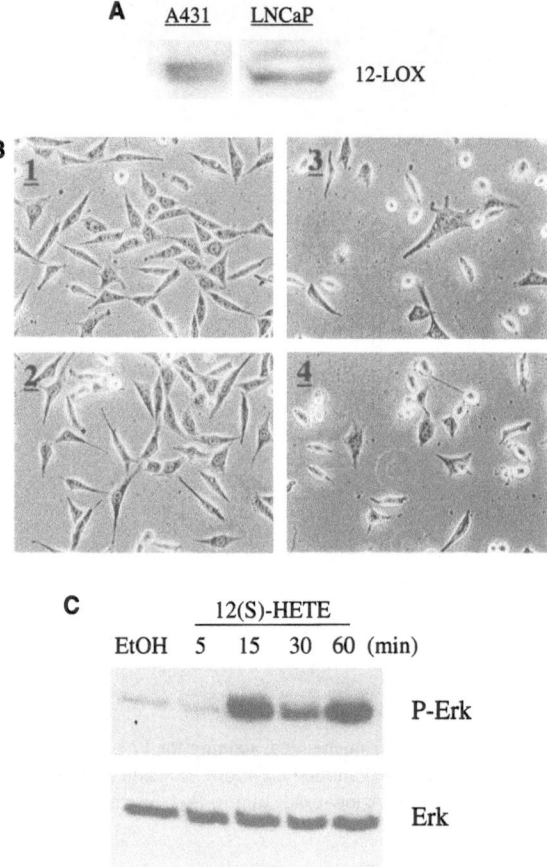

Figure 3. Expression of 12-LOX in LNCaP cells and its involvement in cell survival. A, Immunoblot analysis of 12-LOX expression in LNCaP cells. A431 cells were used as the positive control. The antibody used was obtained from Oxford Biomedical Research Inc (Oxford, MI). B, Inhibition of 12-LOX with baicalein (5 μM) and BHPP (10 μM) induced apoptosis in LNCaP cells. 1, cells treated with DMSO; 2, cells treated with 12(S)-HETE (300 nM); 3, cells treated with baicalein (5 μM); and 4, cells treated with BHPP (10 μM). Pictures were taken 24 h after initiation of treatment. C, Activation of p42/44 MAP kinase by 12(S)-HETE in LNCaP cells. LNCaP cells were serum starved overnight and treated with 300 nM 12(S)-HETE for indicated times. Activation of p42/44 MAP kinase was indicated by the levels of phosphorylated form of Erk (upper panel), in comparison with the level of total Erk protein (bottom panel). As shown, the activation of p42/44 MAP kinase by 12(S)-HETE is evident with 15 min of treatment.

Immunostaining of 18 radical prostatectomy specimens showed a loss of 15-LOX-2 in the majority of prostate adenocarcinomas; 14 of 18 cases showed loss of 15-LOX-2 in >25% of the tumor (mean, 74.9% negative for 15-LOX-2; range, 38.9–100%). Incubation of paired pure benign and pure malignant prostate tissue from the same radical prostatectomies with exogenous arachidonic acid showed that 15-HETE formation was markedly reduced (>90%) or undetectable in incubations of prostate adenocarcinoma [17]. In a subsequent study, they determined the frequency with which 15-LOX-2 immunostaining is reduced in CaP. They found 15-LOX-2 immunostaining was completely absent in 23 of 70 tumors, and negative staining in more than 50% of the tumor in 45 of 70 cases. In contrast, positive stainings for 15-LOX-2 was uniformly observed in secretory cells of benign glands. Further they found the extent of reduced 15-LOX-2 immunostaining correlated with tumor differentiation. In 16 cases with multifocal tumors or different foci of the same tumor with different grades, the higher-grade foci had significantly reduced 15-LOX-2 expression compared with the lower-grade foci. They did not find any significant correlation between 15-LOX-2 immunostaining and serum PSA or pathologic stage. In a subset of 27 cases, 15-LOX-2 expression in high-grade prostatic intraepithelial neoplasia (HGPIN) glands was significantly reduced compared with benign glands. These data show that in contrast to the uniform expression of 15-LOX-2 in differentiated secretory cells of benign prostate, reduced 15-LOX-2 is a common alteration in CaP, and this correlates with tumor cell differentiation [47].

B. Stimulation of tumor growth by overexpression of 15-LOX-1

Kelavkar et al. [48] studied the effect of overexpression of 15-LOX-1 on PC-3 cell growth *in vitro* and *in vivo*. The proliferation rates of PC-3 cells were correlated with the level of 15-LOX-1. The 15-LOX-1 inhibitor, PD146176, demonstrated a dose-dependent inhibition of proliferation. In addition, overexpression of 15-LOX-1 enhanced the ability of PC-3 cells to grow in an anchorage-independent manner in a soft agar colony formation assay. Further, they found that PC-3 cells with high levels of 15-LOX-1 formed tumors more frequently and gave rise to larger tumors than their vector controls or PC-3 parental cells. This study suggests a contributory role for 15-LOX-1 in prostate tumor growth and progression [48].

However, caution should be exercised in correlating 13(S)-HODE with the increased PC-3 proliferation observed in 15-LOX-1 transfected cells. The 13(S)-HODE stimulation of PC-3 cell proliferation observed in this study was achieved at a concentration of $34 \mu M$, a level not likely to be achieved

by endogenous production in tumor cells, even in 15-LOX-1 transfected cells. Therefore, the biological activities of 13(S)-HODE observed at this pharmacological concentration may not be physiologically relevant. In addition, 13(S)-HODE, in nanomolar levels, counteracts on an equimolar basis the biological activities of 12(S)-HETE such as stimulation of tumor cell motility and invasion [37]. Therefore, it is unknown whether 13(S)-HODE, at physiologically relevant levels, stimulates or inhibits tumor cell proliferation. Finally, 13(S)-HODE is a natural ligand for PPARγ [49]. Numerous synthetic and natural ligands for PPARγ have been shown to induce apoptosis in tumor cells. Therefore, it is possible that 13(S)-HODE can induce apoptosis in tumor cells through activation of PPARγ, as shown in the case of 15(S)-HETE as described below.

C. Induction of apoptosis in prostate cancer cells by 15(S)-HETE through PPARγ

It has been shown that some bioactive lipids from the COX pathway (i.e. 15-deoxy-$\Delta^{12,14}$-PGJ_2) and the LOX pathway (i.e. 15-HETE and 13-HODE) are ligands for PPARγ [50]. Many synthetic and natural ligands for PPARγ have been shown as apoptogens for a number of cells [51]. In prostate cancer cells, it has been reported that PPARγ ligands such as troglitazone, inhibited PC-3 cell growth in a dose-dependent manner with ED50 of 3×10^{-7} M. Further, oral adminstration of troglitazone (500 mg/kg/day) produced significant inhibition of PC-3 tumor growth ($P = 0.01$) in immunocompromised mice [52].

Shappell et al. [53] investigated the ability of 15(S)-HETE to activate PPARγ-dependent transcription and modulate proliferation of PC-3 cells. They found that 15(S)-HETE caused a dose-dependent inhibition of PC-3 proliferation in a 14-day soft agar colony-forming assay with IC_{50} of $30 \mu M$. In PC-3 cells transiently transfected with a luciferase reporter linked to a PPAR response element, $10 \mu M$ 15(S)-HETE could effect an approximately 2–3-fold induction of PPARγ-dependent transcription, suggesting that 15-LOX-2-derived 15(S)-HETE may function as an endogenous ligand for PPARγ in the prostate. Therefore, reduced expression of 15-LOX-2 and reduced endogenous production of 15(S)-HETE may contribute to increased proliferation and reduced differentiation in PC [53]. However, once again, considering that high μM doses

68

of 15(S)-HETE were used, these results should be interpreted with caution.

In summary, studies so far suggest divergent roles for 15-LOX-1 and 15-LOX-2 in the progression of human prostate cancer. While the expression of 15-LOX-1 is positively correlated with prostate tumor progression, the levels of 15-LOX-2 are reduced as prostate cancer progresses to a more advanced stage. While 15-LOX-1 stimulates prostate cancer cell growth *in vitro* and tumor growth *in vivo*, 15(S)-HETE reduced prostate cancer cell proliferation possibly through acting as a PPARγ ligand. It should be noted that 13(S)-HODE, the linoleate product of 15-LOX-1, is also a PPARγ ligand. One would expect that similar to 15(S)-HETE, 13(S)-HODE activates PPARγ and reduces the proliferation of tumor cells. Yet, increased endogenous production of 13(S)-HODE in PC-3 cells seems to have no detrimental effect on their proliferation. In contrast, it actually stimulated PC-3 cell growth [48]. These seeming contradictory findings mandate further study to elucidate the exact functional roles played by 15-LOX-1 and 15-LOX-2 and their bioactive lipid products in prostate cancer progression.

VII. Conclusions and final remarks

In the past several years, eicosanoids have emerged as key regulators for prostate cancer progression. Several enzymes involved in biosynthesis of eicoasnoids, such as COX-2, 12-LOX, and 15-LOX-1, have been found up-regulated during the initiation and progression of prostate cancer; while others such as 15-LOX-2 have been found to be down-regulated during the progression of prostate tumor to a more malignant stage. While more studies are needed to resolve many pitfalls and unanswered issues as mentioned earlier, several lines of evidence suggest that the up-regulation of COX-2, 12-LOX, and 15-LOX-1 in prostate cancer is related to the increased tumor angiogenesis and growth. First, selective COX-2 inhibitors such as NS398 were found to inhibit the growth of PC-3 tumors by decreasing tumor angiogenesis and VEGF expression [12,13]. Second, overexpression of 12-LOX in PC-3 cells stimulates tumor angiogenesis and growth *in vivo* [31]. Third, expression of 15-LOX-1 in PC-3 cells was also found stimulatory for tumor angiogenesis and growth [48]. Finally, we found selective inhibition of 12-LOX reduced tumor growth and angiogenesis in a SCID-hu bone model (Nie and Honn, unpublished results). While more studies are needed to define the role of

COX-2, 12-LOX, 5-LOX, 15-LOX-1, and 15-LOX-2 in prostate cancer progression, the data from above pharmacological and molecular biological investigations suggest stimulatory roles for COX-2, 12-LOX, and 15-LOX-1 in tumor angiogenesis and growth. Therefore, inhibition of these enzymes may represent a promising approach to halt or reverse the progression of prostate cancer.

Acknowledgements

This work was supported by NIH CA-29997, United States Army Research Program DAMD 17-98-1-8502, and an award from Cap CURE Foundation (to K.V.H.).

References

1. Norrish AE, Skeaff CM, Arribas GL, Sharpe SJ, Jackson RT: Prostate cancer risk and consumption of fish oils: A dietary biomarker-based case-control study. Br J Cancer 81: 1238–1242, 1999
2. Gupta S, Srivastava M, Ahmad N, Bostwick DG, Mukhtar H: Over-expression of cyclooxygenase-2 in human prostate adenocarcinoma. Prostate 42: 73–78, 2000
3. Lee LM, Pan CC, Cheng CJ, Chi CW, Liu TY: Expression of cyclooxygenase-2 in prostate adenocarcinoma and benign prostatic hyperplasia. Anticancer Res 21:1291–1294, 2001
4. Yoshimura R, Sano H, Masuda C, Kawamura M, Tsubouchi Y, Chargui J, Yoshimura N, Hla T, Wada S: Expression of cyclooxygenase-2 in prostate carcinoma. Cancer 89: 589–596, 2000
5. Kirschenbaum A, Klausner AP, Lee R, Unger P, Yao S, Liu XH, Levine AC: Expression of cyclooxygenase-1 and cyclooxygenase-2 in the human prostate. Urology 56: 671–676, 2000
6. Uotila P, Valve E, Martikainen P, Nevalainen M, Nurmi M, Harkonen P: Increased expression of cyclooxygenase-2 and nitric oxide synthase-2 in human prostate cancer. Urol Res 29: 23–28, 2001
7. Subbarayan V, Sabichi AL, Llansa N, Lippman SM, Menter DG: Differential expression of cyclooxygenase-2 and its regulation by tumor necrosis factor-alpha in normal and malignant prostate cells. Cancer Res 61: 2720–2726, 2001
8. Tjandrawinata RR, Dahiya R, Hughes-Fulford M: Induction of cyclo-oxygenase-2 mRNA by prostaglandin E2 in human prostatic carcinoma cells. Br J Cancer 75: 1111–1118, 1997
9. Liu XH, Yao S, Kirschenbaum A, Levine AC: NS398, a selective cyclooxygenase-2 inhibitor, induces apoptosis and down-regulates bcl-2 expression in LNCaP cells. Cancer Res 58: 4245–4249, 1998

10. Hsu AL, Ching TT, Wang DS, Song X, Rangnekar VM, Chen CS: The cyclooxygenase-2 inhibitor celecoxib induces apoptosis by blocking Akt activation in human prostate cancer cells independently of Bcl-2. J Biol Chem 275: 11397–11403, 2000

11. Lim JT, Piazza GA, Han EK, Delohery TM, Li H, Finn TS, Buttyan R, Yamamoto H, Sperl GJ, Brendel K, Gross PH, Pamukcu R, Weinstein IB: Sulindac derivatives inhibit growth and induce apoptosis in human prostate cancer cell lines. Biochem Pharmacol 58: 1097–1107, 1999

12. Liu XH, Kirschenbaum A, Yao S, Stearns ME, Holland JF, Claffey K, Levine AC: Upregulation of vascular endothelial growth factor by cobalt chloride-simulated hypoxia is mediated by persistent induction of cyclooxygenase-2 in a metastatic human prostate cancer cell line. Clin Exp Metastasis 17: 687–694, 1999

13. Liu XH, Kirschenbaum A, Yao S, Lee R, Holland JF, Levine AC: Inhibition of cyclooxygenase-2 suppresses angiogenesis and the growth of prostate cancer *in vivo*. J Urol 164: 820–825, 2000

14. Tsujii M, Kawano S, DuBois RN: Cyclooxygenase-2 expression in human colon cancer cells increases metastatic potential. Proc Natl Acad Sci USA 94: 3336–3340, 1997

15. Attiga FA, Fernandez PM, Weeraratna AT, Manyak MJ, Patierno SR: Inhibitors of prostaglandin synthesis inhibit human prostate tumor cell invasiveness and reduce the release of matrix metalloproteinases. Cancer Res 60: 4629–4637, 2000

16. Gupta S, Srivastava M, Ahmad N, Sakamoto K, Bostwick DG, Mukhtar H: Lipoxygenase-5 is overexpressed in prostate adenocarcinoma. Cancer 91: 737–743, 2001

17. Shappell SB, Boeglin WE, Olson SJ, Kasper S, Brash AR: 15-lipoxygenase-2 (15-LOX-2) is expressed in benign prostatic epithelium and reduced in prostate adenocarcinoma. Am J Pathol 155: 235–245, 1999

18. Anderson KM, Seed T, Vos M, Mulshine J, Meng J, Alrefai W, Ou D, Harris JE: 5-Lipoxygenase inhibitors reduce PC-3 cell proliferation and initiate nonnecrotic cell death. Prostate 37: 161–173, 1998

19. Ghosh J, Myers CE: Inhibition of arachidonate 5-lipoxygenase triggers massive apoptosis in human prostate cancer cells. Proc Natl Acad Sci USA 95: 13182–13187, 1998

20. Dixon RA, Diehl RE, Opas E, Rands E, Vickers PJ, Evans JF, Gillard JW, Miller DK: Requirement of a 5-lipoxygenase-activating protein for leukotriene synthesis. Nature 343: 282–284, 1990

21. Vickers PJ: 5-Lipoxygenase-activating protein (FLAP). J Lipid Mediat Cell Signal 12: 185–194, 1995

22. Datta K, Biswal SS, Xu J, Towndrow KM, Feng X, Kehrer JP: A relationship between 5-lipoxygenase-activating protein and bcl-xL expression in murine pro-B lymphocytic FL5.12 cells. J Biol Chem 273: 28163–28169, 1998

23. Datta K, Biswal SS, Kehrer JP: The 5-lipoxygenase-activating protein (FLAP) inhibitor, MK886, induces apoptosis independently of FLAP. Biochem J 340: 371–375, 1999

24. Kehrer JP, Biswal SS, La E, Thuillier P, Datta K, Fischer SM, Vanden Heuvel JP: Inhibition of peroxisome-proliferator-activated receptor (PPAR)alpha by MK886. Biochem J 356: 899–906, 2001

25. Honn KV, Tang DG, Gao X, Butovich IA, Liu B, Timar J, Hagmann W: 12-lipoxygenases and 12(S)-HETE: Role in cancer metastasis. Cancer Metastasis Rev 13: 365–396, 1994

26. Hagmann W, Gao X, Zacharek A, Wojciechowski LA, Honn KV: 12-Lipoxygenase in Lewis lung carcinoma cells: Molecular identity, intracellular distribution of activity and protein, and Ca(2+)-dependent translocation from cytosol to membranes. Prostaglandins 49: 49–62, 1995

27. Chen YQ, Duniec ZM, Liu B, Hagmann W, Gao X, Shimoji K, Marnett LJ, Johnson CR, Honn KV: Endogenous 12(S)-HETE production by tumor cells and its role in metastasis. Cancer Res 54: 1574–1579, 1994

28. Liu B, Marnett LJ, Chaudhary A, Ji C, Blair IA, Johnson CR, Diglio CA, Honn KV: Biosynthesis of 12(S)-hydroxyeicosatetraenoic acid by B16 amelanotic melanoma cells is a determinant of their metastatic potential. Lab Invest 70: 314–323, 1994

29. Silletti S, Timar J, Honn KV, Raz A: Autocrine motility factor induces differential 12-lipoxygenase expression and activity in high- and low-metastatic K1735 melanoma cell variants. Cancer Res 54: 5752–5756, 1994

30. Gao X, Grignon DJ, Chbihi T, Zacharek A, Chen YQ, Sakr W, Porter AT, Crissman JD, Pontes JE, Powell IJ, Honn KV: Elevated 12-lipoxygenase mRNA expression correlates with advanced stage and poor differentiation of human prostate cancer. Urology 46: 227–237, 1995

31. Nie D, Hillman GG, Geddes T, Tang K, Pierson C, Grignon DJ, Honn KV: Platelet-type 12-lipoxygenase in a human prostate carcinoma stimulates angiogenesis and tumor growth. Cancer Res 58: 4047–4051, 1998

32. Connolly JM, Rose DP: Enhanced angiogenesis and growth of 12-lipoxygenase gene-transfected MCF-7 human breast cancer cells in athymic nude mice. Cancer Lett 132: 107–112, 1998

33. Timar J, Tang D, Bazaz R, Haddad MM, Kimler VA, Taylor JD, Honn KV: PKC mediates 12(S)-HETE-induced cytoskeletal rearrangement in B16a melanoma cells. Cell Motil Cytoskeleton 26: 49–65, 1993

34. Ulbricht B, Hagmann W, Ebert W, Spiess E: Differential secretion of cathepsins B and L from normal and tumor human lung cells stimulated by 12(S)-hydroxyeicosatetraenoic acid. Exp Cell Res 226: 255–263, 1996

35. Timar J, Bazaz R, Kimler V, Haddad M, Tang DG, Robertson D, Tovari J, Taylor JD, Honn KV: Immunomorphological characterization and effects of 12-(S)-HETE on a dynamic intracellular pool of the alpha IIb beta 3-integrin in melanoma cells. J Cell Sci 108: 2175–2186, 1995

36. Honn KV, Grossi IM, Diglio CA, Wojtukiewicz M, Taylor JD: Enhanced tumor cell adhesion to the subendothelial matrix resulting from 12(S)-HETE-induced endothelial cell retraction. FASEB J 3: 2285–2293, 1989

37. Liu B, Khan WA, Hannun YA, Timar J, Taylor JD, Lundy S, Butovich I, Honn KV: 12(S)-hydroxyeicosatetraenoic acid and 13(S)-hydroxyoctadecadienoic acid regulation of protein kinase C-alpha in melanoma cells: Role of receptor-mediated hydrolysis of inositol phospholipids. Proc Natl Acad Sci USA 92: 9323–9327, 1995.

70

38. Szekeres CK, Tang K, Trikha M, Honn KV: Eicosanoid activation of extracellular signal-regulated kinase1/2 in human epidermoid carcinoma cells. J Biol Chem 275: 38831–38841, 2000

39. Szekeres CK, Trikha M, Nie D, Honn KV: Eicosanoid 12(S)-HETE activates phosphatidylinositol 3-kinase. Biochem Biophys Res Commun 275: 690–695, 2000

40. Liu B, Maher RJ, Hannun YA, Porter AT, Honn KV: 12(S)-HETE enhancement of prostate tumor cell invasion: Selective role of PKC alpha. J Natl Cancer Inst 86: 1145–1151, 1994

41. Tang DG, Chen YQ, Honn KV: Arachidonate lipoxygenases as essential regulators of cell survival and apoptosis. Proc Natl Acad Sci USA 93: 5241–5246, 1996

42. Nie D, Tang K, Diglio C, Honn KV: Eicosanoid regulation of angiogenesis: Role of endothelial arachidonate 12-lipoxygenase. Blood 95: 2304–2311, 2000

43. Brash AR, Boeglin WE, Chang MS: Discovery of a second 15S-lipoxygenase in humans. Proc Natl Acad Sci USA 94: 6148–6152, 1997

44. Spindler SA, Sarkar FH, Sakr WA, Blackburn ML, Bull AW, LaGattuta M, Reddy RG: Production of 13-hydroxyoctadecadienoic acid (13-HODE) by prostate tumors and cell lines. Biochem Biophys Res Commun 239: 775–781, 1997

45. Kelavkar UP, Badr KF: Effects of mutant p53 expression on human 15-lipoxygenase-promoter activity and murine 12/15-lipoxygenase gene expression: Evidence that 15-lipoxygenase is a mutator gene. Proc Natl Acad Sci USA 96: 4378–4383, 1999

46. Kelavkar UP, Cohen C, Kamitani H, Eling TE, Badr KF: Concordant induction of 15-lipoxygenase-1 and mutant p53 expression in human prostate adenocarcinoma: Correlation with Gleason staging. Carcinogenesis 21: 1777–1787, 2000

47. Jack GS, Brash AR, Olson SJ, Manning S, Coffey CS, Smith JA Jr, Shappell SB: Reduced 15-lipoxygenase-2 immunostaining in prostate adenocarcinoma: Correlation

with grade and expression in high-grade prostatic intraepithelial neoplasia. Hum Pathol 31: 1146–1154, 2000

48. Kelavkar UP, Nixon JB, Cohen C, Dillehay D, Eling TE, Badr KF: Overexpression of 15-lipoxygenase-1 in PC-3 human prostate cancer cells increases tumorigenesis. Carcinogenesis 22: 1765–1773, 2001

49. Han KH, Chang MK, Boullier A, Green SR, Li A, Glass CK, Quehenberger O: Oxidized LDL reduces monocyte CCR2 expression through pathways involving peroxisome proliferator-activated receptor gamma. J Clin Invest 106: 793–802, 2000

50. Forman BM, Chen J, Evans RM: Hypolipidemic drugs, polyunsaturated fatty acids, and eicosanoids are ligands for peroxisome proliferator-activated receptors alpha and delta. Proc Natl Acad Sci USA 94: 4312–4317, 1997

51. Kawahito Y, Kondo M, Tsubouchi Y, Hashiramoto A, Bishop-Bailey D, Inoue K, Kohno M, Yamada R, Hla T, Sano H: 15-deoxy-delta(12,14)-PGJ(2) induces synoviocyte apoptosis and suppresses adjuvant-induced arthritis in rats. J Clin Invest 106: 189–197, 2000

52. Kubota T, Koshizuka K, Williamson EA, Asou H, Said JW, Holden S, Miyoshi I, Koeffler HP: Ligand for peroxisome proliferator-activated receptor gamma (troglitazone) has potent antitumor effect against human prostate cancer both *in vitro* and *in vivo*. Cancer Res 58: 3344–3352, 1998

53. Shappell SB, Gupta RA, Manning S, Whitehead R, Boeglin WE, Schneider C, Case T, Price J, Jack GS, Wheeler TM, Matusik RJ, Brash AR, Dubois RN: 15S-Hydroxyeicosatetraenoic acid activates peroxisome proliferator-activated receptor gamma and inhibits proliferation in PC3 prostate carcinoma cells. Cancer Res 61: 497–503, 2001

Address for offprints: Kenneth V. Honn, Department of Radiation Oncology, 431 Chemistry Bldg., Wayne State University, Detroit, MI 48202, USA; *Tel:* (313)577-1018; *Fax:* (313)577-0798; *e-mail:* k.v.honn@wayne.edu

Contribution of the androgen receptor to prostate cancer predisposition and progression

Grant Buchanan[1], Ryan A. Irvine[2], Gerhard A. Coetzee[2] and Wayne D. Tilley[1]
[1]*Department of Medicine, University of Adelaide and Hanson Institute, Adelaide, SA, Australia;*
[2]*Departments of Urology and Preventive Medicine, University of Southern California Keck School of Medicine, Norris Cancer Center, Los Angeles, CA, USA*

Key words: androgen-signaling axis, CAG, GGC, mutation, androgen-ablation therapy

Abstract

Although prostate cancer is heterogeneous in its etiology and progression, androgen signaling through the androgen receptor (AR) appears to be involved in all aspects of the disease, from initiation to development of treatment resistance. Lifetime exposure to a constitutively more active AR, encoded by AR alleles as defined by two translated polymorphic microsatellites (CAG and GGC), results in a significant increase in prostate cancer risk. The AR gene is amplified or a target for somatic gain-of-function mutations in metastatic prostate cancer. Gain-of-function AR gene mutations may result in inappropriate activation of the AR, thereby contributing to the failure of conventional androgen-ablation treatments. In cases where no genetically altered receptors are observed, altered signaling through the AR, achieved by cross-talk with other signaling pathways (e.g. kinase-mediated pathways) and/or inappropriate expression of coregulatory proteins, may contribute to disease progression. Thus, the AR-signaling axis contributes to many aspects of prostate cancer, including initiation, progression and resistance to current forms of therapy. This recognition represents a paradigm shift in our understanding of the molecular mechanisms involved in progression of prostate cancer, and provides insight into novel AR-targeted therapies which ultimately may be more effective than current forms of androgen ablation.

Introduction

The development and maintenance of the normal prostate gland requires a functional androgen-signaling axis [1,2]. The primary components of this axis include testicular biosynthesis and transport of testosterone to target tissues, conversion of testosterone to its more active metabolite 5α-dihydrotestosterone (DHT), maturation of the androgen receptor (AR) to its ligand-binding competent form, and the subsequent transcriptional regulation of AR target genes. Through the AR, the androgen-signaling axis mediates diverse cellular functions in the prostate including differentiation, morphogenesis, angiogenesis, proliferation and apoptosis [1–5].

Prostate tumorigenesis also requires a functional androgen-signaling axis, the components of which form the principal targets of androgen-ablation therapies that inhibit the growth of prostate cancer. For patients who are either diagnosed with or subsequently develop metastatic disease, the only treatment option is androgen ablation (i.e., orchidectomy, treatment with LHRH agonists/antagonists and/or AR antagonists [6,7]). Despite an initial good response in 80–90% of patients with metastatic disease, androgen ablation is essentially palliative and disease progression eventually ensues [7,8]. Resistance to androgen ablation is not necessarily due to loss of androgen sensitivity, but may develop as a consequence of a deregulated androgen-signaling axis resulting from amplification or mutation of the AR gene, or ligand-independent activation (LIA) of the AR by growth factors and cytokines ([9–11]; reviewed in [12–14]).

Recent evidence suggests that the AR is involved in many phases of prostate cancer biology, including genetic predisposition (due to the existence of polymorphic variants), disease progression, and the development of resistance to androgen-ablation therapies. In this review, we document the contribution of the AR to each of these phases of prostate cancer.

M.L. Cher, K.V. Honn and A. Raz (eds.), Prostate Cancer: New Horizons in Research and Treatment, 71–87.
© 2002 *Kluwer Academic Publishers.*

Androgen receptor structure and function

The AR gene is located on the long arm of the X chromosome at Xq11–12, and comprises 8 exons that encode a protein of approximately 110 kDa (Figure 1). The AR can be broadly defined in terms of three distinct functional domains: a large amino-terminal transactivation domain (NTD) containing at least two strong constitutive transactivation functions; a DNA-binding domain (DBD); and a carboxy-terminal ligand-binding domain (LBD) that contains a highly conserved ligand-dependent transactivation function (AF-2) (Figure 1; [15]). The large NTD is encoded in its entirety by exon 1 of the gene and contains two polymorphic trinucleotide microsatellites, CAG and GGC, which encode variable-length polyglutamine (poly-Q) and polyglycine (poly-G) tracts, respectively, in the receptor (Figure 1). The CAG and GGC microsatellites have a normal size distribution of 6–39

and 7–20 repeats respectively [16,17]. The CAG and GGC microsatellites have expanded during primate evolution [18,19]. The Old World marmoset, drill and macaque monkeys, for example, possess only 3, 8 and 7 uninterrupted AR-CAG repeats, respectively [18], and the macaque and the prosimian lemur possess only 6 and 2 uninterrupted AR-GGC repeats, respectively [19]. Rubinsztein et al. [20] have shown that human microsatellite repeats statistically are more likely to be longer than their primate counterparts, suggesting that phylogenetic microsatellite expansion may be reflective of a mutational bias in favor of longer repeat lengths specifically in humans. A directional expansion of coding microsatellite repeats could be tolerated evolutionarily until it significantly alters function of the receptor such that reproduction is compromised.

Expansion of the CAG microsatellite to 40 or more repeats causes a rare, X-linked, adult onset, neurodegenerative disorder called spinal and bulbar

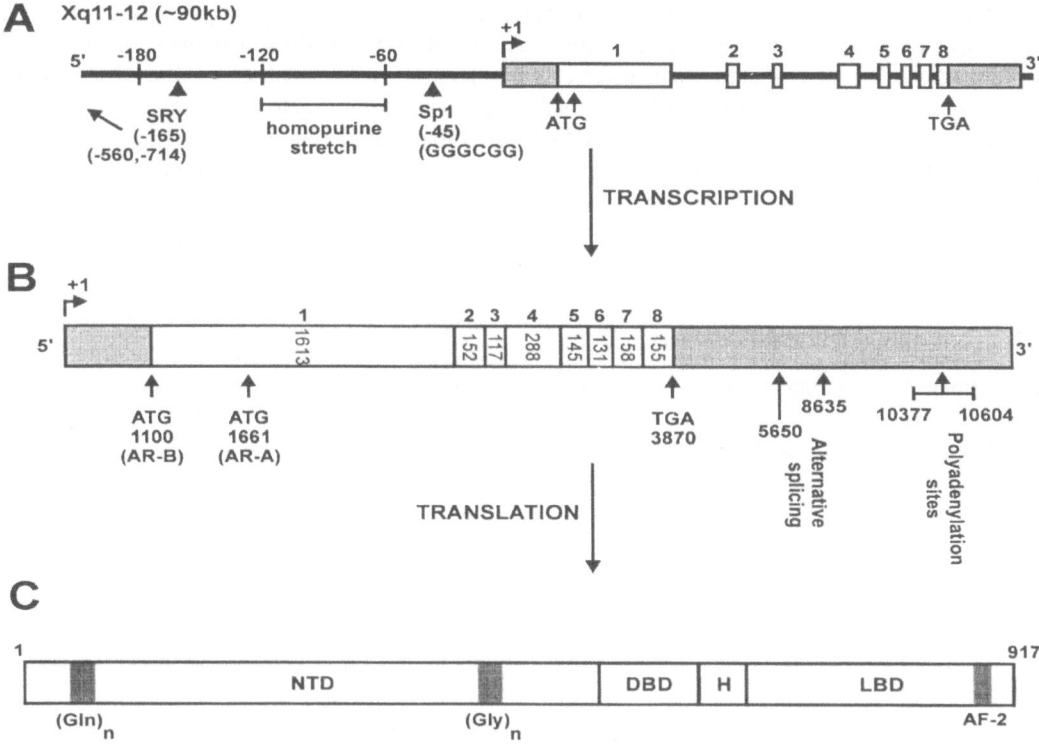

Figure 1. Transcription and translation of the AR. (A) Schematic representation of the AR gene structure on chromosome Xq11–12 showing important binding sites for SRY and SP1 transcription factors. Individual exons are separated by up to 16 kb of intronic sequence. (B) AR mRNA transcript showing alternative splice and polyadenylation sites. Translation is primarily directed from the first of two initiating methionine residues. (C) Structure of the predominant (AR-B) form of the AR. Indicated are the NTD, the DBD, the hinge region (H) and LBD. The positions of the three polymeric amino acid stretches in the NTD and the activation function, AF-2 in the LBD are shown (shaded).

muscular atrophy (SBMA) or Kennedy's disease [21,22]. In addition to progressive muscle weakness and atrophy due to loss of brain stem and spinal cord motor neurons, men with this disorder frequently present with symptoms of partial androgen insensitivity (i.e., gynecomastia and testicular atrophy), indicative of aberrant AR function [23,24]. Receptor proteins encoded by SBMA AR alleles have normal androgen-binding affinities but reduced transactivation capacity compared to wild-type AR [25,26]. Indeed, an inverse relationship between AR transactivation activity and CAG repeat length has been well-established over a CAG size range encompassing normal AR alleles [27–30].

Following translation of the AR, conformational maturation of steroid receptors by a multi-protein chaperone heterocomplex is essential for the acquisition of ligand-binding competence [31]. The specific details of this process for the AR are poorly defined, but in general, it requires at least three heat shock proteins, Hsp40, Hsp70 and Hsp90, and the co-chaperones p23 and Hop [31]. In the final stages of receptor maturation, Hsp90 becomes directly associated with the receptor LBD in a process stabilized by p23, and with one of the tetratricopeptide repeat (TPR) containing proteins which include the immunophilins FKBP51/52 and CyP40, and the protein–serine phosphatase, PP5 [31]. The interaction of the co-chaperone p23 with Hsp90 is an absolute requirement for heterocomplex stabilization of unliganded nuclear receptors [31]. Although many TPR containing proteins appear to have a similar affinity for Hsp90, they exhibit specific preferences for different steroid receptors, and may play a role in hormone action by altering the affinity and specificity for ligand. It is thought that the Hsp90-containing heterocomplex dynamically associates with steroid receptors to maintain them in a conformation that, although unstable, has a high affinity for ligand binding [31]. Following hormone binding in the cytoplasm, the Hsp90-containing heterocomplex is dissociated and the steroid receptor is rapidly translocated into the nucleus.

In the nucleus, the AR dimerizes and binds in the major groove of the DNA double-helix at specific DNA sequences called androgen response elements (AREs). The DNA bound AR dimer recruits a multi-protein complex containing members of the basal transcription machinery (e.g. TFIIF) and additional essential proteins termed cofactors, which act to up-regulate (coactivators) or inhibit (corepressors) target gene expression [32]. Chromatin remodeling occurs via targeted histone acetylation by recruited coactivators, resulting in the stable assembly of the pre-initiation transcriptional complex and enhanced rates of transcription initiation by RNA polymerase II [32]. Following ligand dissociation, the AR is shuttled back to the cytoplasm where it can re-associate with Hsp90 and ligand, subsequently undergoing multiple rounds of nucleocytoplasmic recycling and gene activation [33].

The DBD of steroid receptors contains two zinc finger motifs and a short C-terminal extension that form part of the hinge region [34,35]. Conserved amino acids in the second zinc finger of the DBD ('D' box) form a dimerization interface between steroid receptor monomers. The specificity of steroid receptors is determined at the level of DNA binding by conserved amino acids in the α-helix of the first zinc finger ('P' box) which contact specific base pairs in steroid receptor response elements [34]. Despite their diverse biological effects, the 'P' boxes of class I steroid receptors (i.e., AR and the corresponding receptors for glucocorticoids (GR), mineralocorticoids and progestins) are almost identical and the core DBD, which includes both zinc fingers, shares up to 73% identity [35]. However, sequence differences in the C-terminal extensions, which diverge considerably between steroid receptors (approximately 30% identity), may confer receptor selectivity for particular target sequences by allowing alternative modes of DNA binding [36]. Response elements for steroid receptors generally consist of hexameric half-sites arranged as either inverted repeats (symmetrically arranged palindromes) or direct repeats separated by three nucleotides. A recent analysis of AR-regulated genes has shown that the AR-responsive half-sites arranged as inverted repeats may induce head-to-head dimerization of the receptor, while the polarity of direct repeats may lead to head-to-tail dimerization [37–39]. These two distinct classes of AREs mediate cooperativity of AR binding and the unique regulation of target genes [40].

The contribution of AR-CAG size variation to prostate cancer risk

In 1992, Edwards et al. [16] reported the allelic frequency distribution of AR-CAG repeat size in different US racial–ethnic populations as part of a larger survey of genetic variation in a series of different trimeric and tetrameric tandem repeats. Among African-Americans, the frequency of AR alleles with less than 22 CAG repeats was 65%, as compared to 53% in Caucasians and 34% in Asian-Americans. On the basis of these observations, we hypothesized that AR-CAG repeat length might be associated with the higher risk of prostate cancer in African-Americans, and the intermediate and low risk in Caucasions and Asian-Americans respectively, and that enhanced transcriptional activity of receptors with a shorter AR-CAG allele could promote tumorigenesis by enhancing prostatic epithelial cell turnover [41].

In 1995 we directly tested this hypothesis in a pilot case-control study comprising 68 prostate cancer patients and 123 control subjects [42]. In agreement with Edwards et al. [16] there was a prevalence of short AR-CAG alleles in African-American vs. Caucasian and Asian controls. In addition, modest though not statistically significant enrichment of short AR-CAG alleles was observed in the Caucasian prostate cancer patients. These findings were extended in an expanded follow-up study that showed a significantly higher prevalence of short AR-CAG alleles among prostate

cancer patients, especially among those with advanced disease (Table 1; [43]). In addition to our studies, Hakimi et al. [44] identified a subgroup of patients diagnosed with advanced prostate cancer who had shorter AR-CAG repeats. Hardy et al. [45] furthermore, demonstrated an association between age of onset and AR-CAG repeat length.

Subsequently, several well-designed matched case-control studies demonstrated an approximate 2-fold increased prostate cancer risk, decreased age of onset and/or increased risk of advanced disease for reduced AR-CAG repeat length (Table 1). Giovannucci et al. [17] used a population selected from the Physicians Health Study that included 587 prostate cancer cases and 588 matched controls. The large sample size of this study allowed the authors to stratify cases by tumor grade and stage. A highly significant inverse correlation between AR-CAG repeat length and risk of developing prostate cancer was observed when repeat size was analyzed as a semi-continuous variable. Short AR-CAG alleles also correlated with an increased risk of having

Table 1. Studies evaluating the roles of the AR CAG and/or GGC microsatellites in prostate cancer risk, progression, and age at onset.

Study	Subjects	AR CAG repeat correlation with PCa			AR GGC repeat correlation with PCa		
		Risk	Stage/grade	Age at onset	Risk	Stage/grade	Age at onset
Pilot studies							
Irvine et al., 1995 [42]	US Caucasian	Yes	N/A	N/A	Yes	N/A	N/A
Hardy et al., 1996 [45]	US Caucasian	N/A	No	Yes	N/A	N/A	N/A
Ingles et al., 1997 [43]	US Caucasian	Yes	Yes	N/A	N/A	N/A	N/A
Hakimi et al., 1997 [44]	US Caucasian	Yes	Yes	No	Yes	No	No
Matched case-control studies							
Giovannucci et al., 1997 [17]	US Caucasian	Yes	Yes	No	N/A	N/A	N/A
Standford et al., 1997 [46]	US Caucasian	Yes	No	Yes	Yes	No	Yes
Platz et al., 1998 [53]	US Caucasian	N/A	N/A	N/A	Yes	N/A	N/A
Hsing et al., 2000 [47]	Chinese	Yes	No	No	Yes	No	No
Beilin et al., 2001 [30]	Australian White	No	No	Yes	N/A	N/A	N/A
Other studies							
Ekman et al., 1999 [49]	Swedish White	Yes	N/A	N/A	N/A	N/A	N/A
Edwards et al., 1999 [50]	British Caucasian	No	No	N/A	Yes	No	N/A
Correa-Cerro et al., 1999 [51]	French/German White	No	No	No	No	No	No
Bratt et al., 1999 [52]	Swedish White	No	Yes	Yes	N/A	N/A	N/A
Lange et al., 2000 [53]	US Caucasian (high risk)	No	No	No	N/A	N/A	N/A
Nam et al., 2000 [54]	Canadian	N/A	Yes	N/A	N/A	N/A	N/A
Latil et al., 2001 [55]	French White	No	No	Yes	N/A	N/A	N/A
Modugno et al., 2001 [56]	US Caucasian	Yes	N/A	N/A	N/A	N/A	N/A
Miller et al., 2001 [57]	US Caucasian	No	N/A	N/A	No	N/A	N/A
Panz et al., 2001 [58]	S. Africans (Black & White)	Yes	Yes	N/A	N/A	N/A	N/A

N/A, not applicable or not assessed; Yes, association between polymorphism and listed parameter; No, no significant association detected between polymorphism and listed parameter.

advanced disease, defined as a high-stage or high-grade tumor at diagnosis [17]. In another study, Stanford et al. [46] analyzed AR-CAG repeat length and prostate cancer risk in 301 prostate cancer cases and 277 matched controls [46]. They noted only a small increase in the frequency of AR-CAG alleles with less than 22 repeats in cancer patients compared with controls. Nevertheless, when AR-CAG repeat size was examined as a continuous variable, an overall age-adjusted relative odds of developing prostate cancer of 0.97 was observed for each additional CAG. More recently, Hsing et al. [47] reported that AR-CAG alleles were significantly shorter in prostate cancer patients compared to controls among Shanghai Chinese. This study is important as it was the first to demonstrate this association in a population group other than Caucasian. In a recent case-control study in an Australian Caucasian population [48], no association was observed between AR-CAG repeat length and prostate cancer risk, but a significant effect on the age of onset was observed. In other studies (Table 1), associations between AR-CAG repeat length and prostate cancer risk were not consistently observed, possibly due to small sample sizes, population differences and/or failure to appropriately match cases and controls [49–58].

While the consistent finding of the epidemiologic studies discussed above has provided evidence for an association between AR-CAG repeat length and prostate cancer risk, those studies did not address the molecular mechanisms underlying changes in receptor activity with length variation of the poly-Q tract (encoded by the polymorphic CAG repeat). As stated above, *in vitro* transient cotransfection studies have shown that ARs with longer poly-Q repeats have normal ligand-binding affinities but lower transactivation activities [25–28,48]. Protein expression levels are unlikely to account for this effect since they have been found to be similar for ARs containing between 9 and 42 poly-Q repeats [29]. However, two studies have reported that AR constructs with longer repeat lengths (CAG-50–52) are unstable and undergo accelerated degradation, potentially in a ligand-dependent manner [29,59]. The poly-Q size effect in AR transactivation activity observed in most *in vitro* studies is thought to be mediated, at least in part, through altered functional interactions with cofactors. In transient cotransfection experiments, the p160 coactivators, GRIP1, AIB1 and SRC-1 exaggerate the relative difference in AR transactivation activity with altered poly-Q length [29]. As the p160 coactivators bind to regions of the AR NTD distinct from the poly-Q tract, the size effect may be mediated by steric hindrance of p160–receptor interactions when poly-Q length is increased [29]. The RAS related G-protein, Ran/ARA24, which binds to the AR NTD in the region of the poly-Q, is an AR cofactor that appears to enhance AR activity in a poly-Q size-dependent manner [60]. Given the well-described role for Ran in protein nuclear transport, it is possible that larger poly-Q tracts inhibit the efficiency of Ran-directed AR nuclear import [61]. Clearly, more studies are required to determine whether the effects of other cofactors that act in a cell-, promoter- and/or AR-specific manner can be directly influenced by poly-Q length, and to determine how variation in AR poly-Q length can influence prostate cancer cell growth.

The contribution of AR-GGC size variation to prostate cancer risk

Allelic distributions of the GGC microsatellite are significantly different among racial–ethnic groups [42], with the 16-repeat GGC allele being least prevalent amongst high-risk African-Americans (i.e., 20%) and most prevalent in low-risk Asians (i.e., 70%). This is suggestive of a protective role for this allele in prostate cancer risk. It is possible that the 16-repeat GGC allele encodes an AR containing a poly-G tract of 'optimal' length for normal receptor function in prostatic epithelial cells. While this is speculative, as it is not known whether variation in poly-G length modulates AR activity, a weak though non-significant paucity of the 16-repeat GGC allele was observed among white Caucasian prostate cancer patients compared to control subjects, suggesting that there is enrichment of putative risk alleles (i.e., non-16-repeat GGC alleles) among cases [42].

Because the AR gene is X-linked, with each male inheriting a single maternal copy, it is possible to define a putative AR prostate cancer risk allelotype of short CAG (i.e., <22 repeats) and non-16-repeat GGC. As expected, we observed that the distribution of this allelotype was significantly different among control subjects, with African-Americans and Asians having the highest and lowest prevalence, respectively. Among white Caucasian prostate cancer patients, the <22 CAG/non-16-repeat GGC haplotype conferred a 2-fold increase in risk of prostate cancer, although statistical significance was not reached [42]. Among prostate cancer patients, a nonrandom distribution of CAG and GGC alleles was observed; 66% of patients with a short CAG allele also had a non-16-repeat GGC allele, while only 25% of patients with long CAG alleles had a non-16-repeat GGC allele. As the CAG and GGC microsatellites are in close proximity at the AR locus, it was not surprising to find evidence of linkage disequilibrium between the intragenic markers in patient samples. In contrast, there was no evidence of linkage disequilibirium between control samples when assessed either together or by ethnicity. This indicates that in normal men, either one or both of the microsatellites are hypermutable, resulting in a random distribution of CAG and GGC alleles at the AR locus. Indeed, when the rate of mutation at the CAG microsatellite was measured using single-cell assays of sperm, an exceptionally high rate of 1–4% was observed [62]. Collectively, this data suggests that a non-random subset of CAG and GGC AR alleles occur in men with prostate cancer.

In three matched case-control studies (Table 1), a positive association between AR-GGC repeat length variation and prostate cancer risk was found [47,63,64]. The failure to consistently demonstrate this association in other studies (Table 1), might be due to the lack of statistical power and/or failure to appropriately match cases with controls. A more detailed assessment of the effects of the AR-GGC repeat on prostate cancer risk awaits elucidation of the effects of alterations in poly-G tract length on AR function.

AR and prostate cancer progression: Localized disease

Although the maintenance of AR immunoreactivity has been demonstrated in the majority of prostate tumors in both localized and metastatic disease [65–73], only recently has the role of AR in progression of clinically localized prostate cancer been addressed [71,73]. Henshall et al. [73] reported that AR was expressed in more than 70% of the tumor cells in localized prostate cancer, but that there was a loss of AR immunoreactivity in the adjacent peritumoral stroma which was associated with earlier relapse after radical prostatectomy. Another study by Sweat et al. [71] found no association between AR expression and disease progression in a highly selected cohort of tumors with a Gleason score of 6–9. In a recent study, we found that the level of AR protein in tumor foci determined by video image analysis is a strong predictor of the risk of relapse following radical prostatectomy (unpublished data). While further studies are necessary to determine how AR influences disease progression in clinically

localized prostate cancer, a number of mechanisms have been identified in prostatic tumors that potentially explain the increase in levels of AR immunostaining observed in tumor cells in our study. These mechanisms include amplification of the AR gene [74], changes in the methylation status of the AR promoter and hence transcription of the AR gene [75,76], altered stability of AR mRNA [77] and LIA [11,78]. Irrespective of the mechanism, increased AR levels likely result in altered expression profiles of androgen-regulated proteins, including angiogenic factors, cell adhesion molecules and cell cycle regulators (e.g. vascular endothelial growth factor, integrins and cyclin-dependent kinases and their inhibitors [79–81], which collectively contribute to disease progression.

AR related mechanisms contributing to the failure of androgen-ablation therapy in advanced prostate cancer

Recent studies in clinical prostate cancer have identified several mechanisms that potentially explain how prostate tumors progress following initiation of androgen ablation, including amplification or mutation of the AR gene, and LIA of the AR ([9,82,83]; reviewed in [12,84–86]). These studies suggest that resistance to conventional hormonal therapy is not due to a loss of androgen sensitivity but rather may be a consequence of a deregulated androgen-signaling axis ([87]; reviewed in [84,85]. Although initial studies using the Dunning animal model suggested that loss of AR gene expression could be a mechanism for failure of androgen ablation [88,89], subsequent immunohistochemical studies of clinical prostate cancer have demonstrated that the AR is expressed in essentially all metastatic tumors, including those that continue to grow following androgen ablation [90]. Moreover, amplification of the AR gene has been reported in 22% of prostate cancer metastases [82], and in 23–28% of primary tumors following androgen deprivation [74,91]. An average 2-fold increased level of both AR and PSA proteins has been reported in prostate tumor samples with AR gene amplification compared to samples where no AR amplification was found [9,83]. Increased AR levels may augment the sensitivity of the androgen-signaling axis, and has the potential to contribute to disease progression during the course of androgen ablation.

The first indication that AR gene mutations might contribute to the failure of androgen-ablation therapies came from studies of the androgen-responsive human prostate cancer cell line, LNCaP. The AR in LNCaP cells contains a single amino acid substitution (Thr–Ala877) that facilitates inappropriate activation by glucocorticoids, progestins, adrenal androgens, estradiol and the anti-androgen hydroxyflutamide [92,93]. Subsequently, somatic missense mutations have been detected throughout the AR coding sequence at frequencies of up to 50% in advanced primary tumors and metastatic deposits (reviewed in [12,94]). These mutations consistently result in receptors that exhibit decreased specificity of ligand-binding and enhanced receptor activation by androgens and non-classical ligands compared to wild-type AR (wtAR; reviewed in [85,95]). More recently in collaboration with Dr Norman Greenberg at Baylor College of Medicine, Houston, TX, we reported the identification of AR gene mutations in the autochthonous transgenic adenocarcinoma of mouse prostate (TRAMP) model [96]. Analogous to the findings in clinical prostate cancer, AR gene mutations detected in TRAMP tumors also result in receptors that contribute to altered androgen signaling [96].

Structural and functional collocation of AR variants

We recently reported that nearly 80% of missense AR gene mutations identified in clinical prostate cancer cluster to discrete regions of the receptor that collectively span less than 15% of the coding sequence ([85]; Figure 2; Table 2).

Ligand-binding domain variants. In the LBD, mutations collocate to (i) the 'signature sequence', a conserved 20-amino-acid region of nuclear receptors involved in ligand recognition and specificity [97], (ii) AF-2, a binding site for the p160 cofactors, and (iii) a region at the boundary of the hinge and LBD containing a 4-amino-acid tetrapeptide (^{668}QPIF^{671}) that may define a protein–protein interaction surface. Many of the AR gene mutations identified in the LBD of the AR in the TRAMP model occur in the same three regions as mutations in clinical prostate cancer. For example, a Phe–Ile671 mutation identified in an intact TRAMP mouse collocated to the ^{668}QPIF^{671} tetrapeptide with mutations identified human prostate cancer [10]. AR gene mutations identified in both clinical prostate cancer and TRAMP tumors

in this region exhibit a 2–4-fold greater transactivation activity in response to DHT, non-classical ligands and hydroxyflutamide compared to wtAR (Figure 3A; [10]), without altering ligand-binding kinetics, receptor levels or DNA-binding capacity. Homology modeling revealed that the ^{668}QPIF^{671} tetrapeptide residues form a potential protein–protein interaction surface that is markedly disrupted by the naturally occurring mutations, providing a mechanism that could explain the observed gain in transcriptional activity [10].

Another AR missense mutation identified in the TRAMP model, Phe–Ser697, is located adjacent to the signature sequence. The Ser697 AR variant exhibits markedly reduced transactivation responses to progesterone and 17β-estradiol, but enhanced response to R1881 compared to wtAR (Figure 3B; [96]). These results are consistent with the role of the signature sequence in ligand recognition and specificity, and with previous reports of mutations in this region in clinical disease (reviewed in [12,85]). Analysis of the Thr–Ala877 AR variant, identified in a significant proportion of clinical prostate tumors and in the human prostate cancer cell line, LNCaP, has confirmed that this mutation exhibits increased transactivation activity in response to progesterone, 17β-estradiol, adrenal androgens and hydroxyflutamide compared to wtAR (Figure 3C; [98]). The recently determined AR-LBD crystal structure [99,100] allowed us to use homology modeling to demonstrate that this mutation results in changes to the shape and volume of the ligand-binding pocket such that bulkier ligands like progesterone can be accommodated [96].

DNA-binding domain variants. Five somatic missense mutations have been identified in clinical prostate tumors that collocate to a 14-amino-acid region at the carboxyl-terminal end of the first zinc finger motif in the DBD of the AR [101,102]. The effect of each of these mutations is unknown, but none of the codons in which they occur have been reported to contain mutations that cause receptor inactivation in the clinical syndrome of androgen insensitivity. Mutations in the AR-DBD have been shown to selectively affect transactivation and transrepression functions of the AR on different promoters despite a reduced DNA-binding ability [103,104], and may represent a predisposing factor for male breast cancer [105]. Due to the high homology of the DBD across members of the nuclear receptor superfamily, the cell and promoter specificity of different receptors is, in part,

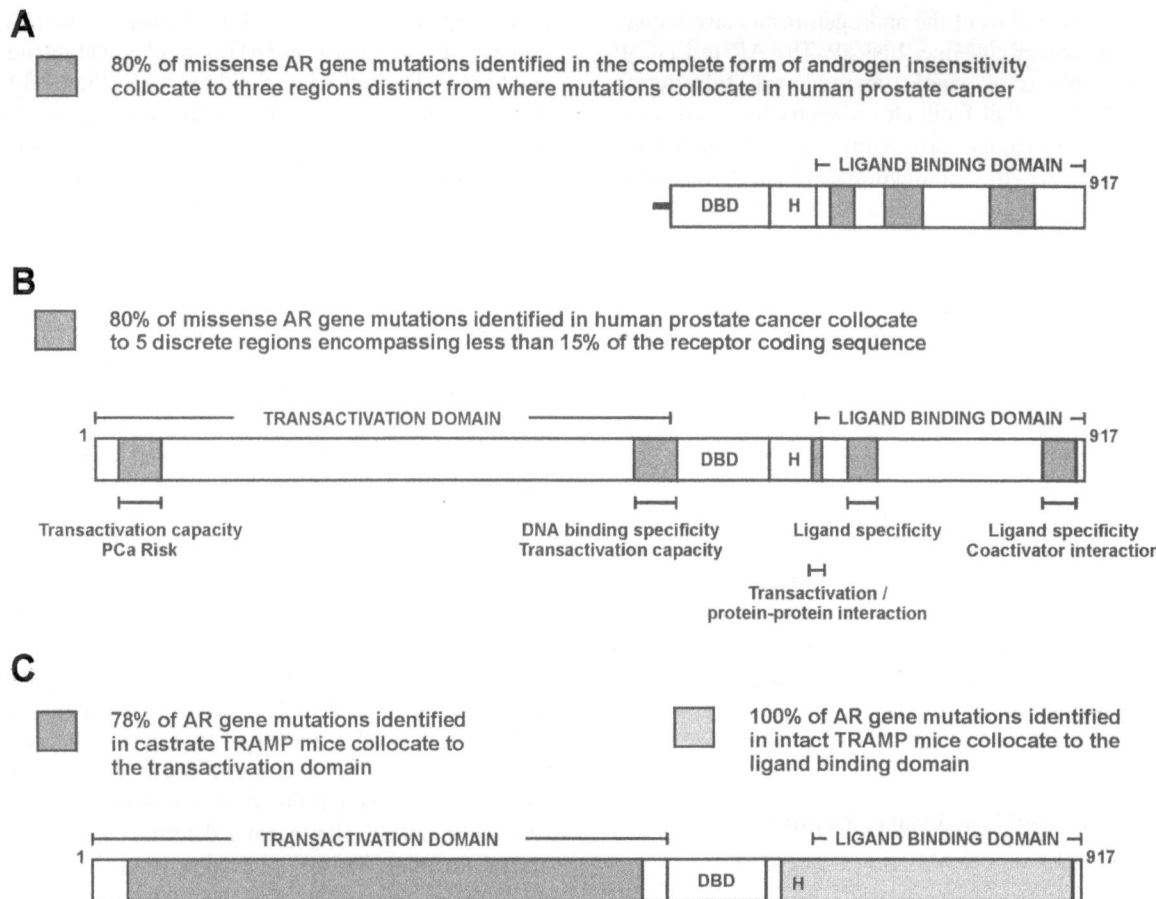

Figure 2. Collocation of AR variants. (A) Collocation of 80% of inactivating AR gene mutations detected in the clinical syndrome of complete androgen insensitivity. (B) Collocation of 80% of AR gene mutations detected in clinical prostate cancer to five discrete regions of the receptor (shaded), which account for less than 15% of the coding sequence. (C) AR gene mutations detected in prostate tumors derived from the TRAMP model segregate to the amino-terminal transactivation domain or to the LBD in castrated and intact mice respectively.

mediated by only a few changes in DBD sequence [106]. It has been speculated that mutations in the DBD could result in AR variants that bind to response elements normally specific for other nuclear receptors [105], leading to inappropriate activation or repression of growth regulatory pathways. In an analogous manner, mutations in androgen receptor response elements have been shown to increase the sensitivity of the enhancer for the glucocorticoid receptor [107]. Modeling experiments suggest that residues in the AR-DBD could form a protein interaction surface [105], and several AR coactivators that interact with the DBD in a ligand-dependent manner [108–110] are predicted to alter receptor activity via local chromatin remodeling [108], interaction with components of the transcriptional machinery [109], or inhibiting nuclear

export [111]. It is also possible that mutations in the DBD of the AR gene identified in prostate cancer could alter the affinity of receptor binding to response elements, resulting in altered expression of a range of target genes regulated by the AR.

Amino-terminal transactivation domain variants. Nearly half of the AR gene mutations identified in clinical prostate cancer are located in the NTD of the receptor. AR gene mutations in this domain have also been identified in the TRAMP model and, analogous to the observations for the LBD, these mutations cluster with those identified in clinical prostate cancer to discrete regions within the NTD that are implicated in receptor function. The main regions of collocation in the NTD are (i) within and adjacent to the poly-Q tract

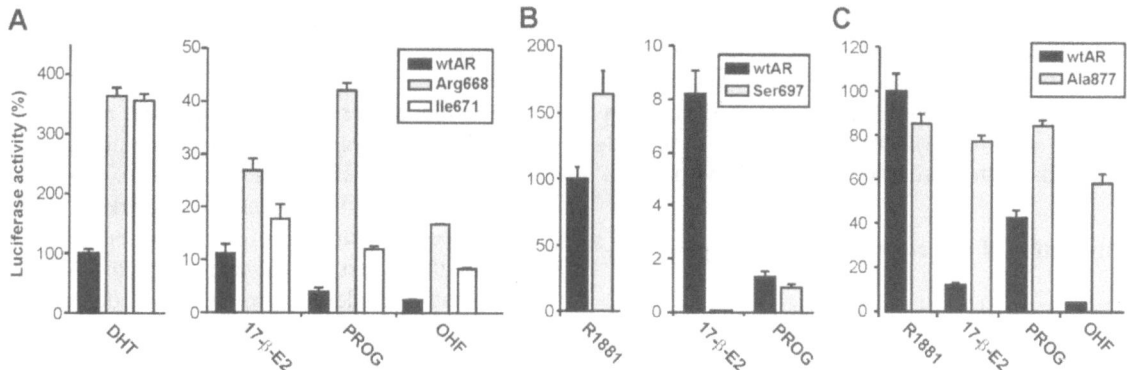

Figure 3. Transactivation capacity of AR variants identified in tumors derived from clinical prostate cancer (Arg668, Ala877) and TRAMP mice (Ile671, Ser697). Transactivation assays were performed in the human prostate cancer cell line, PC-3 with the minimal androgen-responsive probasin promoter, tk81-PB3 as previously described (10). Data is expressed as a percentage of the luciferase activity induced by wtAR in the presence of 1 nM DHT, and represents the mean (±sem) of 3–7 independent experiments. (A) Mutations occurring in [688]QPIF[671] residues. Treatment was with 1 nM of either DHT, 17β-estradiol (17β-E2), or progesterone (PROG), or with 1 μM hydroxyflutamide (OHF). (B) Mutation occurring adjacent to the signature sequence. Treatment was with 1 nM R1881 or 10 nM of either 17β-E2 or PROG. (C) LNCaP AR variant in the region of AF-2. Treatment was with 1 nM of R1881 or 10 nM of either 17β-E2 or PROG, or with 1000 nM OHF.

(codons 54–78), which as discussed above has been implicated in modulating receptor activity and prostate cancer risk, and (ii) a region amino-terminal to the DBD (codons 502–535) known to modulate the transactivation capacity of the receptor in both ligand-dependent and ligand-independent manner (i.e., a LIA function or LIAF) [112,113] (Figure 2).

Somatic contractions in the CAG repeat of the AR gene, which potentially increase AR activity in a subpopulation of cells and thereby contribute to disease progression, have been identified in three independent studies of clinical prostate tumors [114–116]. In addition, we have recently identified a somatic mutation within the CAG repeat of the AR gene in a primary prostate tumor that results in interruption of the polyglutamine repeat by two leucine residues. This AR variant has a 2–4-fold greater ability to transactivate target genes compared to wtAR in the presence of physiological concentrations of DHT [117]. Four additional somatic mutations have been identified in or adjacent to the CAG repeat region of the AR gene in human prostate cancer [101], but have not yet been characterized. Further analysis of inherited and somatic alterations in this region of the AR gene in prostate cancer is warranted to determine the contribution of this motif to AR activity, and its potential to influence the development and/or progression of the disease.

A second region of the NTD where amino acid substitutions have been identified in hormone-refractory prostate tumors is the LIAF. In a recent study, we examined the complete coding sequence of the AR gene for mutations in metastatic tissue biopsies from 12 patients who exhibited the clinical syndrome of steroid-hormone and anti-antiandrogen withdrawal response to hydroxyflutamide. Four of seven mutations identified in the tumor samples collocated to a small carboxyl-terminal portion (codons 502–535) of the NTD of the AR. An additional mutation (Asp–Gly526) previously identified in our studies of primary prostate tumors [101], and another identified in the TRAMP model [96], collocate to this region of the AR. This carboxyl-terminal region of the amino-terminal domain of the AR is known to modulate the transactivation capacity of the receptor in both a ligand-dependent and ligand-independent manner [112,113], and has recently been shown to be involved in direct interactions with the p160 coactivators and the transcription regulator p300/CBP [29,118,119]. This region of the NTD also contains the binding site for the receptor accessory factor (RAF), which enhances the specific DNA binding of rat AR [120]. Further evidence in support of the LIAF region being important in AR transactivation has been provided by recent studies demonstrating that mutation of Ser513, which is located in a consensus MAP kinase phosphorylation site, partially inhibits LIA of the receptor by HER-2/*neu*. Collectively, these observations suggest that the LIAF region may contain an interaction surface for accessory proteins that promote ligand-independent transactivation, and that mutations in this region may alter the ability of the receptor to respond to these and other cofactors, thereby altering the transactivation capacity of the AR in a manner that could provide a growth advantage to prostate cancer cells in an appropriate hormonal environment.

Contribution of cofactors to AR signaling

Two additional AR NTD missense mutations (Met–Thr265; Pro–Ser268; [101]) identified in clinical prostate cancer are located in close proximity to two mutations (Ala–Thr234; Glu–Gly236; [96]) identified in TRAMP tumors. Characterization of the Glu–Gly236 substitution revealed that the variant receptor had increased transactivation function compared to wtAR in response to R1881 and 17β-estradiol only in the presence of the coactivator, ARA70, and increased response to R1881 but not 17β-estradiol in the presence of the coactivator, ARA160 [96]. Similarly, Gregory et al. [121] have shown that over-expression of the p160 coactivators, TIF2/GRIP1 and SRC-1, observed in recurrent tumors from CWR22 human prostate xenografts and clinical prostate cancer, increases AR transactivation capacity at physiological concentrations of non-classical ligands (adrenal androgens, estradiol and progesterone). Similarly, Ye *et al.* [143] have shown that coactivators (e.g. ARA70, ARA160) can enhance the androgenic activity of 17β-estradiol and hydroxyflutamide, suggesting that the effect of agonists and antiandrogens can be modulated by accessory proteins. Collectively, these findings suggest that the phenotype of some AR gene mutations may only be apparent in the presence of the appropriate milieu of coregulators, and that altered expression and/or structure of AR accessory proteins in prostate cancer cells could provide another mechanism contributing to the recurrent growth of prostate tumors in an androgen-depleted environment.

Ligand-independent activation of the AR

Another potentially important mechanism contributing to the failure of androgen ablation is LIA of the AR. The AR can be activated in the absence of ligand by growth factors (keratinocyte growth factor, insulin-like growth factor-1 and epidermal growth factor), cytokines (Interleukin-6), protein kinase-A, components of the MAP kinase pathway (MEKK1), differentiation agents such as butyrate and other factors that directly or indirectly increase intracellular kinase activity or decrease phosphatase activity (reviewed in [84]).

Aberrant expression of growth factor receptors also contributes to development and progression of prostate cancers [12,85]. HER2 (neu/c-erbB-2), a transmembrane glycoprotein member of the epidermal growth factor receptor family, is overexpressed in carcinomas of the breast, ovary, and stomach [17,42,122]. Unlike other epidermal growth factor receptor members, HER2 has intrinsic tyrosine kinase activity and mediates signal transduction in the absence of ligand [123]. Recent studies suggest that HER2 expression is increased in hormone-refractory prostate tumors compared to earlier stages of disease [124,125]. Over-expression of HER2 in androgen-responsive prostate cancer cell lines enhances AR transactivation of androgen-regulated genes such as PSA, in a ligand-independent manner, and increases cell survival during androgen deprivation [11,126]. Although the mechanism involved in HER2 modulation of AR transactivation has not been fully characterized, HER2 expression is associated with activation of MAP kinase and Akt (protein kinase B) pathways which have been implicated in LIA of the AR [11,78]. It was recently shown that the tyrosine kinase receptor, HER-2/*neu*, can promote LIA of the AR via both the PI3K/Akt and MAP kinase pathways [78,127]. In those studies, LIA by HER-2/*neu* could be partially blocked by an inhibitor of the PI3K Akt pathway [78], or mutation of AR-Ser513, which is located in a consensus MAP kinase phosphorylation site. HER-2/*neu* activation of Akt results in binding of Akt to the AR and phosphorylation of the receptor at two residues (Ser212, Ser791). Another study demonstrated that a specific inhibitor of protein kinase A could block LIA of the AR induced by butyrate [127]. These data suggest that both ligand-dependent and ligand-independent signals converge upon the AR, with at least three signal transduction pathways having the potential to activate the AR.

Tumor cells with increased HER2 expression and high AR may have a selective growth advantage. For example HER2 activation of an Akt–AR pathway [11,78,126] may confer a clonal advantage by promoting cancer cell survival via the androgen-signaling axis [78] or by the induction of Akt-dependent pathways [123]. In a recent study using prostate cancer xenograft models, Herceptin (a monoclonal antibody directed against activated HER2) monotherapy resulted in anti-proliferative activity in androgen-dependent LNCaP and CWR22 tumors, but no significant growth inhibition was observed in androgen-independent CWR22 tumors [128]. The lack of response of the androgen-independent tumors to Herceptin in the presence of androgen indicates that signaling through the AR is a requisite for Herceptin response in these prostate tumors [128]. Thus, patients with elevated levels of both HER2 and AR immunostaining may benefit from early treatment targeting both the AR and HER2 signaling cascades.

Therapy selects for AR gene mutations with a phenotype permissive for growth

In the late 1980s, Labrie et al. [129] reported that administration of LHRH agonists in combination with hydroxyflutamide (androgen blockade; CAB) could prolong survival of patients with metastatic prostate cancer by about 17 months. However, subsequent reports were conflicting, and currently most patients initially are treated with monotherapy, usually LHRH agonists. Indeed, a recent systematic review of CAB, encompassing 20 individual trials and more than 6000 patients, concluded that CAB results in only a modest increase in survival compared to monotherapy alone, but is more likely to be associated with adverse events and reduced quality of life [130]. Recent evidence regarding the mechanisms contributing to therapy failure (see above) suggests that combinational approaches with LHRH agonists and receptor antagonists cannot completely abrogate androgen action, and may select for cells with a growth state permissive for a particular hormonal environment. The potential clinical importance of a therapy-mediated selective pressure is illustrated by the syndrome of steroid-hormone and anti-antiandrogen withdrawal, which is characterized by tumor regression and decreasing serum levels of PSA when treatment with an anti-androgen, progestational agent or estrogen is selectively discontinued at a time of clinical progression [131]. A withdrawal response has been observed in up to 30% of patients with hormone-refractory prostate cancer when treatment with the anti-androgen, hydroxyflutamide is terminated [131–133], and has also been documented following withdrawal of the AR antagonists, nilutamide and bicalutamide, the estrogens, diethylstilbestrol and megestrol acetate, and the progestational agent, chlormadinone acetate [134–139]. Withdrawal responses have been reported at a higher incidence following combined therapy, consisting of castration or LHRH agonists in combination with an AR antagonist, compared to antagonist alone,

leading the authors to conclude that prolonged exposure to antiandrogens was the predominant factor in the withdrawal response rather than a low level of androgens [135,140]. In one study, inhibition of adrenal steroid production with ketoconazole following discontinuation of antiandrogen therapy resulted in a higher proportion of patients (55%) exhibiting a withdrawal response and an increased duration of response [141] than reported for withdrawal of the antiandrogen alone [140].

Selection for AR gene mutations with a phenotype permissive for growth is also evident from a number of other studies. AR gene mutations detected in patients who were treated with hydroxyflutamide in conjunction with androgen-ablation therapy result in receptors exhibiting a marked increase in activity in response to hydroxyflutamide, but not to DHT or other androgenic ligands [142]. In the TRAMP model, we recently reported that different hormonal environments result in the selection of AR variants with mutations in distinctly different regions of the receptor [96]. In tumors derived from TRAMP mice at 24–28 weeks of age, 7/7 of the missense AR gene mutations identified in the amino-terminal transactivation domain were derived from mice castrated at 12 weeks of age, whereas 6/8 of the mutations identified in the LBD were from intact animals ([96]; Figure 2C). Moreover, 4/9 of the mutations identified in castrated TRAMP mice resulted in receptors with increased transactivation function in the absence of ligand [96]. Therefore, AR gene mutations identified in prostate cancer could provide a selective growth advantage given the appropriate hormonal environment, resulting in the re-emergence of tumor growth during the course of hormone-ablation therapies. In addition, AR gene amplification and overexpression of the AR has been reported in hormone-refractory prostate cancer following monotherapy but not in primary prostate tumors [9], suggesting an alternative mechanism by which hormonal therapies could select for cells with an ability to maintain growth during treatment.

Conclusions

Collectively, the above evidence suggests that AR signaling plays a key role in many phases of prostate cancer biology. Carefully matched case-control and other studies suggest that length variation of the AR-CAG and AR-GGC polymorphic microsatellite repeats contributes to prostate cancer risk, and may also influence age of onset and tumor pathology, by altering AR transcriptional activity and/or interaction with AR coregulators. AR gene mutations have frequently been reported in clinical prostate cancer and consistently exhibit a gain-of-function phenotype that, along with AR gene amplification and/or activation of the AR by growth factors and cytokines, could facilitate continued AR signaling in an androgen-depleted environment. Thus, resistance to androgen ablation and survival of prostate cancer cells is not necessarily due to the evolution of a growth state that circumvents the androgen-signaling axis, but could be explained in part by increased activity of the AR in the presence of native ligands, inappropriate activation of the AR by non-classical ligands due to mutations in the AR gene or inappropriate expression of AR coregulators, or ligand-independent mechanisms. This represents a paradigm shift in our understanding of hormone-refractory prostate cancer. Further analysis of AR target genes and how their transcription is influenced by non-classical ligands, AR coregulators or variation of the polymorphic AR-CAG and AR-GGC repeats is necessary in order to develop new treatment strategies that target androgen signaling, irrespective of the structure and level of expression of the receptor. This potentially could result in a more complete blockade of androgen signaling, which would represent a significant advance in the treatment of metastatic prostate cancer by preventing or delaying the onset of resistance to androgen-ablation therapies.

Acknowledgements

GB and WDT supported by grants from the National Health and Medical Research Council of Australia, the Anti-Cancer Foundation of South Australia. RAI and GAC supported by grants from the NIH/NCI (R01CA84890) and the United States Department of Defense (DAMD17-00-1-0102).

References

1. Roy AK, Lavrovsky Y, Song CS, Chen S, Jung MH, Velu NK, Bi BY, Chatterjee B: Regulation of androgen action. Vitam Horm 55: 309–352, 1999
2. Kokontis JM, Liao S: Molecular action of androgen in the normal and neoplastic prostate. Vitam Horm 55: 219–307, 1999
3. Tilley WD, Marcelli M, Wilson JD, McPhaul MJ: Characterization and expression of a cDNA encoding the human androgen receptor. Proc Natl Acad Sci USA 86: 327–331, 1989
4. O'Malley B: The steroid receptor superfamily: More excitement predicted for the future. Mol Endocrinol 4: 363–369, 1990
5. Stewart RJ, Panigrahy D, Flynn E, Folkman J: Vascular endothelial growth factor expression and tumor angiogenesis are regulated by androgens in hormone responsive human prostate carcinoma: Evidence for androgen dependent destabilization of vascular endothelial growth factor transcripts. J Urol 165: 688–693, 2001
6. Santen RJ: Clinical review 37: Endocrine treatment of prostate cancer. J Clin Endocrinol Metab 75: 685–689, 1992
7. Thenot S, Charpin M, Bonnet S, Cavailles V: Estrogen receptor cofactors expression in breast and endometrial human cancer cells. Mol Cell Endocrinol 156: 85–93, 1999
8. Kozlowski JM, Ellis WJ, Grayhack JT: Advanced prostatic carcinoma: Early v's late endocrine therapy. In: Andriole GL, Catalona WJ (eds) The Urologic Clinics of North America. WB Saunders Company, Philadelphia, 1991, pp 15–24
9. Linja MJ, Savinainen KJ, Saramaki OR, Tammela TL, Vessella RL, Visakorpi T: Amplification and overexpression of androgen receptor gene in hormone-refractory prostate cancer. Cancer Res 61: 3550–3555, 2001
10. Buchanan G, Yang M, Nahm SJ, Han G, Moore N, Bentel JM, Matusik RJ, Horsfall DJ, Marshall VR, Greenberg NM, Tilley WD: Mutations at the boundary of the hinge and ligand binding domain of the androgen receptor confer increased transactivation function. Mol Endocrinol 15: 46–56, 2000
11. Yeh S, Lin HK, Kang HY, Thin TH, Lin MF, Chang C: From HER2/Neu signal cascade to androgen receptor and its coactivators: A novel pathway by induction of androgen target genes through MAP kinase in prostate cancer cells. Proc Natl Acad Sci USA 96: 5458–5463, 1999
12. Bentel JM, Tilley WD: Androgen receptors in prostate cancer. J Endocrinol 151: 1–11, 1996
13. Sadar MD, Hussain M, Bruchovsky N: Prostate cancer: Molecular biology of early progression to androgen independence. Endocr Relat Cancer 6: 487–502, 1999
14. Jenster G: The role of the androgen receptor in the development and progression of prostate cancer. Semin Oncol 26: 407–421, 1999
15. Kallio PJ, Pakvimo JJ, Janne OA: Genetic regulation of androgen action. Prostate (Suppl 6): 45–51, 1996
16. Edwards A, Hammond HA, Jin L, Caskey CT, Chakraborty R: Genetic variation at five trimeric and tetrameric tandem repeat loci in four human population groups. Genomics 12: 241–253, 1992
17. Giovannucci E, Stampfer MJ, Krithivas K, Brown M, Dahl D, Brufsky A, Talcott J, Hennekens CH, Kantoff PW: The CAG repeat within the androgen receptor gene and its relationship to prostate cancer. Proc Natl Acad Sci USA 94: 3320–3323, 1997

18. Rubinsztein DC, Leggo J, Coetzee GA, Irvine RA, Buckley M, Ferguson-Smith MA: Sequence variation and size ranges of CAG repeats in the Machado-Joseph disease, spinocerebellar ataxia type 1 and androgen receptor genes. Hum Mol Genet 4: 1585–1590, 1995

19. Choong CS, Kemppainen JA, Wilson EM: Evolution of the primate androgen receptor: A structural basis for disease. J Mol Evol 47: 334–342, 1998

20. Rubinsztein DC, Leggo J, Goodburn S, Barton DE, Ferguson-Smith MA: Haplotype analysis of the delta 2642 and (CAG)n polymorphisms in the Huntington's disease (HD) gene provides an explanation for an apparent 'founder' HD haplotype. Hum Mol Genet 4: 203–206, 1995

21. La Spada AR, Wilson EM, Lubahn DB, Harding AE, Fischbeck KH: Androgen receptor gene mutations in X-linked spinal and bulbar muscular atrophy. Nature 352: 77–79, 1991

22. La Spada AR, Roling DB, Harding AE, Warner CL, Spiegel R, Hausmanowa-Petrusewicz I, Yee WC, Fischbeck KH: Meiotic stability and genotype-phenotype correlation of the trinucleotide repeat in X-linked spinal and bulbar muscular atrophy. Nat Genet 2: 301–304, 1992

23. Arbizu T, Santamaria J, Gomez JM, Quilez A, Serra JP: A family with adult spinal and bulbar muscular atrophy, X-linked inheritance and associated testicular failure. J Neurol Sci 59: 371–382, 1983

24. Nagashima T, Seko K, Hirose K, Mannen T, Yoshimura S, Arima R, Nagashima K, Morimatsu Y: Familial bulbospinal muscular atrophy associated with testicular atrophy and sensory neuropathy (Kennedy–Alter–Sung syndrome). Autopsy case report of two brothers. J Neurol Sci 87: 141–152, 1988

25. Mhatre AN, Trifiro MA, Kaufman M, Kazemi-Esfarjani P, Figlewicz D, Rouleau G, Pinsky L: Reduced transcriptional regulatory competence of the androgen receptor in X-linked spinal and bulbar muscular atrophy. Nat Genet 5: 184–188, 1993

26. Chamberlain NL, Driver ED, Miesfeld RL: The length and location of CAG trinucleotide repeats in the androgen receptor N-terminal domain affect transactivation function. Nucleic Acids Res 22: 3181–3186, 1994

27. Kazemi-Esfarjani P, Trifiro MA, Pinsky L: Evidence for a repressive function of the long polyglutamine tract in the human androgen receptor: Possible pathogenetic relevance for the (CAG)n-expanded neuronopathies. Hum Mol Genet 4: 523–527, 1995

28. Tut TG, Ghadessy FJ, Trifiro MA, Pinsky L, Yong EL: Long polyglutamine tracts in the androgen receptor are associated with reduced trans-activation, impaired sperm production, and male infertility. J Clin Endocrinol Metab 82: 3777–3782, 997

29. Irvine RA, Ma H, Yu MC, Ross RK, Stallcup MR, Coetzee GA: Inhibition of p160-mediated coactivation with increasing androgen receptor polyglutamine length. Hum Mol Genet 9: 267–274, 2000

30. Beilin J, Ball EM, Favaloro JM, Zajac JD: Effect of the androgen receptor CAG repeat polymorphism on transcriptional activity: Specificity in prostate and non-prostate cell lines. J Mol Endocrinol 25: 85–96, 2000

31. Pratt WB, Toft DO: Steroid receptor interactions with heat shock protein and immunophilin chaperones. Endocr Rev 18: 306–360, 1997

32. Jenster G, Spencer TE, Burcin MM, Tsai SY, Tsai MJ, O'Malley BW: Steroid receptor induction of gene transcription: A two-step model. Proc Natl Acad Sci USA 94: 7879–7884, 1997

33. Tyagi RK, Lavrovsky Y, Ahn SC, Song CS, Chatterjee B, Roy AK: Dynamics of intracellular movement and nucleocytoplasmic recycling of the ligand-activated androgen receptor in living cells. Mol Endocrinol 14: 1162–1174, 2000

34. Mader S, Leroy P, Chen JY, Chambon P: Multiple parameters control the selectivity of nuclear receptors for their response elements. Selectivity and promiscuity in response element recognition by retinoic acid receptors and retinoid X receptors. J Biol Chem 268: 591–600, 1993

35. Schoenmakers E, Alen P, Verrijdt G, Peeters B, Verhoeven G, Rombauts W, Claessens F: Differential DNA binding by the androgen and glucocorticoid receptors involves the second Zn-finger and a C-terminal extension of the DNA-binding domains. Biochem J 341: 515–521, 1999

36. Schoenmakers E, Verrijdt G, Peeters B, Verhoeven G, Rombauts W, Claessens F: Differences in DNA binding characteristics of the androgen and glucocorticoid receptors can determine hormone-specific responses. J Biol Chem 275: 12290–12297, 2000

37. Luisi BF, Xu WX, Otwinowski Z, Freedman LP, Yamamoto KR, Sigler PB: Crystallographic analysis of the interaction of the glucocorticoid receptor with DNA. Nature 352: 497–505, 1991

38. Rastinejad F, Perlmann T, Evans RM, Sigler PB: Structural determinants of nuclear receptor assembly on DNA direct repeats. Nature 375: 203–211, 1995

39. Gronemeyer H, Moras D: Nuclear receptors. How to finger DNA. Nature 375: 190–191, 1995

40. Reid KJ, Hendy SC, Saito JL, Sorensen P, Nelson CC: Two classes of androgen receptor elements mediate cooperativity through allosteric interactions. J Biol Chem 2000

41. Coetzee GA, Ross RK: Re: Prostate cancer and the androgen receptor. J Natl Cancer Inst 86: 872–873, 1994

42. Irvine RA, Yu MC, Ross RK, Coetzee GA: The CAG and GGC microsatellites of the androgen receptor gene are in linkage disequilibrium in men with prostate cancer. Cancer Res 55: 1937–1940, 1995

43. Ingles SA, Ross RK, Yu MC, Irvine RA, La Pera G, Haile RW, Coetzee GA: Association of prostate cancer risk with genetic polymorphisms in vitamin D receptor and androgen receptor. J Natl Cancer Inst 89: 166–170, 1997

44. Hakimi JM, Schoenberg MP, Rondinelli RH, Piantadosi S, Barrack ER: Androgen receptor variants with short glutamine or glycine repeats may identify unique subpopulations of men with prostate cancer. Clin Cancer Res 3: 1599–1608, 1997

45. Hardy DO, Scher HI, Bogenreider T, Sabbatini P, Zhang ZF, Nanus DM, Catterall JF: Androgen receptor CAG repeat lengths in prostate cancer: Correlation with age of onset. J Clin Endocrinol Metab 81: 4400–4405, 1996

84

46. Stanford JL, Just JJ, Gibbs M, Wicklund KG, Neal CL, Blumenstein BA, Ostrander EA: Polymorphic repeats in the androgen receptor gene: Molecular markers of prostate cancer risk. Cancer Res 57: 1194–1198, 1997

47. Hsing AW, Gao YT, Wu G, Wang X, Deng J, Chen YL, Sesterhenn IA, Mostofi FK, Benichou J, Chang C: Polymorphic CAG and GGN repeat lengths in the androgen receptor gene and prostate cancer risk: A population-based case-control study in China. Cancer Res 60: 5111–5116, 2000

48. So CW, Dong S, So CK, Cheng GX, Huang QH, Chen SJ, Chan LC: The impact of differential binding of wild-type RARalpha, PML-. Leukemia 14: 77–83, 2000

49. Ekman P, Gronberg H, Matsuyama H, Kivineva M, Bergerheim US, Li C: Links between genetic and environmental factors and prostate cancer risk. Prostate 39: 262–268, 1999

50. Edwards SM, Badzioch MD, Minter R, Hamoudi R, Collins N, Ardern-Jones A, Dowe A, Osborne S, Kelly J, Shearer R, Easton DF, Saunders GF, Dearnaley DP, Eeles RA: Androgen receptor polymorphisms: Association with prostate cancer risk, relapse and overall survival. Int J Cancer 84: 458–465, 1999

51. Correa-Cerro L, Wohr G, Haussler J, Berthon P, Drelon E, Mangin P, Fournier G, Cussenot O, Kraus P, Just W, Paiss T, Cantu JM, Vogel W: (CAG)nCAA and GGN repeats in the human androgen receptor gene are not associated with prostate cancer in a French-German population. Eur J Hum Genet 7: 357–362, 1999

52. Bratt O, Borg A, Kristoffersson U, Lundgren R, Zhang QX, Olsson H: CAG repeat length in the androgen receptor gene is related to age at diagnosis of prostate cancer and response to endocrine therapy, but not to prostate cancer risk. Br J Cancer 81: 672–676, 1999

53. Lange EM, Chen H, Brierley K, Livermore H, Wojno KJ, Langefeld CD, Lange K, Cooney KA: The polymorphic exon 1 androgen receptor CAG repeat in men with a potential inherited predisposition to prostate cancer. Cancer Epidemiol Biomarkers Prev 9: 439–442, 2000

54. Nam RK, Elhaji Y, Krahn MD, Hakimi J, Ho M, Chu W, Sweet J, Trachtenberg J, Jewett MA, Narod SA: Significance of the cag repeat polymorphism of the androgen receptor gene in prostate cancer progression. J Urol 164: 567–572, 2000

55. Latil AG, Azzouzi R, Cancel GS, Guillaume EC, Cochan-Priollet B, Berthon PL, Cussenot O: Prostate carcinoma risk and allelic variants of genes involved in androgen biosynthesis and metabolism pathways. Cancer 92: 1130–1137, 2001

56. Modugno F, Weissfeld JL, Trump DL, Zmuda JM, Shea P, Cauley JA, Ferrell RE: Allelic variants of aromatase and the androgen and estrogen receptors: Toward a multigenic model of prostate cancer risk. Clin Cancer Res 7: 3092–3096, 2001

57. Miller EA, Stanford JL, Hsu L, Noonan E, Ostrander EA: Polymorphic repeats in the androgen receptor gene in high-risk sibships. Prostate 48: 200–205, 2001

58. Panz VR, Joffe BI, Spitz I, Lindenberg T, Farkas A, Haffejee M: Tandem CAG repeats of the androgen receptor gene and prostate cancer risk in black and white men. Endocrine 15: 213–216, 2001

59. Butler R, Leigh PN, McPhaul MJ, Gallo JM: Truncated forms of the androgen receptor are associated with polyglutamine expansion in X-linked spinal and bulbar muscular atrophy. Hum Mol Genet 7: 121–127, 1998

60. Hsiao PW, Lin DL, Nakao R, Chang C: The linkage of Kennedy's neuron disease to ARA24, the first identified androgen receptor polyglutamine region-associated coactivator. J Biol Chem 274: 20229–20234, 1999

61. Rush MG, Drivas G, D'Eustachio P: The small nuclear GTPase Ran: How much does it run? Bioessays 18: 103–112, 1996

62. Zhang L, Leeflang EP, Yu J, Arnheim N: Studying human mutations by sperm typing: Instability of CAG trinucleotide repeats in the human androgen receptor gene. Nat Genet 7: 531–535, 1994

63. Lu S, Tsai SY, Tsai MJ: Molecular mechanisms of androgen-independent growth of human prostate cancer LNCaP-AI cells. Endocrinology 140: 5054–5059, 1999

64. Platz EA, Giovannucci E, Dahl DM, Krithivas K, Hennekens CH, Brown M, Stampfer MJ, Kantoff PW: The androgen receptor gene GGN microsatellite and prostate cancer risk. Cancer Epidemiol Biomarkers Prev 7: 379–384, 1998

65. Tilley WD, Lim-Tio SS, Horsfall DJ, Aspinall JO, Marshall VR, Skinner JM: Detection of discrete androgen receptor epitopes in prostate cancer by immunostaining: Measurement by color video image analysis. Cancer Res 54: 4096–4102, 1994

66. Prins GS, Sklarew RJ, Pertschuk LP: Image analysis of androgen receptor immunostaining in prostate cancer accurately predicts response to hormonal therapy. J Urol 159: 641–649, 1998

67. Sadi MV, Barrack ER: Image analysis of androgen receptor immunostaining in metastatic prostate cancer. Heterogeneity as a predictor of response to hormonal therapy. Cancer 71: 2574–2580, 1993

68. Takeda H, Akakura K, Masai M, Akimoto S, Yatani R, Shimazaki J: Androgen receptor content of prostate carcinoma cells estimated by immunohistochemistry is related to prognosis of patients with stage D2 prostate carcinoma. Cancer 77: 934–940, 1996

69. Pertschuk LP, Schaeffer H, Feldman JG, Macchia RJ, Kim YD, Eisenberg K, Braithwaite LV, Axiotis CA, Prins G, Green GL: Immunostaining for prostate cancer androgen receptor in paraffin identifies a subset of men with a poor prognosis. Lab Invest 73: 302–305, 1995

70. Pertschuk LP, Macchia RJ, Feldman JG, Brady KA, Levine M, Kim DS, Eisenberg KB, Rainford E, Prins GS, Greene GL: Immunocytochemical assay for androgen receptors in prostate cancer: A prospective study of 63 cases with long-term follow-up. Ann Surg Oncol 1: 495–503, 1994

71. Sweat SD, Pacelli A, Bergstralh EJ, Slezak JM, Bostwick DG: Androgen receptor expression in prostatic intraepithelial neoplasia and cancer. J Urol 161: 1229–1232, 1999

72. Kattan MW, Wheeler TM, Scardino PT: Postoperative nomogram for disease recurrence after radical prostatectomy for prostate cancer. J Clin Oncol 17: 1499–1507, 1999

73. Henshall SM, Quinn DI, Lee CS, Head DR, Golovsky D, Brenner PC, Delprado W, Stricker PD, Grygiel JJ, Sutherland RL: Altered expression of androgen receptor in the malignant epithelium and adjacent stroma is associated with early relapse in prostate cancer. Cancer Res 61: 423–427, 2001

74. Koivisto P, Kononen J, Palmberg C, Tammela T, Hyytinen E, Isola J, Trapman J, Cleutjens K, Noordzij A, Visakorpi T, Kallioniemi OP: Androgen receptor gene amplification: A possible molecular mechanism for androgen deprivation therapy failure in prostate cancer. Cancer Res 57: 314–319, 1997

75. Jarrard DF, Kinoshita H, Shi Y, Sandefur C, Hoff D, Meisner LF, Chang C, Herman JG, Isaacs WB, Nassif N: Methylation of the androgen receptor promoter CpG island is associated with loss of androgen receptor expression in prostate cancer cells. Cancer Res 58: 5310–5314, 1998

76. Kinoshita H, Shi Y, Sandefur C, Meisner LF, Chang C, Choon A, Reznikoff CR, Bova GS, Friedl A, Jarrard DF: Methylation of the androgen receptor minimal promoter silences transcription in human prostate cancer. Cancer Res 60: 3623–3630, 2000

77. Yeap BB, Krueger RG, Leedman PJ: Differential posttranscriptional regulation of androgen receptor gene expression by androgen in prostate and breast cancer cells. Endocrinology 140: 3282–3291, 1999

78. Wen Y, Hu MC, Makino K, Spohn B, Bartholomeusz G, Yan DH, Hung MC: HER-2/neu promotes androgen-independent survival and growth of prostate cancer cells through the Akt pathway. Cancer Res 60: 6841–6845, 2000

79. Ruohola JK, Valve EM, Karkkainen MJ, Joukov V, Alitalo K, Harkonen PL: Vascular endothelial growth factors are differentially regulated by steroid hormones and antiestrogens in breast cancer cells. Mol Cell Endocrinol 149: 29–40, 1999

80. Goldberg YP, Kalchman MA, Metzler M, Nasir J, Zeisler J, Graham R, Koide HB, O'Kusky J, Sharp AH, Ross CA, Jirik F, Hayden MR: Absence of disease phenotype and intergenerational stability of the CAG repeat in transgenic mice expressing the human Huntington disease transcript. Hum Mol Genet 5: 177–185, 1996

81. Lu S, Tsai SY, Tsai MJ: Regulation of androgen-dependent prostatic cancer cell growth: Androgen regulation of CDK2, CDK4, and CKI p16 genes. Cancer Res 57: 4511–4516, 1997

82. Bubendorf L, Kononen J, Koivisto P, Schraml P, Moch H, Gasser TC, Willi N, Mihatsch MJ, Sauter G, Kallioniemi OP: Survey of gene amplifications during prostate cancer progression by high-throughout fluorescence in situ hybridization on tissue microarrays. Cancer Res 59: 803–806, 1999

83. Koivisto PA, Helin HJ: Androgen receptor gene amplification increases tissue PSA protein expression in hormone-refractory prostate carcinoma. J Pathol 189: 219–223, 1999

84. Jenster G: Ligand-independent activation of the androgen receptor in prostate cancer by growth factors and cytokines. J Pathol 191: 227–228, 2000

85. Buchanan G, Greenberg NM, Scher HI, Harris JM, Marshall VR, Tilley WD: Collocation of androgen receptor gene mutations in prostate cancer. Clin Cancer Res 7: 1273–1281, 2001

86. Grossmann ME, Huang H, Tindall DJ: Androgen receptor signaling in androgen-refractory prostate cancer. J Natl Cancer Inst 93: 1687–1697, 2001

87. Wong CI, Zhou ZX, Sar M, Wilson EM: Steroid requirement for androgen receptor dimerization and DNA binding. Modulation by intramolecular interactions between the NH2-terminal and steroid-binding domains. J Biol Chem 268: 19004–19012, 1993

88. Quarmby VE, Beckman WCJ, Cooke DB, Lubahn DB, Joseph DR, Wilson EM, French FS: Expression and localization of androgen receptor in the R-3327 Dunning rat prostatic adenocarcinoma. Cancer Res 50: 735–739, 1990

89. Tilley WD, Wilson CM, Marcelli M, McPhaul MJ: Androgen receptor gene expression in human prostate carcinoma cell lines. Cancer Res 50: 5382–5386, 1990

90. Culig Z, Hobisch A, Hittmair A, Peterziel H, Cato AC, Bartsch G, Klocker H: Expression, structure, and function of androgen receptor in advanced prostatic carcinoma. Prostate 35: 63–70, 1998

91. Koivisto P, Visakorpi T, Kallioniemi OP: Androgen receptor gene amplification: A novel molecular mechanism for endocrine therapy resistance in human prostate cancer. Scand J Clin Lab Invest (Suppl 226): 57–63, 1996

92. Veldscholte J, Ris-Stalpers C, Kuiper GG, Jenster G, Berrevoets C, Claassen E, van Rooij HC, Trapman J, Brinkmann AO, Mulder E: A mutation in the ligand binding domain of the androgen receptor of human LNCaP cells affects steroid binding characteristics and response to antiandrogens. Biochem Biophys Res Commun 173: 534–540, 1990

93. Zhao XY, Malloy PJ, Krishnan AV, Swami S, Navone NM, Peehl DM, Feldman D: Glucocorticoids can promote androgen-independent growth of prostate cancer cells through a mutated androgen receptor. Nat Med 6: 703–706, 2000

94. Buchanan G, Tilley WD: Androgen Receptor Structure and Function in Prostate Cancer. In: Li JJ, Darling JR, Li SA (eds) Hormonal Carcinogenesis III, Springer-Verlag, New York, 2000, pp 333–341

95. Gelmann EP: Androgen receptor mutations in prostate cancer. Cancer Treat Res 87: 285–302, 1996

96. Han G, Foster BA, Mistry S, Buchanan G, Harris JM, Tilley WD, Greenberg NM: Hormone status selects for spontaneous somatic androgen receptor variants that demonstrate specific ligand and cofactor dependent activities in autochthonous prostate cancer. J Biol Chem 276: 11204–11213, 2001

97. Wurtz JM, Bourguet W, Renaud JP, Vivat V, Chambon P, Moras D, Gronemeyer H: A canonical structure for the ligand-binding domain of nuclear receptors. Nat Struct Biol 3: 206, 1996

86

98. Veldscholte J, Berrevoets CA, Ris-Stalpers C, Kuiper GG, Jenster G, Trapman J, Brinkmann AO, Mulder E: The androgen receptor in LNCaP cells contains a mutation in the ligand binding domain which affects steroid binding characteristics and response to antiandrogens. J Steroid Biochem Mol Biol 41: 665–669, 1992

99. Matias PM, Donner P, Coelho R, Thomaz M, Peixoto C, Macedo S, Otto N, Joschko S, Scholz P, Wegg A, Basler S, Schafer M, Egner U, Carrondo MA: Structural evidence for ligand specificity in the binding domain of the human Androgen receptor: Implications for pathogenic gene mutations. J Biol Chem 275: 26164–26171, 2000

100. Sack JS, Kish KF, Wang C, Attar RM, Kiefer SE, An Y, Wu GY, Scheffler JE, Salvati ME, Krystek SR, Weinmann R, Einspahr HM: Crystallographic structures of the ligand-binding domains of the androgen receptor and its T877A mutant complexed with the natural agonist dihydrotestosterone. Proc Natl Acad Sci USA 98: 4904–4909, 2001

101. Tilley WD, Buchanan G, Hickey TE, Bentel JM: Mutations in the androgen receptor gene are associated with progression of human prostate cancer to androgen independence. Clin Cancer Res 2: 277–285, 1996

102. Marcelli M, Ittmann M, Mariani S, Sutherland R, Nigam R, Murthy L, Zhao Y, DiConcini D, Puxeddu E, Esen A, Eastham J, Weigel NL, Lamb DJ: Androgen receptor mutations in prostate cancer. Cancer Res 60: 944–949, 2000

103. Aarnisalo P, Santti H, Poukka H, Palvimo JJ, Janne OA: Transcription activating and repressing functions of the androgen receptor are differentially influenced by mutations in the deoxyribonucleic acid-binding domain. Endocrinology 140: 3097–3105, 1999

104. Bruggenwirth HT, Boehmer AL, Lobaccaro JM, Chiche L, Sultan C, Trapman J, Brinkmann AO: Substitution of Ala564 in the first zinc cluster of the deoxyribonucleic acid (DNA)-binding domain of the androgen receptor by Asp, Asn, or Leu exerts differential effects on DNA binding. Endocrinology 139: 103–110, 1998

105. Poujol N, Lobaccaro JM, Chiche L, Lumbroso S, Sultan C: Functional and structural analysis of R607Q and R608K androgen receptor substitutions associated with male breast cancer. Mol Cell Endocrinol 130: 43–51, 1997

106. Rundlett SE, Miesfeld RL: Quantitative differences in androgen and glucocorticoid receptor DNA binding properties contribute to receptor-selective transcriptional regulation. Mol Cell Endocrinol 109: 1–10, 1995

107. Verrijdt G, Schoenmakers E, Haelens A, Peeters B, Verhoeven G, Rombauts W, Claessens F: Change of specificity mutations in androgen-selective enhancers. Evidence for a role of differential DNA binding by the androgen receptor. J Biol Chem 275: 12298–12305, 2000

108. Blanco JG, Minucci S, Lu J, Yang XJ, Walker KK, Chen H, Evans RM, Nakatani Y, Ozato K: The histone acetylase PCAF is a nuclear receptor coactivator. Genes Dev 12: 1638–1651, 1998

109. Moilanen AM, Karvonen U, Poukka H, Yan W, Toppari J, Janne OA, Palvimo JJ: A testis-specific androgen receptor coregulator that belongs to a novel family of nuclear proteins. J Biol Chem 274: 3700–3704, 1999

110. Moilanen AM, Poukka H, Karvonen U, Hakli M, Janne OA, Palvimo JJ: Identification of a novel RING finger protein as a coregulator in steroid receptor-mediated gene transcription. Mol Cell Biol 18: 5128–5139, 1998

111. Poukka H, Karvonen U, Yoshikawa N, Tanaka H, Palvimo JJ, Janne OA: The RING finger protein SNURF modulates nuclear trafficking of the androgen receptor. J Cell Sci 113: 2991–3001, 2000

112. Chamberlain NL, Whitacre DC, Miesfeld RL: Delineation of two distinct type 1 activation functions in the androgen receptor amino-terminal domain. J Biol Chem 271: 26772–26778, 1996

113. Gao T, Marcelli M, McPhaul MJ: Transcriptional activation and transient expression of the human androgen receptor. J Steroid Biochem Mol Biol 59: 9–20, 1996

114. Schoenberg MP, Hakimi JM, Wang S, Bova GS, Epstein JI, Fischbeck KH, Isaacs WB, Walsh PC, Barrack ER: Microsatellite mutation (CAG24–>18) in the androgen receptor gene in human prostate cancer. Biochem Biophys Res Commun 198: 74–80, 1994

115. Watanabe M, Ushijima T, Shiraishi T, Yatani R, Shimazaki J, Kotake T, Sugimura T, Nagao M: Genetic alterations of androgen receptor gene in Japanese human prostate cancer. Jpn J Clin Oncol 27: 389–393, 1997

116. Wallen MJ, Linja M, Kaartinen K, Schleutker J, Visakorpi T: Androgen receptor gene mutations in hormone-refractory prostate cancer. J Pathol 189: 559–563, 1999

117. Yang M, Raynor M, Neufing PJ, Buchanan G, Tilley WD: Disruption of the polyglutamine tract results in increased ligand-induced transcriptional activity of the androgen receptor. Proc Amer Ass Canc Res 40 (Abstract 2699): 408, 1999

118. Ma H, Hong H, Huang SM, Irvine RA, Webb P, Kushner PJ, Coetzee GA, Stallcup MR: Multiple signal input and output domains of the 160-kilodalton nuclear receptor coactivator proteins. Mol Cell Biol 19: 6164–6173, 1999

119. Fronsdal K, Engedal N, Slagsvold T, Saatcioglu F: CREB binding protein is a coactivator for the androgen receptor and mediates cross-talk with AP-1. J Biol Chem 273: 31853–31859, 1998

120. Kupfer SR, Marschke KB, Wilson EM, French FS: Receptor accessory factor enhances specific DNA binding of androgen and glucocorticoid receptors. J Biol Chem 268: 17519–17527, 1993

121. Gregory CW, He B, Johnson RT, Ford OH, Mohler JL, French FS, Wilson EM: A mechanism for androgen receptor-mediated prostate cancer recurrence after androgen deprivation therapy. Cancer Res 61: 4315–4319, 2001

122. Kantoff P, Giovannucci E, Brown M: The androgen receptor CAG repeat polymorphism and its relationship to prostate cancer. Biochim Biophys Acta 1378: C1–C5, 1998

123. Zhou BP, Hu MC, Miller SA, Yu Z, Xia W, Lin SY, Hung MC: HER-2/neu blocks tumor necrosis factor-induced apoptosis via the Akt/NF-kappaB pathway. J Biol Chem 275: 8027–8031, 2000

124. Signoretti S, Montironi R, Manola J, Altimari A, Tam C, Bubley G, Balk S, Thomas G, Kaplan I, Hlatky L, Hahnfeldt P, Kantoff P, Loda M: Her-2-neu expression

and progression toward androgen independence in human prostate cancer. J Natl Cancer Inst 92: 1918–1925, 2000

125. Osman I, Scher HI, Drobnjak M, Verbel D, Morris M, Agus D, Ross JS, Cordon-Cardo C: HER-2/neu (p185neu) protein expression in the natural or treated history of prostate cancer. Clin Cancer Res 7: 2643–2647, 2001

126. Craft N, Shostak Y, Carey M, Sawyers CL: A mechanism for hormone-independent prostate cancer through modulation of androgen receptor signaling by the HER-2/neu tyrosine kinase. Nat Med 5: 280–285, 1999

127. Sadar MD, Gleave ME: Ligand-independent activation of the androgen receptor by the differentiation agent butyrate in human prostate cancer cells. Cancer Res 60: 5825–5831, 2000

128. Agus DB, Scher HI, Higgins B, Fox WD, Heller G, Fazzari M, Cordon-Cardo C, Golde DW: Response of prostate cancer to anti-Her-2/neu antibody in androgen-dependent and -independent human xenograft models. Cancer Res 59: 4761–4764, 1999

129. Labrie F, Dupont A, Cusan L, Gomez J, Emond J, Monfette G: Combination therapy with flutamide and medical (LHRH agonist) or surgical castration in advanced prostate cancer: 7-year clinical experience. J Steroid Biochem Mol Biol 37: 943–950, 1990

130. Schmitt B, Bennett C, Seidenfeld J, Samson D, Wilt T: Maximal androgen blockade for advanced prostate cancer. Cochrane Database Syst RevCD001526, 2000

131. Kelly WK, Slovin S, Scher HI: Steroid hormone withdrawal syndromes. Pathophysiology and clinical significance. Urol Clin North Am 24: 421–431, 1997

132. Kelly WK, Scher HI: Prostate specific antigen decline after antiandrogen withdrawal: The flutamide withdrawal syndrome. J Urol 149: 607–609, 1993

133. Small EJ, Srinivas S: The antiandrogen withdrawal syndrome. Experience in a large cohort of unselected patients with advanced prostate cancer. Cancer 76: 1428–1434, 1995

134. Huan SD, Gerridzen RG, Yau JC, Stewart DJ: Antiandrogen withdrawal syndrome with nilutamide. Urology 49: 632–634, 1997

135. Nieh PT: Withdrawal phenomenon with the antiandrogen casodex. J Urol 153: 1070–1072, 1995

136. Small EJ, Carroll PR: Prostate-specific antigen decline after casodex withdrawal: Evidence for an antiandrogen withdrawal syndrome. Urology 43: 408–410, 1994

137. Bissada NK, Kaczmarek AT: Complete remission of hormone refractory adenocarcinoma of the prostate in response to withdrawal of diethylstilbestrol. J Urol 153: 1944–1945, 1995

138. Dawson NA, McLeod DG: Dramatic prostate specific antigen decrease in response to discontinuation of megestrol acetate in advanced prostate cancer: Expansion of the antiandrogen withdrawal syndrome. J Urol 153: 1946–1947, 1995

139. Akakura K, Akimoto S, Furuya Y, Ito H: Incidence and characteristics of antiandrogen withdrawal syndrome in prostate cancer after treatment with chlormadinone acetate. Eur Urol 33: 567–571, 1998

140. Scher HI, Kelly WK: Flutamide withdrawal syndrome: Its impact on clinical trials in hormone-refractory prostate cancer. J Clin Oncol 11: 1566–1572, 1993

141. Small EJ, Baron A, Bok R: Simultaneous antiandrogen withdrawal and treatment with ketoconazole and hydrocortisone in patients with advanced prostate carcinoma. Cancer 80: 1755–1759, 1997

142. Taplin ME, Bubley GJ, Ko YJ, Small EJ, Upton M, Rajeshkumar B, Balk SP: Selection of androgen receptor mutations in prostate cancers treated with androgen antagonists. Cancer Res 59: 2511–2515, 1999

143. Yeh S, Kang HY, Miyamoto H, Nishimura K, Chang HC, Ting HJ, Rahman M, Lin HK, Fujimoto N, Hu YC, Mizokami A, Huang KE, Chang C: Differential induction of androgen receptor transactivation by different androgen receptor coactivators in human prostate cancer DU145 cells. Endocrine 11: 195–202, 1999

Address for offprints: Wayne D. Tilley, Dame Roma Mitchell Cancer Research Laboratories, University of Adelaide, Hanson Institute, PO Box 14, Rundle Mall, SA 5000, Australia; *Tel:* 61-8-8222 3033, *Fax:* 61-8-8222 3035; *e-mail:* wayne.tilley@imvs.sa.gov.au

Regulation of apoptosis in prostate cancer

Sushma Gurumurthy[1], Krishna Murthi Vasudevan[2] and Vivek M. Rangnekar[1,2,3,4]
[1]Graduate Center for Toxicology, [2]Department of Microbiology and Immunology, [3]Department of Radiation Medicine, [4]L.P. Markey Cancer Center, University of Kentucky, Lexington, KY, USA

Key words: prostate cancer, apoptosis, genes

Abstract

Transformation and malignant progression of prostate cancer is regulated by the inability of prostatic epithelial cells to undergo apoptosis rather than by increased cell proliferation. The basic apoptotic machinery of most prostate cancer cells is intact and the inability to undergo apoptosis is due to molecular alterations that result in failure to initiate or execute apoptotic pathways. This review discusses the role of anti-apoptotic proteins such as Bcl-2/Bcl$_{XL}$, NF-κB, IGF, caveolin, and Akt, and pro-apoptotic molecules such as PTEN, p53, Bin1, TGF-β, and Par-4 that can regulate progression of prostate cancer. In addition to highlighting the salient features of these molecules and their relevance in apoptosis, this review provides an appraisal of their therapeutic potential in prostate cancer. Molecular targeting of these proteins and/or their innate pro- or anti-apoptotic pathways, either singly or in combination, may be explored in conjunction with conventional and currently available experimental strategies for the treatment of both hormone-sensitive and hormone-resistant prostate cancer.

Introduction

Deregulation of cell proliferation in conjunction with the suppression of apoptosis constitutes a minimal common platform for the initiation and progression of most neoplastic lesions [1]. However, inhibition of apoptosis rather than enhanced cellular proliferation is the critical pathophysiological factor that contributes to the development of prostatic adenocarcinoma [2]. Cells of the normal adult prostate or those constituting primary prostate cancer are dependent on androgen for survival and proliferation. Upon withdrawal of androgen the rate of apoptosis overtakes the rate of cell proliferation, thereby causing involution of the normal prostate and regression of the tumor [3]. This observation has contributed to the establishment of androgen-ablation as the mainstay form of treatment for prostate cancer. The natural history of prostate cancer, however, follows a pattern of progression from localized disease that is androgen-dependent to more advanced, invasive and metastatic disease, which is often associated with loss of androgen-dependence [4,5]. As androgen-ablation treatment targets the androgen-dependent cells, the heterogeneous presence of androgen-independent prostatic cancer

cells within the tumor leads to development of an androgen-independent disease in about 30% of the patients within about 3 years of treatment [6]. The development of androgen-independent prostate cancer is a consequence of lack of an apoptotic response to androgen-ablation owing to mechanisms that allow survival of the cells within primary or metastatic tumors [7,8]. Androgen-independent cells contain intact cell death programs but they fail to initiate or execute these programs in response to conventional modes of treatment, thereby tilting the balance in favor of cell proliferation [9]. The potential to induce apoptosis by overriding the roadblocks created by the anti-apoptotic mechanisms in androgen-independent or metastatic cells is, thus, one of the salient traits indispensable to any effective therapeutic regimen of prostate cancer. This review highlights the molecular mechanisms that may contribute to the anti-apoptotic roadblocks to treatment and further identifies potential molecular approaches that may be exploited to circumvent or override these anti-apoptotic mechanisms in prostate cancer cells. Following an introduction of the general features of apoptosis that are common to mammalian cells, this review describes the salient characteristics of anti-apoptotic molecules such as Bcl-2/Bcl$_{XL}$, NF-κB,

M.L. Cher, K.V. Honn and A. Raz (eds.), Prostate Cancer: New Horizons in Research and Treatment, 89–107.
© 2002 *Kluwer Academic Publishers.*

IGF, caveolin and Akt, and pro-apoptotic molecules such as PTEN, p53, Bin1, TGF-β, and Par-4 that serve to regulate the progression of prostate cancer (Table 1). Finally, the concluding remarks emphasize the untapped potential of these molecular targets in prostate cancer therapy.

General features of apoptosis

Apoptosis is characterized by stereotypic morphological changes, evident in the nucleus where chromatin condenses to compact geometric figures accompanied by cytoplasmic shrinkage, phosphatidylserine

(PS) exposure on the cell membrane, zeiosis and formation of apoptotic bodies [10,11]. The molecular and biochemical pathways involved in apoptosis (Figure 1) can be broadly grouped as 'private' pathways and 'common' pathways. The private pathways reflect the usage of distinct early cascades of molecular events that are activated specifically depending on the type of exogenous insult such as tumor necrosis factor (TNF), ionizing or ultraviolet radiation, or growth factor- or androgen-withdrawal, and cell type involved. The private pathways induced by diverse insults converge on a common pathway comprising of a set of molecular components collectively known as caspases that activate a cascade of proteolytic events

Table 1. Regulators of apoptosis in prostate cancer

Protein	Function	Significance in prostate cancer	Reference
Bcl-2	Anti-apoptotic protein.	Over-expressed in 70% androgen-independent prostate cancers, contributes to chemoresistance and metastasis.	[9]
Bcl_{XL}	Anti-apoptotic protein.	Over-expressed in all prostate cancers, contributes to chemoresistance. Over-expressed in prostate cancer cell line DU-145.	[30]
Bax	Pro-apoptotic protein.	Loss of expression in DU-145 cells.	[47]
NF-κB	Anti-apoptotic transcription factor, induces apoptosis inhibitors, IAPs, Bcl_{XL} and metastatic proteins, VEGF, IL-8.	Elevated activity in androgen-independent prostate cancer cells PC-3, DU-145. Contributes to invasiveness and chemoresistance.	[51,60,50]
IKK	IκB kinase, increases NF-κB activity by promoting degradation of IκB.	Constitutively active in the PC-3 and DU-145 cells.	[51]
IκB	Binds to p65 and retains it in the cytoplasm.	Found to be up-regulated by androgen receptor (AR) in androgen-dependent prostate cancer cells.	[56]
Caveolin	Integral membrane protein, involved in various signaling and transport processes.	Over-expressed in metastatic prostate cancer in rat and humans. Inhibits c-myc induced apoptosis, and interacts with AR to promote androgen-independence.	[75,72]
IGF-I	Growth factor, provides mitogenic stimulus to prostate cancer. Anti-apoptotic protein.	IGF-I elevated in some cases of prostate cancer. IGF-IR promotes invasion and metastasis.	[61]
Akt	Pro-survival/anti-apoptotic kinase. Phosphorylation-mediated activation of IKK and inactivation of Bad, caspase-9.	Akt-3 isoform promotes metastatic progression. Involved in signaling cross-talk with the AR that contributes to androgen-independence.	[80,82]
PTEN	Tumor suppressor, phosphatase activity inhibits activation of Akt.	Silenced through methylation of promoter, and deletion. Deleted in LNCaP and PC-3 cells. Replenishment induces apoptosis.	[85]
p53	Tumor suppressor, transcription factor, pro-apoptotic protein.	Inactivated in advanced prostate cancers, mainly bone metastases. Deleted in PC-3 and DU-145 cells.	[91]
Bin1	Tumor suppressor, c-myc interacting protein.	Deleted in metastatic disease, reduced expression in PC-3 and DU-145 cells. Ectopic expression induces apoptosis in cancer cells.	[106]
TGF-β	Cell secretory growth factor, causes growth inhibition and apoptosis in normal prostate.	Loss of TGF-β sensitivity leads to prostate cancer. Loss of TGF-β receptors seen in prostate cancers.	[116,119]
Par-4	Pro-apoptotic protein induced by apoptotic stimuli.	Ectopic Par-4 induces apoptosis, selectively, in androgen-independent prostate cancer cells and causes tumor regression.	[15,20]

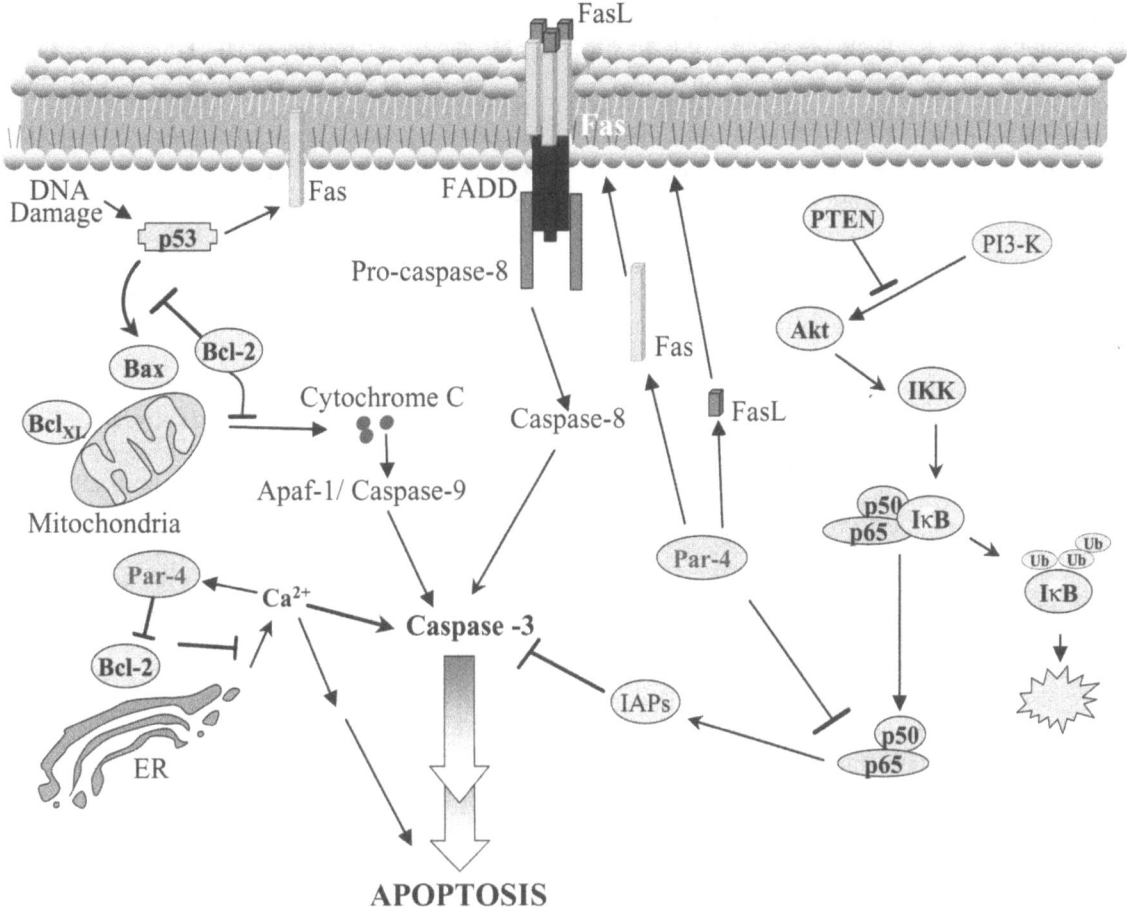

Figure 1. Pro- and anti-apoptotic pathways in the prostate. Apoptosis is initiated by activation of private pathways that are specific to the type of apoptotic insult or activator. Most private pathways culminate in activation of the effector caspases, which induce cell death. Private pathways: (a) receptor-mediated, for example binding of FasL to its receptor Fas triggers binding of FADD to the receptor and activates the common cell death pathway following caspase-8 activation; (b) mitochondrial initiation, triggered by apoptotic insults such as DNA damage, is associated with release of cytochrome C, Apaf and activation of caspase-9, and is prevented by Bcl-2 members Bcl-2 and Bcl$_{XL}$ and (c) release of Ca^{2+} from the endoplasmic reticulum (ER) leading to activation of caspases as well as Ca^{2+} dependent endonucleases. Most private pathways result in activation of caspase-3 which causes cell death by activation of death mediators such nucleases and translocases and by degradation of structural and survival proteins. Pro-apoptotic proteins such as p53 or Par-4 activate different private pathways by promoting trafficking Fas to the cell membrane and inhibition of Bcl-2 or NF-κB. Anti-apoptotic proteins Akt and NF-κB block apoptosis by up-regulation of the IAP family of proteins, which inhibit the activity of various caspases. *Abbreviations*: FADD: Fas Associated Death Domain, FasL: Fas ligand, Par-4: Prostate apoptosis response-4, IAP: Inhibitor of Apoptosis proteins.

leading to nucleosomal DNA fragmentation. The private pathways of apoptosis can be generally categorized into: (a) the extrinsic pathway that involves ligation of the cell surface death receptors such as Fas/CD95, TNF-R1, or TRAIL by their corresponding ligand leading to binding and activation of the death domain protein FADD and caspase-8; or (b) the intrinsic pathway, triggered by ionizing or ultraviolet radiation or by agents that elevate intracellular Ca^{2+} that causes alterations in the mitochondria leading

to at least three different cell death pathways [11]. The first of these mitochondrial pathways involves classical apoptosis by cytochrome C release into the cytosol; the second involves necrotic programed cell death mediated by release of reactive oxygen species; and the third involves the release of apoptosis inducing factor leading to paraptosis, which does not involve nucleosomal DNA fragmentation. Both pro- and anti-apoptotic members of the Bcl-2 family of proteins are localized on the outer mitochondrial membrane, where

92

they compete to regulate the release of cytochrome C. The functional predominance of pro-apoptotic molecules results in the cytosolic release of cytochrome C, which associates with Apaf-1 and pro-caspase-9 to form the apoptosome. The death receptor-mediated and mitochondrial/apoptosome-mediated pathways converge at the level of downstream effector caspases, mainly caspase-3. Further downstream of caspase-3 activation, the apoptotic program branches into a multitude of subprograms, the end result of which is ordered dismantling and removal of the cell corpse [10,11]. It is important to note that the extrinsic pathway downstream of caspase-8, depending on the cell type, converges either directly on caspase-3 or indirectly on caspase-3 via the mitochondrial activation pathway.

Caspases are a group of cysteine-containing proteases that specifically cleave aspartate-containing domains in the downstream target caspases, so as to activate them, or in the case of pro-survival cellular substrates so as to inactivate them [12]. As many as 14 caspases have been identified and classified as initiator caspases and effector caspases. The initiator caspases, such as caspase-2, -8, -9, and -10 are activated by various apoptotic signals, and upon activation they in turn cleave and activate downstream effector caspases. The effector caspases, such as caspase-3, -6, and -7 target specific cellular protein substrates to either activate or inactivate them [10,12]. For example, caspase-3 activates endonucleases, responsible for nucleosomal DNA fragmentation, and scramblase, an enzyme responsible for flipping of PS to the outer leaflet of the cell membrane [13].

Several alternative caspase-3-independent cell death programs have been described recently [11]. These are usually mediated by serine proteases like calpain and cathepsin but may be switched on by death receptor activation or mitochondrial engagement as in classical apoptosis. The relevance of these alternate forms of apoptosis has not been addressed in prostate cancer cells but may be of interest considering the prominent role played by Ca^{2+} in androgen-ablation-induced apoptosis in the prostate.

Cell surface changes that allow recognition and removal of the apoptotic cell are now considered the most important set of events in apoptosis. PS is expressed on the inner leaflet of the membrane bilayer in normal cells. Caspase-activation of the enzyme scramblase and Ca^{2+} inhibition of translocase [13] leads to permanent expression of PS on the cell surface. This change on the apoptotic cell surface is recognized by the PS receptor, PSR. Physical interaction of PS and PSR leads to engulfment of the apoptotic cell by professional phagocytic cells and also most neighboring tissue cells.

Both androgen-dependent and -independent prostate cancer cells have an intact apoptotic machinery [14]. For instance, the androgen-independent PC-3, DU-145, and the androgen-dependent LNCaP prostate cancer cells are differentially sensitive to Fas, TNF, or TRAIL induced apoptosis that is induced predominantly by activating caspase-8, -7, and -3 and release of cytochrome C. Resistance to apoptosis is due to alterations that block the apoptotic pathways at various levels. Androgen-independent prostate cancer cells fail to initiate apoptosis upon androgen-withdrawal owing to their inability to elevate intracellular Ca^{2+}. Over-expression of anti-apoptotic proteins Bcl-2 and Bcl_{XL}, constitutive activation of pro-survival proteins such as Akt and NF-κB, loss or inactivation of tumor suppressors such as p53, PTEN, and Bin1, all lead to inhibition of apoptosis [15]. These alterations along with others accumulate with the progression of the tumor, thereby contributing to the advancement of the localized cancer to androgen-independent metastasis.

Intracellular Ca^{2+}

Intracellular Ca^{2+} is an important signaling intermediate essential for apoptosis of both normal prostatic cells and prostate cancer cells following androgen-ablation [16]. Several chemotherapeutic agents also induce the release of intracellular Ca^{2+} to cause apoptosis. Withdrawal of androgen triggers the release of Ca^{2+} from the endoplasmic reticulum (ER); this is followed by a release-activated influx of extracellular Ca^{2+} resulting in rapid elevation of cytosolic Ca^{2+}. This further activates a series of Ca^{2+} dependent proteins, such as calmodulin, that initiate downstream apoptotic pathways. Support for the involvement of Ca^{2+} in androgen-induced apoptosis comes from the observation that agents that directly mobilize Ca^{2+} such as calcium ionophore ionomycin trigger apoptosis in rat or human prostatic cells and mimic regression of the prostate by hormone-ablation. Thapsigargin (TG), an irreversible inhibitor of sarcoplasmic/endoplasmic reticulum Ca^{2+} ATPase (SERCA) pump evokes a similar response. TG causes depletion of intracellular ER Ca^{2+} stores, resulting in elevation of cytosolic Ca^{2+}. Androgen-independent prostate cancer cells fail to undergo apoptosis post-androgen-ablation due to their inability to elevate intracellular Ca^{2+} [9]. Treatment with calcium ionophores or TG can activate apoptosis in androgen-independent prostate cancer cells. Dunning R-3327 AT3, a highly metastatic androgen-independent rat cell line, shows sustained elevation of Ca^{2+} upon treatment with ionomycin, and within 24 h the cells begin to fragment genomic DNA and undergo apoptosis [17]. The exact mechanism by which androgen-ablation results in the release of ER Ca^{2+} stores is not known. Release of intracellular Ca^{2+} activates Ca^{2+}-dependent protein calmodulin; activated calmodulin then binds plasma membrane Ca^{2+} ATPase pump resulting in the capacitative influx of extracellular Ca^{2+}. The entry of extracellular Ca^{2+} is essential for induction of apoptosis. The ability of nifedepine, a Ca^{2+} channel blocker, to delay prostate involution after androgen-ablation further supports this theory. Recently Wertz and Dixit showed that release of ER stores of Ca^{2+} is necessary and sufficient to induce apoptosis and the release activated influx of extracellular Ca^{2+} provides a synergistic elevation of Ca^{2+} and enhances the apoptotic events [18]. The increase in intracellular Ca^{2+}, induced either by hormone-withdrawal or TG treatment, results in epigenetic reprograming with an increase in expression of pro-apoptotic genes such as α-prothymosin, c-myc, and GADD153 [9,16,19], and prostate apoptosis response genes (Par) most notably Par-4 [20].

Intracellular Ca^{2+} elevation induces apoptosis through multiple subprograms dictated by downstream Ca^{2+}-dependent enzymes. Wyllie [21] has identified the role of Ca^{2+}/Mg^{2+}-dependent endonucleases involved in fragmentation of genomic DNA. Moreover, a Ca^{2+}-dependent endonuclease DNAse I is known to participate in apoptotic DNA degradation. Direct activation of Ca^{2+} proteases, calpain and nuclear scaffold protease mediate the degradation of cell integrity proteins fodrin and lamin, respectively [22]. Importantly, Ca^{2+} plays a critical role in maintaining the expression of PS on the outer membrane that is essential for clearance of the apoptotic cell corpse. This key role of Ca^{2+} involves the direct inhibition of the enzyme translocase, thereby preventing the translocation of PS back to the inner leaflet of the cell membrane [22]. Ca^{2+} is also capable of activating caspase-3, -7, and caspase-3-like activity necessary for nucleosomal DNA fragmentation and other morphological changes [18,23]. These observations imply that intracellular Ca^{2+} plays an integral role in the apoptosis of normal prostatic cells as well as prostate cancer cells.

Bcl-2 and Bcl$_{XL}$

The Bcl-2 family comprises a group of proteins with highly conserved regions of homology that serve to function either as pro-apoptotic or anti-apoptotic molecules [24]. An interaction between Bcl-2 family members to form hetero- or homo-dimers dictates their pro- or anti-apoptotic role [25–27]. However, recent studies suggest that Bcl-2 family members can independently regulate susceptibility to apoptosis [28]. Several members of the Bcl-2 family are often involved in prostate cancer, the most prominent being Bcl-2 and Bcl$_{XL}$. Bcl-2 is a known protooncogene whose over-expression results in malignant transformation in several cancers [29]. Extensive studies have established Bcl-2 as a major player involved in prostate cancer progression and development of androgen-independence and metastasis. Bcl$_{XL}$ is a relatively new member of the Bcl-2 family and less was known about its role in cancers until recently. Several investigators have now found that Bcl$_{XL}$ behaves similar to Bcl-2 in many aspects of prostate cancer progression [30].

Bcl-2 and Bcl$_{XL}$ are anti-apoptotic proteins with similar mechanism of action in preventing apoptosis. They are localized to the outer mitochondrial membrane, ER and nuclear membrane [31]. They act to regulate mitochondrial membrane potential and volume, and can block the apoptosis-inducing release of cytochrome C and apoptosis inhibitory factor into the cytoplasm [32–36]. In addition, Bcl-2 and Bcl$_{XL}$ may also suppress apoptosis in a cytochrome C-independent manner [37], perhaps because of their ability to inhibit cytotoxin-induced caspase-3 activity and subsequent poly (ADP-ribose) polymerase cleavage and lamin B1 degradation [30,38]. Both Bcl-2 and Bcl$_{XL}$ can inhibit apoptosis induced by release of intracellular Ca^{2+} from the ER or by causing a reduction in the nuclear buildup of intranuclear Ca^{2+} levels after the initiation of apoptosis [39]. Bcl-2 and Bcl$_{XL}$ have been found to be over-expressed in prostate cancer [40]. The functional consequence of their over-expression is suppression of apoptosis and not enhancement of cell proliferation. Over-expression of Bcl-2 and Bcl$_{XL}$ enables prostate cancer cells to resist apoptosis induced by androgen-withdrawal, physiological death inducers such as TRAIL, or chemotherapeutic agents.

In the normal prostate gland, Bcl-2 expression is restricted to the basal epithelial cells of the glandular epithelium that are resistant to androgen-deprivation [41]. This may be the origin of androgen-independent cells that emerge post-hormone withdrawal. By contrast, androgen-sensitive secretory glandular epithelial cells do not express Bcl-2. Androgen down-regulates the expression of Bcl-2, and Bcl-2 is up-regulated following withdrawal of androgen [9]. Correspondingly, most androgen-dependent tumors are also Bcl-2 negative. Interestingly, Bcl-2 is expressed in 70% of androgen-independent tumors and only in 34% of bone metastases of hormone-refractory patients [42], whereas Bcl_{XL} is positive in 100% of the prostate adenocarcinoma cases studied. The exact reason for this differential pattern of expression is not known; however, it appears that over-expression of Bcl-2 and Bcl_{XL} may be the key factors enabling prostate cancer cells to survive in androgen-deprived environments [43], allowing the selection of androgen-independent prostate cancer cells. In a study that included patients with metastatic stage D1 and D2 disease and eight Dunning R-3327 rat prostate cancer sublines, Furuya et al. [44] have shown that detectable Bcl-2 expression correlates with aggressive behavior of the tumor.

Bcl-2 and Bcl_{XL} have been demonstrated to block apoptosis induced by physiological agents such as TRAIL and biochemical inducers such as the protein kinase inhibitor staurosporine (STS) in PC-3, DU-145 and LNCaP prostate cancer cells [45,46]. However, PC-3 cells are resistant to STS treatment when compared to LNCaP, owing to endogenous over-expression of Bcl_{XL}, that results in failure to release cytochrome C or to activate caspase-3 and -9 [47]. Down-regulation of endogenous Bcl_{XL} with the use of an antisense oligonucleotide restores sensitivity to apoptosis in PC-3 cells. Another prostate cancer cell line DU-145, on the other hand, is resistant to STS-induced apoptosis owing to the lack of expression of pro-apoptotic Bcl-2 family member Bax, underscoring the importance of other Bcl-2 family members and their significance in prostate cancer apoptosis [46].

One of the biggest hurdles in the treatment of prostate cancer after hormone-depletion is the emergence of androgen-independent cells that are highly resistant to conventional forms of therapy including androgen-ablation, ionizing radiation and chemotherapy. Since Bcl-2 and Bcl_{XL} are involved in the development of androgen-independence, they may very well contribute to resistance to therapy; and there is a huge body of literature supporting this theory (cited in reference [30]). Recently, Lebedeva et al. [30], engineered LNCaP and PC-3 cells to over-express Bcl_{XL} and showed that this desensitized the cells to the effects of cytotoxic chemotherapeutic agents. They then down-regulated endogenous levels of both Bcl_{XL} and Bcl-2 or only Bcl_{XL} and demonstrated marked increase in chemosensitivity in both cases. As the increase in chemosensitivity was comparable, they concluded that Bcl-2 has little or no cytoprotective role in chemodesensitization. Conversely, several chemotherapeutic agents are known to induce apoptosis through the transcriptional down-regulation or phosphorylation-mediated inactivation of Bcl-2 and Bcl_{XL} [48]. p53 is a tumor suppressor and pro-apoptotic protein that is frequently inactivated in advanced and metastatic prostate cancer. It is known to induce apoptosis by down-regulation of Bcl-2. Bcl-2 in turn is known to block apoptosis and is often over-expressed in metastatic prostate cancer. Based on these observations, it is possible to speculate that Bcl-2 expression and inactivation of p53 may confer considerable growth advantage in prostate cancer [40]. In a study to address this theory, McDonnell et al. [42] examined the expression patterns of Bcl-2 and p53 in bone marrow biopsy specimens from stage D prostate cancer patients. The results revealed that the occurrence of p53 mutations and Bcl-2 over-expression are independent genetic processes in advanced prostate cancers.

Based on these observations, it is clear that Bcl-2 and Bcl_{XL} play an important role in prostate cancer progression, androgen-independence and metastasis, making them ideal targets for single or combination therapy. In fact, several researchers have developed therapeutic approaches with Bcl-2 family members. These include the use of adenoviral constructs over-expressing pro-apoptotic member Bax and the use of peptides of the BH3 homology domain that act as dominant-negative inhibitors of Bcl-2 and Bcl_{XL} anti-apoptotic functions. Importantly, based on current literature, it appears that Bcl_{XL} may be the dominant player in progression of prostate cancer. Bcl-2 is over-expressed in some but not all androgen-independent and metastatic tumors. By contrast, Bcl_{XL} expression is seen in almost all cases of prostate cancer. It is also the natural cause of resistance to apoptosis induced by physiological as well as chemotherapeutic agents. Ectopic over-expression of Bcl-2 in prostate cancer cell lines was used to prove its ability to transform cells to the androgen-independent phenotype and to prove chemoresistance. But given the close structural, localization and functional similarity between Bcl-2 and Bcl_{XL}, Bcl-2 could very easily mimic the effect of Bcl_{XL}. Further, several tumors over-express both Bcl-2 and Bcl_{XL}. Does the ratio of Bcl-2 to Bcl_{XL} influence the aggressive trait of the tumor? Another aspect that is unknown is the mechanism by which these proteins promote the progression of the hormone-dependent prostate cancer to the hormone-independent phenotype. One possibility is that they may offer protection against spontaneous apoptosis that could occur when putative mutations responsible for androgen-independence induce DNA damage. Unraveling these puzzles will be critical to the design of therapeutic strategies for androgen-independent prostate cancers.

NF-κB

NF-κB is a transcriptional activator with potent anti-apoptotic functions implicated in oncogenesis and resistance to various therapeutic agents [49]. In prostate cancer, NF-κB contributes to the progression to androgen-independence and increased invasive and metastatic properties [50,51]. The NF-κB family of transcription factors is comprised of five heterodimeric members including p65 (Rel A), p50, p52, c-Rel, and RelB. They are characterized by the presence of the Rel homology domain required for DNA binding and for interaction with the inhibitory IκB proteins. The transcriptional activity of NF-κB is regulated by a tight complex network involving the interplay of several proteins whose dysregulation results in aberrant activation of NF-κB leading to expression of an array of anti-apoptotic and pro-survival proteins that contribute to oncogenesis. The ability of NF-κB to function as a DNA-binding transcription factor is regulated at two distinct levels: (a) entry into the nucleus for DNA binding, and (b) activation of the transcription function by phosphorylation of key serine residues. Cytoplasmic retention of the subunits is maintained by the IκB family proteins; IκB physically interacts with p65 to mask the nuclear localization sequence, thereby retaining it in the cytoplasm. IκB levels serve an important mode of regulation of NF-κB transcriptional activity. Phosphorylation of IκB by the upstream IκB kinase (IKK) complex leads to rapid ubiquitin-mediated degradation of IκB and liberation of NF-κB, so it can enter the nucleus and bind to its DNA motif. IKK can be activated by several kinases such as Akt and PKC [49]. In addition to IκB-dependent regulation, NF-κB activity is positively modulated by signaling events that result in direct phosphorylation of the NF-κB subunits. Several kinases have been implicated in phosphorylation of specific amino acid residues of NF-κB such as PKCζ,

PKA, and CKII. When either or both of these regulatory steps are deregulated, NF-κB transcriptional activity is elevated, as often noticed in several cancers [52].

NF-κB contributes to oncogenesis and resistance to chemotherapy by its ability to suppress cell death pathways [49,53]. NF-κB increases the expression of anti-apoptotic proteins, TRAF-1 and TRAF-2, and IAP group of proteins that inhibit caspase-8-mediated cell death [54]. Bcl-2 family members A1/Bfl1, IEX, Bcl$_{XL}$, and Bcl-2 are other anti-apoptotic proteins induced by NF-κB [49]. NF-κB can also abrogate p53-mediated apoptosis by competing for nuclear coactivators such as p300/CBP [55].

Low basal levels of NF-κB are detected in normal prostatic epithelial cells and androgen-dependent cell line LNCaP [15,50,51]. Androgen-independent prostate cancer cells PC-3 and DU-145, on the other hand, have aberrantly elevated NF-κB activity. In addition, PC-3 and DU-145 cells have constitutively active IKK, which activates NF-κB; this may explain the aberrant NF-κB activity. LNCaP cells, however, have minimal IKK activity [51]. Thus, NF-κB is constitutively activated in the hormone-insensitive prostate tumor cell lines PC-3 and DU-145, but not in the hormone-responsive LNCaP cell line or normal prostate epithelial cells. It is well known that NF-κB and the androgen receptor (AR) inversely regulate each other due to competition for coactivators. Another possible mechanism of AR regulation is by up-regulation of IκB [56]. AR inhibits the expression of NF-κB target genes such as IL-6 through the up-regulation of IκB. It is not very clear whether or not elevation of NF-κB leads to androgen-independence.

NF-κB is often activated by several physiological and chemotherapeutic agents and ionizing radiation. Disproportionate elevation of NF-κB activity contributes to resistance of the tumor to conventional forms of therapy. PC-3 and DU-145 prostate cancer cells are resistant to treatment with TNF [57]. In a recent study, Sumitomo et al. [58] demonstrated that inhibition of NF-κB using pyrrolidine dithiocarbamate and NF-κB decoy increased sensitivity of these cells to TNF. Moreover, NF-κB is activated by several chemotherapeutic agents such as doxorubicin, vincristine, paclitaxel, and this may render the tumors resistant to further therapy [59]. To combat this self-defeating elevation of NF-κB by anti-neoplastic agents, novel strategies are being considered so that NF-κB can be inhibited simultaneously with administration of the chemotherapeutic agent.

The constitutive activation of NF-κB in prostate tumor cells increases the expression of anti-apoptotic proteins, thereby decreasing the effectiveness of anti-tumor therapy and contributing to the development of the malignant phenotype. Evidence that NF-κB contributes to the invasive behavior of prostate cancer cells is provided in a recent study [60], where the NF-κB levels of PC-3 sublines with varying levels of invasiveness were investigated. The most highly invasive PC-3 sublines show approximately 2-fold increase in NF-κB DNA binding as well as elevated transcription activity. Invasiveness could be blocked by IκB super-repressor [60]. In another study, Huang et al. [50] show that NF-κB promotes angiogenesis, invasion, and metastasis by increasing the transcription of angiogenic genes such as IL-8, VEGF, and MMP-9. They use the metastatic cell line PC-3M transfected with IκB or a vector to induce orthotopic tumors in nude mice and demonstrate that IκB-expressing tumors had slow growth and low metastatic ability. Although potential NF-κB-regulated genes such as IL-8, VEGF, and MMP-9 have been implicated in progression of the metastatic phenotype, the precise contribution of these proteins as well as that of IAP or other targets of NF-κB needs further functional evaluation. Importantly, data from clinical specimens of prostate cancer are essential to corroborate the significance of NF-κB and its downstream anti-apoptotic target genes in clinical prostate cancer.

IGF

Insulin-like growth factor-I (IGF-I) contributes to the development of prostate cancer by stimulating cell proliferation and by inhibiting apoptosis [61]. The IGF axis consists of the insulin-like growth factor receptor 1 (IGF-IR), ligands IGF-I and -II, and IGF-binding proteins, which modulate IGF action [62]. IGF-IR when activated by its ligands, protects many different cell types from a wide range of pro-apoptotic insults. The protective effect of the IGF-IR against cell death has been confirmed by the finding that down-regulation of the IGF-IR by antisense strategies, dominant-negative mutants, or triple-helix formation causes massive apoptosis of cells, especially when the cells are growing in anchorage-independent conditions. The IGF-IR is known to activate several signaling pathways. Ligand binding activates its major substrate, IRS-1, which activates phosphatidylinositol 3-kinase (PI3K). PI3K then activates the Akt/protein kinase B. This pathway is responsible for the anti-apoptotic effects of IGF-IR. However, IGF-IR has two alternative pathways: (a) the mitogen-activated protein kinase pathway originating from another major substrate of the IGF-IR, the Shc protein, and (b) the mitochondrial translocation of Raf-1. The activation of the Akt/protein kinase B pathway in response IGF-I results in phosphorylation of BAD. Phosphorylated Bad is no longer capable of being heterodimerized with Bcl_{XL} at membrane sites, is sequestered into the cytosol, bound to 14.3.3, and is inactivated as a cell death promoting protein. Interestingly, for cell survival, it is sufficient that any two of these three pathways be operative to exert protection from apoptosis [63].

In vitro studies have demonstrated that prostatic epithelial cells respond to the mitogenic activity of IGF-I [64]. Moreover, tumors of the prostate cancer cell line PC-3 have a significantly lower proliferation rate in IGF-I-deficient hosts than in IGF-I-expressing hosts. One cohort study and two case-control studies in men have shown positive associations between prostate cancer risk and circulating IGF-I level [65,66]. Prostate cancer risk is increased in men with elevated plasma IGF-I. This association is particularly strong in younger men, suggesting that circulating IGF-I may be specifically involved in the early pathogenesis of prostate cancer. In addition to its pro-survival and anti-apoptotic functions discussed so far, IGF-IR together with IRS promotes the invasiveness and metastasis of prostate tumor cells and it does so in a unique fashion. Although IGF-IR is not an absolute requirement for normal growth, it is a strict requirement for anchorage-independent growth [67,68]. Human prostatic tumor cells stably expressing a dominant-negative mutant of IGF-IR are not inhibited when grown in monolayer, but they fail to form colonies in soft agar or tumors in mice [61]. This differential effect on normal growth (cells in monolayer cultures) and abnormal growth (anchorage-independent growth) indicates that targeting of IGF-IR is a promising strategy for cancer therapy. Several prostate cancer cells are characterized with a PTEN mutation, modest levels of IGF-IR and lack of IRS-1. The loss of activation of the PI3K activation function of IRS-1, is compensated in these cells by the mutation in PTEN, an inhibitor of PI3K. As IRS-1 enhances cell attachment to the substrate, by extinguishing IRS-1, the cancer cells would decrease their attachment to the substrate and increase motility, thus favoring invasion and metastasis. These characteristics together favor the metastatic spread of prostatic cancer cells without decreasing their growth potential [61].

Caveolin

Caveolin is a 21–24 kDa integral membrane protein present in caveolae that are enriched with cholesterol, glycosphingolipid, and lipid-mediated signaling proteins [69]. The primary function of caveolin in normal cells is membrane trafficking of non-clathrin-dependent endocytosis and intracellular cholesterol transport. Caveolin has been shown to bind and modulate several protein kinases and to associate with endothelial nitric oxide synthase [70]. Recent *in vivo* and *in vitro* studies have shown that caveolin binds and directly interacts with a variety of signaling molecules via a modular protein domain termed the caveolin-scaffolding domain. Caveolin inhibits the activity of both tyrosine and serine/threonine kinases, including src family tyrosine kinases, epidermal growth factor receptor neu, mitogen-activated protein kinase (MEK1), extra-cellular signal regulated kinase-2 (ERK2), protein kinase C (PKC), and protein kinase A [70].

Caveolin serves as a tumor suppressor and as a pro-apoptotic protein in several tumors such as those of the breast and lung [71]. By contrast, caveolin has emerged as an important, albeit controversial, player in prostate cancer development and progression. Caveolin is over-expressed in prostate cancers, where it is believed to promote cell survival and metastasis [72]. This function of caveolin is attributed to inhibition of c-myc or of androgen-withdrawal-induced apoptosis in prostate cancer cells [72]. Caveolin is over-expressed in both mouse and human prostate tumors [73]. In tumor cells derived from the mouse prostate reconstitution model, the expression of caveolin is linked to hormone-resistant metastatic prostate cancer [73]. The findings of the study suggests that caveolin regulates androgen-responsiveness in prostate cancer because a positive correlation was noted between expression of caveolin and progression of cancer in tumor samples from prostate cancer patients [73]. Caveolin is a downstream effector of testosterone-mediated survival; moderate levels of caveolin promote both survival and metastatic pathways in both human and mouse prostate tumor cells [74]. Caveolin can, in fact, substitute for testosterone to promote the survival of prostate cancer cells *in vitro* and *in vivo*. It has been shown that caveolin enhances ligand-dependent activation of the AR. AR co-localizes to caveolin-rich regions on the cell membrane and has been shown by co-immunoprecipitation studies to physically interact with the caveolin [75]. The interaction may play a role in the conversion of androgen-dependent cells to androgen-independent phenotype. Studies using stable transfection of antisense caveolin showed that reduced levels of caveolin triggers apoptosis following withdrawal of androgen [76]. It has also been shown that over-expression of caveolin inhibits c-myc-induced apoptosis in LNCaP prostate cancer cells by direct physical interaction with c-myc [72]. From these findings it may appear that the anti-apoptotic role of caveolin is critical for its metastatic function. Caveolin may offer a promising target for therapy if convincingly shown to support the progression of prostate cancer.

Another possible mechanism by which caveolin may promote progression is by conferring resistance to chemotherapy. Over-expression of caveolin is associated with a multi-drug resistant phenotype independent of P-glycoprotein in human cancer cell lines from several different tumor types [77]. Moreover, caveolin may regulate multiple signal transduction pathways including Ca^{2+} and mitogen-activated protein kinases in a cell type- and context-specific fashion [70]. Clearly, further studies are essential to define the prognostic value of caveolin in prostate cancer.

Akt

The Akt/PKB kinase controls many of the intracellular processes that are dysregulated in human cancer; including the suppression of apoptosis and anoikis, and the induction of cell cycle progression [78]. Akt is activated via the PI3K signaling pathway. Akt is dysregulated in a variety of tumors by several different mechanisms: by over-expression of protein; by constitutive activation in tumors harboring mutant Ras oncogenes; or by inactivation of the inhibitory phosphatase, PTEN. The anti-apoptotic role of Akt is attributed to its ability to phosphorylate and inactivate death effector proteins such as Bad and caspase-9 [79]. Additionally, through phosphorylation and activation of the IKK complex, Akt activates NF-κB transcriptional activity, which constitutes the additional wave of resistance to apoptosis via its death inhibitory target genes like IAPs. Three isoforms of Akt have been identified: Akt-1, -2, and -3. Selective up-regulation of Akt-3 RNA expression has been reported in hormone-independent prostate cancer cell lines raising the possibility that Akt-3 expression may be increased with prostate tumor progression. However, all three of the

Akt isoforms have been found to be expressed in normal prostate and tumor tissues. Based on these findings, it seems that tumorigenesis may not involve a dramatic shift in the RNA expression patterns of the three Akt isoforms [80].

Elevated Akt activity is responsible for development of androgen refractory status in prostate cancer [81]. Upon withdrawal of androgen, LNCaP cells initially arrest in G1 and then trans-differentiate into neuroendocrine-like cells that eventually resume androgen-independent proliferation. Both acute and chronic androgen-ablation results in an increase in basal levels of PI3K and Akt activities, which are sustained throughout the androgen-independent progression process. Under these conditions, inhibition of PI3K, pharmacologically or with ectopic expression of PTEN, arrests cell proliferation and blocks progression to the androgen-independent state. Akt also confers resistance to apoptosis by other apoptotic effectors such as TRAIL [82]. Prostate cancer cells expressing the highest level of constitutively active Akt are more resistant to apoptosis by TRAIL than those expressing the lowest level. Down-regulation of constitutively active Akt by PI3K inhibitors, wortmannin and LY294002, reverse cellular resistance to TRAIL. Conversely, transfection of constitutively active Akt into cells with low Akt activity increases Akt activity and attenuates TRAIL-induced apoptosis. Inhibition of TRAIL sensitivity occurs at the level of BID cleavage, as caspase-8 activity is not affected [82].

A specific role for Akt in prostate cancer through its ability to inhibit AR transcriptional activity has been reported [83]. AR functions as a transcriptional activator upon binding to its ligand, and Akt can repress the transactivation of AR target genes presumably by phosphorylation of AR at Ser-210 and Ser-790 leading to its inactivation. A constitutive activating mutation at Ser-210 results in the reversal of Akt-mediated suppression of the transactivation function of AR. Activation of the PI3K/Akt pathway results in the suppression of AR target genes, such as p21, and this may involve the inhibition of the interaction between AR and its coregulators.

PTEN

PTEN is a tumor suppressor with phosphatase activity located in the region on chromosome 10q, that is often deleted in many tumors including advanced

prostate cancer [37,84,85]. PTEN specifically inhibits the activation of Akt/PKB serine/threonine kinase by blocking the signal transduction pathway mediated by PI3K. PTEN expression is lost in more than 50% of the advanced prostate cancers, through methylation-mediated transcriptional silencing or PTEN deletion [86]. Mutation or loss of expression of PTEN in prostate cancer cell lines such as LNCaP and PC-3 cells results in constitutive activation of Akt kinase-dependent anti-apoptotic pathways that render the prostate cancer cells resistant to apoptosis. Adenoviral-mediated reintroduction of PTEN in LNCaP prostate cancer cells, which do not express endogenous PTEN, results in induction of apoptosis [85]. Moreover, insertion of functional chromosome 10 in rat prostate carcinoma cells inhibits the subsequent development of tumor metastases [87]. Additionally, PTEN has been shown to impair TNF-induced activation of Akt and the IKK complex. Transient expression of PTEN-suppressed IKK activation and TNF-induced NF-κB DNA binding and transactivation in DU-145 prostate cancer cells [88], underscoring the possible importance of PTEN loss in dysregulation of NF-κB activity in prostate cancer.

p53

Among the molecules that play a role in the regulation of apoptosis, p53 has emerged as one of the leading stars [89]. p53 is a transcriptional regulator equipped with multiple functions, including activation of cell cycle arrest, apoptosis, senescence, and differentiation. p53 protein functions as a transcriptional activator or repressor, depending upon the promoter context [90]. It can up-regulate downstream target genes, such as p21/waf1, IGF binding protein-3, bax and fas/apo1, implicated in growth inhibition and apoptotic cell death and can down-regulate anti-apoptotic genes such as Bcl-2 [89].

Mutations of p53 are uncommon in primary prostate cancer, but occur frequently in advanced disease [91]. Mutations involving p53 are, therefore, regarded as late events during multi-step prostate carcinogenesis. In fact, recent studies suggest that mutations in *p53* gene lead to hormone-refractory prostate cancer. Compared to wild-type p53, mutant p53 protein is stably expressed, and is therefore readily detectable by immunohistochemistry for prognostic significance. Elevated p53 protein was present in 16 of 17 hormone-refractory specimens (94%), 4 of 8 untreated metastatic tumors (50%) and 6 of 27 primary untreated tumors (22%) [91]. In another study, DNA analysis of representative specimens with elevated p53 confirmed *p53* gene alterations in 9 of 11 cases (82%). This study revealed a clear progression of increased p53 alteration from untreated primary to hormone-refractory disease [92]. Buttyan et al. [93], have confirmed these observations. These investigators created stable variants of the androgen-responsive, wild-type p53-expressing LNCaP cells by transfection with expression vectors designed to reduce expression or function of wild-type p53. The transfectants were then tested for their ability to form tumors in castrated male nude mice. LNCaP transfectants that expressed dominant-negative p53 were readily able to form tumors in castrated male nude mice whereas parental LNCaP cells or control-transfected LNCaP cells were not [93]. Thus, it appears that loss of wild-type p53 function can contribute to the hormone-resistance of prostate cancer cells.

p53 does not seem to be involved in apoptosis of prostate cancer cells following androgen-ablation [94]. The role of the *p53* gene in the programed cell death pathway induced by androgen-ablation in p53 null mice was studied by Berges et al. [94]. There was an identical induction of apoptosis in prostate cells upon castration in both wild-type p53 mice and p53 deficient (null) mice. Several *in vitro* studies utilizing p53-negative prostate cancer cells PC-3 and TSU-Pr1 have documented that these cells readily undergo apoptosis induced by a variety of chemotherapeutic agents [95], suggesting the presence of p53-independent pathway(s) for induction of apoptosis in prostate cancer. For example, apoptosis induced by immediate early genes like EGR-1 (early growth response-1) and Par-4 in prostate cancer cells are p53-independent [15,96]. On the other hand, Michael Cohen et al. [57] have shown the involvement of p53 in TNF-induced apoptosis in LNCaP cells. These cells are sensitive to TNF treatment and express wild-type p53; TNF treatment results in the accumulation of p53 and up-regulation of p21/waf1. LNCaP transfectants LN-56 that overexpress dominant-negative p53, are highly resistant to apoptosis induced by TNF. Moreover, TNF-induced apoptosis in LNCaP cells is accompanied by caspase-dependent proteolysis of p21/waf1 and Rb. Apoptosis is significantly attenuated in LN-56, which lack wild-type p53 function. Accumulation of p53 in TNF-treated LNCaP cells is decreased in the presence of the caspase inhibitor Z-VAD-FMK, suggesting a role for activated caspases in acceleration of p53 response.

In summary, these results indicate that p53 is involved in TNF-mediated apoptosis in LNCaP [57].

The p53 homolog p63 encodes different isotypes that are able to either transactivate p53 reporter genes (TAp63) or act as p53-dominant-negative mutants (ΔNp63) [97]. The *p63* gene is expressed in the regenerative epithelial compartments of several organs. In the normal epidermis, hair follicles, and stratified squamous cell cultures, p63 is restricted to cells with a high proliferative potential and is absent in cells undergoing terminal differentiation [97]. The *p63* gene is, thus, likely associated with tissue renewal as a regulator of the tissue stem cell phenotype. Prostate basal cells, but not secretory or neuroendocrine cells, express p63. In addition, prostate basal cells in culture predominantly express the ΔNp63α isotype. In contrast, p63 protein is not detected in human prostate adenocarcinomas. Finally, and most importantly, p63-null mice do not develop the prostate [98]. These findings indicate that p63 is required for prostate development. Furthermore, p63 immunohistochemistry may be a valuable tool in the differential diagnosis of benign *versus* malignant prostatic lesions [98,99]. However, even though full-length p63 has been shown to induce apoptosis, its role in prostate cancer apoptosis still remains to be elucidated.

p73 is another p53 homolog capable of mediating apoptotic cell death [100]. Additionally, p73 can activate some, but not all of the p53 target genes. No mutations of p73 are found in prostate cancer [101]. Variable expression of p73 may be associated with prostate tumor growth: expression analysis showed that p73 is down-regulated in 42% of the cases and up-regulated in 31% of prostate cancer cases [102]. However, the relevance of p73 in prostate cancer cell apoptosis is yet to be established.

Bin1

Bin1 is a nucleo-cytoplasmic adaptor protein with features of a tumor suppressor that was identified through its ability to interact with c-myc, and inhibit malignant transformation by c-myc [103–105]. The human *Bin1* gene is located at chromosome 2q14 within a region that is frequently deleted in metastatic prostate cancer [106]. Because the proto-oncogene c-myc is often activated in tumors that have progressed to metastatic status, the events that promote this process are of considerable significance.

RNA and immunohistochemical analyses indicate that Bin1 is expressed in most primary tumors, even at slightly elevated levels relative to benign tissues, but that it is frequently missing or inactivated by aberrant splicing in metastatic tumors and androgen-independent tumor cell lines [106]. Ectopic expression of Bin1 suppresses the growth of prostate cancer lines *in vitro* [106]. These findings support the candidacy of Bin1 as the chromosome 2q prostate tumor suppressor gene.

Bin1 engages a caspase-independent cell death process, characterized by cell shrinkage, substratum detachment, extensively vacuolated cytoplasm, and non-nucleosomal DNA degradation [107]. Cells in all phases of the cell cycle are susceptible to death, and p53 and Rb are dispensable for this action of Bin1. Notably, Bin1 does not activate caspases and the broad-spectrum caspase inhibitor Z-VAD-FMK does not block cell death [107]. Consistent with the lack of caspase involvement, dying cells lack nucleosomal DNA cleavage and nuclear lamina degradation. Moreover, neither Bcl-2 nor dominant inhibition of the Fas pathway can rescue the cells from Bin1 action. AEBSF, a serine protease inhibitor that inhibits apoptosis by c-myc potently suppresses apoptosis by Bin1 [107]. Loss of Bin1 may promote malignancy by blunting death penalties associated with oncogene activation. Additionally, Bin1 does not induce cell death in normal and non-transformed cells and is an effective inducer of apoptosis in tumor cells where c-myc is amplified [105]. As c-myc is often amplified in prostate cancer, these observations offer mechanistic insight into the role of Bin1 in prostate cancer cell apoptosis.

TGF-β

TGF-β plays a critical role in controlling proliferation and apoptosis in prostate epithelial cells [108]. The TGF-β family consists of 3 isoforms, which are involved in a variety of biological processes; TGF-β1 is the most abundant isoform expressed in the prostate gland. TGF-β signaling results from interaction of TGF-β with its cell surface receptors type-I (RI) and type-II (RII). Upon ligand binding, RI is activated by RII phosphorylation to propagate signals to downsteam substrates such as the SMAD family of proteins. TGF-β1 plays a multi-functional role in tumorigenesis. It inhibits the growth of various malignant cells especially those of epithelial cell origin, by arresting them in the G1 phase of the cell cycle [109]. Moreover, in many different cell types, TGF-β induces apoptosis [110,111].

In the normal prostate gland, TGF-β1 counteracts the action of growth stimulating factors such as EGF/TGF-α and bFGF on epithelial and stromal cells, respectively [112]. *In vitro*, TGF-β inhibits proliferation and induces apoptosis in normal prostate cells of both rat and human origin [113]. TGF-β1 up-regulates the levels of cyclin-dependent inhibitors like p15, p21, and p27, and thus causes growth arrest of the prostate epithelial cells in the G1 phase of the cell cycle [114]. It also induces apoptosis in prostate epithelial cells *in vivo*, even in the presence of physiological levels of androgen [110,115]. Prostate cancer cells, however, evade TGF-β-induced growth arrest and apoptosis by loss of functional TGF-β receptors.

Prostate tumor cells of both human and rat origin often show reduced sensitivity to TGF-β1-induced growth inhibition when compared to normal prostatic epithelial cells [3,116]. DU-145 and PC-3 cells are inhibited by TGF-β1, while LNCaP cells are totally resistant [117]. Loss of TGF-β sensitivity has been demonstrated to be due to loss of TGF-β1 receptor expression in the prostate tumor cells. Similarly, in transgenic mice carrying dominant-negative TGF-β RII, there is an absence of apoptosis in the ventral prostate lobes [118]. Ectopic re-expression of TGF-β RII in LNCaP prostate cancer cells restores the sensitivity to TGF-β1 resulting in growth arrest and apoptosis induction [119]. Additionally, the transfected LNCaP/TGF-β RII cells exhibit decreased tumorigenicity through down-regulation of Bcl-2 expression and induction of caspase-1 expression [119].

The molecular mechanisms underlying TGF-β-mediated growth suppression in prostate cancer cells are less well understood. It has been shown that TGF-β negatively regulates the androgen signaling through the downstream activation of Smad3, which represses transcriptional activity of AR by directly binding to it [120]. Recent findings suggest that the levels of Smad are reduced in prostate tumor compared to the normal prostate, suggesting that decreased Smad expression may constitute an alternate means of escaping sensitivity to TGF-β, thereby favoring tumor progression [108]. Thus, restoration of sensitivity to TGF-β by various means may provide a valuable approach to combat prostate cancer growth.

Par-4

Par-4 is a pro-apoptotic gene that can induce apoptosis in prostate cancer cells [15]. The *par-4* gene was first isolated by differential screening for genes that are up-regulated when androgen-independent prostate cancer cells are induced to undergo apoptosis upon treatment with ionomycin or TG [20]. Par-4 expression is specifically up-regulated by the action of apoptotic agents and not with growth-stimulatory, growth-arresting or necrotic agents. Abrogation of endogenous Par-4 expression with an antisense oligomer or function with a dominant-negative mutant inhibits apoptosis by exogenous insults, indicating that Par-4 induction is necessary for apoptosis [121]. While endogenous Par-4 is essential to sensitize prostate cancer cells to apoptosis, over-expression of ectopic Par-4 is sufficient to induce cell death in prostate cancer cells by apoptosis [15].

The precise physiological function of endogenous Par-4 is not known. However, Par-4 is known to interact with several proteins and to modulate various signal transduction pathways. The interaction partners of Par-4 include atypical protein kinase C isoforms PKCζ and PKCι/λ, Wilm's tumor suppressor protein WT1 and Dlk/Zip kinase [122–124]. These interactions are mediated by the leucine zipper domain in the carboxy-terminus of Par-4, and regulate the anti-survival and pro-apoptotic functions of Par-4. Over-expression of PKCζ abrogates Par-4-induced apoptosis. Growth arrest, which is a reversible form of growth inhibition, provides protection from apoptosis and allows survival of target cells. WT1 enhances growth arrest and provides protection from apoptosis; co-expression of ectopic Par-4 relieves the anti-apoptotic effects of WT1 and enhances apoptosis [123].

Par-4 influences several signaling pathways. In fibroblasts, Par-4 is down-regulated by oncogenic-Ras, -Raf, or -Src, but when restored, Par-4 inhibits ERK1/ERK2 expression and activity, and thereby abrogates oncogene-induced cellular transformation [125,126]. Additionally, Par-4 can up-regulate p38 kinase activity. Simultaneous down-regulation of ERK activity and up-regulation of p38 kinase activity are considered important in the induction of an apoptotic program by Par-4 in response to ultraviolet radiation [127]. Moreover, Par-4 inhibits the transcriptional activity of NF-κB and AP-1 [122,128,129].

In the normal prostate gland, Par-4 is expressed in the mesenchyme surrounding the ventral part of the prostate and the basal glandular epithelial cells but is absent in adjacent differentiated ductal cells, implying that Par-4 expression is decreased during differentiation. Ductal cells of the prostate gland do not undergo apoptosis unless they are deprived of hormonal stimula-tion, such as by castration. Upon testosterone-ablation caused by castration, ductal cells undergo apoptosis, which peaks at day 3. Par-4 levels increase in ductal cells of the rat prostate on day 1 and day 3 post-castration and diminish by day 5, suggesting that Par-4 induction is an early and transient event in apoptosis of prostate ductal cells [130]. By contrast, Bcl-2 is expressed in the ductal cells and the levels are decreased after androgen-withdrawal [131]. Consistently, an inverse correlation between Par-4 and Bcl-2 expression is noticed in human prostate tumors. Par-4 but not Bcl-2 is detected in the primary and metastatic prostate tumors. Xenografts of human androgen-dependent CWR22 tumors are immunoreactive for Par-4 but not Bcl-2, whereas the androgen-independent CWR22R tumors show mutually exclusive patterns of expression, with pockets that stain for Bcl-2 but not Par-4 [131]. Qiu et al. [131] have shown that ectopic expression of Par-4 can down-regulate Bcl-2 expression and that replenishment of Bcl-2 abrogates Par-4-dependent sensitization to apoptosis by other insults.

It is now clear that Par-4 is sufficient to directly induce apoptosis in prostate cancer cells and cause tumor regression [15]. It functions even in the presence of potential protective mechanisms such as high NF-κB activity, Bcl$_{XL}$ or Bcl-2 or in the absence of wild-type p53 or PTEN function. Ectopic expression of Par-4 is sufficient to induce apoptosis in androgen-independent prostate cancer cells PC-3, DU-145, and TSU-Pr but not in androgen-dependent LNCaP cells or normal prostate epithelial cells. Par-4 induces apoptosis by a unique co-parallel activation of a pro-death pathway together with the inhibition of a pro-survival pathway. Par-4 activates the pro-death FasL–Fas–FADD–caspase-8 pathway by effecting the translocation of Fas and FasL to the cell membrane, and in parallel it inhibits the pro-survival transcriptional activity of NF-κB. Par-4 does not inhibit the ability of NF-κB to bind to DNA but abrogates the transcriptional activity of NF-κB, thereby presumably preventing the expression of NF-κB-regulated anti-apoptotic genes. The inhibition of NF-κB alone with IκB or activation of the Fas pathway alone are not sufficient to induce apoptosis; but when the IκB and Fas are introduced together they mimic Par-4-induced apoptosis. This implies that each pathway is essential but not sufficient to accomplish apoptosis of the prostate cancer cells. Par-4 selectively kills prostate cancer cells such as PC-3 and DU-145 that show high levels of NF-κB activity. Androgen-dependent prostate cancer cells such as LNCaP or normal prostate epithelial cells, which have low NF-κB

102

activity are not affected by Par-4. Par-4 utilizes this unique mechanism to cause regression of subcutaneous [15] and orthotopic tumors (Herman et al. unpublished observations) in animal models. Because elevated NF-κB activity correlates with an increase in the aggressive traits of several cancers [49,51,52] and because Par-4 does not cause apoptosis of normal or non-transformed cells, Par-4 is an ideal molecule for therapeutic intervention.

Conclusions

Prostate cancer cells develop multiple apoptosis blocking strategies during the various stages of progression from normal epithelial cells to androgen-dependent tumor cells, and further onto malignant androgen-independent tumor cells. Therefore, while designing therapeutic strategies one has to take into account the complex interplay of anti-apoptotic machinery that the cells possess. Therapeutic intervention of prostate cancer requires the identification of the network of roadblocks in the apoptotic pathways and designing molecular approaches to dismantle them. Several molecules identified in this review, and in particular, p53, PTEN, and Par-4 satisfy the necessary criteria of prospective candidates for prostate cancer therapy. They induce apoptosis in cancer cells using a multifaceted approach where several different apoptotic pathways are activated. Moreover, these molecules are selective in their apoptotic action on tumor cells. While androgen-dependent cells can be eliminated by androgen-ablation, a combinatorial approach of androgen-ablation and gene therapy with Par-4, for instance, will not only obliterate the residual prostate cancer cells following radical prostatectomy, but will also induce apoptosis in the emerging androgen-independent cancer cell population. Further studies using such combinatorial approaches may be essential to elucidate the relevance of co-expression of the pro-apoptotic molecules in conjunction with conventional or experimental forms of treatment for prostate cancer. Such a combinatorial approach will not only augment the kinetics of apoptosis-induction in the tumors but may also help target cells that develop resistance to any one of the approaches. Emerging trends in micro-array-based approaches can be very useful in creating a molecular fingerprint of each tumor so as to identify molecular predictors of progression for prognostic value, and further develop susceptibility profiles for each of the

apoptosis-producing genes. Such profiles may be useful for predicting the usefulness of combinatorial therapeutic protocols for prostate cancer.

The challenge posed by metastatic prostate cancer to treatment options is particularly noteworthy. Gene carrier systems that will allow accurate delivery of the gene to micro- and macro-metastatic lesions, especially to the bone, are essential for the success of prostate cancer gene therapy. Recent experiments have utilized the PSA promoter or the osteocalcin promoter to ensure expression of candidate genes in prostate cancer cells or associated bone stromal osteoblasts to reduce intraosseus growth of prostate cancer cells in animal models ([132] and references cited therein). Further refinement of the delivery reagents and expression tools will lead to the availability of targeted approaches that can evaluate the potential of the above genes for therapy of prostate cancer.

Acknowledgement

VMR was supported by NIH grants CA60872 and CA84511.

References

1. Evan GI, Vousden KH: Proliferation, cell cycle and apoptosis in cancer. Nature 411: 342–348, 2001
2. Tu H, Jacobs SC, Borkowski A, Kyprianou N: Incidence of apoptosis and cell proliferation in prostate cancer: Relationship with TGF-beta1 and bcl-2 expression. Int J Cancer 69: 357–363, 1996
3. Denmeade SR, Lin XS, Isaacs JT: Role of programmed (apoptotic) cell death during the progression and therapy for prostate cancer. Prostate 28: 251–265, 1996
4. Lu-Yao GL, McLerran D, Wasson J, Wennberg JE: An assessment of radical prostatectomy. Time trends, geographic variation, and outcomes. The Prostate Patient Outcomes Research Team. JAMA 269: 2633–2636, 1993
5. Small EJ, Reese DM, Vogelzang NJ: Hormone-refractory prostate cancer: An evolving standard of care. Semin Oncol 26: 61–67, 1999
6. Isaacs JT, Lundmo PI, Berges R, Martikainen P, Kyprianou N, English HF: Androgen regulation of programmed death of normal and malignant prostatic cells. J Androl 13: 457–464, 1992
7. Huang A, Gandour-Edwards R, Rosenthal SA, Siders DB, Deitch AD, White RW: p53 and bcl-2 immunohistochemical alterations in prostate cancer treated with radiation therapy. Urology 51: 346–351, 1998
8. Denmeade SR, Isaacs JT: Activation of programmed (apoptotic) cell death for the treatment of prostate cancer. Adv Pharmacol 35: 281–306, 1996

9. Denmeade SR, Tombal B, Isaacs JT: Apoptotic pathways in prostate cancer. In: Mattson MP, Estus S, Rangnekar VM (eds) Programmed Cell Death, Volume II: Advances in Cell Aging and Gerontology, Vol 6, Elsevier B.V., Amsterdam, Netherlands, 2001, pp 23–54

10. Hengartner MO: The biochemistry of apoptosis. Nature 407: 770–776, 2000

11. Leist M, Jaattela M: Four deaths and a funeral: From caspases to alternative mechanisms. Nat Rev Mol Cell Biol 2: 589–598, 2001

12. Thornberry NA, Lazebnik Y: Caspases: Enemies within. Science 281: 1312–1316, 1998

13. Henson PM, Bratton DL, Fadok VA: The phosphatidylserine receptor: A crucial molecular switch? Nat Rev Mol Cell Biol 2: 627–633, 2001

14. Rokhlin OW, Bishop GA, Hostager BS, Waldschmidt TJ, Sidorenko SP, Pavloff N, Kiefer MC, Umansky SR, Glover RA, Cohen MB: Fas-mediated apoptosis in human prostatic carcinoma cell lines. Cancer Res 57: 1758–1768, 1997

15. Chakraborty M, Qiu SG, Vasudevan KM, Rangnekar VM: Par-4 drives trafficking and activation of Fas and FasL to induce prostate cancer cell apoptosis and tumor regression. Cancer Res 61: 7255–7263, 2001

16. Furuya Y, Lundmo P, Short AD, Gill DL, Isaacs JT: The role of calcium, pH, and cell proliferation in the programmed (apoptotic) death of androgen-independent prostatic cancer cells induced by thapsigargin. Cancer Res 54: 6167–6175, 1994

17. Martikainen P, Kyprianou N, Tucker R, Isaacs JT: Programmed death of nonproliferating androgen-independent prostatic cancer cells. Cancer Res 51: 4693–4700, 1991

18. Wertz IE, Dixit VM: Characterization of calcium release-activated apoptosis of LNCaP prostate cancer cells. J Biol Chem 275: 11470–11477, 2000

19. Lin XS, Denmeade SR, Cisek L, Isaacs JT: Mechanism and role of growth arrest in programmed (apoptotic) death of prostatic cancer cells induced by thapsigargin. Prostate 33: 201–207, 1997

20. Sells SF, Wood DP Jr, Joshi-Barve SS, Muthukumar S, Jacob RJ, Crist SA, Humphreys S, Rangnekar VM: Commonality of the gene programs induced by effectors of apoptosis in androgen-dependent and -independent prostate cells. Cell Growth Differ 5: 457–466, 1994

21. Wyllie AH: Glucocorticoid-induced thymocyte apoptosis is associated with endogenous endonuclease activation. Nature 284: 555–556, 1980

22. McConkey DJ, Orrenius S: The role of calcium in the regulation of apoptosis. Biochem Biophys Res Commun 239: 357–366, 1997

23. Juin P, Pelletier M, Oliver L, Tremblais K, Gregoire M, Meflah K, Vallette FM: Induction of a caspase-3-like activity by calcium in normal cytosolic extracts triggers nuclear apoptosis in a cell-free system. J Biol Chem 273: 17559–17564, 1998

24. Gross A, McDonnell JM, Korsmeyer SJ: BCL-2 family members and the mitochondria in apoptosis. Genes Dev 13: 1899–1911, 1999

25. Yin XM, Oltvai ZN, Korsmeyer SJ: BH1 and BH2 domains of Bcl-2 are required for inhibition of apoptosis and heterodimerization with Bax. Nature 369: 321–323, 1994

26. Hanada M, Aime-Sempe C, Sato T, Reed JC: Structure-function analysis of Bcl-2 protein. Identification of conserved domains important for homodimerization with Bcl-2 and heterodimerization with Bax. J Biol Chem 270: 11962–11969, 1995

27. Yang E, Zha J, Jockel J, Boise LH, Thompson CB, Korsmeyer SJ: Bad, a heterodimeric partner for Bcl-$_{XL}$ and Bcl-2, displaces Bax and promotes cell death. Cell 80: 285–291, 1995

28. Knudson CM, Korsmeyer SJ: Bcl-2 and Bax function independently to regulate cell death. Nat Genet 16: 358–363, 1997

29. Reed JC, Cuddy M, Slabiak T, Croce CM, Nowell PC: Oncogenic potential of bcl-2 demonstrated by gene transfer. Nature 336: 259–261, 1988

30. Lebedeva I, Rando R, Ojwang J, Cossum P, Stein CA: Bcl-xL in prostate cancer cells: Effects of overexpression and down-regulation on chemosensitivity. Cancer Res 60: 6052–6060, 2000

31. Krajewski S, Tanaka S, Takayama S, Schibler MJ, Fenton W, Reed JC: Investigation of the subcellular distribution of the bcl-2 oncoprotein: Residence in the nuclear envelope, endoplasmic reticulum, and outer mitochondrial membranes. Cancer Res 53: 4701–4714, 1993

32. Vander Heiden MG, Chandel NS, Williamson EK, Schumacker PT, Thompson CB: Bcl$_{XL}$ regulates the membrane potential and volume homeostasis of mitochondria. Cell 91: 627–637, 1997

33. Kim CN, Wang X, Huang Y, Ibrado AM, Liu L, Fang G, Bhalla K: Overexpression of Bcl-$_{XL}$ inhibits Ara-C-induced mitochondrial loss of cytochrome C and other perturbations that activate the molecular cascade of apoptosis. Cancer Res 57: 3115–3120, 1997

34. Kluck RM, Bossy-Wetzel E, Green DR, Newmeyer DD: The release of cytochrome C from mitochondria: A primary site for Bcl-2 regulation of apoptosis. Science 275: 1132–1136, 1997

35. Yang J, Liu X, Bhalla K, Kim CN, Ibrado AM, Cai J, Peng TI, Jones DP, Wang X: Prevention of apoptosis by Bcl-2: Release of cytochrome C from mitochondria blocked. Science 275: 1129–1132, 1997

36. Minn AJ, Kettlun CS, Liang H, Kelekar A, Vander Heiden MG, Chang BS, Fesik SW, Fill M, Thompson CB: Bcl-$_{XL}$ regulates apoptosis by heterodimerization-dependent and -independent mechanisms. EMBO J 18: 632–643, 1999

37. Li F, Srinivasan A, Wang Y, Armstrong RC, Tomaselli KJ, Fritz LC: Cell-specific induction of apoptosis by microinjection of cytochrome C. Bcl-$_{XL}$ has activity independent of cytochrome C release. J Biol Chem 272: 30299–30305, 1997

38. Ibrado AM, Huang Y, Fang G, Liu L, Bhalla K: Overexpression of Bcl-2 or Bcl-$_{XL}$ inhibits Ara-C-induced CPP32/Yama protease activity and apoptosis of human acute myelogenous leukemia HL-60 cells. Cancer Res 56: 4743–4748, 1996

104

39. Marin MC, Fernandez A, Bick RJ, Brisbay S, Buja LM, Snuggs M, McConkey DJ, von Eschenbach AC, Keating MJ, McDonnell TJ: Apoptosis suppression by bcl-2 is correlated with the regulation of nuclear and cytosolic Ca^{2+}. Oncogene 12: 2259–2266, 1996

40. Bruckheimer EM, Gjertsen BT, McDonnell TJ: Implications of cell death regulation in the pathogenesis and treatment of prostate cancer. Semin Oncol 26: 382–398, 1999

41. McDonnell TJ, Troncoso P, Brisbay SM, Logothetis C, Chung LW, Hsieh JT, Tu SM, Campbell ML: Expression of the protooncogene bcl-2 in the prostate and its association with emergence of androgen-independent prostate cancer. Cancer Res 52: 6940–6944, 1992

42. McDonnell TJ, Navone NM, Troncoso P, Pisters LL, Conti C, von Eschenbach AC, Brisbay S, Logothetis CJ: Expression of bcl-2 oncoprotein and p53 protein accumulation in bone marrow metastases of androgen independent prostate cancer. J Urol 157: 569–574, 1997

43. Raffo AJ, Perlman H, Chen MW, Day ML, Streitman JS, Buttyan R: Overexpression of bcl-2 protects prostate cancer cells from apoptosis *in vitro* and confers resistance to androgen depletion *in vivo*. Cancer Res 55: 4438–4445, 1995

44. Furuya Y, Krajewski S, Epstein JI, Reed JC, Isaacs JT: Expression of bcl-2 and the progression of human and rodent prostatic cancers. Clin Cancer Res 2: 389–398, 1996

45. Rokhlin OW, Guseva N, Tagiyev A, Knudson CM, Cohen MB: Bcl-2 oncoprotein protects the human prostatic carcinoma cell line PC3 from TRAIL-mediated apoptosis. Oncogene 20: 2836–2843, 2001

46. Marcelli M, Marani M, Li X, Sturgis L, Haidacher SJ, Trial JA, Mannucci R, Nicoletti I, Denner L: Heterogeneous apoptotic responses of prostate cancer cell lines identify an association between sensitivity to staurosporine-induced apoptosis, expression of Bcl-2 family members, and caspase activation. Prostate 42: 260–273, 2000

47. Li X, Marani M, Mannucci R, Kinsey B, Andriani F, Nicoletti I, Denner L, Marcelli M: Overexpression of Bcl-$_{XL}$ underlies the molecular basis for resistance to staurosporine-induced apoptosis in PC-3 cells. Cancer Res 61: 1699–1706, 2001

48. Blagosklonny MV, Giannakakou P, el-Deiry WS, Kingston DG, Higgs PI, Neckers L, Fojo T: Raf-1/bcl-2 phosphorylation: A step from microtubule damage to cell death. Cancer Res 57: 130–135, 1997

49. Mayo MW, Baldwin AS: The transcription factor NF-κB: Control of oncogenesis and cancer therapy resistance. Biochim Biophys Acta 1470: M55–M62, 2000

50. Huang S, Pettaway CA, Uehara H, Bucana CD, Fidler IJ: Blockade of NF-κB activity in human prostate cancer cells is associated with suppression of angiogenesis, invasion, and metastasis. Oncogene 20: 4188–4197, 2001

51. Palayoor ST, Youmell MY, Calderwood SK, Coleman CN, Price BD: Constitutive activation of IκB kinase alpha and NF-κB in prostate cancer cells is inhibited by ibuprofen. Oncogene 18: 7389–7394, 1999

52. Rayet B, Gelinas C: Aberrant rel/NF-κB genes and activity in human cancer. Oncogene 18: 6938–6947, 1999

53. Beg AA, Sha WC, Bronson RT, Baltimore D: Constitutive NF-κB activation, enhanced granulopoiesis, and neonatal lethality in I kappa B alpha-deficient mice. Genes Dev 9: 2736–2746, 1995

54. Wang CY, Mayo MW, Korneluk RG, Goeddel DV, Baldwin AS Jr: NF-κB antiapoptosis: Induction of TRAF1 and TRAF2 and c-IAP1 and c-IAP2 to suppress caspase-8 activation. Science 281: 1680–1683, 1998

55. Webster GA, Perkins ND: Transcriptional cross talk between NF-κB and p53. Mol Cell Biol 19: 3485–3495, 1999

56. Keller ET, Chang C, Ershler WB: Inhibition of NFκB activity through maintenance of IkappaBalpha levels contributes to dihydrotestosterone-mediated repression of the interleukin-6 promoter. J Biol Chem 271: 26267–26275, 1996

57. Rokhlin OW, Gudkov AV, Kwek S, Glover RA, Gewies AS, Cohen MB: p53 is involved in tumor necrosis factor-alpha-induced apoptosis in the human prostatic carcinoma cell line LNCaP. Oncogene 19: 1959–1968, 2000

58. Sumitomo M, Tachibana M, Nakashima J, Murai M, Miyajima A, Kimura F, Hayakawa M, Nakamura H: An essential role for nuclear factor kappa B in preventing TNF-alpha-induced cell death in prostate cancer cells. J Urol 161: 674–679, 1999

59. Das KC, White CW: Activation of NF-κB by antineoplastic agents. Role of protein kinase C. J Biol Chem 272: 14914–14920, 1997

60. Lindholm PF, Bub J, Kaul S, Shidham VB, Kajdacsy-Balla A: The role of constitutive NF-κB activity in PC-3 human prostate cancer cell invasive behavior. Clin Exp Metastasis 18: 471–479, 2000

61. Reiss K, Wang JY, Romano G, Furnari FB, Cavenee WK, Morrione A, Tu X, Baserga R: IGF-I receptor signaling in a prostatic cancer cell line with a PTEN mutation. Oncogene 19: 2687–2694, 2000

62. Baserga R: The contradictions of the insulin-like growth factor 1 receptor. Oncogene 19: 5574–5581, 2000

63. Peruzzi F, Prisco M, Morrione A, Valentinis B, Baserga R: Anti-apoptotic signaling of the insulin-like growth factor-I receptor through mitochondrial translocation of c-Raf and Nedd4. J Biol Chem 276: 25990–25996, 2001

64. Reiss K, Valentinis B, Tu X, Xu SQ, Baserga R: Molecular markers of IGF-I-mediated mitogenesis. Exp Cell Res 242: 361–372, 1998

65. Stattin P, Bylund A, Rinaldi S, Biessy C, Dechaud H, Stenman UH, Egevad L, Riboli E, Hallmans G, Kaaks R: Plasma insulin-like growth factor-I, insulin-like growth factor-binding proteins, and prostate cancer risk: A prospective study. J Natl Cancer Inst 92: 1910–1917, 2000

66. Chan JM, Stampfer MJ, Giovannucci E, Gann PH, Ma J, Wilkinson P, Hennekens CH, Pollak M: Plasma insulin-like growth factor-I and prostate cancer risk: A prospective study. Science 279: 563–566, 1998

67. Ludwig T, Eggenschwiler J, Fisher P, D'Ercole AJ, Davenport ML, Efstratiadis A: Mouse mutants lacking the type 2 IGF receptor (IGF2R) are rescued from perinatal

lethality in Igf2 and Igf1r null backgrounds. Dev Biol 177: 517–535, 1996

68. Baserga R: The IGF-I receptor in cancer research. Exp Cell Res 253: 1–6, 1999

69. Smart EJ, Graf GA, McNiven MA, Sessa WC, Engelman JA, Scherer PE, Okamoto T, Lisanti MP: Caveolins, liquid-ordered domains, and signal transduction. Mol Cell Biol 19: 7289–7304, 1999

70. Shaul PW, Anderson RG: Role of plasmalemmal caveolae in signal transduction. Am J Physiol 275: L843–L851, 1998

71. Razani B, Schlegel A, Liu J, Lisanti MP: Caveolin-1, a putative tumour suppressor gene. Biochem Soc Trans 29: 494–499, 2001

72. Timme TL, Goltsov A, Tahir S, Li L, Wang J, Ren C, Johnston RN, Thompson TC: Caveolin-1 is regulated by c-myc and suppresses c-myc-induced apoptosis. Oncogene 19: 3256–3265, 2000

73. Yang G, Truong LD, Timme TL, Ren C, Wheeler TM, Park SH, Nasu Y, Bangma CH, Kattan MW, Scardino PT, Thompson TC: Elevated expression of caveolin is associated with prostate and breast cancer. Clin Cancer Res 4: 1873–1880, 1998

74. Li L, Yang G, Ebara S, Satoh T, Nasu Y, Timme TL, Ren C, Wang J, Tahir SA, Thompson TC: Caveolin-1 mediates testosterone-stimulated survival/clonal growth and promotes metastatic activities in prostate cancer cells. Cancer Res 61: 4386–4392, 2001

75. Lu ML, Schneider MC, Zheng Y, Zhang X, Richie JP: Caveolin-1 interacts with androgen receptor. A positive modulator of androgen receptor mediated transactivation. J Biol Chem 276: 13442–13451, 2001

76. Nasu Y, Timme TL, Yang G, Bangma CH, Li L, Ren C, Park SH, DeLeon M, Wang J, Thompson TC: Suppression of caveolin expression induces androgen sensitivity in metastatic androgen-insensitive mouse prostate cancer cells. Nat Med 4: 1062–1064, 1998

77. Yang CP, Galbiati F, Volonte D, Horwitz SB, Lisanti MP: Upregulation of caveolin-1 and caveolae organelles in Taxol-resistant A549 cells. FEBS Lett 439: 368–372, 1998

78. Chan TO, Rittenhouse SE, Tsichlis PN: AKT/PKB and other D3 phosphoinositide-regulated kinases: Kinase activation by phosphoinositide-dependent phosphorylation. Annu Rev Biochem 68: 965–1014, 1999

79. Khwaja A: Akt is more than just a Bad kinase. Nature 401: 33–34, 1999

80. Zinda MJ, Johnson MA, Paul JD, Horn C, Konicek BW, Lu ZH, Sandusky G, Thomas JE, Neubauer BL, Lai MT, Graff JR: AKT-1, -2, and -3 are expressed in both normal and tumor tissues of the lung, breast, prostate, and colon. Clin Cancer Res 7: 2475–2479, 2001

81. Lin HK, Yeh S, Kang HY, Chang C: Akt suppresses androgen-induced apoptosis by phosphorylating and inhibiting androgen receptor. Proc Natl Acad Sci USA 98: 7200–7205, 2001

82. Thakkar H, Chen X, Tyan F, Gim S, Robinson H, Lee C, Pandey SK, Nwokorie C, Onwudiwe N, Srivastava RK: Pro-survival function of akt/protein kinase b in prostate cancer cells. Relationship with trail resistance. J Biol Chem 276: 38361–38369, 2001

83. Murillo H, Huang H, Schmidt LJ, Smith DI, Tindall DJ: Role of PI3K signaling in survival and progression of LNCaP prostate cancer cells to the androgen refractory state. Endocrinology 142: 4795–4805, 2001

84. Steck PA, Pershouse MA, Jasser SA, Yung WK, Lin H, Ligon AH, Langford LA, Baumgard ML, Hattier T, Davis T, Frye C, Hu R, Swedlund B, Teng DH, Tavtigian SV: Identification of a candidate tumour suppressor gene, MMAC1, at chromosome 10q23.3 that is mutated in multiple advanced cancers. Nat Genet 15: 356–362, 1997

85. Davies MA, Koul D, Dhesi H, Berman R, McDonnell TJ, McConkey D, Yung WK, Steck PA: Regulation of Akt/PKB activity, cellular growth, and apoptosis in prostate carcinoma cells by MMAC/PTEN. Cancer Res 59: 2551–2556, 1999

86. Whang YE, Wu X, Suzuki H, Reiter RE, Tran C, Vessella RL, Said JW, Isaacs WB, Sawyers CL: Inactivation of the tumor suppressor PTEN/MMAC1 in advanced human prostate cancer through loss of expression. Proc Natl Acad Sci USA 95: 5246–5250, 1998

87. Murakami YS, Albertsen H, Brothman AR, Leach RJ, White RL: Suppression of the malignant phenotype of human prostate cancer cell line PPC-1 by introduction of normal fragments of human chromosome 10. Cancer Res 56: 2157–2160, 1996

88. Gustin JA, Maehama T, Dixon JE, Donner DB: The PTEN tumor suppressor protein inhibits tumor necrosis factor-induced nuclear factor kappa B activity. J Biol Chem 276: 27740–27744, 2001

89. Vousden KH: p53: Death star. Cell 103: 691–694, 2000

90. Ludwig RL, Bates S, Vousden KH: Differential activation of target cellular promoters by p53 mutants with impaired apoptotic function. Mol Cell Biol 16: 4952–4960, 1996

91. Navone NM, Troncoso P, Pisters LL, Goodrow TL, Palmer JL, Nichols WW, von Eschenbach AC, Conti CJ: p53 protein accumulation and gene mutation in the progression of human prostate carcinoma. J Natl Cancer Inst 85: 1657–1669, 1993

92. Heidenberg HB, Sesterhenn IA, Gaddipati JP, Weghorst CM, Buzard GS, Moul JW, Srivastava S: Alteration of the tumor suppressor gene p53 in a high fraction of hormone refractory prostate cancer. J Urol 154: 414–421, 1995

93. Burchardt M, Burchardt T, Shabsigh A, Ghafar M, Chen MW, Anastasiadis A, de la Taille A, Kiss A, Buttyan R: Reduction of wild type p53 function confers a hormone resistant phenotype on LNCaP prostate cancer cells. Prostate 48: 225–230, 2001

94. Berges RR, Furuya Y, Remington L, English HF, Jacks T, Isaacs JT: Cell proliferation, DNA repair, and p53 function are not required for programmed death of prostatic glandular cells induced by androgen ablation. Proc Natl Acad Sci USA 90: 8910–8914, 1993

95. Bowen C, Voeller HJ, Kikly K, Gelmann EP: Synthesis of procaspases-3 and -7 during apoptosis in prostate cancer cells. Cell Death Differ 6: 394–401, 1999

96. Ahmed MM, Sells SF, Venkatasubbarao K, Fruitwala SM, Muthukkumar S, Harp C, Mohiuddin M, Rangnekar VM: Ionizing radiation-inducible apoptosis in the absence of

p53 linked to transcription factor EGR-1. J Biol Chem 272: 33056–33061, 1997

97. Yang A, Kaghad M, Wang Y, Gillett E, Fleming MD, Dotsch V, Andrews NC, Caput D, McKeon F: p63, a p53 homolog at 3q27-29, encodes multiple products with transactivating, death-inducing, and dominant-negative activities. Mol Cell 2: 305–316, 1998

98. Signoretti S, Waltregny D, Dilks J, Isaac B, Lin D, Garraway L, Yang A, Montironi R, McKeon F, Loda M: p63 is a prostate basal cell marker and is required for prostate development. Am J Pathol 157: 1769–1775, 2000

99. Parsons JK, Gage WR, Nelson WG, De Marzo AM: p63 protein expression is rare in prostate adenocarcinoma: Implications for cancer diagnosis and carcinogenesis. Urology 58: 619–624, 2001

100. Jost CA, Marin MC, Kaelin WG Jr: p73 is a human p53-related protein that can induce apoptosis. Nature 389: 191–194, 1997

101. Yokomizo A, Mai M, Bostwick DG, Tindall DJ, Qian J, Cheng L, Jenkins RB, Smith DI, Liu W: Mutation and expression analysis of the p73 gene in prostate cancer. Prostate 39: 94–100, 1999

102. Takahashi H, Fukutome K, Watanabe M, Furusato M, Shiraishi T, Ito H, Suzuki H, Ikawa S, Hano H: Mutation analysis of the p51 gene and correlation between p53, p73, and p51 expressions in prostatic carcinoma. Prostate 47: 85–90, 2001

103. Elliott K, Sakamuro D, Basu A, Du W, Wunner W, Staller P, Gaubatz S, Zhang H, Prochownik E, Eilers M, Prendergast GC: Bin1 functionally interacts with Myc and inhibits cell proliferation via multiple mechanisms. Oncogene 18: 3564–3573, 1999

104. Sakamuro D, Elliott KJ, Wechsler-Reya R, Prendergast GC: BIN1 is a novel MYC-interacting protein with features of a tumour suppressor. Nat Genet 14: 69–77, 1996

105. DuHadaway JB, Sakamuro D, Ewert DL, Prendergast GC: Bin1 mediates apoptosis by c-Myc in transformed primary cells. Cancer Res 61: 3151–3156, 2001

106. Ge K, Minhas F, Duhadaway J, Mao NC, Wilson D, Buccafusca R, Sakamuro D, Nelson P, Malkowicz SB, Tomaszewski J, Prendergast GC: Loss of heterozygosity and tumor suppressor activity of Bin1 in prostate carcinoma. Int J Cancer 86: 155–161, 2000

107. Elliott K, Ge K, Du W, Prendergast GC: The c-Myc-interacting adaptor protein Bin1 activates a caspase-independent cell death program. Oncogene 19: 4669–4684, 2000

108. Bruckheimer EM, Kyprianou N: Apoptosis in prostate carcinogenesis. A growth regulator and a therapeutic target. Cell Tissue Res 301: 153–162, 2000

109. Hocevar BA, Howe PH: Mechanisms of TGF-beta-induced cell cycle arrest. Miner Electrolyte Metab 24: 131–135, 1998

110. Martikainen P, Kyprianou N, Isaacs JT: Effect of transforming growth factor-beta 1 on proliferation and death of rat prostatic cells, Endocrinology 127: 2963–2968, 1990

111. Oberhammer F, Bursch W, Tiefenbacher R, Froschl G, Pavelka M, Purchio T, Schulte-Hermann R: Apoptosis is induced by transforming growth factor-beta 1 within 5 hours in regressing liver without significant fragmentation of the DNA. Hepatology 18: 1238–1246, 1993

112. Russell PJ, Bennett S, Stricker P: Growth factor involvement in progression of prostate cancer. Clin Chem 44: 705–723, 1998

113. Danielpour D, Kadomatsu K, Anzano MA, Smith JM, Sporn MB: Development and characterization of nontumorigenic and tumorigenic epithelial cell lines from rat dorsal-lateral prostate. Cancer Res 54: 3413–3421, 1994

114. Robson CN, Gnanapragasam V, Byrne RL, Collins AT, Neal DE: Transforming growth factor-beta1 up-regulates p15, p21 and p27 and blocks cell cycling in G1 in human prostate epithelium. J Endocrinol 160: 257–266, 1999

115. Kyprianou N, Isaacs JT: Identification of a cellular receptor for transforming growth factor-beta in rat ventral prostate and its negative regulation by androgens. Endocrinology 123: 2124–2131, 1988

116. Steiner MS: Transforming growth factor-beta and prostate cancer. World J Urol 13: 329–336, 1995

117. Wilding G, Zugmeier G, Knabbe C, Flanders K, Gelmann E: Differential effects of transforming growth factor beta on human prostate cancer cells in vitro. Mol Cell Endocrinol 62: 79–87, 1989

118. Kundu SD, Kim IY, Yang T, Doglio L, Lang S, Zhang X, Buttyan R, Kim SJ, Chang J, Cai X, Wang Z, Lee C: Absence of proximal duct apoptosis in the ventral prostate of transgenic mice carrying the C3(1)-TGF-beta type II dominant negative receptor. Prostate 43: 118–124, 2000

119. Guo Y, Kyprianou N: Restoration of transforming growth factor beta signaling pathway in human prostate cancer cells suppresses tumorigenicity via induction of caspase-1-mediated apoptosis. Cancer Res 59: 1366–1371, 1999

120. Hayes SA, Zarnegar M, Sharma M, Yang F, Peehl DM, ten Dijke P, Sun Z: SMAD3 represses androgen receptor-mediated transcription. Cancer Res 61: 2112–2118, 2001

121. Sells SF, Han SS, Muthukkumar S, Maddiwar N, Johnstone R, Boghaert E, Gillis D, Liu G, Nair P, Monnig S, Collini P, Mattson MP, Sukhatme VP, Zimmer SG, Wood DP Jr, McRoberts JW, Shi Y, Rangnekar VM: Expression and function of the leucine zipper protein Par-4 in apoptosis. Mol Cell Biol 17: 3823–3832, 1997

122. Diaz-Meco MT, Municio MM, Frutos S, Sanchez P, Lozano J, Sanz L, Moscat J: The product of par-4, a gene induced during apoptosis, interacts selectively with the atypical isoforms of protein kinase C. Cell 86: 777–786, 1996

123. Johnstone RW, See RH, Sells SF, Wang J, Muthukkumar S, Englert C, Haber DA, Licht JD, Sugrue SP, Roberts T, Rangnekar VM, Shi Y: A novel repressor, par-4, modulates transcription and growth suppression functions of the Wilms' tumor suppressor WT1. Mol Cell Biol 16: 6945–6956, 1996

124. Page G, Kogel D, Rangnekar V, Scheidtmann KH: Interaction partners of Dlk/ZIP kinase: Co-expression of Dlk/ZIP kinase and Par-4 results in cytoplasmic retention and apoptosis. Oncogene 18: 7265–7273, 1999

125. Qiu SG, Krishnan S, el-Guendy N, Rangnekar VM: Negative regulation of Par-4 by oncogenic Ras is essential

for cellular transformation. Oncogene 18: 7115–7123, 1999

126. Barradas M, Monjas A, Diaz-Meco MT, Serrano M, Moscat J: The downregulation of the pro-apoptotic protein Par-4 is critical for Ras-induced survival and tumor progression. EMBO J 18: 6362–6369, 1999

127. Berra E, Municio MM, Sanz L, Frutos S, Diaz-Meco MT, Moscat J: Positioning atypical protein kinase C isoforms in the UV-induced apoptotic signaling cascade. Mol Cell Biol 17: 4346–4354, 1997

128. Nalca A, Qiu SG, El-Guendy N, Krishnan S, Rangnekar VM: Oncogenic Ras sensitizes cells to apoptosis by Par-4. J Biol Chem 274: 29976–29983, 1999

129. Diaz-Meco MT, Lallena MJ, Monjas A, Frutos S, Moscat J: Inactivation of the inhibitory kappaB protein kinase/nuclear factor kappaB pathway by Par-4 expression potentiates tumor necrosis factor alpha-induced apoptosis. J Biol Chem 274: 19606–19612, 1999

130. Boghaert ER, Sells SF, Walid AJ, Malone P, Williams NM, Weinstein MH, Strange R, Rangnekar VM: Immunohisto-chemical analysis of the proapoptotic protein Par-4 in normal rat tissues. Cell Growth Differ 8: 881–890, 1997

131. Qiu G, Ahmed M, Sells SF, Mohiuddin M, Weinstein MH, Rangnekar VM: Mutually exclusive expression patterns of Bcl-2 and Par-4 in human prostate tumors consistent with down-regulation of Bcl-2 by Par-4. Oncogene 18: 623–631, 1999

132. Matsubara S, Wada Y, Gardner TA, Egawa M, Park MS, Hsieh CL, Zhau HE, Kao C, Kamidono S, Gillenwater JY, Chung LW: A conditional replication-competent adenoviral vector, Ad-OC-E1a, to cotarget prostate cancer and bone stroma in an experimental model of androgen-independent prostate cancer bone metastasis. Cancer Res 61: 6012–6019, 2001

Address for offprints: Vivek M. Rangnekar, Combs Building Rm. 303, University of Kentucky, 800 Rose Street, Lexington, KY, USA; *Tel:* 859-257-2677; *Fax:* 859-257-9608; *e-mail:* vmrang01@pop.uky.edu

On the role of cell surface carbohydrates and their binding proteins (lectins) in tumor metastasis

Elieser Gorelik[1], Uri Galili[2] and Avraham Raz[3]
[1]University of Pittsburgh Cancer Institute and Department of Pathology, Pittsburgh, PA; [2]Department of Cardiovascular-Thoracic Surgery, Rush University, Chicago, IL; [3]Karmanos Cancer Institute, Wayne State University, Detroit, MI, USA

Key words: metastasis, carbohydrate, glycoprotein, lectin, galectin

Abstract

This review focuses on the recent advances in investigations of the role of cell surface carbohydrates in tumor metastasis. It also summarizes the results of extensive studies of endogenous lectins, their structure, carbohydrate specificity and biological functions with the major emphasis on the significance of lectin–cell surface carbohydrate interactions in a metastatic process. Numerous data demonstrate that malignant transformation is associated with various and complex alterations in the glycosylation process. Some of these changes might provide a selective advantage for tumor cells during their progression to more invasive and metastatic phenotype. Cell glycosylation depends on the expression and function of various glycosyltransferases and glycosidases. Recently, transfection of genes encoding various glysosyltransferases gene in sense and antisense orientation helped to bring direct evidence that changes in cell surface carbohydrates are important for the metastatic behavior of tumor cells. Cell surface carbohydrates affect tumor cell interactions with normal cells or with the extracellular matrix during metastatic spread and growth. These interactions can be mediated via tumor cell carbohydrates and their binding proteins known as endogenous lectins. The family of the discovered endogenous lectins is rapidly expanding. The number of C-type lectins has reached 50 and at least 10 galectins have been identified. The biological significance of the endogenous lectins and their possible role in tumor growth and metastasis formation has started to unravel. Some lectins recognize the 'foreign' patterns of cell surface carbohydrates expressed by microorganisms and tumor cells, and play a role in innate and adaptive immunity. It was shown that lectins affect tumor cell survival, adhesion to the endothelium or extracellular matrix, as well as tumor vascularization and other processes that are crucial for metastatic spread and growth.

1. Introduction

Mammalian cells have an effective glycosylation machinery that includes glycosyltransferases and glycosidases. The sum activities of these enzymes determine the glycosylation patterns of proteins and lipids. Carbohydrates have an immense potential for encoding biological information [1–3]. Properties of peptides are primarily dependent on the number and sequences of amino acids. In contrast, carbohydrates might provide broader variations that depend not only on the number and sequences of monomeric units but also on the position and anomeric configuration (α or β) of the glucosidic units and the occurrence of branch points. Thus, two molecules of a single monosaccharide can join to form 11 different disaccharides, whereas two single amino acids can form one dipeptide. Four different monosaccharides can form 35,560 distinct tetrasaccharides, but four different amino acids can form only 24 tetrapeptides [3]. The heterogeneity and branching of oligosaccharides might yield a further level of structural and functional diversity compared to peptides and lipids.

Carbohydrates can be associated with proteins or lipids and form glycoproteins, glycolipids or glycosaminoglycans. Oligosaccharide chains link to protein by two types of linkages: (a) through C-1 binding of N-acetylgalactosamine to the hydroxyl of threonine or serine, via glycosidic bond (O-link chain), or (b) through binding of N-acetylglucosamine

M.L. Cher, K.V. Honn and A. Raz (eds.), Prostate Cancer: New Horizons in Research and Treatment, 109–141.
© 2002 Kluwer Academic Publishers.

to the amide side chain of an asparagine (N-link chain). The asparagine that have linked carbohydrate chains are those with the sequence Asn-X-Ser (Thr)-. Carbohydrate domains of glycoproteins and glycolipids are synthesized by a series of hierarchically organized glycosyltransferases within the endoplasmic reticulum and Golgi apparatus. In addition, glycosidases can remove some carbohydrates and thus modify carbohydrate portion of the glycoconjugates [1].

The importance of cell surface carbohydrates is particularly evident from the finding of their variation in expression during embryonic development and cell differentiation. Numerous data has been accumulated showing that malignant transformation is also associated with various alterations in the expression of cell surface carbohydrates, that might indicate that carbohydrates play a role in malignant transformation. Moreover, it has been suggested that cell surface carbohydrates might determine the ability of malignant cells to form distant metastases in various anatomical locations [4–7].

Analysis of the significance of protein glycosylation revealed that glycosylation of proteins can affect their folding, intracellular trafficking and localization, the rate of degradation and determine their organizational framework within cytoplasm, membranes and extracellularly [1,2]. Glycosylation of lipids was found to affect membrane rigidity and the function of membrane proteins such as growth factor receptors and integrins [8–10]. Carbohydrate chains on proteins and lipids seems to play an important role in the cell-to-cell interactions and interactions of cells with extracellular matrix and soluble molecules [1,2,11].

It is believed that some of these interactions are mediated via binding of the carbohydrate portion of the glycoconjugates to specific proteins. Proteins that selectively bind to a specific carbohydrate structure are generally known as lectins (from the Latin legere, to select or choose). Initially lectins were isolated from various plants [3]. These proteins have no enzymatic activity and are distinct from the immunoglobulins (antibodies) that also could bind carbohydrates. Usually, lectins are oligomeric proteins with several carbohydrate-binding sites per molecule. The ability of plant lectins to bind sugars and to induce aggregation of cells of various origins was known for a century. However, much of the research interest in lectins started in 1960 when Peter Nowel found that the phytoheamagglutinin (PHA) lectin isolated from the red kidney bean is able to induce proliferation of peripheral blood lymphocytes. This simple observation

had paramount importance in various aspects of cell biology. Before 1960, chromosomal analysis in human and animals cells was almost exclusively restricted to analysis of malignant cells, since they are highly mitotic and chromosomal analysis could be performed only on dividing cells at the metaphase stage. Thus stimulation of proliferation of human peripheral blood lymphocytes with PHA laid a ground for human chromosome analysis and human cytogenetics. Secondly, it was soon discovered that PHA as well as Con A lectins exclusively stimulate the proliferation of T lymphocytes, whereas PWM lectin is mitogenic for T plus B lymphocytes [12,13]. Based on this observation, evaluation of lymphocyte responses to lectin stimulation became a useful approach for evaluation of functional activity of lymphocytes and immunological status in human and animal studies [12].

Analysis of lectin–carbohydrate interactions helped to identify the carbohydrates that specifically bind to certain lectins. Lectin-binding analysis became a useful tool for the analysis of cell surface carbohydrate profiles of normal and malignant cells. Investigations of the interactions between lectins and cell surface carbohydrates of various normal and malignant cells revealed that these interactions could induce various biological effects, including stimulation of cell proliferation or cell death [14,15]. Crosslinking of cell surface carbohydrates by lectins can lead to cytoskeleton reorganization [16], protein-tyrosine phosphorylation [17], trigger superoxide/H_2O_2 and granule enzyme release from neutrophils [18]. Human or animal lymphocytes incubated with PHA or Con A lectins become highly cytotoxic and are able to kill various normal and malignant cell targets. This cytotoxicity was termed lectin dependent cell-mediated cytotoxicity (LDCC) [12,13]. Some lectins are able to kill normal or malignant cells directly in the absence of lymphocytes. Lectin-mediated cytotoxicity and selection of malignant cells for resistance to the cytotoxic effects of lectins was widely used for the analysis of the carbohydrate changes that were associated with lectin resistance as well as with the biosynthesis of carbohydrates [19]. Moreover, lectin-resistant cell variants with changed carbohydrate structure became a very useful tool for investigation of the role of cell surface carbohydrates in tumor growth and metastasis formation [7, 20–22].

It is worth nothing that, initially, the analysis of various lectin-mediated biological effects was performed *in vitro* using human or animal cells and plant-derived lectins. These studies obviously raise the question of whether the observed lectin-mediated effects are *in vitro* artifacts or they represent processes that also occur *in vivo* in mammals. Recently, it became apparent that lectins exist not only in plants but also in all living organisms including microorganisms, insects, animals and humans. The number of the discovered animal lectins increases every year. Studies on mammalian lectins reported no homology with plant lectins, suggesting that lectins are essential for the existence of living organisms and, therefore, were independently reinvented by nature. The biological significance of these endogenous lectins is a subject of extensive investigations. The obtained information implies that endogenous lectins play an important role in various biological processes such as host defense immunity, inflammation, cell proliferation and cell death, trafficking normal leukocytes as well as malignant cells and their spread and metastatic growth [23–28].

The possible involvement of endogenous lectins in metastasis formation could be an outcome of their interactions with cell surface carbohydrates. Several excellent reviews on the role of cell surface carbohydrates in tumor and metastasis formation have been previously published [4,5,7,29]. Recently, studies in this field have progressed substantially as a result of novel approaches such as transfection of genes coding various glucosyltransferases and glycosidases in sense and antisense orientation. We feel there is a need to summarize the most recent advances in this area. In addition, we tried to assess the significance of carbohydrate changes for metastasis formation in the light of their possible interactions with endogenous lectins. Studies of endogenous lectins became multidirectional and show their immense importance in various biological mechanisms, including metastatic spread and growth. Therefore, we attempted to summarize the accumulated data related to the structure of, endogenous lectins their interactions with oligosaccharides and their significance, particularly in regulation of tumor metastasis formation.

2. Alterations of cell surface carbohydrates in malignant cells

Numerous experimental data accumulated for the last several decades on extensive investigations of various human and experimental tumors, revealed that malignant transformation is associated with various changes in cell glycosylation. Tumor cells display aberrant patterns of glycosylation in carbohydrates linked to ceramides (glycolipids and glycosphingolipids

inserted in the lipid bilayer) and carbohydrates linked to cell surface proteins (glycoproteins) [4,5,7,29,30]. The information on carbohydrate alterations identified in glycolipids has been more accurate than that in glycoproteins, because a specific glycolipid can be isolated and structurally defined, whereas carbohydrates of glycoproteins are always heterogeneous [4]. Analysis of tumor cell glycolipids revealed that the major glycosylation changes are based on two different mechanisms: blockage of carbohydrate synthesis or neosynthesis. Several different chemotypes of aberrant glycosylation were identified in tumor cells that were associated without or with accumulation of precursor of ganglio- and globo-series structures [4]. Gangliosides are sialic acid-containing glycosphingolipids that are primarily expressed in the plasma membrane, and play an important role in cell growth and differentiation. GD3 ganglioside overexpression was observed in many tumors of neuroectodermal or epithelial origin such as glioma, medulloblastoma, neuroblastoma, melanoma, head and neck tumors, breast cancer and teratomas [4,31–33]. An increase in the ganglioside content and the accumulation of more complex gangliosides observed in various tumors makes them immunogenic, and gangliosides could serve as a tumor antigen recognized by immune system. Monoclonal antibodies (Mabs) against GD3 in human melanomas and acute non-lymphocytic leukemia [34], GD2 in human neuroectodermal tumors [35], Gg3 in Hodgkin's lymphoma and Gb3 in Burkitt's lymphoma [36,37] have been generated and have been used in the clinical trials.

It is believed that ganglioside accumulation in tumor cells stimulates tumor growth by affecting growth factor receptor or the function of integrins [4]. However, recent studies brought new insights into the possible mechanisms by which gangliosides might regulate tumor growth. It was found that exogenous GD3 gangliosides added *in vitro* could stimulate vascular endothelial growth factor (VEGF) production by tumor cells [38]. Using a corneal vascularization model, it was demonstrated that the effect of gangliosides on the neoangiogenesis depends on the ratio between GM3 : GD3. Stimulation or inhibition of angiogenesis was induced by decreased or increased GM3 : GD3 ratio, respectively [39].

Tumor vascularization is essential for tumor growth [40]. The importance of gangliosides in tumor growth and regulation of VEGF production and tumor vascularization was recently confirmed using the gene transfection technique. GM3 ganglioside is an important precursor of more complex gangliosides. GM3 can be converted to GM2 in the a-series by GM2-synthase or in GD3 in the b-series by GD3-synthase. Transfection of murine EPEN cell line that expresses only GM3 ganglioside with the GM2-synthase cDNA resulted in the production of complex gangliosides such as GM2, GM1 and GD1a. In parallel, increase in tumor growth of the transfected cells was observed [33]. This increase in tumor formation by EPEN cells transfected with the GM2-synthase cDNA was found to be a result of increased VEGF production and tumor vascularization [33].

To inhibit GD3 expression, a rat F-11 cell line was transfected with antisense GD3-synthase cDNA. Antisense-transfected tumor cells showed a reduction in the expression of GD3 that paralleled with the reduction in tumor growth [31]. Suppression of GD3 gangliosides by antisense GD3-synthase cDNA transfection was associated with inhibition of VEGF production and tumor vascularization [31]. Thus, the observed changes in ganglioside expression by tumor cells might affect VEGF production, tumor vascularization and tumor growth.

Analysis of cell surface carbohydrates in tumors from cancer patients and experimental animals showed that the most common changes in glycoproteins of tumor cells are associated with the presence of larger, more branched N-linked oligosaccharides [6,7,41]. The β1-6GlcNAc-branched N-glycans are tri- or tetra-antenna-like oligosaccharides that represent a subset of the complex-type N-glycans. Increased β1-6 branching of N-linked oligosaccharides in tumor cells can be detected by an increase in L-PHA lectin binding [6,7,41]. Increased β1-6 branching of N-linked oligosaccharides is a result of increase of GlcNAcβ1-6Manα1-6Manβ branching at the trimannosyl core of complex-type oligosaccharides that is due to the increased activity of N-acetylglucosomyltransferase V (GlcNAc-TV) that is also known as MGAT5 (mannoside acetyl glucosaminyl transferase 5). GlcNAc-TV catalyzes the transfer of N-acetylglucosamine from UDP-N-acetylglucosamine to α6-D-mannoside to produce the β1-6 linked branching of N-glycan oligosaccharides, which controls the polylactosamine content. Increased β1-6 branching of N-linked oligosaccharides could be found in the early stage of carcinogenesis induced by oncogenes v-src, H-ras, v-fps or by oncogenic viruses [42–45]. Malignant transformation is associated with an increased expression of the GlcNAc-TV gene. This gene is 155 kb long, contains 17 exons

and is regulated at the level of transcription by multiple promoters. Two cis-acting elements have been identified, each of them containing an Ets-1 binding site (5′-GGA-3) [46]. Further analysis of the regulation of the GlcNAc-TV gene expression showed that it could be inhibited with herbimycin A, suggesting that src kinase could be involved in the regulation of GlcNAc-TV gene expression [47]. The src stimulation of the GlcNAc-TV gene was abrogated by transfection with a dominant-negative mutant of the Raf kinase or Ets-2, indicating the involvement of Ets transcription factors in the regulation of this gene. The src-responsive element was located to a 250 base pair region containing two overlapping Ets sites. Thus the observed stimulatory effects of the src kinase on GlcNAc-TV gene expression are dependent on Ets [47]. Ets-1 transcription factor was also involved in the regulation of matrix metalloproteinases (MMPs) that are important for tumor invasion and tumor-induced angiogenesis [48]. Some data based on the analysis of human colon carcinoma cell lines showed that cell lines having K-ras mutations manifested increased β1-6GlcNAc branching. In these cell lines, the level of branching correlated with the level of ras-GTP activity. In contrast, cell lines that express wild type of K-ras showed no elevation of β1-6 branching. These results suggest that β1-6 branching is linked to K-ras activation [49].

The increased β1-6 branching of N-linked oligosaccharides can provide additional lactosamine antennae for the terminal capping by sialic acid, resulting in an increase in tumor cell sialylation [7]. Branching of O-linked oligosaccharides may affect tumor cell sialylation as well. Increase in tumor cell sialylation is common for various tumors. This could also be due to an increase in sialyltransferase activity [50,51]. Using mice transgenic for the SV40 large T antigen under the control of a liver-specific promoter (antithrombin III promoter), the glycosylation changes were investigated during hepatocellular carcinoma formation [52]. Serum glycoproteins and liver cell membranes manifested a substantial increase in α2,6 sialylation even at the earliest stage of hepatocellular carcinoma formation as a result of increased activity of the galactoside: α2,6 sialyltransferase (α2,6ST) [52]. A similar increase in the galactoside α2,6ST activity was observed in rat fibroblast transfected with the c-Ha-ras oncogene [53].

An increased body of evidence has indicated that changes in the expression of the histo-blood ABO and Lewis group antigens are also common for various types of malignancies [30]. The blood group antigens are present not only on erythrocytes but also on various nucleated cells of different histological origin. These antigens represent carbohydrate structures that are built up by sequential addition of sugar residues onto an oligosaccharide precursor, catalyzed by specific glycosyltransferases [54]. $\alpha 1,2$ fucosyltransferase ($\alpha 1,2$FT) catalyzes a transglycosylation reaction between the nucleotide sugar donor guanosine diphosphate-fucose (GDP-Fuc) and oligosaccharide acceptors to generate the H blood group antigen with the terminal structure Fuc$\alpha 1$-2Gal$\beta 1$-3GlcNAc-R, or Fuc$\alpha 1$-2Gal$\beta 1$-4GlcNAc-R [54]. These oligosaccharides can be further converted into A and B blood group antigens by linking either an N-acetylgalactosamine or a galactose to the penultimate galactose, respectively [54].

Elevated level of H antigen and $\alpha 1,2$FT was found in human colon adenocarcinomas that was associated with poor prognosis [55]. The level of A and B antigen expression in tumor cells displays a wide range of variation. Reduction or complete loss of histo-blood group A and B antigens has been found in various human malignancies such as lung, gastrointestinal, cervical cancer, oral and bladder carcinomas [56–59]. It was found that the level of decreased expression of A/B in lung and cervical malignancies are correlated with their invasive and metastatic properties [60,61]. A similar correlation was found in oral and bladder carcinomas [57,62]. Furthermore, a decrease or loss of both A and B carbohydrate structures was correlated with reduced survival of patients with lung cancer [63]. These differences in survival could be attributed to the higher invasive and metastatic properties of tumor cells with reduced expression of A and B carbohydrates [64].

To determine whether these parameters are cause related, Ichikawa et al. [65] transfected human colon carcinoma HRT18 and gastric carcinoma MKN74 cell lines with cDNAs of blood group A or B transferases. Transfected cells expressing A and B antigens showed a significant reduction in Matrigel-dependent haptotactic motility [65]. This motility is largely controlled by integrin chains $\alpha 3$, $\alpha 6$ and $\beta 1$. Antibodies against these integrins can also inhibit haptotactic motility of the parental cells [65]. It was found that in tumor cells transfected with the A and B transferases, $\alpha 3$, $\alpha 6$ and $\beta 1$ integrin chains were heavily A- and B-glycosylated, whereas parental cells integrins expressed H epitope [65]. Thus, A and B glycosylation of the integrin receptors may be responsible for the changes in haptotactic motility of the transfected cells. It was shown that

N-glycosylation of integrin is essential for the correct assembly of α and β subunits and their function [8].

To further assess the significance of A and B antigen expression, Ichikawa et al. [64] separated human SW480 and HT29 cells expressing histo-blood group A into A-positive and A-negative sub populations, using the panning procedure. These cells manifested significant differences in their Matrigel-dependent haptotactic motility. A-negative tumor cells showed higher level of haptotactic motility than A-positive cells. No differences in the integrin expression were found. However, a reduction in haptotactic motility of A-positive cells was associated with A-glycosylation of $\alpha 3$, $\alpha 6$ and $\beta 1$ chains of integrin receptors. In addition, A-negative cells showed not only increased motility but also increased rate of *in vitro* proliferation [64]. It was proposed that observed association between expression of A antigen and cell proliferation is based on the following possibilities: (a) a common transcription factor that controls both cell proliferation and A/B transferase gene expression is induced during tumor progression; (b) A/B glycosylation of some growth factors (e.g. EGF, TGF-β) might affect their function [64].

Recently, the expression of Lewis blood group antigens and their isomers in various human malignancies became a subject of extensive investigations. These studies were stimulated by findings that sialyl Le^a (sLe^a) and sialyl Le^x (sLe^x) antigen could serve as a ligand of endogenous C-type lectin named selectins. Le^x, Le^y, sLe^x and polymeric forms of these molecules are synthesized based on polylactosamine type 2 chains (Gal$\beta 1$-4GlcNAc$\beta 1$-3) by substitution with fucose and sialic acid, whereas synthesis of Le^a and sLe^a depends on the presence of polylactosamine type 1 chains (Gal$\beta 1$-3GlcNAc$\beta 1$-3) [54].

Studies using immunohistochemical staining of tumors showed that normal breast epithelial cells do not express sLe^a and sLe^x molecules, whereas expression of these molecules was increased in primary breast carcinoma lesions [66]. In general, numerous studies indicate that Lewis antigens are synthesized *de novo* or overexpressed in a majority of human carcinomas of the colon, bladder, breast and lungs, and are often associated with the advanced forms of malignancies [67–69]. Furthermore, some studies indicate that the level of expression of sLe might have a prognostic value in cancer patients. Patients with colon carcinoma showed a positive correlation between sLe^x expression and poor prognosis [68,70].

sLe^x and sLe^a, associated with glycoproteins, can be present in N-glycans or O-glycans [69]. Thus, it was of interest to determine whether N- or O-type association of these carbohydrates more closely correlates with tumor progression. The synthesis of sLe^x and sLe^a depends on the function of β1,6-N-acetylglucosaminyltransferase (C2GnT) [29]. Immunohistochemical analysis of sLe^a and sLe^x and expression of C2GnT in human colorectal specimens revealed that C2GnT was expressed in 63% of the cancer tissues studied, whereas no expression of C2GnT was found in normal mucosa of all the 46 patients. About 68% of colorectal cancer cells expressing sLe^a and 58% of cells expressing sLe^x contained mRNA for C2GnT. sLe^a and sLe^x on the cell surface of these carcinoma cells were expressed in O-glycans [69]. When expression of C2GnT, as well as sLe^a and sLe^x, was evaluated in colorectal carcinomas, it was concluded that C2GnT expression closely correlates with the vessel invasion and with the depth of tumor invasion. These data suggest that expression of sLe^a and sLe^x in O-glycans is associated with lymphatic and venous invasions [69]. Furthermore, a comparative analysis of sLe^a and sLe^x expression by tumor cells from primary and metastatic lesions showed obvious differences in the expression of sLe^x and/or sLe^a in most patients [71,72]. The importance of sLe^x and sLe^a in metastasis formation will be discussed later (see section 3.2.1).

In summary, alterations of cell surface carbohydrates are often observed as a result of malignant transformation. These changes are usually found both in human as well as in experimental tumors, and they can be detected in the earliest stages of malignant transformation. The often observed association between changes in tumor cell glycosylation and survival time of cancer patients suggests that alterations in tumor cell glycosylation patterns are not accidental but an important part of tumor progression toward more malignant phenotype.

2.1. Cell surface carbohydrate in primary and metastatic cells

The histochemical analysis of carbohydrate expression by human tumor cells derived from the primary and metastatic lesions showed obvious differences, suggesting that changes in the expression of cell surface carbohydrates by metastatic cells might be a contributing factor in metastasis formation [5–7,30,67,68]. This possibility is further supported by a comparative analysis of carbohydrate expression in experimental tumors with different metastatic potentials. Several reports showed a positive correlation between the levels of cell surface sialylation and metastatic ability of various experimental tumors. Using 29 murine and rat cell lines, Yogeeswaran and Salk [73] found a positive correlation between the metastatic ability of these lines and their total sialic acid content. Similarly, highly metastatic variant (ESb) of Eb T-lymphoma of DBA/2 mice showed higher level of cell membrane sialylation than the parental low metastatic tumor cells [74,75]. Selection of ESb cells for their plastic adherence resulted in a loss of their metastatic potential and, in parallel, the selected plastic adherent sub-line (ESb-M) manifested a reduction in cell surface sialylation. When the metastatic revertants from ESb-M were isolated from the spleen (ESb-MR) or the brain (ESb-MBR) of tumor bearing mice, the increase in the metastatic ability of these revertants was associated with an increase in their sialylation [74,75]. A similar association between the levels of cell surface sialylation and metastatic potentials was reported in various sub-lines of MDAY-D2 lymphoma cells [74].

The correlation between cell surface sialylation and metastatic potentials of tumor cells is not absolute and in some cell lines the degree of sialylation does not correlate with metastasis formation [76]. The distribution of sialic acid on specific N- or O-linked oligosaccharides rather than the total quantity of sialic acid may affect the metastatic properties of these cells. Analysis of B16 melanoma sub-lines with high and low metastatic potentials showed no differences in the total levels of sialic acid, but showed differences in the position of the sialic residues. In high metastatic sub-lines more α2-3 sialylation in SAα2-3Galβ1-4GlcNAc oligosaccharides was observed, whereas in low metastatic cell lines higher sialylation was found in SAα2-6Galβ1-4GlcNAc and SAα2-3Galβ1-3GalNAc chains [77].

Metastatic potential of tumor cells was also associated with increased β1-6 branching of the N-linked oligosaccharides [43,44,78]. Increased β1-6 branching increases the number of Galβ1-4GlcNAc structures that can be sialylated, resulting in a total increase in cell surface sialylation. Some evidence indicates that increased GlcNAc branching might lead not only to a quantitative increase in sialylation but also to an increase in α2-3-linked sialic residues. It is believed that an elevated level of α2-3 sialylation increases the metastatic potentials of tumor cells [79].

Thus several lines of evidence indicate a strong correlation between cell membrane carbohydrates and metastatic properties of tumor cells.

2.2. Inhibitors of glycosylation and metastasis formation

To obtain a more direct confirmation on the role of carbohydrates in metastatic behavior of tumor cells, it is imperative to modify the expression of surface carbohydrates and evaluate the effect of these changes on the metastatic ability of tumor cell. Such studies have been performed using various inhibitors of glycosylation [80,81]. Tunicamycin inhibits the initial steps in glycosylation by blocking the transfer of the preassembled Glc3Man9GlcNAc2 unit from dolichol phosphate to Asn-X-Ser/Thr sequence of glycoproteins. Castanospermine, deoxynojirimycin and 1,6-epi-cyclophellitol are α-glucosidase inhibitors and prevent removal of terminal glucose residues, leading to production of high mannose oligosaccharides with terminal glucose residues. This may inhibit intracellular movement of glycoproteins or their function. Mannostatin, 1-deoxymannojirimycin and swainsonine are the Golgi α-mannosidase I and II inhibitors [80,81].

Basically all experiments showed that in vitro pretreatment of tumor cells or in vivo treatment with inhibitors of glycosylation resulted in a profound inhibition of metastasis formation [82,83]. Swainsonine has been the most extensively investigated [83,84]. Analysis of the mechanisms of anti-metastatic effects of these inhibitors revealed that swainsonine suppressed β1-6GlcNAc branching, reduced adhesion of the treated cells to endothelial cells and inhibited tumor cell invasion. This inhibition of invasiveness was found to be a result of increase in TIMP-1 and decrease in collagenase IV expression [85]. Castanospermine treatment of v-fms-transformed tumor cells resulted in an accumulation of immature forms of the v-fms-transformed glycoproteins and inhibitions of tumor formation [86]. Swainsonine showed low toxicity in vivo and was able to inhibit experimental and spontaneous metastasis as well as local tumor growth of murine or xeno-transplanted human tumors [83]. However, further studies showed that inhibitors of glycosylation seem to have a variety of pleotropic effects and thus could affect cell properties independent of the process of glycosylation. Furthermore, it was found that swainsonine is able to stimulate NK cells, activate macrophages and stimulate T lymphocyte proliferation [87]. Swainsonine protected mice had their survival increased their survival after toxic doses of chemotherapeutic drugs, and increased bone marrow recovery in these mice by stimulation of the hematopoietic stem cell differentiation [88]. The anti-tumor and anti-metastatic effects of swansonine were abrogated in immuno deficient or immuno depressed mice, suggesting that these effects are mostly mediated via stimulation of the host's immune system [87].

2.3. Cell surface carbohydrates and metastatic properties of tumor cells selected for resistance to lectins

The ability of plant lectins to recognize the specific carbohydrate structure was widely used for analysis of the cell surface of normal and malignant cells. In addition, lectin binding to malignant cells or to glycoproteins separated on SDS-polyacrylamide slab gels were utilized in order to identify differences in carbohydrate structure of metastatic and non-metastatic tumor cells [89,90]. The comparative analysis of lectin binding to tumor cells revealed some differences in binding of Con A, WGA and SBA lectins to low and high metastatic lines of B16 melanoma [89]. Analysis of various cell lines or clones of RAW117 lymphoma showed a correlation between reduction of Con A-binding sites and metastatic potentials, whereas no correlation was observed between binding of WGA and metastatic properties of the tested cells [91,92]. These differences in lectin binding reflect some differences in the expression of cell surface carbohydrates by tumor cells with different metastatic potentials.

In parallel with their ability to bind and induce aggregation of normal or malignant cells, some lectins were found to be highly cytotoxic. Lectins, such as Con A, PHA, WGA, RIC, LCA and GS1B$_4$ are able to kill normal or malignant cells at relatively low concentrations [93]. To exert their cytotoxic effect, lectins have to bind to specific oligosaccharides expressed by cell surface glycoproteins or glycolipids. Thus, cells that do not express the specific carbohydrates would be resistant to cytotoxic action of lectin. Lack of certain carbohydrate structure recognizable by the lectin can be due to a defect at specific points in the oligosaccharide biosynthesis or processing pathway. It was found that the frequency of the glycosylation mutant cell variants resistant to lectins is very low, but can be increased following mutagenic treatments [19]. Selected lectin-resistant cell variants were found to be a useful experimental model for studying oligosaccharide biosynthesis, intracellular transport and stability of glycoproteins, investigation of the role of carbohydrates in cell-to-cell interactions, tumor growth and metastasis formation [19]. Various cell lines, such as B16 melanoma, MDAY-D2 lymphoma, FLC leukemia, Raw117H103LL lymphoma, 3LL Lewis lung carcinoma were used for the selection of cell variants resistant to WGA lectin. WGA exerts toxicity by binding to sialic acid and/or β-GlcNAc residues. It is expected that WGA-resistant variant would show changes in the expression of the binding carbohydrates. Indeed, in most cases, the WGA resistance was associated with a loss of WGA-binding carbohydrates [19].

The metastatic ability of WGA-resistant cell variants has been widely tested. WGA-resistant cell variant Wa-4 was selected from B16 melanoma. Wa-4 cells, in comparison to parental B16 melanoma cells, showed loss of sialic acid and metastatic ability. A reduction in cell membrane sialylation was the result of a 60-fold increase in α1,3FT activity and replacement of sialic acid by fucose as the terminal residues on the N-acetyllactosamine chain [22]. Studies with WGA-resistant cell variants of MDAY-D2 lymphoma helped to identify several types of mutants [20,79]. A class 1 mutant of MDAY-D2 line that was selected for resistance to WGA showed a decrease in sialic acid and galactose expression with a parallel reduction in its metastatic potentials. These changes were found to be caused by a defect in UDP-Gal transport into the Golgi, capping N-linked structures with GlcNAc, resulting in the generation of truncated glycolipids and O-linked oligosaccharides [20,79]. A similar defect in sugar donor transport led to loss of sialic acid and galactosyl epitopes in human melanoma selected for resistance to WGA that paralleled with the reduced ability of these melanoma cells to form metastases in nude mice [94]. The class 2 glycosylation mutants of MDAY-D2 cells expressed NeuNGc as terminal residues instead of NeuNAc, without detectable changes in the complex-type oligosaccharides. The class 2 mutation did not affect the metastatic property of MDAY-D2 cells [20].

The class 3 glycosylation mutant of MDAY-D2 lymphoma cells which was selected for resistance to L-PHA, resulted in a reduction of the GlcNAc-TV activity and in β1-6 branched structures with a parallel decrease in their tumorigenic and metastatic properties [43]. These data support other findings described above on the significance of sialic acid and β1-6 branching of N-linked oligosaccharides in regulation of metastatic properties of tumor cells. However, selection of tumor cells for resistance to lectin was not always found to be associated with loss of metastatic properties. For example, WGA-resistant variants (class 2 mutants) of MDAY-D2 lymphoma showed no changes in their metastatic potential [20]. Selection of RAW117H10 lymphoma cells for resistance to Con A resulted in an increase of their metastatic properties. It is note worthy that the selection of the same cells for resistance to WGA reduced their ability to metastasize [92].

2.4. Glycosyltransferase gene transfection: Effects on cell surface carbohydrate expression and metastatic properties of tumor cells

The observed differences in the expression of cell surface carbohydrates by high and low metastatic cell lines suggest, but not prove, the involvement of cell surface carbohydrates in the metastatic process. The tested cell lines or clones may be different not only in cell surface carbohydrates but also in other properties controlling metastatic potential. Similarly, inhibition of tumor cell glycosylation by various inhibitors could be nonspecific and other cellular properties and mechanisms could be affected. Moreover, it is impossible to determine which particular carbohydrates are responsible for the observed changes in the metastatic behavior of tumor cells when a broad inhibition of the glycosylation processes is induced. Lectin-resistant tumor cell lines were useful tools in an investigation of the role of cell surface carbohydrates in metastasis formation. However, some cautions in the interpretation of these data should be taken. In various studies selection of lectin-resistant variants was performed after treatment with the mutagenic agent, such as ethyl methane sulfonate (EMS). Later it was found that EMS treatment increases tumor cell immunogenicity that might affect the ability of tumor cell to form metastasis [95].

Recently, in order to evaluate the significance of cell surface carbohydrates in the metastatic process, a new approach has been utilized. The changes in surface carbohydrates are likely to be associated with a selective process for the emergence of tumor cells with metastatic potential. The biosynthetic basis for such changes is alterations in the activity of various glycosyltransferases. These enzymes are responsible for addition of carbohydrate units in a sequential manner to the growing oligosaccharide chains on glycolipids and glycoproteins. While the glycosyltransferases which synthesize the core portion of the oligosaccharide, up to the mannosyl residues of N-linked oligosaccharides, are located in the endoplasmic reticulum, the enzymes synthesizing the outer portion of the complex carbohydrate chain (i.e. N-acetyllactosaminyl portion and the 'capping' units such as sialic acid, fucose and galactose) are located within the Golgi apparatus and the trans-Golgi compartment. These enzymes bind to the acceptor residue on the carbohydrate chain (e.g. N-acetyllactosamine $Gal\beta1$-4GlcNAc-R) and link to it a sugar unit from a sugar nucleotide (e.g. CMP-SA or UDP-Gal) [1,11]. Increasing number of genes coding the glycosyltransferases have been recently sequenced. Transfection of genes encoding glycosyltransferases or glycosidases represents a new approach that might help to evaluate more directly the significance of cell surface carbohydrates in regulation of metastatic properties of tumor cells.

2.4.1. $\alpha1,3$ galactosyltransferase cDNA transfection and metastatic properties of murine melanomas

Analysis of the pattern of lectin binding by B16 melanoma cells revealed that these cells do not react with SBA, PNA and VV lectins as well as with the $GS1B_4$ lectin. The SBA, PNA and VV lectin-binding sites are actually present in these cells but they are blocked by sialic acid and can be detected only after neuraminidase treatment [89,96–99]. No $GS1B_4$ binding was observed after neuraminidase treatment of B16 melanoma cells. The ligand for $GS1B_4$ lectin has been previously shown to be the carbohydrate structure $Gal\alpha1$-3Galβ1-4GlcNAc-R (termed the α-gal epitope) [100]. This epitope is synthesized in the Golgi apparatus by the enzyme $\alpha1,3$ galactosyltransferase ($\alpha1,3GT$) and expressed in all mammals except humans, apes and Old World monkey. Due to the mutation in the $\alpha1,3GT$ gene, humans, apes and Old World monkey do not express α-gal epitopes but they produce large amounts of a natural antibody against α-gal epitopes [101]. Anti-gal antibody is responsible for the hyperacute rejection of the organ and tissue transplanted into human from the discordant animals, like pigs that express high levels of α-gal epitopes [102,103]. Analysis of numerous normal and malignant cell murine tumors of different histological origin showed that they express α-gal epitopes. However, murine melanomas such as B16, JB/RH, JB/MS as well as Cloudman S91 melanoma do not express α-gal epitopes [96–99]. Lack of α-gal epitopes in BL6 cells is the result of down-regulation of the $\alpha1,3GT$ gene [97,99]. To test the possible involvement of α-gal epitopes in metastasis formation, BL6, JB/RH and JB/MS melanoma cell lines were transfected with

murine $\alpha1,3GT$ cDNA [97]. Transfection of melanoma cells with the $\alpha1,3GT$ gene resulted in the appearance of α-gal epitopes. In parallel, the transfected cells expressed SBA, PNA and VV lectin-binding sites [97]. The appearance of these lectin-binding carbohydrates was the indirect outcome of the $\alpha1,3GT$ gene transfection, and resulted from decreased sialylation of the carbohydrate chains. The reason for this decrease is that $\alpha1,3GT$ competes with $\alpha2,3ST$ or $\alpha2,6ST$ for capping of the same acceptor, N-acetyllactosamine (i.e. $Gal\beta1$-4GlcNAc-R) within the Golgi apparatus. Thus when $\alpha1,3GT$ caps the N-acetyllactosamine with terminal α-gal residue to form $Gal\alpha1$-3Galβ1-4GlcNAc-R, sialyltransferases are unable to cap the same acceptor with sialic acid [104]. This decreases the sialylation of N-acetyllactosamine and prevents masking of many SBA, PNA and VV binding epitopes [97].

In parallel with alterations in cell membrane carbohydrates, transfection of $\alpha1,3GT$ cDNA into BL6, JB/RH and JB/MS melanoma cells substantially reduced their metastatic ability. It seems unlikely that this reduction in metastasis formation was due to the changes in their immunogenicity or sensitivity to NK cell-mediated immunity, because these cells still showed low number of metastasis in immuno competent as well as in immuno suppressed (X-irradiated) mice [97].

2.4.2. Effect of sense and antisense fucosyltransferase cDNAs transfection on tumorigenic and metastatic properties of tumor cells

The effect of $\alpha1,3GT$ gene transfection raised the question of whether the observed reduction in metastatic properties of melanoma cells is specifically associated with the expression of the terminal α-gal or can other carbohydrates in the same position on N-linked carbohydrate chain have similar inhibitory effect on metastasis formation. To test this, the effect of $\alpha1,2FT$ gene transfection and capping of N-acetyllactosamine with $\alpha1,2$ fucose on metastatic properties of BL6 melanoma cells was investigated [98]. $\alpha1,2FT$ catalyzes a transglycosylation reaction between the nucleotide sugar substrate GDP-Fuc and oligosaccharide acceptors to generate the H blood group antigen, also known as O. In mice, H determinants are expressed during embryonic development, in adult intestinal or endometrial epithelium [105]. Alterations in fucose metabolism and tumor cell fucosylation have been previously demonstrated, and they were associated with tumorigenic and metastatic properties of some murine tumor cell lines [106]. However, the particular fucosylated structures associated with metastatic properties remain unknown.

BL6 melanoma cells were transfected with the human α1,2FT cDNA (FUT1) resulting in the appearance of the H determinants recognized by UEA-I lectin. The metastatic properties of the transfected cells significantly reduced in parallel [98]. This effect was not immunologically mediated and α1,2FT-transfected BL6 melanoma cells showed lower metastatic ability both in immuno competent C57BL/6 and immuno deficient nude mice [98]. The result of α1,3GT or α1,2FT gene transfection might indicate that loss of metastatic potential by BL6 melanoma cells is due to the appearance of α-gal epitopes (Galα1-3Galβ1-4GlcNAc-R) or fucosyl epitopes (Fucα1-2Galβ1-4GlcNAc-R). However, this might be a result of other carbohydrate changes associated with the expression of these epitopes, particularly, changes in cell surface sialylation. Indeed, appearance of α-gal or fucosyl epitopes in BL6 melanoma cells transfected with the α1,3GT or α1,2FT gene resulted in a decrease in sialic acid residues on the N-linked carbohydrate chains of glycoproteins and glycolipids [98].

It is believed that at least five different enzymes in mammalian cells (α1,3GT, α1,2FT, α2,3ST, α2,6ST and β1,3-N-acetylglucoaminyltransferase) compete for the common acceptor on complex-type N-linked oligosaccharides [104]. Reduction in cell surface sialylation in BL6 melanoma cells transfected with α1,3GT or α1,2FT genes is likely to be the result of competition between α1,2FT or α1,3GT and sialyltransferases for a common acceptor, N-acetyllactosamine. Thus, capping of N-acetyllactosamine with fuc or gal residues prevents capping with sialic acid, resulting in reduction of sialylation of N-linked carbohydrate chains of glycoproteins and/or glycolipids. The positive correlation between the cell surface sialylation and metastatic ability of various cell lines has been previously demonstrated [73–75]. However, it still remains unclear whether changes in sialic acid or concomitant changes in expression of α-gal or H epitopes are responsible for the observed decline in metastatic properties of tumor cells.

When rat colon carcinoma cells were transfected with the human α1,2FT (FUT1) cDNA, the transfected cells showed increase in their tumorigenicity following their transplantation into nude mice [107]. Metastatic properties of these cells were not investigated.

As presented above, transfection of glucosyltransferase genes into tumor cells that do not express these genes can be a useful approach for investigation of the role of cell surface carbohydrates in metastasis formation. For the same purpose, it will also be important to specifically inhibit the expression of certain carbohydrates and assess its effect on the metastatic potential of tumor cells. Previously this was attempted using various chemical inhibitors of glycosylation [80,81]. To induce more specific inhibition of cell surface glycosylation, the antisense technology has been used [108–110].

In human, α1,2FTs are encoded by two genes (FUT1 and FUT2) [105,111]. Similarly in rat, α1,2FTs are encoded by two genes (termed FTA and FTB) that are homologous to human FUT1 and FUT2 [112]. α1,2FT catalyzes a transglycosylation reaction between the nucleotide sugar substrate GDP-Fuc and oligosaccharide acceptors to generate the H blood group antigen. In rats, four types of oligosaccharide acceptors have been identified: an N-acetylglucosamine (with terminal type 1 (Galβ1-3GlcNAc-) and type 2 (Galβ1-4GlcNAc-)) or an N-acetylgalactosamine (type 3 (Galβ1-3GalNAcα1-R) and type 4 (Galβ1-3GalNAc$\beta\alpha$1-R)) [54]. In chemically induced rat colon carcinoma PBOb cells, FTA and FTB are expressed at the same level and these cells express H antigen type 2 recognized by UEA-1 as well as type 1, 3 and 4 recognized by LM137/276 mab [108]. When PBOb cells were transfected with antisense FTB cDNA, the transfected cells showed a marked reduction in the expression of H antigen type 1, 2 and 3 that paralleled the change in fucosylation of variant of CD44 – the product of exon V6. A test of their tumorigenic potentials showed a reduction in their ability to grow in syngeneic rats [108].

To assess the possible involvement of α1,2FT encoded by the FTA gene in the regulation of tumorigenicity and metastatic ability, PBOb cells were transfected with antisense FTA [110]. Transfection resulted in a decrease of α1,2FT activity and a reduction of H type 2 expression detected by UEA-I lectin with no changes in the expression of type 1,3 and 4 H antigen. PBOb colon carcinoma cells that lost type 2 H antigen expression showed increased tumor growth in immuno competent syngeneic rats with no changes in their metastatic ability. When antisense FTA-transfected cells and control PBOb cells were inoculated into immuno deficient SCID mice no differences in their growth were observed, suggesting that increased tumor growth of antisense FTA-transfected cells in immuno competent rats might be due to a reduction in their immunogenicity [110]. Thus, antisense transfection of FTB inhibited H antigen type 1,3 and 4 expression and tumor growth of PBOb cells, whereas antisense transfection of FTA inhibited H antigen type 2 that was associated with increased growth of PBOb tumor [108,110]. These differences in tumor growth might be associated with changes in tumor cell immunogenicity.

In addition to $\alpha1,2FT$, several other fucosyltransferases are involved in fucosylation of the glycoconjugates. Several human $\alpha1,3FT$ genes have been identified (FUT3-7) that encode several tissue-specific fucosyltransferase (FUC-TIII-VII) [113]. $\alpha1,3/\alpha1,4FT$ gene (also known as FUT3) encodes fucosyltransferase that catalyzes transglycosylation reactions leading to the expression of sLe^a and sLe^x blood group structures which serve as ligands for E-selectin [114]. B16F10 melanoma cells express neither E-selectin nor its ligands [115]. When transfected with a cDNA encoding $\alpha1,3/4FT$, the E-selectin ligand appeared on these cells but this did not affect their ability to form metastases in normal C57BL/6 mice. However, in the E-selectin transgenic mice, B16F10 melanoma cells expressing E-selectin ligand formed numerous liver metastases. The parental B10F10 cells failed to develop metastasis in the liver both in normal or E-selectin transgenic mice [115].

To further assess the role of selectin ligand sLe^x and sLe^a in the regulation of metastatic properties of tumor cells, antisense FUT3 has been transfected into human colon carcinoma cells (HT-29LMM) that express higher levels of FUT3 transcript, $\alpha1,3/\alpha1,4FT$ activity and sLe^x and sLe^a [109]. HT-29LMM was isolated from metastatic lesion resulting from intra-splenic injections of HT-29 cells into nude mice [116]. Transfection of antisense FUT3 into HT-29LMM cells resulted in loss of FUT3 transcript, $\alpha1,3/\alpha1,4FT$ activity and expression of sLe^x and sLe^a. While the parental HT-29LMM cells formed numerous metastasis in the liver after intra-splenic injections, no metastases were found in mice inoculated with antisense-transfected HT-29LMM cells [109].

$\alpha1,6FT$ catalyzes $\alpha1,6$ fucosylation of N-glycans. Overexpression of $\alpha1,6FT$ was found in some but not all hepatomas [117]. Fucosylation of α-fetoprotein in hepatoma patients is an indicator of poor prognosis [118]. However, the role of $\alpha1,6FT$ in hepatoma progression remains unclear. To receive more direct experimental support of the role of $\alpha1,6FT$ in metastasis formation, Miyoshi et al. [117] transfected a human hepatoma line Hep3B with the $\alpha1,6FT$ gene.

The transfected cells showed high levels of $\alpha1,6FT$ activity without changes in their invasiveness. Two-dimensional electrophoresis followed by LCA lectin binding, which preferentially recognizes $\alpha1,6$ fucose in N-glycans, showed fucosylation of several glycoproteins (M_r 50,000–150,000, pI 4.8–5.5). It was found that $\alpha5$ chain of VLA-5 integrin was highly fucosylated. The adhesion of the transfected hepatoma cells to normal hepatocytes or non-parenchymal liver cells was inhibited. In parallel, metastatic ability of these cells was significantly impaired [117].

2.4.3. Alterations of metastatic properties of tumor cells by $\beta1,6$-N-acetylglucosaminyl-transferase gene transfection.

The increase in the $\beta1$-6 branches is the most common alteration in cell surface carbohydrates during malignant transformation [6,7,43]. Synthesis of the elongated $\beta1$-6 branches is catalyzed by $\beta1,6$-N-acetylglucosaminyltransferase (GnT-V; EC 2.4.1.155). It was demonstrated that metastatic potentials of experimental or human tumors are positively correlated with GnT-V activity [6,7,43]. In an attempt to obtain more direct confirmation of the involvement of $\beta1$-6 branches in the regulation of the metastatic potentials of tumor cells, Yoshimura et al. [119] transfected B16F10 melanoma cells with the cDNA encoding $\beta1,4$-N-acetylglucosaminyltransferase (GnT-III; EC 2.4.1.144). GnT-III competes with GnT-V for the same substrate on the tri-antennary structure of N-linked oligosaccharides and once a bisecting GlcNAc residue is added to the core mannose by GnT-III, it prevents the formation of triantennary structure by GnT-V. The GnT-III-transfected B16F10 melanoma cells showed a high expression of GnT-III without the inhibition of GnT-V which in fact was slightly elevated [119]. The transfected cells showed an increase in binding to E-PHA that has high affinity for bisected oligosaccharides and reduced reactivity with L-PHA which binds specifically to GlcNAc residues on the $\beta1$-6 branches of tri- or tetra-antennary carbohydrate chains. Reduction in the $\beta1$-6 branches on GnT-III-transfected B16F10 melanoma cells was associated with reduction of their ability to form pulmonary metastases after i.v. inoculation [119].

Similarly, human K562 cells were transfected with the GnT-III gene and their ability to grow and form metastasis in nude mice was analyzed [120]. The GnT-III-transfected K562 cells showed an increase in binding of PHA-E and a decrease in binding of PHA-L and DSA lectins, suggesting an increase of bisecting GlcNAc on the N-oligosaccharides, while tri- or tetra-antennary structures were decreased. This was also confirmed by a decrease in binding of Con A lectin that has affinity for the core mannose of bi-antennary structures of complex-type and high-mannose-type N-glycans. A reduction in β1-6 branching of N-linked oligosaccharides reduces lactosamine antennae for the terminal capping by sialic acid, leading to a reduction in tumor cell sialylation. Indeed, the GnT-III-transfected K562 cells showed a reduction in terminal sialic acid as reflected by a substantial decrease in their binding to LFA lectin [120].

When GnT-III gene-transfected K562 cells were inoculated s.c. into nude mice, no local growth was observed but numerous metastatic foci in the spleen were found [120]. This discrepancy in the effect of GnT-III gene transfection in B16F10 melanoma and K562 leukemia cells can be explained based on the following findings. K562 cells are highly sensitive to NK cell-mediated cytotoxicity, but GnT-III gene transfection rendered K562 cells resistant to NK cell-mediated cytotoxicity *in vitro* [120]. These data suggest that eventually K562 cells have all potentials for metastatic growth, and NK cells are predominately responsible for the elimination of these cells and prevention of metastasis formation. NK resistance of GnT-III-transfected K562 cells increased their survival and their ability to form metastatic lesions. This conclusion is also supported by the experiments in which NK-depleted mice were used. When nude mice were treated with anti-asialo GM1 antibody it resulted in the elimination of NK cell activity. In NK-depleted nude mice even parental K562 cells were able to survive and metastasize into the spleen. B16F10 melanoma cells are NK resistant and there is no evidence that the GnT-III gene transfection changed their NK sensitivity. Indeed, low metastatic ability of GnT-III gene-transfected B16F10 cells was retained in the NK-depleted mice [119]. Inhibition of metastatic properties of B16F10 melanoma cells transfected with the GnT-III gene was in parallel with reduction in their invasiveness and adhesion to laminin and collagen. The mechanisms responsible for these changes remain unclear and were attributed to the possible changes in the N-glycosylation of the integrins [119].

2.4.4. Sialidase cDNA transfection and metastasis formation

Transfection of galactosyltransferase or fucosyltransferase genes resulted in synthesis of the terminal galactose and fucose, as well as in reduction of the terminal sialic acid and sialylation of cell surface carbohydrates. Similar transfection with the GnT-III gene leads to a reduction in the β1-6 branching of N-linked oligosaccharides reducing lactosamine antennae for the terminal capping by sialic acid. Several lines of evidence indicate that cell surface sialylation positively correlates with the metastatic ability of tumor cells [73–75]. The expression of sialic acid residues depends not only on the activity of sialyltransferase but also on sialidase that can cleave sialic acid in different linkages. In rats, four types of sialidase have been identified based on their subcellular localization, catalytic activity and immunological properties [121]. Cytosolic sialidase hydrolyzes glycoproteins, oligosaccharides and gangliosides at neutral pH. BL6 melanoma cells do not express cytosolic type of sialidase [122]. To evaluate whether overexpression of sialidase might affect sialylation of glycoconjugates and metastasis formation, BL6 melanoma cells were transfected with a cytosolic sialidase cDNA. The stable transfected BL6 cells showed a significant reduction in their lung colonization. Similarly, sialidase transfection reduced the ability of BL6 melanoma cells to form spontaneous metastasis in immuno competent C57BL/6 and immuno deficient nude mice [122]. Total sialic acid content was slightly reduced without changes in sialidase-released sialic acids in BL6 melanoma cells transfected with sialidase gene. Invasiveness and cell motility of sialidase-transfected cells was impaired without changes in their adhesion to laminin, collagen IV and fibronectin. Lectin flow cytometry and lectin blotting did not detect any changes in cell surface or intracellular glycoprotein sialylation. However, these cells showed about 50% reduction in the GM3 ganglioside content and an increase in the lactosylceramide level probably as a result of GM3 desialylation. Based on the findings that intracellular GM3 is associated with the cytoskeleton, it was suggested that GM3 desialylation in the sialidase-transfected B16 melanoma cells leads to alteration of cytoskeleton functions reflected in the impairment of cell motility, invasiveness and metastasis formation [122].

It is note worthy that transfection of BL6 melanoma cells with sialidase gene did not affect their growth *in vitro* and *in vivo*. However, similar transfection of the cytosolic sialidase gene into a human epidermis carcinoma cell A431 increased their rate of proliferation that was associated with a decrease in GM3 level with little changes in protein sialylation. Increased cell growth rate of sialidase gene-transfected A431 was in parallel with enhanced EGF receptor tyrosine autophosphorylation [123]. Metastatic properties of these cells were not tested.

2.4.5. Inhibition of GD3 ganglioside expression by the antisense GD3-synthase gene and metastatic property of tumor cells

Ganglioside GD3 is often overexpressed in various malignancies [5]. GD3 is synthesized as a result of conversion of GM3 by CMP-sialic acid: α2,8ST (GD3-synthase; EC 2.4.99.8). To assess the possible role of GD3 ganglioside in tumor growth and metastasis formation, the antisense vector against the GD3-synthase gene was transfected into a rat F-11 cell line [5,31,32,124]. The transfected cells showed almost 10 times reduction of GD3 that was associated with a substantial inhibition of tumor growth in nude mice. It is of importance to note that *in vitro* growth of these cells was only slightly reduced, suggesting that observed tremendous inhibition of tumor growth *in vivo* can hardly be explained by the reduced proliferative ability of the tumor cells. *In vivo* inhibition of tumor growth was found to be a result of inhibition of VEGF production and tumor vascularization [32]. Furthermore, a substantial difference in the metastatic ability of the tested cell lines was observed. The parental F-11 tumor cells were highly metastatic and after i.v. inoculation metastatic nodules were found in the ovaries, breast, uterus, oviducts, kidneys and bladder but not in lungs or liver. All 12 mice inoculated with the parental F-11 tumor cells have multiple and large metastatic nodules in these organs. In contrast, after inoculation of the antisense GD3-transfected F-11 cell, only two out of eight mice developed metastases. Both of these two mice had a single metastatic nodule in the ovary. These nodules were very small in comparison to those formed by the parental F-11 cells [124]. Loss of metastatic ability by the antisense GD3-transfected F-11 cells was in parallel with a reduction in their invasiveness and cell motility. It is most likely that a reduction in the number and size of metastatic nodules is a result of inhibition of VEGF gene expression and VEGF production found in these cells [32].

2.5. Glycosyltransferase gene knockout mice: A new tool for investigation of the role of cell carbohydrates in tumor growth and metastasis formation

Recently, glycosyltransferase-deficient mice have been generated as a new tool for investigation of the

biological significance of cell carbohydrates in embryogenesis, tissue development and function as well as their role in carcinogenesis and metastasis formation.

α1,3GT knock out mice are healthy and fertile [125]. These mice are very useful in the analysis of the role of α-gal epitopes and anti-gal antibody in the acute rejection of xenografts that mimic the situation in the clinical practice when human recipients are transplanted with animal tissues or organs.

β1,4GT knockout mice were born normally and were fertile. However, their epithelial cell proliferation of the skin and small intestine was enhanced, and cell differentiation in the intestinal villi was abnormal. These mice showed growth retardation and early death [126]. So far no studies of metastasis formation using these knockout mice have been performed.

Increased β1-6GlcNAc branching is the most typical carbohydrate change associated with malignant transformation and metastasis formation [6,7,43,44]. β1-6GlcNAc branching is catalyzed by GlcNAc-TV, also known as MGAT5. MGAT5-deficient mice were generated by targeted gene mutation in embryonic stem cells [127]. MGAT5-deficient mice showed no MGAT5 catalytic activity and MGAT5 products were undetectable. Mice were viable without obvious abnormalities. However, more detailed analysis of these mice revealed some deficiency in leukocyte recruitment into the site of inflammation, T cell reactivity and nurturing behavior [127]. To investigate the role of β1-6GlcNAc branching in the primary carcinogenesis and metastasis formation, MGAT5-deficient mice were crossed with PyMT transgenic mice that express the viral oncogene Polyomavirus middle T antigen in mammary epithelium. PyMT transgenic mice started to develop breast tumor at 8 weeks of age, and at age 16 weeks 50% of the mammary pads had tumors. In PyMT MGAT5$-/-$ mice tumors developed later, so 50% incidence of tumors in these mice was found at age 24 weeks. Furthermore, growth of these tumors was slower and formation of spontaneous lung metastasis was substantially inhibited. This reflected in lower numbe of nodules and their smaller size. The histological analysis of mammary tissues revealed no impairment in tumor initiation as indicated by multi-focal tumor formation in PyMT MGAT5Z$-/-$ and PyMT MGAT5$+/+$ mice. The observed differences in tumor and metastasis is formation is probably due to reduced proportion of the proliferating cells. Growth of breast tumor cells from PyMT MGAT5$-/-$ mice on fibronectin-coated cover slip showed impaired membrane ruffling, actin stress fiber networks with paxillin in a punctate distribution of focal adhesions beneath the cells. In the PyMT MGAT5+/− cells paxillin was very concentrated in ruffled edges, with fine radial actin fibers extending into the cells. The amount of phoshorylated and non-phosphorylated PKB was reduced in malignant cells from PyMT MGAT5−/− mice. Similar changes were observed in fibroblasts from MGAT5−/− mice, suggesting that the MGAT5 null mutation affects focal adhesion in the absence of an oncogene [127].

Overall, studies with MGAT5-deficient mice and experiments with transfection of the genes coding glycosyltransferases or sialidase have provided additional and more direct confirmation of the importance of carbohydrates in the regulation of metastatic properties of tumor cells. However, mechanisms by which carbohydrates might control the metastatic properties of tumor cells remain unclear. Some data suggest that carbohydrate changes and associated changes in metastatic potentials of tumor cells is mostly due to changes in the function of adhesion molecules, growth factor receptors or cell motility. Several lines of evidence indicate that cell surface carbohydrates might affect metastasis formation via their interactions with the proteins known as endogenous lectins.

3. Endogenous lectins

Lectins i.e. carbohydrate-binding proteins were originally found in plants and were widely used for the analysis of carbohydrate structure and function in normal and malignant cells [3]. Investigations of the interactions between plant lectins and cell surface carbohydrates of various normal and malignant cells revealed, that these interactions could induce various biological effects and prompted the search for the presence of endogenous lectins in vertebrates. In the 1970s it became apparent that lectins are widely presented in all living organisms [3,25,26]. Animal lectins although share no structural homology to plant lectins do show similar specificity to carbohydates. Thus, the genes for animals' lectin were probably reinvented during evolution by nature since lectin-carbohydrate interactions were essential for the existence and development of complex multiorgan organisms. This stimulated Cooper and Barondes to entitle their review 'God must love galectins; he made so many of them' [128].

C-type lectins. The animal lectins have been divided into several categories among which are the C- and S-type lectins [24–26,128]. C-type lectins are Ca^{2+} dependent and exist as cell bound or in secreted form. C-type lectins contain one or more carbohydrate recognition domains (CRDs), and about 50 lectins which have thus far been identified in avian and mammals, all include a Ca^{2+} binding domain and a hydrophobic core [26,129].

The collectin family of C-type lectin includes a group of collagenous lectins that are present in mammalian serum, pulmonary and gastrointestinal secreted milieu. This group includes mannose binding proteins (MBPs), conglutinin and pulmonary surfactant SP-A and SP-D. MBP was initially identified on the cell surface of rabbit and rat liver, and its secreted form was isolated from the serum of animals and humans, and two types of MBP (MBP-A and MBP-C) have been identified [26,129]. MBPs contain carbohydrate binding region, a cystein-rich NH_2-terminus domain that stabilizes the α-helix structure of the collagen-like domain. Collagen-like domain shows a structural homology with the complement C1q and is able to activate the classical complement pathway in the absence of antigen–antibody complexes. Serum containing MBPs may bind to the oligomannose sequences of the glycoconjugates present on the cell surface of bacteria and fungi, and activate the complement and thus contribute to the elimination of the bacterial, and fungal infections.

Pulmonary collectins, also known as surfactant proteins (SP-A and SP-D), are trimeric containing three CRD and the basic trimers of SP-A and SP-D could form higher-order multimeric structures. SP-A is commonly composed of six trimers (octadecamers) and similar to MBP is organized as a bouquet containing two to six building blocks, each of which consists of a trimer of the constituent polypeptide resembling the C1q component of the complement. However, SP-A is unable to activate the complement [130]. SP-D usually forms a larger structure of four or more trimeric CRD heads forming cruciform structure [130,131]. All of the collectins bind mannose with high affinity and have relatively low affinity for glucose. In contrast to MBP, SP-D has a relatively strong affinity for maltose and glucose with low affinity for GlcNAc [131,132]. Collectins might play a role in the pattern recognition of invaded bacteria and respiratory viruses [132].

Mannose receptor (MR), a C-type lectin, is a prototype of a newer family of multi-lectin receptor proteins. This family includes the phospholipase A_2 (PLA_2) receptor, a dendritic cell receptor (DEC-205) and MP-like multi-lectin receptor [133]. MR is a 180 kDa transmembrane protein present on the surface of macrophages, dendritic cells and hepatic sinusoidal endothelium (HSE) [133,134]. MR contains a series of eight tandem lectin-like CRDs. CRDs 4 and 5 form a protease-resistant ligand-binding core capable of binding carbohydrate ligands with high affinity. CRDs 4–8 are required for high affinity binding to their natural ligands such as yeast mannan. Only CRD-4 retains its sugar-binding activity when expressed in isolation. In spite of the fact that CRD-4 of MR and MBP-A and MBP-C have only 25–28% sequence identity, they manifest similar carbohydrate specificity and are able to bind mannose, fucose and GlcNAc [133]. Site-directed mutagenesis combined with NMR and molecular modeling helped to identify the orientation of monosaccharides bound to CRD-4 of MR. GlcNAc binds to CRD-4 of MR in the same orientation as in CRD of MBP-C. Mannose binding to CRD-4 is rotated by 180° relative to GlcNAc binding. Fucose binds to CRD-4 in the same orientation seen in MBP-C [135]. Since MR that is expressed by both dendritic cells and macrophages are antigen presenting cells, it is believed that MR is involved in eliciting specific immune responses [133].

Another group of C-type lectins includes L-, E- and P-selectins that are encoded by genes located on human and murine chromosome 1. All selectins share a similar structure that includes an extracellular C-type lectin domain, a single epidermal growth (EGF)-like domain, and two to nine short consensus repeat (SCR) units homologous to complement binding proteins, a transmembrane domain, and a cytoplasmic tail [27,136,137]. The selectins are closely related having about 40% identity in the SCR domains and up to 65% identity in the CRD and EGF domains (137). L-selectin is constitutively expressed on leukocytes expressing high levels of functional ligands for both E- and P-selectins expressed by endothelial cells. The interaction between selectins and their ligands mediates the rolling of leukocytes on endothelium at sites of tissue injury or inflammation with subsequent tight binding to endothelium via integrin–ligand interactions and further extravasation [137]. L-selectin is also involved in the regulation of lymphocytes trafficking into lymph nodes by their binding to specialized high endothelial venules (HEV) of lymph nodes. L-selectin has a higher expression on the cell surface of naïve T lymphocytes in comparison to activated and memory T lymphocytes. Naïve T lymphocytes show no functional ligands for the endothelial selectins.

P-selectin is rapidly induced on the surface of endothelial cells or platelets following their activation with several agonists such as histamine or thrombin. P-selectin binds to myeloid cells and to a subset of T cells. E-selectin is expressed primarily on endothelial cells following activation with pro-inflammatory cytokines such as IL-1 or TNF. E-selectin mediates the adhesion of myeloid cells and of a subset of memory T cells [137]. Numerous experimental data indicate that selectins might play a role in migration not only of leukocytes but also malignant cells and thus controlling the metastatic spread of various malignant cells [137].

The common feature of most of the selectin ligands is a lactosamine backbone of either type 1 (Galβ1-3GlcNAc) or type 2 (Galβ1-4GlcNAc) expressing sialylated and fucosylated oligosaccharides such as sLe^x and sLe^a or their sulfated equivalents [27]. These carbohydrates are usually found at the non-reducing termini of N- or O-linked oligosaccharides, or on glycosphingolipids. L- and P-selectin, but not E-selectin, also bind sulfatide, heparin, heparan sulfate proteoglycans, fucoidin and dextran sulfate. In addition to sharing common carbohydrate ligands, the selectins have a limited number of distinct high affinity glycoprotein ligands. L-selectin binds to different heavily glycosylated mucin-like proteins on mouse HEV in lymph nodes: GlyCAM-1, CD34, MAdCAM-1, as well as to induced ligands on activated vascular endothelium. P-selectin binds to P-selectin glycoprotein ligand-1 (PSGL-1) that is expressed on normal and malignant myeloid cells, as well as on cells of lymphoid and dendritic origin. An E-selectin ligand-1 (ESL-1) was identified on mouse myelomonocytic cells. In addition to CRD domain, the EGF and SCR domains of the selectins play a role in cell adhesion to endothelium. This is implied from the findings that deletion of either EGF or SCR domains of L- or E-selectin abolished or reduced the binding activity of selectins [27]. Using a panel of chimeras selectins created by exchange of only the CRDs between L- and P-selectin revealed that the CRD determines specificity. Chimeras selectins with exchanged CRD portion between L-selectin and EGF domain from P-selectin were found to display a dual specificity and binding to ligands of both L- and P-selectins [138].

NK cells' C-type lectins are a distinct group of type-II transmembrane proteins that contain CRD at the COOH terminus linked by neck region of various lengths to a transmembrane domain and cytoplasmic tail. This group includes NKR-P1, Ly49, NKG2 receptors that are mostly, but not exclusively, expressed by

NK cells. NKR-P1 lectin is a signaling molecule that is involved in the activation of NK cells' lytic machinery [139]. Ly49 that is expressed by murine NK cells contains at least five membranes, Ly49A, Ly49B and Ly49C that are involved in the down-regulation of NK cells' activity following their interaction with MHC class I molecules of the target cells. NKG2 is the human homologue of Ly49 that also includes several members (NKG2-A, -C and -D). NKG2 is expressed by human NK cells and also inhibits NK cell activity following its interaction with MHC class I molecules on the target cells [139].

Based on the CRD sequences NK cell lectins could be separated into distinct groups [139]. The sequence alignments and cluster analysis of CRDs of NK cell lectins revealed that typical structures of the C-type lectin CRD are only partially conserved in the NK cell receptors [130]. The differences are related to the lack of conservation of both polar (Ca^{2+}-ligation) residues and hydrophobic residues in loops 3 and 4 in the CRD of NK cell receptor. The similarity and differences between the typical C-type lectins and NK cell receptors suggest an evolutionary divergence from a common ancestral gene [130]. Several other molecules such as CD72 (a pan B cell marker), CD23 (low affinity Fc receptor for IgE) may also be classified as C-type-like receptors [130,139].

Galectins. A group of lectins known as the Ca^{2+} independent S-type lectins were termed galectins [24–26,128]. To date, 10 galectins have been identified; all bind N-acetyllactosamine (Galβ1-nGlcNAc-R) primarily via recognition of the β-gal unit. The CRDs of galectins are mainly encoded by three exons that show about 20–40% identity. Based on the CRD structure, galectins are divided into three groups. Galectins-1, -2, -5, -7 and -10 contain a single CRD. Galectins-4, -6, -8 and -9 are tandem repeat-type composed of two homologous CRDs. Galectin-3 is a chimera-type containing the COOH terminal CRD, the amino-terminal of 12 residues, and a collagen like domain of Pro-Gly-Tyr rich repeats [24]. Galectins are located both intracellularly and extracellularly. They are also secreted in soluble form. Galectins have been found to be involved in various processes, including cell adhesion, cell growth regulation, apoptosis, inflammation, immune function, embryogenesis, pre RNA splicing, angiogenesis and tumor metastasis formation [23,24,28,128,140].

Galectin-1 is a homodimer of 14 kD subunits, able to bind various glycoproteins: laminin, fibronectin, lysosome-associated membrane proteins (LAMPs) as well as the hematopoietic cell surface membrane proteins CD43 and CD45. Galectin-1 is highly expressed by human thymic epithelial cells and is involved in the binding of thymocytes to thymic epithelial cells [23]. It was recently demonstrated that galectin-1 and galectin-9 are able to induce apoptosis of thymocytes [141]. It was suggested that the expression of galectin-1 and galectin-9 by thymic epithelial cells might play an important role in the selection of T lymphocytes during their maturation in the thymus.

Galectin-3 is 31 kD β-gal-binding protein that is widely expressed in different normal and malignant cells [24,128,142–144]. Galectin-3 is localized on the cell surface as well as in intracellular space such as the cytoplasm or the nuclear matrix, and is secreted by a non-classical pathway. Numerous glycoproteins are capable of interacting with galectin-3, including laminin, lysosomal-associated proteins, Mac-2 binding protein, carcinoembryonic antigen, Fc receptor for IgE and mucin [24,128,142]. Galectin-3 is also able to bind single-stranded DNA and RNA – a binding that is not inhibited by lactose, implying that this binding is not mediated by the CRD domain [145,146].

Malignant transformation of rat normal embryonic fibroblasts or NIH-3T3 cells is associated with an increase in galectin-3 expression [147]. Conversely, differentiation of K-1735 murine melanoma cells induced by retinoic acid or cAMP resulted in its down-regulation [148]. Several reports showed that the expression of galectin-3 correlates with neoplastic progression in various malignancies such as head and neck cancer, cancer of thyroid and gastric or anaplastic large-cell lymphoma [149–151]. There are reports that galectin-3 was down-regulated in carcinomas of the ovary, utrerus and breast compared to normal counterparts [152–154].

3.1. The biological significance of endogenous lectins

An increasing body of evidence indicates that endogenous lectins might play a role in a vast variety of biological processes such as cell proliferation and programmed cell death, cell adhesion, immune system function, inflammation, tumor growth and metastasis formation.

3.1.1. Endogenous lectins and immune system
Broad selectivity of monosaccharide-binding site and the geometrical arrangement of multiple CRD in the

lectins provide a basis for the discriminative recognition between self and non-self [130]. Thus, endogenous lectins are able to recognize the carbohydrate patterns expressed by the invading microorganisms. Therefore, endogenous lectins are important part of the host's defense immunity against invading bacteria or fungi [130]. Endogenous lectins are able to (a) perform direct killing of these microorganisms as a part of innate defense mechanisms; (b) help to phagocytize the invaded microorganisms by macrophages and dendritic cells; (c) phagocytized bacteria could be killed, their proteins will be processed and small peptides that are associated with the MHC molecules can be presented to T lymphocytes, resulting in induction of the specific immune responses. Thus, lectins play a role in innate and adaptive immunity.

MBP is a distinct example of a protective lectin [133,155–157]. It was found that the CRD of MBP is capable of binding to the oligomannose on cell surface oligosacharides of various bacteria and fungi. The collagen-like domain of MBP has structural homology to C1q component of the complement system. Thus, the binding of MBP to bacteria triggers complement fixation by activating the MBP-associated serine proteases (MASP-1 and MASP-2) that are associated with an N-terminal collagenous domain. Activated MASPs subsequently cleave and activate downstream components of the complement leading to destruction of the invaded microorganism [155,157]. MBP is able to activate both the classical and alternative complement pathways [133,157]. In addition, binding of serum MBP to bacteria and activation of complement leads to the formation of C3b and C5b fragments that increase opsonization and phagocytosis and the clearance of bacteria by macrophages [156]. Moreover, some data showed that MBP binding to bacteria could directly stimulate the phagocytosis of MBP opsonized bacteria by monocytes and neutrophils [133,156]. The significance of MBPs in the defense system is strongly supported by finding of individuals with MBP deficiency. MBP deficiency impairs their defense, manifesting in an increase of their susceptibility to the infections [133]. MBP deficiency is found to be the result of at least three mutations within the collagen-like domain of MBP. The impairment of the mutated MBP is a result of replacement of Arg-52 to Cys, Gly-54 to Asp or Gly-57 to Glu in the collagen domain that inhibit oligomerization of the structural unit of MBP and consequently abolish its ability to activate the complement. In addition, these mutations are associated with a reduced level of MBP in serum [133]. Reduced serum level of MBP

was attributed to impaired secretion of MBP resulting from mutations in the collagen-like domain [158].

Other collectins, such as surfactant proteins SP-A and SP-D are also important in host's innate immunity, particularly in the host's protection from pulmonary infections. It was shown that SP-A enhances respiratory virus clearance. SP-A deficient mice manifested increased susceptibility to group B streptococcal infection [159,160].

Another endogenous lectin, MR that is expressed on the cell surface of macrophage and dendritic cells is able to recognize a wide range of Gram-negative and Gram-positive bacteria, yeasts, parasites and mycobacterium [133]. Binding of MR to these microorganisms helps their phagocytosis by macrophages and dendritic cells, both of which are potent antigen presenting cells [133,134]. Phagocytosis of various microorganisms via MR expressed by these cells might increase processing of the phagocytized proteins, formation of small peptides that bind to MHC class I or class II molecules. This leads to their presentation to T cells and stimulation of antibacterial immune responses. Thus, collectins, MBP and MR are involved in the host protection against invading microorganisms. Although these data indicate that these lectins play a role in protection against pathogenic infections, it seems likely that they are also able to recognize and eliminate malignant cells with altered carbohydrate structure.

Additional confirmation of the role of lectins in immunity comes from studies of NK cell C-type lectins that are well known for their ability to regulate NK cell-mediated lysis. Some lectins such as NKR-P1 activate and some as Ly49 in mice and NKG2 in human suppress the cytolytic activity of NK cells. Although some data indicate that these lectins retain their ability to bind sugars, however, there is no good evidence that carbohydrate recognition by these lectins is important for their function.

3.1.2. Apoptotic and antiapoptotic effects of endogenous lectins

Analysis of the interactions between plant lectins and mammalian cells revealed that these lectins could induce various biological effects, including stimulation of cell proliferation or induction of cell death. Stimulation of human and animal T lymphocyte proliferation and production of various lymphokines by some lectins such as PHA and Con A was found to be the result of lectin binding and activation of T cell receptor. Furthermore, lectin-stimulated lymphocytes become highly cytotoxic and are capable of killing various malignant cells, a phenomenon known as LDCC [12]. Some lectins such as ricin (RIC), abrin, Con A, PHA, WGA, GS1A$_4$, GS1B$_4$ and LCA are able to kill various normal and malignant cells directly in the absence of the lymphocytes. Analysis of the mechanisms of this cytotoxicity revealed that lectins are killing cells which act via apoptosis induction [93,161].

Based on the analysis of the mechanisms of plant lectin cytotoxicity against murine or human tumor cells, some predictions have been made [93,161]: (a) some endogenous animal lectins may also be cytotoxic to normal or malignant cells; (b) endogenous lectins with cytotoxic activity may represent a primitive mechanism for the elimination of aberrant somatic cells as well as invading microorganisms; (c) since alteration of cell membrane carbohydrates is a common feature of malignant cells, lectin-mediated cytotoxicity might play a role in the host's anti-tumor and anti-metastatic defense.

Recent findings confirmed that some endogenous animal lectins are cytotoxic. It was reported that galectin-1 in human and galectin-9 in mice are able to induce apoptosis of thymocytes [141,162,163]. Galectin-1 and galectin-9 are expressed by thymic epithelial cells in human and mice, respectively. Analysis of sensitivity of human thymocytes to galectin-1-induced apoptosis revealed the high sensitivity of two distinct populations of immature thymocytes: double positive thymocytes expressing relatively low levels of CD4, CD8 and not expressing CD3 and CD69 (CD3$^-$, Cd4^{lo}, CD8^{lo}, CD69$^-$). These cells represent the non-selected population of thymocytes, and these could die because they are not positively selected in the thymus. It was suggested that the death of these thymocytes is triggered by galectin-1 [162]. The second population of thymocytes CD3^{int}, CD4^{lo}, CD8^{lo}, CD69$^-$ that corresponds to thymocytes after negative selection was also found to be sensitive to galectin-1-induced apoptosis. It is note worthy that antibodies to CD3 could potentiate thymocyte sensitivity to galectin-1-induced apoptosis, suggesting that galectin-1 expressed by thymic epithelial cells might serve as a second signal needed for intrathymic selection of thymocytes [162]. It was shown that galectin-1 preferentially kills proliferating cells such as dividing thymocytes or PHA blasts [162].

In mice, the thymic epithelial cells express galectin-9 that was shown to be effective in the induction of apoptosis of murine thymocytes [141]. However, the precise population of murine thymocytes with maximum sensitivity to galectin-9-induced apoptosis was not identified. Recombinant galectin-9 induces homotypic aggregation of thymocytes that can be achieved at a concentration of 2.5–20 µM, whereas apoptosis can be induced at 10 times lower concentrations (0.25–2.5 µM) [141]. The carbohydrate recognition is important for the initiation of apoptosis induced by galectin-1 and galectin-9. This is implied from the finding that such apoptosis can be blocked with 0.2 M lactose [141,162].

The precise mechanisms of galectin-induced apoptosis remain unclear. It was suggested that galectin-9 induces apoptosis by binding glycoconjugate receptor on the thymocytes after secretion from thymic epithelium [141]. Alternatively, galectin-1 or galectin-9 expressed on thymic epithelium might induce apoptosis of thymocytes by binding to the counter receptor(s) such as leukosialin (CD43) or leukocyte common antigen CD45 [162].

These data indicate that galectin-1 and galectin-9 are involved in the physiological process of natural T lymphocyte selection in the thymus. Galectin-1 is probably involved in the regulation of immune response. Indeed, treatment of Lewis rats with recombinant galectin-1 abrogated the development of autoimune encephalomyelitis in these animals [164]. The cytotoxic activity of galectin-1 and galectin-9 was not limited by killing normal thymocytes but was also exerted against malignant cells. Recombinant galectin-1 was found to be efficient in triggering apoptotic death of the human T cell line MOLT-4 and Jurkat as well as several human B lymphoid cell lines, including Burkitt's lymphoma cells [162]. Although the galectin-mediated killing of malignant cells was demonstrated in vitro, the involvement of galectins in elimination of tumor cells in vivo needs further exploration.

The experiments with galectin-3 showed that it is unable to induce apoptosis. On the contrary, galectin-3 has anti-apoptotic effect [165,166]. Indeed, transfection of human T cell leukemia cells Jurkat E6-1 with galectin-3 cDNA rendered them resistant to Fas-antibody-mediated apoptosis [165]. Galectin-3, in contrast to other galectins, contains the NWGR motif in the C-terminus, whereas in other members of galectin family the corresponding sequence at that region is XWGXEER. The NWGR motif is also present in Bcl-2 and was found to be primarily responsible for the anti-apoptotic effect of both galectin-3 and Bcl-2 [165, 166]. Substitution of glycine to alanine in the NWGR motif abrogated the anti-apoptotic effect of galectin-3 [166]. In galectin-1 the overlapping motif is AWGT, whereas galectin-9 contains QWGP and SWGQ in the N- and C-terminal carbohydrate binding domains, respectively. These differences may be associated with the lack of anti-apoptotic ability in galectin-1 and galectin-9 [166]. However, it is unclear which sequences are of prime importance for the apoptotic properties of galectin-1 and galectin-9.

3.1.3. Endogenous lectins in cell-to-cell and cell-extracellular matrix interactions

Another aspect of the biological effects of endogenous lectins is associated with their involvement in cell-to-cell or cell–extracellular matrix interactions and cell migration. Galectin-1 was found to be able to bind laminin, fibronectin, CD43 and CD45 on T lymphocytes and β-lactosamine-containing glycolipid. Galectin-3 binds laminin, carcinoembryonic antigen, LPS, Fc receptors for IgE, Mac-2 binding protein [162,167–169]. Galectins could increase the adhesion of normal and malignant cells and form homotypic and heterotypic cell–cell interactions [170,171]. Survival of various normal cells largely depends on their ability to adhere to the extracellular matrix. Prevention of such adhesion triggers apoptosis in these cells. This form of apoptosis is known as anoikis [172]. It is believed that integrins play a key role in providing a survival signal and prevention of anoikis. However, some data showed an involvement of galectin-3 in cell protection from anoikis [173].

The most compelling data of the involvement of lectins in cell–cell interactions that affect metastasis formation are based on studies of selectins and their ligands. These studies will be discussed below.

3.2. Endogenous lectins and metastasis formation

3.2.1. Selectin–ligand interactions in metastasis formation

Line finding of P- and E-selectin expression by endothelial cells and the selectin ligand by tumor cells stimulated interest in whether selectin–ligand interactions play a role in formation of metastatic tumors. Numerous studies of the human normal and malignant tissue showed that sLe^x and sLe^a are overexpressed in a majority of human carcinomas of the colon, bladder, breast and lungs. Overexpression of sLe^x and sLe^a is often associated with the advanced forms of malignancies [66–69]. Some studies indicate that the level of expression of selectin ligand might have a prognostic value in cancer patients [68,70]. Furthermore, a

comparative analysis of sLe^a and sLe^x expression by tumor cells from primary and metastatic lesions indicated that the expression of sLe^x and/or sLe^a was higher in metastatic lesions in most patients [71,72].

The importance of selectin–ligand interactions in metastasis formation was supported by experiments in which human colon carcinoma KM12-HX was selected for different expression of sLe^x. Cells with high expression of sLe^x showed increased ability to bind to endothelial cells and metastasize into liver [174]. Using the opposite approach namely, selection of colon carcinoma OCUC-LM for high ability to metastasize into liver, it was found that the metastatic variant expresses a higher level of sLe^x than parental cell line [175]. Blocking of sLe^a with specific antibody resulted in an inhibition of metastasis formation by human pancreatic adenocarcinomas in nude mice [176].

Association between selectin ligand expression and metastatic potentials was extensively investigated using various experimental tumor models. The expression of sLe^a and sLe^x was compared in human lung adenocarcinoma lines with different metastatic ability. sLe^a and sLe^x expression was higher in human lung adenocarcinoma line HAL-8Luc that is capable of forming experimental metastasis in the lungs of nude mice than in HAL-24Luc cells that failed to form lung foci after i.v. inoculation into nude mice. Only metastatic line HAL-8Luc showed a significant adherence to E-selectin expressed in human endothelial cell. This adhesion was blocked by anti-E-selectin mAb as well as by mAb against sLe^x [177].

When human colon cancer cell line (LM) was injected into the spleen of nude mice a liver metastasis developed. Tumor cells derived from the liver metastasis were again inoculated into the spleen of nude mice and such procedure was repeated five times. Tumor cells after three and five selective procedures (termed LM-H3 and LM-H5, respectively) expressed 3 and 4.5 times, respectively, higher levels of sLe^a than the parental LM cells. These experiments indicate that selection for higher metastatic ability is associated with an increased expression of sLe^a [175].

H-59 sub-line was selected from murine 3LL Lewis lung carcinoma for the ability to metastasize into the liver [178]. M-27 line failed to metastasize to liver and adhered to the rTNF activated endothelial cells, whereas H-59 line showed high adhesion to the rTNF-α activated endothelial cells. This adhesion was blocked in the presence of anti-E-selectin mAb. When mice inoculated with H-59 cells were treated with mAb against E-selectin the number of developed liver metastasis was reduced by 97% , suggesting that E-selectin is important for the development of liver metastasis by H-59 cells [178]. Normal endothelial cells express very low or not detectable level of E- and P-selectins. The ability of anti-E-selectin mAb to inhibit metastasis formation following i.v. inoculation of tumor cells indicates that inoculation of tumor cell is associated with the up-regulation of E-selectin by endothelium [178]. This might be the result of tumor cell-induced production of IL-1 and/or TNF that are known to be able to up-regulate the expression of E- and P-selectins in endothelial cells. Indeed, intrasplenic/portal route of inoculation of H-59 liver metastasizing lung carcinoma cells or B16F1 melanoma cells resulted in the up-regulation of IL-1 and TNF messages by liver cells [179]. IL-1 and TNF messages were detected 30–60 min after inoculation of H-59 cells, reaching a pick at 4–6 h and declined to basal levels 24 h later. IL-1/TNF mRNA induction by B16F1 melanoma cells was delayed (4–6 h after inoculation) and short lived (no message for these cytokines was found after 8 h). In parallel, E-selectin mRNA transcript in the liver was detected 2 h after H-59 cell inoculation and disappeared 24 h later. B16F1 cells were also able to induce E-selectin message but this effect was comparatively late and more transient. It is of interest to note that M-27 cells that failed to form metastasis in the liver also failed to induce IL-1/TNF as well as E-selectin expression. *In situ* hybridization demonstrated that E-selectin expression in response to tumor cell inoculation was in the HSE [179].

These studies suggest that tumor cells up-regulate the expression of E-selectin by endothelium, and the ability of tumor cells to induce E-selectin expression correlates with the metastatic potential of tumor cells. However, this correlation was demonstrated following intra-splenic tumor cell inoculation and induction of E-selectin by HSE with consecutive formation of liver metastasis. It remains unclear whether i.v. inoculated tumor cells are also able to induce E-selectin expression and whether it correlates with tumor cell ability to form pulmonary metastasis.

The importance of E-selectin in metastasis formation was further supported by experiments in which a soluble form of E-selectin was used. Soluble E-selectin (fusion product E-selectin-immunoglobulin) was able to inhibit lung colonization by i.v. inoculated human colon carcinoma cells, HT-29 [180]. This inhibition was observed in nude mice in which E-selectin expression by endothelium was induced by cytokine treatment. In parallel, *in vitro* experiments showed that soluble E-selectin inhibited HT-29 binding to activated endothelial cells, and *in vivo* it blocked the retention of the i.v. inoculated HT29 cells in the lungs [180]. It is of note that although HT-29 cells express ligands capable of binding both E- and L-selectin, only soluble E-selectin had anti-metastatic effect, whereas soluble L-selectin showed no effect on metastasis formation [180].

Recently Fukuda et al. [181] using phage peptide libraries identified a small peptide IELLQAR that binds anti-Lewis A antibody as well as to E-, P- and L-selectins in a calcium-dependent manner. Phage harboring this peptide as well as synthetic IELLQAR peptide inhibited the binding of sLe^x and sLe^a to E-selectin. This peptide inhibited binding of human lung tumor HL-60 cells expressing sLe^x to E-selectin. Similarly, E-selectin binding of B16FTIIIM melanoma cells that express sLe^x after transfection with α1,3FT was also inhibited by IELLQAR peptide. Moreover, when mice were i.v. inoculated with IELLQAR peptide and 20 min later with B16FTIIIM melanoma or HL-60 cells, metastasis formation in the lungs was significantly inhibited [181]. These results further confirm the importance of E-selectin–ligand interaction in metastasis formation.

An additional confirmation for the importance of E-selectin-sLe interactions in metastasis formation was provided by the gene transfection experiments. B16F10 melanoma cells express neither E-selectin nor its ligands. Biancone et al. [115] transfected B16F10 melanoma with a cDNA encoding α1-3/4FT and found that the transfected cells expressed sLe^a, but not sLe^x. Expression of sLe^a, however, did not affect the ability of B16F10 cells to form metastases in normal C57BL/6 mice. It might be known that normal non-activated endothelium does not express or expresses low level of E-selectin. Therefore metastasis formation was tested in the E-selectin transgenic mice [115]. Two types of the E-selectin transgenic mice were used in these experiments (tines and tangelos mice). Tines mice contain a full-length murine E-selectin cDNA under the chicken β-actin promoter that induces the expression of E-selectin in all tested organs (liver, kidney, brain, heart, muscle, spleen and intestine). Tangelos mice contain a transgene containing a cDNA encoding only the extracellular domain of E-selectin under the control of the α1 anti-trypsin promoter. In these mice a soluble E-selectin has been produced. B16F10 melanoma cells that do not express E-selectin ligand after i.v. inoculation into normal and E-selectin (TgnES and TgEsol) transgenic mice generated the same number of pulmonary metastases and no metastasis was found in other organs [115]. The α1-3/4FT-transfected B16F10 (B16F10ft) cells also formed only pulmonary metastases in normal C57BL/6 mice, whereas in TngES mice they developed large infiltrating tumor masses in liver and small tumors in the lungs. However, in TngEsol mice producing soluble form of E-selectin, B16F10ft cells formed only small tumor nodules in lungs and liver. Liver metastases in TngEsol, in contrast to TngES mice, were well-delineated and non-infiltrated [115]. It is possible that the differences in the size of liver metastases in TgnES and TgnEsol might be due to the differences in E-selectin expression in these mice. Immunohistochemical analysis showed that in TgnES mice E-selectin was predominantly expressed by the endothelium of liver sinusoids and venules with low expression by hepatocytes. In contrast, in TgnEsol mice E-selectin was expressed by hepatocytes but not endothelium. Although TgnES mice endothelium of cardiac and skeletal muscle, as well as of different organs highly expressed E-selectin, no metastases in these anatomical locations were found. The metastasis formation in the liver of these mice was attributed to the relatively low shear forces in the sinusoids and venules of the liver in comparison to other organs. These low shear forces did not interfere with tumor cell attachment and further strong adhesion to endothelium, extravasation and formation of liver metastasis [115].

B16F1 melanoma cells were transfected with the α1,3FT cDNA and then they were sorted into three groups based on the level of sLe^x expression: B16F1 cells with high (H), moderate (M) and negative (N) for sLe^x expression [182]. Cells with high sLe^x expression (B16F1FTIII.H) bound E-selectin better than did B16F1 cells with a moderate expression of sLe^x (B16F1FTIII.M). However, after i.v. inoculation, B16F1FTIII.H melanoma cells with high sLe^x expression were equal to sLe^x negative B16F1III.N melanoma cells in their ability to form metastatic nodules in the lungs [182]. In contrast, B16F1FTIII.M cells with a moderate expression of sLe^x produced more metastatic nodules in the lungs than B16F1 cells that lacked sLe^x (B16F1FTIII.N). Increased metastatic ability of B16F1FTIII.M cells was inhibited by preincubation of these cells with anti-sLe^x antibody, indicating that the newly expressed molecule in the transfected cells is responsible for increased metastatic potential of these cells [182]. It was surprising that B16F1 melanoma cells expressing high level of sLe^x (B16F1FTIII.H) after transfection with α1,3FTIII

cDNA showed no increase in metastasis formation in normal C57BL/6 mice. However, when metastatic properties of these cells were tested in the NK-deficient beige mice or in the NK-depleted C57BL/6 mice, B16F1FTIII.H cells formed more pulmonary metastasis than did B16F1FTIII.N cells [182]. These results imply that B16F1 melanoma cells with high expression of sLe^x became sensitive to NK cell-mediated cytotoxicity, resulting in the destruction of the i.v. inoculated tumor cells and abrogation of the prometastatic effect of E-selectin-sLe^x interactions. Therefore no difference in the total number of metastasis in the lungs were found after inoculation of B16F1FTIII.H and B16F1FTIII.N melanoma cells into normal mice [182]. These results also illustrate the importance of testing the metastasis formation in immuno deficient or immuno suppressed mice, as changes in cell surface carbohydrate might affect not only the ability of tumor cells to migrate and settle in different anatomical location but also their ability to survive the host's immune responses.

P-selectin is expressed by activated platelets and endothelial cells [27]. On the other hand P-selectin ligands are constitutively expressed by various human tumor cells [183]. This creates a possibility for interactions of P-selectin on the platelets and endothelial cells with the ligands on the intravascular migrated metastatic tumor cells. The involvement of P-selectin in metastasis formation was recently evaluated using P-selectin knock out mice. Kim et al. have generated double null mutant mice by backcrossing of P-selectin-deficient mice with RAG2 knock out mice. RAG2 null mice are deficient in T and B lymphocytes but have normal NK cell activity. These mice are unable to reject the transplanted human tumor cells. When LS180 cells were inoculated i.v., 7 of 9 RAG$-/-$, P-selectin$+/+$ versus 2 of 9 of RAG$-/-$, P-selectin$-/-$ mice developed progressively growing tumors in the cervical lymph nodes and surrounding tissues. In the lungs microscopic metastatic foci were found in 8 of 9 P-selectin$+/+$ mice and in only 1 of 9 P-selectin$-/-$ mice [184]. These results imply that the expression of P-selectin is beneficial for metastasis formation. This could be due to the increase in platelet–tumor cell aggregation. When tumor cell–platelet interactions in P-selectin$+/+$ and P-selectin$-/-$ mice were analyzed, it was found that thrombin activated platelets from P-selectin$+/+$ mice formed numerous aggregates with LS180 cells. When tumor cells were pretreated with O-sialoglycoprotein endopeptidase (OSGP), an enzyme that selectively cleaves mucin from the cell surfaces and thus removes

P-selectin ligands, tumor cells-platelet aggregation was inhibited. Platelets from P-selectin-deficient mice did not form rosetting with tumor cells. Similarly, in P-selectin positive mice immunohistochemical analysis of lung sections after i.v. inoculation of LS180 cells, revealed numerous tumor cells that were almost completely covered by platelets. In contrast, in P-selectin-deficient mice very few platelets were associated with tumor cells in the lung vasculature [184]. When distribution of i.v. inoculated radiolabeled LS180 cells was analyzed it was found that a significantly more number of tumor cells were deposited in the lungs, liver and kidney of P-selectin+/+ than P-selectin−/− mice [184]. If less radiolabeled tumor cells were found in P-selectin−/− mice 3 h after i.v. inoculation the question is where are these cells? Tumor cells entering into the blood stream interact with various cellular and non-cellular components of the blood that might result in the activation of the coagulation system [185]. It leads to the formation of platelet–tumor cell aggregation and fibrin deposition on tumor cell surface. It might create tumor microemboli, facilitating their deposition in distant organs and enhance the formation of the metastatic foci [185]. In addition, fibrin deposition and clustering of tumor cells with platelets creates a shield that protects tumor cells from destruction by NK and other cytotoxic cells and help tumor cells to establish distant metastasis [186,187]. Therefore, prevention of blood coagulation by various anticoagulant agents such as heparin or warfarin all result in a substantial inhibition of metastasis formation [186]. Similarly, platelet depletion or inhibition of their activation also might inhibit the formation of pulmonary metastases [185,186]. This inhibition largely depends on the presence of active NK cells and was almost completely abrogated in NK cell-depleted mice [186]. Thus the observed reduction in tumor cell survival and metastasis formation in P-selectin−/− mice could be attributed to reduced tumor cell–platelet aggregation and more efficient elimination of uncovered tumor cells in P-selectin deficient mice.

L-selectin is expressed by leukocytes and was found to be important for their homing as a result of L-selectin interaction with its ligand on the endothelial cells. While naïve T lymphocytes express relatively high level of L-selectin and migrate into lymph nodes, activated T lymphocytes express low or no L-selectin and have a higher ability to migrate into the site of inflammation. When T lymphocytes from the tumor bearing mice were restimulated *in vitro* and selected for their expression of L-selectin, they showed different

therapeutic efficacy against established metastasis. The anti-tumor T lymphocytes with a low level of L-selectin were highly efficient in the eradication of pulmonary and brain metastasis after i.v. adoptive transfer. In contrast, T lymphocytes with a high level of L-selectin or non-separated T lymphocytes had substantially lower therapeutic efficacy [188,189].

3.3. Galectins and metastasis

Galectins are expressed on normal and malignant cells as well as by extracellular matrix or exist in soluble form. Malignant cells are characterized by various changes in cell surface carbohydrates and changes in the expression of galectins [142]. Increased expression of galectin-3 correlates with neoplastic progression in some malignancies such as head and neck cancer, cancer of thyroid, gastric or anaplastic large-cell lymphoma, tumors in the central nervous system [149–151]. In contrast, galectin-3 was found to be down-regulated in carcinomas of the ovary, uterus, and breast compared with the normal counterparts [152–154]. Changes in the expression of galectin-3 by tumor cells might affect their interactions with the corresponding ligands on normal and malignant cells, and their ability to grow locally or metastasize into various anatomical locations. This possibility is supported by experiments in which the expression of galectin-3 was modified by gene transfection. Low metastatic colon cancer cells (LS174T) were transfected with galectin-3 cDNA and acquired a more metastatic phenotype after inoculation into spleen or cecum of nude mice [190]. When high metastatic colon cancer lines (LSLiM6 and HM7) were transfected with the antisense galectin-3 cDNA, resulted in a reduced galectin-3 expression and metastatic ability [190].

Analysis of galectin-3 expression in five human breast carcinoma lines showed that three of these cell lines that were able to grow in nude mice expressed galectin-3, whereas two lines that failed to grow in nude mice showed no galectin-3 expression [191]. When non-tumorigenic cells were transfected with the galectin-3 cDNA, the cells manifested an increased ability of anchorage-independent growth and became tumorigenic in nude mice. Furthermore, one clone (11-9-1-4) that showed the highest ability to grow in nude mice was also able to form metastasis in lymph nodes [191]. No correlation between galectin-1 and tumorigenicity of these cell lines was found [191].

It is still unclear how galectin-3 was able to increase the ability of these lines to develop progressively growing tumors in nude mice. Galectin-3 is not an oncogene and the investigated lines were originally derived from an already malignant tumor. It is possible that the expression of the transfected galectin-3 in the non-tumorigenic line provides better conditions for tumor cell survival, proliferation and metastatic spread in nude mice. This may be the result of interaction of galectin-3 with its natural ligands. It was found that galectin-3-transfected cells in comparison to the parental breast carcinoma cells displayed an increased adherence to laminin and collagen type IV that paralleled with an increased invasion of matrigel [192]. This possibility is supported by findings that exogenous galectin-3 enhanced the ability of human breast carcinoma cells to invade the basement membrane [193]. In addition, the increased ability of galectin-3-transfected breast carcinoma cell lines to grow and metastasize in nude mice can be attributed to the anti-apoptotic effect of galectin-3 [166]. Thus overexpression of galectin-3 in the transfected cells may increase their survival and ability to grow and develop metastasis in nude mice. If it is correct, it is expected that metastatic cells might have a higher expression of galectin-3 than non-metastazing cells. Accordingly, the analysis of galectin-3 expression in the low and high metastatic cell variants of experimental tumors such as K-1735 melanoma, UV-2237 fibrosarcoma and A-31 angiosarcoma showed a positive correlation between the expression of galectin-3 and the metastatic ability of these cell lines [142,147]. To show that this correlation is cause related, the weakly metastatic clone of UV-2237 fibrosarcoma was transfected with the galectin-3 cDNA. The transfected cells showed a substantial increase in their metastatic potential [194].

The possible involvement of galectin-3 in metastasis formation is further supported by experiments in which *in vitro* preincubation of B16 melanoma cells and UV-2237 fibrosarcoma cells with anti-galectin-3 mab before their i.v. inoculation significantly decreased the number of developed pulmonary metastasis [195]. Galectin-3 might also affect tumor cell adhesion, formation of homotypic or heterotypic aggregation and their invasiveness [128,144,192]. The involvement of galectin-3 as well as other lectins in metastasis formation might be due to interactions between the lectins expressed by tumor cells and carbohydrate portion of putative glycoconjugates expressed by normal cells or extracellular matrix. Similarly, lectins expressed by normal cells might interact with the carbohydrates on tumor cells during tumor cell migration, extravasation and tumor growth in a new anatomic location. If this

assumption is correct then one could expect that simple sugars could compete with the natural ligand for binding to the endogenous lectin and affect metastasis formation. Indeed, several studies support this possibility. Infusion of D-galactose and arabinogalactan significantly inhibited the formation of experimental liver metastasis by the murine L-1 sarcoma cells [196]. Similarly, methyl-α-D-lactoside and lacto-N-tetrose inhibited B16 melanoma metastasis formation [197].

The possible involvement of carbohydrate–lectin interactions in the metastatic process is further supported by studies on the effect of natural citrus pectin and pH-modified citrus pectin on metastasis formation [198]. Citrus pectin is a branched complex polysaccharide polymer responsible for the texture of fruit and vegetables containing about 50% of the anhydrogalacturonic acid, 20% of galactose and 15% arabinose. Modification of citrus pectin by pH resulted in the degradation of the main galacturonic acid chain and formation of non-branched carbohydrate chains. When B16F1 melanoma cells were inoculated i.v. together with citric pectin, a three-fold increase in the number of developed pulmonary metastasis was found. In contrast, inoculation of B16F1 cells with pH-modified citrus pectin resulted in a substantial inhibition of metastasis formation [198]. Further analysis revealed that modified citrus pectin inhibited B16F1 melanoma cells adhesion to laminin, whereas original citrus pectin had no effect on tumor cell binding or spreading on to laminin. Modified citrus pectin was also able to inhibit homotypic aggregation of B16F1 melanoma cells. In contrast, citrus pectin enhanced tumor cell aggregation [199]. There is a positive correlation between metastatic potential of tumor cells and their ability to form homotypic aggregates *in vitro*. Tumor cells that aggregate and form clumps produce more experimental pulmonary metastases than non-clumping cells [200].

Formation of tumor cell aggregates (homotypic aggregation) could be mediated via integrin–ligand interactions [201]. Homotypic aggregation could be also a result of intercellular adhesion mediated via interaction between cell–surface lectin of one cell and carbohydrate-containing complementary molecules on adjacent cells. *In vivo*, serum glycoproteins might serve as a bridge between cells inducing their clumping leading to increased embolization in the pulmonary vasculature, and increased formation of pulmonary metastasis following i.v. inoculation of tumor cells. Some observations strongly support the involvement of galectin-3 in cell aggregate formation [170]. These include: (a) exogenous asialofetuin, a glycoprotein rich in terminal β-gal residues, induces homotypic aggregation of tumor cells; (b) this aggregation is inhibited by anti-galectin-3 antibody or its Fab' fragments; (c) when insect cells Sf9, that do not express endogenous galectin-3, were transfected with the cDNA encoding galectin-3, the galectin-3 expressing Sf9 cells underwent homotypic aggregation in the presence of asialofetuin, and (d) homotypic aggregation was substantially inhibited by the competitive sugar lactose, but not with sucrose [170]. Recent studies indicate that galectin-3 is involved in tumor-induced angiogenesis [140]. Galectin-3 stimulates *in vitro* capillary tube formation and chemotaxis of endothelial cells as well as *in vivo* vascularization. It is note worthy that the galectin-3-mediated stimulation of the capillary tube formation and chemotaxis can be inhibited by lactose, a competitive disaccharide, and by modified citrus pectin, a competitive polysaccharide [140]. The involvement of galectin-3 in angiogenesis might be one of the mechanisms by which galectin-3 may affect local tumor growth and metastasis formation.

While these data indicate that galectin-3 might play a role in metastasis formation, the involvement of other galectins in metastatic process remains unclear and needs further investigation.

3.4. MBP and MR in metastasis formation

MBP was found to be highly efficient in the recognition and binding to the carbohydrates expressed by bacteria invading into the blood. Due to its homology to Cr1 of complement, MBP is able to trigger the activation of the classical and alternative pathway of complement, resulting in lysis of the invaded microorganisms [155,157]. MBP does not bind to normal cells, including the circulating blood cells but carbohydrate changes associated with malignant transformation could make tumor cells recognizable by MBP. Some experimental data support this possibility. When mice bearing a human colorectal carcinoma SW1116 were inoculated with the recombinant vaccinia virus containing a human MBP gene a significant inhibited growth of this tumor was observed [202]. It is of interest to note that the mutated form of MBP, which is unable to activate the complement, was equally efficient in the inhibition of SW1116 tumor growth [202]. These results suggest complement independent mechanisms of anti-tumor effect of MBP.

MR is a 175 kDa transmembrane glycoprotein which is expressed by macrophages and dendritic cells. MR is also found on HSE cells, lymphatic endothelial cells

of small intestine and sinusoidal endothelial cells of lymph nodes but not of spleen and thymus [203]. MR contains eight tandem lectin-like CRDs that bind mannose, fucose and GlcNAc [133]. These carbohydrates are abundantly expressed by tumor cells and may facilitate tumor cell interaction with the MR of endothelial cells. Since only particular type of endothelial cells express MR, its interaction with tumor cells might determine the tissue or organ specificity of certain metastasis. Expression of MR is up-regulated following treatment of mice with IL-1 or LPS [204]. When mice were pretreated with IL-1 or LPS, the numbers of liver metastases after intra-splenic inoculation of B16 melanoma cells increased by 73–87%. LPS-induced enhancement of liver metastasis was blocked by the administration of IL-1R antagonist, suggesting that this effect of LPS is mediated via induction of IL-1. It was found that IL-1 and LPS increased the MR activity in HSE, as measured by endocytosis of fluorescein-conjugated ovalbumin. In parallel, in IL-1 and LPS treated mice an increase in adhesion of B16 melanoma cells was observed [204]. However, IL-1 is also able to up-regulate VCAM-1 and E- and P-selectin expression by endothelium. So it remains unclear whether the observed increase in B16 melanoma liver metastasis could be attributed to the stimulation of MR expression or to other adhesion molecules.

Additional studies on the possible involvement of MR in metastasis formation were performed using B16 melanoma cells that were treated with 1-deoximannojirimycin (1-DMM). Treatment of B16 melanoma cells with 1-DMM increased the expression of high mannose-type oligosacharides. After intrasplenic inoculation, 1-DMM-treated B16 melanoma cells generated significantly more liver metastasis than untreated B16 cells. This augmentation was blocked by i.p. inoculation of rIL-1 antagonist [205]. *In vitro* test showed that 1-DMM-treated B16 cells with a higher expression of mannose-type oligosaccharides, were more adhesive to HSE than parental B16 cells. Increased adhesiveness of 1-DMM-treated cells to HSE was blocked by anti-VCAM-1 antibody and by rIL-1 antagonist, suggesting the involvement of IL-1-mediated up-regulation of VCAM-1 in this process. VCAM-1 is a ligand for VLA-4 integrin that is expressed by B16 melanoma cells. Incubation of HSE with mannan and 1-DMM-treated B16 cells resulted in the production of IL-1 by HSE. It was proposed that the binding of tumor cells to MR triggers IL-1 production. Then IL-1 induces VCAM-1 expression by endothelium, resulting in increased adhesion of tumor cells to

HSE cells, tumor arrest in the liver with further extravasation and formation of liver metastasis [205]. It is very likely that MR-induced up-regulation of VCAM-1 on endothelial cells leads to its interaction with VLA-4 expressed by tumor cells and thus further contributing to the observed increase in metastasis formation. The possible involvement of MBP and MR in metastasis formation needs further experimental support.

4. Summary and conclusions

The data accumulated during the last several decades clearly demonstrate that malignant transformation is associated with various and complex alterations in the glycosylation process. The precise mechanisms responsible for these changes and their significance in malignant transformation still remain largely unclear. Malignant transformation is primarily associated with the up-regulation of oncogenes or down-regulation of the tumor suppressor genes. This results in uncontrolled cell proliferation and alterations in the expression of various cellular genes that cause angiogenesis, invade the surrounding tissues, extravasate and form metastatic foci in various anatomical locations. The changes in the expression of cellular genes during malignant transformation depend on the expression of the regulatory transcription factors that control genes regulating cell proliferation or invasiveness as well as some genes encoding glycosyltransferases. This assumption is supported by findings that transcription factor ETS-1 up-regulates the expression of MMP genes that might lead to increased tumor cell invasiveness and stimulate angiogenesis [48]. In parallel, ETS-1 regulates the expression of N-acetylglucosyltransferase V [46,47]. Similarly the her/neu oncogene increases the transcription of N-acetylglucosyltransferase V [206]. Thus, the observed changes in tumor cell glycosylation could be a by-product of the changes associated with the alterations in gene expression during malignant transformation. Some of these changes might provide a selective advantage for tumor cells during their progression to more invasive and metastatic phenotype.

The possible involvement of cell surface carbohydrates in the metastatic process is supported by studies demonstrating major differences in the expression of cell surface carbohydrates between the primary and metastatic tumors in cancer patients and in experimental animals [6,7]. However, these correlative studies suggest rather then prove that metastatic properties of tumor cells are depending on carbohydrate composition of cell surface glycoconjugates. More direct support for importance of cell surface carbohydrates in metastasis formation was obtained when the glycosylation of tumor cells was altered as result of inhibition of glycosylation with various inhibitors, or due to selection of tumor cells for resistance to plant lectins [6,7]. Recently gene transfection technique help to provide a more direct confirmation for the importance of cell carbohydrates in metastasis formation. Transfection of genes encoding various glysosyltransferases gene in sense and antisense orientation helped to bring direct evidence that changes in cell surface carbohydrates are important for the metastatic behavior of tumor cells [31,32,97,98,108–110,117,119, 120, 122]. However, overexpression of the transfected glycosyltransferase induces various carbohydrate changes as a result of changing the balance between galactosyltransferases in the endoplasmic reticulum or in the Golgi apparatus. For example, transfection of galactosyltransferase or fucosyltransferase genes resulted in the appearance of the terminal galactose or fucose, but this is also paralleled with a reduction of sialic acid and cell membrane sialylation. These changes are the result of the competition between the galactosyltransferase or fucosyltransferase with sialyltransferases for the common substrate N-acetyllactosamine. Similarly, transfection with a gene encoding GnT-III leads to competition between GnT-III and GNT-V and prevention of β1-6 branching. A reduction in β1-6 branching of N-linked oligosaccharides reduce lactosamine antennae for the terminal capping by sialic acid, leading to a reduction in tumor cell sialylation. Thus, it needs to be established whether the appearance of new carbohydrates or simultaneous changes in sialic acid expression are important for changes in metastatic ability of the glycosyltransferase gene-transfected cells.

How could changes in tumor cell glycosylation affect the metastatic properties of tumor cells? Analysis of the significance of protein glycosylation revealed that glycosylation could affect folding, localization, as well as functional and structural organization of proteins. Glycosylation could also affect the rate of protein degradation and their organizational framework within cytoplasm, membrane and extracellularly [1,2,11]. The observed changes in tumor cell surface carbohydrates might also affect membrane rigidity, the functional activity of membrane proteins including growth factor receptors and integrins, immunogenicity and sensitivity of tumor cells to natural cell-mediated immunity [8–10,64]. It is believed that the interaction of

134

tumor cells with normal cells or with the extracellular matrix plays an important role during metastatic spread and growth [207,208]. Numerous data indicate that these cell-to-cell or cell–extracellular matrix interactions largely mediated via integrin–ligand interactions could be affected by alterations in the glycosylation of integrins. In addition, these interactions can be mediated via tumor cell carbohydrates and endogenous lectins.

Numerous endogenous lectins have been discovered. The biological significance of the endogenous lectins and their possible role in tumor growth and metastasis formation has started to unravel. Endogenous lectin–carbohydrate interactions can be mediated via carbohydrates on tumor cells and lectins on normal cells such as endothelial cells or lymphocytes as well as soluble lectins. Similarly, lectins on tumor cells may interact with carbohydrates expressed by normal cells. Thus, endogenous lectin–carbohydrate interactions could affect metastatic potentials of tumor cells via a number of mechanisms, including adhesion of tumor cells to endothelium, blood cells or extracellular matrix. The interactions between E- and P-selectins on endothelial cells and sLe^x and sLe^a on tumor cells was found to be important for homing and metastasis formation in some tissues and organs [27,175,178,179,209].

Increasing number of evidence indicates that endogenous lectins such as MBP, surfactant proteins (SP-A and SP-D) and MP play an important role in innate and adoptive immunity [130,139]. However, involvement of these lectins in anti-tumor immunity and prevention of metastasis formation needs more direct experimental confirmation. Some plant lectins are highly cytotoxic and are able to induce apoptosis [93,161]. It is possible that some endogenous lectins can also kill certain normal or malignant cells *in vivo*. If so, lectin-mediated cytotoxicity might represent a primitive non-immunological mechanism of elimination of cells with altered cell membrane carbohydrate composition. Since carbohydrate alterations are common feature of malignant cells, this lectin-mediated cytotoxicity might play a role in the host's anti-tumor and anti-metastatic defense [93,161]. It was shown that galectin-1 in humans and galectin-9 in mice are able to induce apoptosis of certain population of human T lymphocytes during their differentiation in thymus. Moreover, recombinant galectin-1 was capable of inducing apoptosis of human malignant cells such as MOL4 and K562 lymphomas [23,162,163]. However, the possible role of galectin-1 or other putative endogenous lectin in tumor cell elimination needs

to be further established by more direct experimental confirmation.

An opposite role may be assigned to galectin-3, which was found to have an anti-apoptotic effect. Thus, overexpression of galectin-3 by tumor cells provides certain advantage and increase, their survival during metastasis formation [142,147,165,166,194]. In general, involvement of galectin-3 in metastasis formation is well documented. In addition to its anti-apoptotic activity galectin-3 affects cell–cell interactions, tumor cell invasiveness and promotes tumor vascularization [140,170,198].

In summary, recent studies using genetic engineering of tumor cells with the genes encoding various glycosyltransferases and glycosidase brought an additional support of the importance of cell carbohydrates in the regulation of metastatic properties of tumor cells. However, the involved mechanisms still remain obscure. With the discovery of the endogenous lectins the possible interactions between these lectins and their carbohydrate ligands in metastasis formation become extensively explored. Although various aspects of lectin–carbohydrate interactions are far from being completely understood, increasing number of experimental data confirms their importance in metastasis processes. Further investigations are needed to shed more light on the understanding of the biological significance of endogenous lectins, their interactions with cell surface carbohydrates and their role in tumor metastasis formation.

References

1. Opdenakker G, Rudd PM, Ponting CP, Dwek RA: Concepts and principles of glycobiology. Faseb J 7: 1330–1337, 1993
2. Sharon N: Carbohydrates. Sci Am 243: 90–116, 1980
3. Sharon N, Lis H: Lectins as cell recognition molecules. Science 246: 227–234, 1989
4. Hakomori S: Aberrant glycosylation in cancer cell membranes as focused on glycolipids: Overview and perspectives. Cancer Res 45: 2405–2414, 1985
5. Hakomori S: Tumor malignancy defined by aberrant glycosylation and sphingo(glyco)lipid metabolism. Cancer Res 56: 5309–5318, 1996
6. Dennis JW: N-linked oligosaccharide processing and tumor cell biology. Semin Cancer Biol 2: 411–420, 1991
7. Dennis JW: Changes in glycosylation associated with malignant transformation and tumor progression. In: Fukuda M (ed.) Cell Surface Carbohydrates and Cell Development, CRC Press, Boca Raton, 1992, pp 161–194
8. Chammas R, Veiga SS, Line S, Potocnjak P, Brentani RR: Asn-linked oligosaccharide-dependent interaction between laminin and gp120/140. An alpha 6/beta 1 integrin. J Biol Chem 266: 3349–3355, 1991

9. Zheng M, Fang H, Tsuruoka T, Tsuji T, Sasaki T, Hakomori S: Regulatory role of GM3 ganglioside in alpha 5 beta 1 integrin receptor for fibronectin-mediated adhesion of FUA169 cells. J Biol Chem 268: 2217–2222, 1993

10. Akiyama SK, Yamada SS, Yamada KM: Analysis of the role of glycosylation of the human fibronectin receptor. J Biol Chem 264: 18011–18018, 1989

11. Kornfeld RaKS: Structure of glycoproteins and their oligosaccharide units. In: Lennarz W (ed.) The Biochemistry of Glycoproteins and Proteoglycans, Plenum Press, New York, 1980

12. Berke G: In: Paul W (ed.) Fundamental Immunology, Raven Press Ltd, New York, 1989, pp 735–764

13. Bevan MJ, Cohn M: Cytotoxic effects of antigen- and mitogen-induced T cells on various targets. J Immunol 114: 559–565, 1975

14. Kilpatrick D: Use of lectins as mitogens for lymphocytes. In: Rhodes J, Milton J (ed.) Lectins Methods and Protocols, Humana Press, Totowa, 1998, pp 385–392

15. Yu L-G, Phodes J: Mitogenic effects of lectins on epithelial cells. In: Rhodes J, Milton J (ed.) Lectins Methods and Protocols, Humana Press, Totowa, 1998, pp 379–384

16. Carcinci P, Becchetti E, Bodo M: Effects of lectins on cytoskeletal organization in mammalian cells. In: Rhodes J, Milton J (ed.) Lectins Methods and Protocols, Humana Press, Totowa, 1998, pp 407–421

17. Sada K, Yamamura, H: Effect of lectins on protein kinase activity. In: Rhodes J, Milton J (ed.) Lectin Methods and Protocols, Humana Press, Totowa, 1998, pp 423–432

18. Timoshenko AV, Kayser K, Drings P, Andre S, Dong X, Kaltner H, Schneller M, Gabius HJ: Carbohydrate-binding proteins (plant/human lectins and autoantibodies from human serum) as mediators of release of lysozyme, elastase, and myeloperoxidase from human neutrophils. Res Exp Med 195: 153–162, 1995

19. Stanley P: Surface carbohydrate alterations of mutant mammalian cells selected for resistance to plant lectins. In: Lennarz W (ed.) The Biochemistry of Glycoproteins and Proteoglycans, Plenum Press, New York, 1981, pp 161–190

20. Dennis JW: Different metastatic phenotypes in two genetic classes of wheat germ agglutinin-resistant tumor cell mutants. Cancer Res 46: 4594–4600, 1986

21. Tao TW, Burger MM: Lectin-resistant variants of mouse melanoma cells. I. Altered metastasizing capacity and tumorigenicity. Int J Cancer 29: 425–430, 1982

22. Tao TW, Burger MM: Non-metastasising variants selected from metastasising melanoma cells. Nature 270: 437–438, 1977

23. Perillo NL, Marcus ME, Baum LG: Galectins: Versatile modulators of cell adhesion, cell proliferation, and cell death. J Mol Med 76: 402–412, 1998

24. Barondes SH, Cooper DN, Gitt MA, Leffler H: Galectins. Structure and function of a large family of animal lectins. J Biol Chem 269: 20807–20810, 1994

25. Drickamer K, Taylor ME: Biology of animal lectins. Annu Rev Cell Biol 9: 237–264, 1993

26. Drickamer K: Increasing diversity of animal lectin structures. Curr Opin Struct Biol 5: 612–616, 1995

27. Varki A: Selectin ligands. Proc Natl Acad Sci USA 91: 7390–7397, 1994

28. Rabinovich GA: Galectins: An evolutionarily conserved family of animal lectins with multifunctional properties; a trip from the gene to clinical therapy. Cell Death Differ 6: 711–721, 1999

29. Fukuda M: Possible roles of tumor-associated carbohydrate antigens. Cancer Res 56: 2237–2244, 1996

30. Hakomori S: Aberrant glycosylation in tumors and tumor-associated carbohydrate antigens. Adv Cancer Res 52: 257–331, 1989

31. Zeng G, Li DD, Gao L, Birkle S, Bieberich E, Tokuda A, Yu RK: Alteration of ganglioside composition by stable transfection with antisense vectors against GD3-synthase gene expression. Biochemistry 38: 8762–8769, 1999

32. Zeng G, Gao L, Birkle S, Yu R: Suppression of ganglioside GD3 expression in a rat F-11 tumor cell line reduces tumor growth, angiogenesis and vascular endothelial growth factor production. Cancer Res 60: 6670–6676, 2000

33. Manfredi MG, Lim S, Claffey KP, Seyfried TN: Gangliosides influence angiogenesis in an experimental mouse brain tumor. Cancer Res 59: 5392–5397, 1999

34. Pukel CS, Lloyd KO, Travassos LR, Dippold WG, Oettgen HF, Old LJ: GD3, a prominent ganglioside of human melanoma. Detection and characterisation by mouse monoclonal antibody. J Exp Med 155: 1133–1147, 1982

35. Cahan LD, Irie RF, Singh R, Cassidenti A, Paulson JC: Identification of a human neuroectodermal tumor antigen (OFA-I-2) as ganglioside GD2. Proc Natl Acad Sci USA 79: 7629–7633, 1982

36. Nudelman E, Kannagi R, Hakomori S, Parsons M, Lipinski M, Wiels J, Fellous M, Tursz TA: Glycolipid antigen associated with Burkitt's lymphoma defined by a monoclonal antibody. Science 220: 509–511, 1983

37. Kniep B, Monner DA, Burrichter H, Diehl V, Muhlradt PF: Gangliotriaosylceramide (asialo GM2), a glycosphingolipid marker for cell lines derived from patients with Hodgkin's disease. J Immunol 131: 1591–1594, 1983

38. Koochekpour S, Merzak A, Pilkington GJ: Vascular endothelial growth factor production is stimulated by gangliosides and TGF-beta isoforms in human glioma cells in vitro. Cancer Lett 102: 209–215, 1996

39. Ziche M, Morbidelli L, Alessandri G, Gullino PM: Angiogenesis can be stimulated or repressed in vivo by a change in GM3 : GD3 ganglioside ratio. Lab Invest 67: 711–715, 1992

40. Folkman J: Angiogenesis in cancer, vascular, rheumatoid and other disease. Nat Med 1: 27–31, 1995

41. Fernandes B, Sagman U, Auger M, Demetrio M, Dennis JW: Beta 1-6 branched oligosaccharides as a marker of tumor progression in human breast and colon neoplasia (see comments). Cancer Res 51: 718–723, 1991

42. Pierce M, Arango J: Rous sarcoma virus-transformed baby hamster kidney cells express higher levels of asparagine-linked tri- and tetraantennary glycopeptides containing [GlcNAc-beta (1,6)Man-alpha (1,6)Man] and poly-N-acetyllactosamine sequences than baby hamster kidney cells. J Biol Chem 261: 10772–10777, 1986

136

43. Dennis JW, Laferte S, Waghorne C, Breitman ML, Kerbel RS: Beta 1-6 branching of Asn-linked oligosaccharides is directly associated with metastasis. Science 236: 582–585, 1987

44. Dennis JW, Kosh K, Bryce DM, Breitman ML: Oncogenes conferring metastatic potential induce increased branching of Asn-linked oligosaccharides in rat2 fibroblasts. Oncogene 4: 853–860, 1989

45. Yamashita K, Tachibana Y, Ohkura T, Kobata A: Enzymatic basis for the structural changes of asparagine-linked sugar chains of membrane glycoproteins of baby hamster kidney cells induced by polyoma transformation. J Biol Chem 260: 3963–3969, 1985

46. Kang R, Saito H, Ihara Y, Miyoshi E, Koyama N, Sheng Y, Taniguchi N: Transcriptional regulation of the N-acetylglucosaminyltransferase V gene in human bile duct carcinoma cells (HuCC-T1) is mediated by Ets-1 [published erratum appears in J Biol Chem 1999 Jan 1; 274(1): 554]. J Biol Chem 271: 26706–26712, 1996

47. Buckhaults P, Chen L, Fregien N, Pierce M: Transcriptional regulation of N-acetylglucosaminyltransferase V by the src oncogene. J Biol Chem 272: 19575–19581, 1997

48. Vandenbunder B, Queva C, Desbiens X, Wernert N, Stehelin D: Expression of the transcription factor c-Ets1 correlates with the occurrence of invasive processes during normal and pathological development. Invasion Metastasis 14: 198–209, 1994

49. Wojciechowicz DC, Park PY, Paty PB: Beta 1-6 branching of N-linked carbohydrate is associated with K-ras mutation in human colon carcinoma cell lines. Biochem Biophys Res Commun 212: 758–766, 1995

50. Gessner P, Riedl S, Quentmaier A, Kemmner W: Enhanced activity of CMP-neuAc:Gal beta 1-4GlcNAc:alpha 2,6-sialyltransferase in metastasizing human colorectal tumor tissue and serum of tumor patients: Cancer Lett 75: 143–149, 1993

51. Dall'Olio F, Malagolini N, di Stefano G, Minni F, Marrano D, Serafini-Cessi F: Increased CMP-NeuAc:Gal beta 1,4GlcNAc-Rs alpha 2,6 sialyltransferase activity in human colorectal cancer tissues. Int J Cancer 44: 434–439, 1989

52. Pousset D, Piller V, Bureaud N, Monsigny M, Piller F: Increased alpha2,6 sialylation of N-glycans in a transgenic mouse model of hepatocellular carcinoma. Cancer Res 57: 4249–4256, 1997

53. Le Marer N, Laudet V, Svensson EC, Cazlaris H, Van Hille B, Lagrou C, Stehelin D, Montreuil J, Verbert A, Delannoy P: The c-Ha-ras oncogene induces increased expression of beta-galactoside alpha-2, 6-sialyltransferase in rat fibroblast (FR3T3) cells. Glycobiology 2: 49–56, 1992

54. Oriol R, Le Pendu J, Mollicone R: Genetics of ABO, H, Lewis, X and related antigens. Vox Sang 51: 161–171, 1986

55. Sun J, Thurin J, Cooper HS, Wang P, Mackiewicz M, Steplewski Z, Blaszczyk-Thurin M: Elevated expression of H type GDP-L-fucose:beta-D-galactoside alpha-2-L-fucosyltransferase is associated with human colon adenocarcinoma progression. Proc Natl Acad Sci USA 92: 5724–5728, 1995

56. Mandel U, Langkilde NC, Orntoft TF, Therkildsen MH, Karkov J, Reibel J, White T, Clausen H, Dabelsteen E: Expression of histo-blood-group-A/B-gene-defined glycosyltransferases in normal and malignant epithelia: Correlation with A/B-carbohydrate expression. Int J Cancer 52: 7–12, 1992

57. Orntoft TF: Carbohydrate changes in bladder carcinomas. APMIS Suppl 27: 181–187, 1992

58. Lee JS, Ro JY, Sahin AA, Hong WK, Brown BW, Mountain CF, Hittelman WN: Expression of blood-group antigen A–a favorable prognostic factor in non-small-cell lung cancer. N Engl J Med 324: 1084–1090, 1991

59. Yuan M, Itzkowitz SH, Palekar A, Shamsuddin AM, Phelps PC, Trump BF, Kim YS: Distribution of blood group antigens A, B, H, Lewisa, and Lewisb in human normal, fetal, and malignant colonic tissue. Cancer Res 45: 4499–4511, 1985

60. Davidsohn I, Ni LY: Loss of isoantigens A, B, and H in carcinoma of the lung. Am J Pathol 57: 307–334, 1969

61. Davidsohn I, Kovarik S, Ni LY: Isoantigens A, B, and H in benign and malignant lesions of the cervix. Arch Pathol 87: 306–314, 1969

62. Orntoft TF, Meldgaard P, Pedersen B, Wolf H: The blood group ABO gene transcript is down-regulated in human bladder tumors and growth-stimulated urothelial cell lines. Cancer Res 56: 1031–1036, 1996

63. Matsumoto H, Muramatsu H, Shimotakahara T, Yanagi M, Nishijima H, Mitani N, Baba K, Muramatsu T, Shimazu H: Correlation of expression of ABH blood group carbohydrate antigens with metastatic potential in human lung carcinomas. Cancer 72: 75–81, 1993

64. Ichikawa D, Handa K, Hakomori S: Histo-blood group A/B antigen deletion/reduction vs. continuous expression in human tumor cells as correlated with their malignancy. Int J Cancer 76: 284–289, 1998

65. Ichikawa D, Handa K, Withers DA, Hakomori S: Histo-blood group A/B versus H status of human carcinoma cells as correlated with haptotactic cell motility: Approach with A and B gene transfection. Cancer Res 57: 3092–3096, 1997

66. Renkonen J, Paavonen T, Renkonen R: Endothelial and epithelial expression of sialyl Lewis(x) and sialyl Lewis(a) in lesions of breast carcinoma. Int J Cancer 74: 296–300, 1997

67. Miyake M, Taki T, Hitomi S, Hakomori S: Correlation of expression of H/Le(y)/Le(b) antigens with survival in patients with carcinoma of the lung (see comments). N Engl J Med 327: 14–18, 1992

68. Nakamori S, Kameyama M, Imaoka S, Furukawa H, Ishikawa O, Sasaki Y, Kabuto T, Iwanaga T, Matsushita Y, Irimura T: Increased expression of sialyl Lewis x antigen correlates with poor survival in patients with colorectal carcinoma: clinicopathological and immunohistochemical study. Cancer Res 53: 3632–3637, 1993

69. Shimodaira K, Nakayama J, Nakamura N, Hasebe O, Katsuyama T, Fukuda M: Carcinoma-associated expression of core 2 beta-1,6-N-acetylglucosaminyltransferase gene in human colorectal cancer: role of O-glycans in tumor progression. Cancer Res 57: 5201–5206, 1997

70. Irimura T, Nakamori S, Matsushita Y, Taniuchi Y, Todoroki N, Tsuji T, Izumi Y, Kawamura Y, Hoff SD, Cleary KR, et al.: Colorectal cancer metastasis determined by carbohydrate-mediated cell adhesion: role of sialyl-LeX antigens. Semin Cancer Biol 4: 319–324, 1993

71. Sawada R, Tsuboi S, Fukuda M: Differential E-selectin-dependent adhesion efficiency in sublines of a human colon cancer exhibiting distinct metastatic potentials. J Biol Chem 269: 1425–1431, 1994

72. Ikeda Y, Mori M, Kajiyama K, Haraguchi Y, Sasaki O, Sugimachi K: Immunohistochemical expression of sialyl Tn, sialyl Lewis a, sialyl Lewis a-b-, and sialyl Lewis x in primary tumor and metastatic lymph nodes in human gastric cancer. J Surg Oncol 62: 171–176, 1996

73. Yogeeswaran G, Salk PL: Metastatic potential is positively correlated with cell surface sialylation of cultured murine tumor cell lines. Science 212: 1514–1516, 1981

74. Altevogt P, Fogel M, Cheingsong-Popov R, Dennis J, Robinson P, Schirrmacher V: Different patterns of lectin binding and cell surface sialylation detected on related high- and low-metastatic tumor lines. Cancer Res 43: 5138–5144, 1983

75. Fogel M, Altevogt P, Schirrmacher V: Metastatic potential severely altered by changes in tumor cell adhesiveness and cell-surface sialylation. J Exp Med 157: 371–376, 1983

76. Steele JG, Rowlatt C, Sandall JK, Franks LM: Cell surface properties of high- and low-metastatic cell lines selected from a spontaneous mouse lung carcinoma. Int J Cancer 32: 769–779, 1983

77. Passaniti A, Hart GW: Cell surface sialylation and tumor metastasis. Metastatic potential of B16 melanoma variants correlates with their relative numbers of specific penultimate oligosaccharide structures. J Biol Chem 263: 7591–7603, 1988

78. Seberger PJ, Chaney WG: Control of metastasis by Asn-linked, beta1-6 branched oligosaccharides in mouse mammary cancer cells. Glycobiology 9: 235–241, 1999

79. Dennis JW, Laferte S, Fukuda M, Dell A, Carver JP: Asn-linked oligosaccharides in lectin-resistant tumor-cell mutants with varying metastatic potential. Eur J Biochem 161: 359–373, 1986

80. Roberts JD, Klein JL, Palmantier R, Dhume ST, George MD, Olden K: The role of protein glycosylation inhibitors in the prevention of metastasis and therapy of cancer. Cancer Detect Prev 22: 455–462, 1998

81. Goss PE, Baker MA, Carver JP, Dennis JW: Inhibitors of carbohydrate processing: A new class of anticancer agents. Clin Cancer Res 1: 935–944, 1995

82. Humphries MJ, Matsumoto K, White SL, Olden K: Inhibition of experimental metastasis by castanospermine in mice: Blockage of two distinct stages of tumor colonization by oligosaccharide processing inhibitors. Cancer Res 46: 5215–5222, 1986

83. Humphries MJ, Matsumoto K, White SL, Olden K: Oligosaccharide modification by swainsonine treatment inhibits pulmonary colonization by B16-F10 murine melanoma cells. Proc Natl Acad Sci USA 83: 1752–1756, 1986

84. Irimura T, Gonzalez R, Nicolson GL: Effects of tunicamycin on B16 metastatic melanoma cell surface glycoproteins and blood-borne arrest and survival properties. Cancer Res 41: 3411–3418, 1981

85. Korczak B, Dennis JW: Inhibition of N-linked oligosaccharide processing in tumor cells is associated with enhanced tissue inhibitor of metalloproteinases (TIMP) gene expression. Int J Cancer 53: 634–639, 1993

86. Ostrander GK, Scribner NK, Rohrschneider LR: Inhibition of v-fms-induced tumor growth in nude mice by castanospermine. Cancer Res 48: 1091–1094, 1988

87. Humphries MJ, Matsumoto K, White SL, Molyneux RJ, Olden K: Augmentation of murine natural killer cell activity by swainsonine, a new antimetastatic immunomodulator. Cancer Res 48: 1410–1415, 1988

88. Oredipe OA, White SL, Grzegorzewski K, Gause BL, Cha JK, Miles VA, Olden K: Protective effects of swainsonine on murine survival and bone marrow proliferation during cytotoxic chemotherapy. J Natl Cancer Inst 83: 1149–1156, 1991

89. Raz A, McLellan WL, Hart IR, Bucana CD, Hoyer LC, Sela BA, Dragsten P, Fidler IJ: Cell surface properties of B16 melanoma variants with differing metastatic potential. Cancer Res 40: 1645–1651, 1980

90. Irimura T, Nicolson GL: Carbohydrate chain analysis by lectin binding to electrophoretically separated glycoproteins from murine B16 melanoma sublines of various metastatic properties. Cancer Res 44: 791–798, 1984

91. Reading CL, Brunson KW, Torrianni M, Nicolson GL: Malignancies of metastatic murine lymphosarcoma cell lines and clones correlate with decreased cell surface display of RNA tumor virus envelope glycoprotein gp70. Proc Natl Acad Sci USA 77: 5943–5947, 1980

92. Reading CL, Belloni PN, Nicolson GL: Selection and in vivo properties of lectin-attachment variants of malignant murine lymphosarcoma cell lines. J Natl Cancer Inst 64: 1241–1249, 1980

93. Gorelik E: Mechanisms of cytotoxic activity of lectins. Trends Glycoscience and Glycobiology 6: 435–445, 1994

94. Ishikawa M, Dennis JW, Man S, Kerbel RS: Isolation and characterization of spontaneous wheat germ agglutinin-resistant human melanoma mutants displaying remarkably different metastatic profiles in nude mice. Cancer Res 48: 665–670, 1988

95. Frost P, Kerbel RS, Bauer E, Tartamella-Biondo R, Cefalu W: Mutagen treatment as a means for selecting immunogenic variants from otherwise poorly immunogenic malignant murine tumors. Cancer Res 43: 125–132, 1983

96. Gorelik E, Jay G, Kim M, Hearing VJ, DeLeo A, McCoy JP Jr: Effects of H-2Kb gene on expression of melanoma-associated antigen and lectin-binding sites on BL6 melanoma cells. Cancer Res 51: 5212–5218, 1991

97. Gorelik E, Duty L, Anaraki F, Galili U: Alterations of cell surface carbohydrates and inhibition of metastatic property of murine melanomas by alpha 1,3 galactosyltransferase gene transfection. Cancer Res 55: 4168–4173, 1995

98. Gorelik E, Xu F, Henion T, Anaraki F, Galili U: Reduction of metastatic properties of BL6 melanoma cells expressing

138

terminal fucose(alpha)1-2-galactose after alpha1,2-fucosyltransferase cDNA transfection. Cancer Res 57: 332–336, 1997

99. Gorelik E, Kim M, Duty L, Henion T, Galili U: Control of metastatic properties of BL6 melanoma cells by H-2Kb gene: Immunological and nonimmunological mechanisms. Clin Exp Metastasis 11: 439–452, 1993

100. Goldstein IJ, Blake DA, Ebisu S, Williams TJ, Murphy LA: Carbohydrate binding studies on the Bandeiraea simplicifolia I isolectins. Lectins which are mono-, di-, tri-, and tetravalent for N-acetyl-D-galactosamine. J Biol Chem 256: 3890–3893, 1981

101. Galili U, Shohet SB, Kobrin E, Stults CL, Macher BA: Man, apes, and Old World monkeys differ from other mammals in the expression of alpha-galactosyl epitopes on nucleated cells. J Biol Chem 263: 17755–17762, 1988

102. Galili U: Evolution and pathophysiology of the human natural anti-alpha-galactosyl IgG (anti-Gal) antibody. Springer Semin Immunopathol 15: 155–171, 1993

103. Galili U: Interaction of the natural anti-Gal antibody with alpha-galactosyl epitopes: A major obstacle for xenotransplantation in humans (see comments). Immunol Today 14: 480–482, 1993

104. Smith DF, Larsen RD, Mattox S, Lowe JB, Cummings RD: Transfer and expression of a murine UDP-Gal:beta-D-Gal-alpha 1,3-galactosyltransferase gene in transfected Chinese hamster ovary cells. Competition reactions between the alpha 1,3-galactosyltransferase and the endogenous alpha 2,3-sialyltransferase. J Biol Chem 265: 6225–6234, 1990

105. Rajan VP, Larsen RD, Ajmera S, Ernst LK, Lowe JB: A cloned human DNA restriction fragment determines expression of a GDP-L-fucose: beta-D-galactoside 2-alpha-L-fucosyltransferase in transfected cells. Evidence for isolation and transfer of the human H blood group locus. J Biol Chem 264: 11158–11167, 1989

106. Dennis JW, Kerbel RS: Characterization of a deficiency in fucose metabolism in lectin-resistant variants of a murine tumor showing altered tumorigenic and metastatic capacities in vivo. Cancer Res 41: 98–104, 1981

107. Goupille C, Hallouin F, Meflah K, Le Pendu J: Increase of rat colon carcinoma cells tumorigenicity by alpha(1-2) fucosyltransferase gene transfection. Glycobiology 7: 221–229, 1997

108. Labarriere N, Piau JP, Otry C, Denis M, Lustenberger P, Meflah K, Le Pendu J: H blood group antigen carried by CD44V modulates tumorigenicity of rat colon carcinoma cells. Cancer Res 54: 6275–6281, 1994

109. Weston BW, Hiller KM, Mayben JP, Manousos GA, Bendt KM, Liu R, Cusack JC Jr: Expression of human alpha(1,3)fucosyltransferase antisense sequences inhibits selectin-mediated adhesion and liver metastasis of colon carcinoma cells. Cancer Res 59: 2127–2135, 1999

110. Hallouin F, Goupille C, Bureau V, Meflah K, Le Pendu J: Increased tumorigenicity of rat colon carcinoma cells after alpha1,2-fucosyltransferase FTA anti-sense cDNA transfection. Int J Cancer 80: 606–611, 1999

111. Rouquier S, Lowe JB, Kelly RJ, Fertitta AL, Lennon GG, Giorgi D: Molecular cloning of a human genomic region containing the H blood group alpha(1,2)fucosyltransferase gene and two H locus-related DNA restriction fragments. Isolation of a candidate for the human Secretor blood group locus. J Biol Chem 270: 4632–4639, 1995

112. Piau JP, Labarriere N, Dabouis G, Denis MG: Evidence for two distinct alpha(1,2)-fucosyltransferase genes differentially expressed throughout the rat colon. Biochem J 300: 623–626, 1994

113. Cameron HS, Szczepaniak D, Weston BW: Expression of human chromosome 19p alpha(1,3)-fucosyltransferase genes in normal tissues. Alternative splicing, polyadenylation, and isoforms. J Biol Chem 270: 20112–20122, 1995

114. Lowe JB, Kukowska-Latallo JF, Nair RP, Larsen RD, Marks RM, Macher BA, Kelly RJ, Ernst LK: Molecular cloning of a human fucosyltransferase gene that determines expression of the Lewis x and VIM-2 epitopes but not ELAM-1-dependent cell adhesion. J Biol Chem 266: 17467–17477, 1991

115. Biancone L, Araki M, Araki K, Vassalli P, Stamenkovic I: Redirection of tumor metastasis by expression of E-selectin in vivo. J Exp Med 183: 581–587, 1996

116. Price JE, Daniels LM, Campbell DE, Giavazzi R: Organ distribution of experimental metastases of a human colorectal carcinoma injected in nude mice. Clin Exp Metastasis 7: 55–68, 1989

117. Miyoshi E, Noda K, Ko JH, Ekuni A, Kitada T, Uozumi N, Ikeda Y, Matsuura N, Sasaki Y, Hayashi N, Hori M, Taniguchi N: Overexpression of alpha1-6 fucosyltransferase in hepatoma cells suppresses intrahepatic metastasis after splenic injection in athymic mice. Cancer Res 59: 2237–2243, 1999

118. Yamashita F, Tanaka M, Satomura S, Tanikawa K: Prognostic significance of Lens culinaris agglutinin A-reactive alpha-fetoprotein in small hepatocellular carcinomas. Gastroenterology 111: 996–1001, 1996

119. Yoshimura M, Nishikawa A, Ihara Y, Taniguchi S, Taniguchi N: Suppression of lung metastasis of B16 mouse melanoma by N-acetylglucosaminyltransferase III gene transfection. Proc Natl Acad Sci USA 92: 8754–8758, 1995

120. Yoshimura M, Ihara Y, Ohnishi A, Ijuhin N, Nishiura T, Kanakura Y, Matsuzawa Y, Taniguchi N: Bisecting N-acetylglucosamine on K562 cells suppresses natural killer cytotoxicity and promotes spleen colonization. Cancer Res 56: 412–418, 1996

121. Miyagi T, Sagawa J, Konno K, Handa S, Tsuiki S: Biochemical and immunological studies on two distinct ganglioside-hydrolyzing sialidases from the particulate fraction of rat brain. J Biochem (Tokyo) 107: 787–793, 1990

122. Tokuyama S, Moriya S, Taniguchi S, Yasui A, Miyazaki J, Orikasa S, Miyagi T: Suppression of pulmonary metastasis in murine B16 melanoma cells by transfection of a sialidase cDNA. Int J Cancer 73: 410–415, 1997

123. Meuillet EJ, Kroes R, Yamamoto H, Warner TG, Ferrari J, Mania-Farnell B, George D, Rebbaa A, Moskal JR, Bremer EG: Sialidase gene transfection enhances epidermal growth factor receptor activity in an epidermoid carcinoma cell line, A431: Cancer Res 59: 234–240, 1999

124. Zeng G, Gao L, Yu RK: Reduced cell migration, tumor growth and experimental metastasis of rat F-11 cells whose

expression of GD3-synthase is suppressed. Int J Cancer 88: 53–57, 2000

125. Thall AD, Murphy HS, Lowe JB: Alpha 1,3-Galactosyltransferase-deficient mice produce naturally occurring cytotoxic anti-Gal antibodies. Transplant Proc 28: 556–557, 1996

126. Asano M, Furukawa K, Kido M, Matsumoto S, Umesaki Y, Kochibe N, Iwakura Y: Growth retardation and early death of beta-1,4-galactosyltransferase knockout mice with augmented proliferation and abnormal differentiation of epithelial cells. Embo J 16: 1850–1857, 1997

127. Granovsky M, Fata J, Pawling J, Muller WJ, Khokha R, Dennis JW: Suppression of tumor growth and metastasis in Mgat5-deficient mice. Nat Med 6: 306–312, 2000

128. Cooper DN, Barondes SH: God must love galectins; he made so many of them. Glycobiology 9: 979–984, 1999

129. Bezouska K, Crichlow GV, Rose JM, Taylor ME, Drickamer K: Evolutionary conservation of intron position in a subfamily of genes encoding carbohydrate-recognition domains. J Biol Chem 266: 11604–11609, 1991

130. Weis WI, Taylor ME, Drickamer K: The C-type lectin superfamily in the immune system. Immunol Rev 163: 19–34, 1998

131. Sastry K, Ezekowitz RA: Collectins: Pattern recognition molecules involved in first line host defense [published erratum appears in Curr Opin Immunol 1993 Aug; 5(4):566]. Curr Opin Immunol 5: 59–66, 1993

132. White MR, Crouch E, Chang D, Sastry K, Guo N, Engelich G, Takahashi K, Ezekowitz RA, Hartshorn KL: Enhanced antiviral and opsonic activity of a human mannose-binding lectin and surfactant protein D chimera. J Immunol 165: 2108–2115, 2000

133. Stahl PD, Ezekowitz RA: The mannose receptor is a pattern recognition receptor involved in host defense. Curr Opin Immunol 10: 50–55, 1998

134. Stahl P, Schlesinger PH, Sigardson E, Rodman JS, Lee YC: Receptor-mediated pinocytosis of mannose glycoconjugates by macrophages: characterization and evidence for receptor recycling. Cell 19: 207–215, 1980

135. Hitchen PG, Mullin NP, Taylor ME: Orientation of sugars bound to the principal C-type carbohydrate-recognition domain of the macrophage mannose receptor. Biochem J 333: 601–608, 1998

136. Stoolman LM: Adhesion molecules controlling lymphocyte migration. Cell 56: 907–910, 1989

137. Tedder TF, Steeber DA, Chen A, Engel P: The selectins: vascular adhesion molecules. Faseb J 9: 866–873, 1995

138. Tu L, Chen A, Delahunty MD, Moore KL, Watson SR, McEver RP, Tedder TF: L-selectin binds to P-selectin glycoprotein ligand-1 on leukocytes: Interactions between the lectin, epidermal growth factor, and consensus repeat domains of the selectins determine ligand binding specificity. J Immunol 157: 3995–4004, 1996

139. Chambers WH, Adamkiewicz T, Houchins JP: Type II integral membrane proteins with characteristics of C-type animal lectins expressed by natural killer (NK) cells. Glycobiology 3: 9–14, 1993

140. Nangia-Makker P, Honjo Y, Sarvis R, Akahani S, Hogan V, Pienta KJ, Raz A: Galectin-3 induces endothelial cell morphogenesis and angiogenesis. Am J Pathol 156: 899–909, 2000

141. Wada J, Ota K, Kumar A, Wallner EI, Kanwar YS: Developmental regulation, expression, and apoptotic potential of galectin-9, a beta-galactoside binding lectin. J Clin Invest 99: 2452–2461, 1997

142. Raz A, Lotan R: Endogenous galactoside-binding lectins: A new class of functional tumor cell surface molecules related to metastasis. Cancer Metastasis Rev 6: 433–452, 1987

143. Raz A, Carmi P, Raz T, Hogan V, Mohamed A, Wolman SR: Molecular cloning and chromosomal mapping of a human galactoside-binding protein. Cancer Res 51: 2173–2178, 1991

144. Barondes SH, Castronovo V, Cooper DN, Cummings RD, Drickamer K, Feizi T, Gitt MA, Hirabayashi J, Hughes C, Kasai K, et al.: Galectins: A family of animal beta-galactoside-binding lectins [letter]. Cell 76: 597–598, 1994

145. Wang L, Inohara H, Pienta KJ, Raz A: Galectin-3 is a nuclear matrix protein which binds RNA. Biochem Biophys Res Commun 217: 292–303, 1995

146. Dagher SF, Wang JL, Patterson RJ: Identification of galectin-3 as a factor in pre-mRNA splicing. Proc Natl Acad Sci USA 92: 1213–1217, 1995

147. Raz A, Meromsky L, Lotan R: Differential expression of endogenous lectins on the surface of nontumorigenic, tumorigenic and metastatic cells. Cancer Res 46: 3667–3672, 1986

148. Lotan R, Lotan D, Carralero DM: Modulation of galactoside-binding lectins in tumor cells by differentiation-inducing agents. Cancer Lett 48: 115–122, 1989

149. Schoeppner HL, Raz A, Ho SB, Bresalier RS: Expression of an endogenous galactose-binding lectin correlates with neoplastic progression in the colon. Cancer 75: 2818–2826, 1995

150. Gillenwater A, Xu XC, el-Naggar AK, Clayman GL, Lotan R: Expression of galectins in head and neck squamous cell carcinoma. Head Neck 18: 422–432, 1996

151. Bresalier RS, Yan PS, Byrd JC, Lotan R, Raz A: Expression of the endogenous galactose-binding protein galectin-3 correlates with the malignant potential of tumors in the central nervous system. Cancer 80: 776–787, 1997

152. van den Brule FA, Berchuck A, Bast RC, Liu FT, Gillet C, Sobel ME, Castronovo V: Differential expression of the 67-kD laminin receptor and 31-kD human laminin-binding protein in human ovarian carcinomas. Eur J Cancer 8: 1096–1099, 1994

153. van den Brule FA, Buicu C, Berchuck A, Bast RC, Deprez M, Liu FT, Cooper DN, Pieters C, Sobel ME, Castronovo V: Expression of the 67-kD laminin receptor, galectin-1, and galectin-3 in advanced human uterine adenocarcinoma. Hum Pathol 27: 1185–1191, 1996

154. Castronovo V, van den Brule FA, Jackers P, Clausse N, Liu FT, Gillet C, Sobel ME: Decreased expression of galectin-3 is associated with progression of human breast cancer. J Pathol 179: 43–48, 1996

155. Ikeda K, Sannoh T, Kawasaki N, Kawasaki T, Yamashina I: Serum lectin with known structure activates complement through the classical pathway. J Biol Chem 262: 7451–7454, 1987

156. Kuhlman M, Joiner K, Ezekowitz RA: The human mannose-binding protein functions as an opsonin. J Exp Med 169: 1733–1745, 1989

157. Schweinle JE, Ezekowitz RA, Tenner AJ, Kuhlman M, Joiner KA: Human mannose-binding protein activates the alternative complement pathway and enhances serum bactericidal activity on a mannose-rich isolate of Salmonella. J Clin Invest 84: 1821–1829, 1989

158. Heise CT, Nicholls JR, Leamy CE, Wallis R: Impaired secretion of rat mannose-binding protein resulting from mutations in the collagen-like domain. J Immunol 165: 1403–1409, 2000

159. LeVine AM, Bruno MD, Huelsman KM, Ross GF, Whitsett JA, Korfhagen TR: Surfactant protein A-deficient mice are susceptible to group B streptococcal infection. J Immunol 158: 4336–4340, 1997

160. Harrod KS, Trapnell BC, Otake K, Korfhagen TR, Whitsett JA: SP-A enhances viral clearance and inhibits inflammation after pulmonary adenoviral infection. Am J Physiol 277: L580–L588, 1999

161. Kim M, Rao MV, Tweardy DJ, Prakash M, Galili U, Gorelik E: Lectin-induced apoptosis of tumour cells. Glycobiology 3: 447–453, 1993

162. Perillo NL, Uittenbogaart CH, Nguyen JT, Baum LG: Galectin-1, an endogenous lectin produced by thymic epithelial cells, induces apoptosis of human thymocytes. J Exp Med 185: 1851–1858, 1997

163. Perillo NL, Pace KE, Seilhamer JJ, Baum LG: Apoptosis of T cells mediated by galectin-1. Nature 378: 736–739, 1995

164. Offner H, Celnik B, Bringman TS, Casentini-Borocz D, Nedwin GE, Vandenbark AA: Recombinant human beta-galactoside binding lectin suppresses clinical and histological signs of experimental autoimmune encephalomyelitis. J Neuroimmunol 28: 177–184, 1990

165. Yang RY, Hsu DK, Liu FT: Expression of galectin-3 modulates T-cell growth and apoptosis. Proc Natl Acad Sci USA 93: 6737–6742, 1996

166. Akahani S, Nangia-Makker P, Inohara H, Kim HR, Raz A: Galectin-3: A novel antiapoptotic molecule with a functional BH1 (NWGR) domain of Bcl-2 family. Cancer Res 57: 5272–5276, 1997

167. Ohannesian DW, Lotan D, Thomas P, Jessup JM, Fukuda M, Gabius HJ, Lotan R: Carcinoembryonic antigen and other glycoconjugates act as ligands for galectin-3 in human colon carcinoma cells. Cancer Res 55: 2191–2199, 1995

168. Zhou Q, Cummings RD: L-14 lectin recognition of laminin and its promotion of in vitro cell adhesion. Arch Biochem Biophys: 300: 6–17, 1993

169. Ozeki Y, Matsui T, Yamamoto Y, Funahashi M, Hamako J, Titani K: Tissue fibronectin is an endogenous ligand for galectin-1. Glycobiology 5: 255–261, 1995

170. Inohara H, Raz A: Functional evidence that cell surface galectin-3 mediates homotypic cell adhesion. Cancer Res 55: 3267–3271, 1995

171. Inohara H, Akahani S, Koths K, Raz A: Interactions between galectin-3 and Mac-2-binding protein mediate cell-cell adhesion. Cancer Res 56: 4530–4534, 1996

172. Frisch SM, Francis H: Disruption of epithelial cell-matrix interactions induces apoptosis. J Cell Biol 124: 619–626, 1994

173. Kim HR, Lin HM, Biliran H, Raz A: Cell cycle arrest and inhibition of anoikis by galectin-3 in human breast epithelial cells. Cancer Res 59: 4148–4154, 1999

174. Izumi Y, Taniuchi Y, Tsuji T, Smith CW, Nakamori S, Fidler IJ, Irimura T: Characterization of human colon carcinoma variant cells selected for sialyl Lex carbohydrate antigen: liver colonization and adhesion to vascular endothelial cells. Exp Cell Res 216: 215–221, 1995

175. Yamada N, Chung YS, Takatsuka S, Arimoto Y, Sawada T, Dohi T, Sowa M: Increased sialyl Lewis A expression and fucosyltransferase activity with acquisition of a high metastatic capacity in a colon cancer cell line. Br J Cancer 76: 582–587, 1997

176. Kishimoto T, Ishikura H, Kimura C, Takahashi T, Kato H, Yoshiki T: Phenotypes correlating to metastatic properties of pancreas adenocarcinoma in vivo: The importance of surface sialyl Lewis(a) antigen. Int J Cancer 69: 290–294, 1996

177. Martin-Satue M, Marrugat R, Cancelas JA, Blanco J: Enhanced expression of alpha(1,3)-fucosyltransferase genes correlates with E-selectin-mediated adhesion and metastatic potential of human lung adenocarcinoma cells. Cancer Res 58: 1544–1550, 1998

178. Brodt P, Fallavollita L, Bresalier RS, Meterissian S, Norton CR, Wolitzky BA: Liver endothelial E-selectin mediates carcinoma cell adhesion and promotes liver metastasis. Int J Cancer 71: 612–619, 1997

179. Khatib A M, Kontogiannea M, Fallavollita L, Jamison B, Meterissian S, Brodt P: Rapid induction of cytokine and E-selectin expression in the liver in response to metastatic tumor cells. Cancer Res 59: 1356–1361, 1999

180. Mannori G, Santoro D, Carter L, Corless C, Nelson RM, Bevilacqua MP: Inhibition of colon carcinoma cell lung colony formation by a soluble form of E-selectin. Am J Pathol 151: 233–243, 1997

181. Fukuda MN, Ohyama C, Lowitz K, Matsuo O, Pasqualini R, Ruoslahti E, Fukuda MA: Peptide mimic of E-selectin ligand inhibits sialyl Lewis X-dependent lung colonization of tumor cells. Cancer Res 60: 450–456, 2000

182. Ohyama C, Tsuboi S, Fukuda M: Dual roles of sialyl Lewis X oligosaccharides in tumor metastasis and rejection by natural killer cells. Embo J 18: 1516–1525, 1999

183. Stone JP, Wagner DD: P-selectin mediates adhesion of platelets to neuroblastoma and small cell lung cancer. J Clin Invest 92: 804–813, 1993

184. Kim YJ, Borsig L, Varki NM, Varki A: P-selectin deficiency attenuates tumor growth and metastasis. Proc Natl Acad Sci USA 95: 9325–9330, 1998

185. Gasic GJ, Tuszynski GP, Gorelik E: Interaction of the hemostatic and immune systems in the metastatic spread of tumor cells. Int Rev Exp Pathol 29: 173–212, 1986

186. Gorelik E, Bere WW, Herberman RB: Role of NK cells in the antimetastatic effect of anticoagulant drugs. Int J Cancer 33: 87–94, 1984

187. Gorelik E: Augmentation of the antimetastatic effect of anticoagulant drugs by immunostimulation in mice. Cancer Res 47: 809–815, 1987

188. Kagamu H, Shu S: Purification of L-selectin(low) cells promotes the generation of highly potent CD4 antitumor effector T lymphocytes. J Immunol 160: 3444–3452, 1998

189. Kjaergaard J, Shu S: Tumor infiltration by adoptively transferred T cells is independent of immunologic specificity but requires down-regulation of L-selectin expression. J Immunol 163: 751–759, 1999

190. Bresalier RS, Mazurek N, Sternberg LR, Byrd JC, Yunker CK, Nangia-Makker P, Raz A: Metastasis of human colon cancer is altered by modifying expression of the beta-galactoside-binding protein galectin 3. Gastroenterology 115: 287–296, 1998

191. Nangia-Makker P, Thompson E, Hogan C, Ochieng J, Raz A: Induction of tumorigenicity by galectin-3 in a non-tumorigenic human breast carcinoma lines. Int J Oncol 7: 1079–1089, 1995

192. Warfield PR, Makker PN, Raz A, Ochieng J: Adhesion of human breast carcinoma to extracellular matrix proteins is modulated by galectin-3. Inv Metastasis 17: 101–112, 1997

193. Le Marer N, Hughes RC: Effects of the carbohydrate-binding protein galectin-3 on the invasiveness of human breast carcinoma cells. J Cell Physiol 168: 51–58, 1996

194. Raz A, Zhu DG, Hogan V, Shah N, Raz T, Karkash R, Pazerini G, Carmi P: Evidence for the role of 34-kDa galactoside-binding lectin in transformation and metastasis. Int J Cancer 46: 871–877, 1990

195. Meromsky L, Lotan R, Raz A: Implications of endogenous tumor cell surface lectins as mediators of cellular interactions and lung colonization. Cancer Res 46: 5270–5275, 1986

196. Beuth J, Ko HL, Oette K, Pulverer G, Roszkowski K, Uhlenbruck G: Inhibition of liver metastasis in mice by blocking hepatocyte lectins with arabinogalactan infusions and D-galactose. J Cancer Res Clin Oncol 113: 51–55, 1987

197. Oguchi H, Toyokuni T, Dean B, Ito H, Otsuji E, Jones VL, Sadozai KK, Hakomori S: Effect of lactose derivatives on metastatic potential of B16 melanoma cells. Cancer Commun 2: 311–316, 1990

198. Platt D, Raz A: Modulation of the lung colonization of B16-F1 melanoma cells by citrus pectin. J Natl Cancer Inst 84: 438–442, 1992

199. Inohara H, Raz A: Effects of natural complex carbohydrate (citrus pectin) on murine melanoma cell properties related to galectin-3 functions. Glycoconj J 11: 527–532, 1994

200. Raz A, Bucana C, McLellan W, Fidler IJ: Distribution of membrane anionic sites on B16 melanoma variants with differing lung colonising potential. Nature 284: 363–364, 1980

201. Qian F, Vaux D, Weissman I: Expression of the integrin alpha4beta1 on melanoma cells can inhibit the invasive stage of metastasis formation. Cell 77: 335–347, 1994

202. Ma Y, Uemura K, Oka S, Kozutsumi Y, Kawasaki N, Kawasaki T: Antitumor activity of mannan-binding protein in vivo as revealed by a virus expression system: Mannan-binding proteindependent cell-mediated cytotoxicity. Proc Natl Acad Sci USA 96: 371–375, 1999

203. Takahashi K, Donovan MJ, Rogers RA Ezekowitz RA: Distribution of murine mannose receptor expression from early embryogenesis through to adulthood. Cell Tissue Res 292: 311–323, 1998

204. Vidal-Vanaclocha F, Alvarez A, Asumendi A, Urcelay B, Tonino P, Dinarello CA: Interleukin 1 (IL-1)-dependent melanoma hepatic metastasis in vivo; increased endothelial adherence by IL-1-induced mannose receptors and growth factor production in vitro. J Natl Cancer Inst 88: 198–205, 1996

205. Mendoza L, Olaso E, Anasagasti MJ, Fuentes AM, Vidal-Vanaclocha F: Mannose receptor-mediated endothelial cell activation contributes to B16 melanoma cell adhesion and metastasis in liver. J Cell Physiol 174: 322–330, 1998

206. Chen L, Zhang W, Fregien N, Pierce M: The her-2/neu oncogene stimulates the transcription of N-acetylglucosaminyltransferase V and expression of its cell surface oligosaccharide products. Oncogene 17: 2087–2093, 1998

207. Fidler I, Gerstein D, Hart I: The biology of cancer invasion and metastasis. Adv Cancer Res 28: 149–250, 1978

208. Liotta LA: Cancer cell invasion and metastasis. Sci Am 266: 54–59, 62–63, 1992

209. Mannori G, Crottet P, Cecconi O, Hanasaki K, Aruffo A, Nelson RM, Varki A, Bevilacqua MP: Differential colon cancer cell adhesion to E-, P-, and L-selectin: Role of mucin-type glycoproteins. Cancer Res 55: 4425–4431, 1995

Address for offprints: Elieser Gorelik, University of Pittsburgh Cancer Institute, BST, W954, Pittsburgh, PA 15213, USA; *Tel:* (412)-624-0346; *Fax:* (412)-624-7736; *e-mail:* gorelik@pitt.edu

Metastasis suppression in prostate cancer

Erich B. Jaeger[1], Rajeev S. Samant[2] and Carrie W. Rinker-Schaeffer[1]
[1]*The University of Chicago Urology Research Laboratory*, [2]*The Jake Gittlen Cancer Research Institute, Pennsylvania State College of Medicine, PA, USA*

Key words: metastasis, metastasis-suppressor genes, prostate cancer

Abstract

Due to a lack of effective treatments, the development of metastases remains the most lethal aspect of prostate cancer. In order to help overcome this problem there has been an ongoing effort to develop strategies for early intervention. This includes the development of strategies that allow histologic lesions and disseminated cells that are highly likely to cause metastatic disease to be distinguished from those that are not, as well as therapeutic approaches to specifically target bone metastases. Such approaches will be expedited by the identification of genes and signaling cascades that regulate metastatic growth. Genes that specifically suppress metastasis are strong candidates for these studies. This review will focus on metastasis-suppressor genes that have been identified functionally, particularly those found to play a role in prostate cancer, and discuss how the identification and study of these genes has influenced our overall understanding of the metastatic process.

1. What are metastasis-suppressor genes? How might they act?

Metastasis-suppressor genes (MSGs) are genes whose normal functions suppress the formation of spontaneous overt metastases. Thus, their cellular function is distinct from oncogenes, which promote cellular transformation, and tumor suppressor genes, which suppress all tumor growth. In order to form a spontaneous hematogenous metastasis a cell must complete every step in a series of events known as the metastatic cascade [1–3]. The steps involved in this cascade include escape from the primary tumor and invasion into the surrounding tissue, entering and surviving in the bloodstream, arresting and/or extravasating at a secondary site, and finally survival and proliferation at a secondary site. MSGs that block any of these individual steps will block the formation of overt metastases. When efforts to identify MSGs were initiated, it was generally believed that these genes would prevent the escape of cells from the primary tumor, acting on initial steps of the metastatic cascade. This is indeed the case for some of the MSGs identified, as will be discussed below. However, functional studies have also revealed unanticipated and novel biochemical and cellular functions for MSGs in the metastatic cascade [4].

One question of recent debate has been the clinical significance of cancerous cells found in the circulation. Clearly, these cells have passed through the first stages of the metastatic cascade, but the significance of that accomplishment is uncertain. We know, from clinical and experimental studies, that metastasis is a largely inefficient process, with less than 0.1% of cells injected into the circulation successfully forming secondary tumors in experimental models [3,5]. This low percentage has been attributed to low cell survival rates in the circulation and low extravasational rates at the secondary site [6]. The advent of the reverse transcriptase polymerase chain reaction has provided a sensitive means of detecting disseminated cancer cells, but studies have yet to show a consistent correlation between the presence of tumor cells in the circulation or at a metastatic site and future development of disease [7,8]. For example, although detection of prostate-specific antigen mRNA has been correlated with an increased risk of disease recurrence in patients with bone marrow micrometastases, the majority of patients with tumor cell-positive bone marrow samples did not develop recurrent disease within the timeframe of the study [9]. Thus, the ability to screen for markers that would help to predict disease recurrence would be of significant value.

M.L. Cher, K.V. Honn and A. Raz (eds.), Prostate Cancer: New Horizons in Research and Treatment, 143–150.
© 2002 *Kluwer Academic Publishers.*

A growing body of evidence also suggests that the ability of a cell to grow within a vessel may be as important as its ability to extravasate and then grow. The utilization of vital fluorescent dyes and green fluorescent protein, combined with improvements in intravital microscopy, has enabled the observation of single tumor cells in the circulation and at secondary sites *in vivo* [6,10]. In recent studies [11,12], over 95% of injected cells did not survive in the lungs past 14 days, but of those that did, the majority that grew into microscopic metastases went on to form macroscopic metastases. Cells that survived but did not proliferate remained dormant, and hemodynamic destruction of cells arrested in the microcirculation was not a major factor. These findings indicate that the ability of cells to initiate growth at the secondary site is a critical step in the formation of overt metastases. As described in the following sections, work from our laboratories has indicated a new role for MSG function in controlling growth of tumor cancer cells at the metastatic site. Thus, the utility of MSG expression and/or function to predict the ability of disseminated cells to grow into clinically important lesions is the subject of growing interest. A broad review of MSG identification and function has recently been reported by Yoshida et al. [4], but for the purpose of this review we will concentrate upon the potential roles of MSGs in prostate cancer.

2. MSG identification: Differential expression techniques

2.1. Nm23

As mentioned above, some of the MSGs identified to date act at early stages of the metastatic cascade, and many of these were identified using differential gene expression techniques. The first MSG to be identified, *nm23* [13], is one such gene. When transfected into DU145 and MTLn3 prostate cancer cell lines, *nm23* reduces invasiveness, adhesion to extracellular matrix, and colony formation. Transfection of *nm23* mutants lacking the native nucleoside diphosphate kinase activity produced similar results, suggesting that metastasis suppression is independent of this activity [14]. In clinical samples, Gleason score 8–10 tumors exhibit weaker *nm23* staining than lower grade tumors [15]. Protein expression profiles of androgen-stimulated prostate cancer cells have also indicated an up-regulation of *nm23* in response to androgen [16]. At this time, the

mechanism of *nm23* action appears to be related to its kinase activity and its regulation of the Rad and Rac1 GTPases [17]. This regulation may be mediated through the association of *nm23* with the product of the multiple endocrine neoplasia type 1 gene (*MEN1*), menin, which was found to interact with *nm23* in a yeast two-hybrid assay [18].

2.2. Maspin

Several prostate cancer cell lines have little or no maspin/PI5 expression, but show reduced invasiveness and motility following transfection with this gene. Expression of exogenous p53 in prostate cancer cell lines LNCaP, DU145, and PC-3 has also been found to induce maspin expression [19]. Although it does not fit the classic description of a MSG, insofar as its expression can also suppress primary tumor growth, reduction in maspin expression correlates with higher tumor stage and grade, as well as increased risk of disease recurrence following radical prostatectomy. This loss of expression was also correlated with expression of p53 [20]. Early clues as to the mechanism of action of maspin come from studies demonstrating an inhibitory interaction with cell surface-bound urokinase-type plasminogen activator in DU145 cells [21].

2.3. HP1^Hsα and Gelsolin

Differential display methods have implicated other genes that may be involved in prostate cancer metastasis suppression, and some of these candidates are beginning to be tested functionally and examined in clinical disease. In particular, transfection of *HP1*^Hsα into breast cancer cell line MDA-MB-231 reduced the invasive potential of these cells, while examination of clinical samples indicated expression of *HP1*^Hsα is decreased in metastatic tumor tissues [22]. Recently, gelsolin was also found to suppress spontaneous metastasis of melanoma cells, as well as restrict growth in soft agar, retard cell spreading, and reduce chemotactic migration to fibronectin [23]. What role these MSGs may play with regard to prostate cancer remains a subject for investigation.

3. MSG identification: Microcell-mediated chromosomal transfer

In addition to the information gained from cDNA subtraction and differential display studies, microcell-mediated chromosomal transfer (MMCT) has proven to be one of the more successful means of functionally identifying MSGs. MMCT has a demonstrated record of utility and applicability as well. First used to identify tumor suppressor genes, MMCT has grown and evolved into a method that has also aided in the functional identification of genes associated with senescence and gene extinction [4].

MMCT has been most widely used in the identification of prostate cancer MSGs. The rationale behind using the MMCT approach for this purpose was based upon work by Ichikawa et al. [24], who demonstrated that fusion of nonmetastatic and highly metastatic Dunning rat prostate cancer cells produced nonmetastatic hybrid cells. These hybrids, though nonmetastatic, were nonetheless unaffected in terms of tumorigenicity and *in vivo* tumor growth rates. Subsequent studies of the suppressed hybrids suggested that loss of specific chromosomes was associated with the metastatic phenotype. MMCT was thus used to introduce single human chromosomes, tagged with a selectable marker or markers such as neomycin phosphotransferase, into metastatic recipient cells, thereby permitting the localization of MSGs to specific human chromosomes.

To date, MMCT has led to the functional identification of five MSGs – *BrMS-1*, *KiSS-1*, *CD44*, *KAI-1*, and *MKK4* – and prostate cancer metastasis suppressor activities on six additional chromosomes (Table 1). Additional activities that suppress the metastasis of other cancers have also been identified [4]. All of these genes reduce spontaneous metastasis *in vivo* without affecting tumorigenicity or the primary tumor growth rate.

3.1. BRMS-1

Identified most recently [33], *BRMS-1* is located at 11q13.1–q13.2 and has been shown to restore cell–cell communication via gap junctions in MDA-MB-435 breast cancer cells. This effect may be related to an observed up-regulation of connexin 43 expression and concomitant down-regulation of connexin 32 expression, the combination of which leads to a gap junction phenotype more similar to that found in normal breast tissue [34]. The potential role of *BRMS-1* in prostate cancer is currently under investigation.

3.2. KiSS-1

Mapped to chromosome 1q32–41, *KiSS-1* also suppresses metastasis of MDA-MB-435 cells, as well as B16BL6 melanoma cells, and has been found to encode metastin, a ligand of the orphan G-protein-coupled receptor hOT7T175 [35]. *In vitro* studies have demonstrated that metastin inhibits the chemotaxis, invasion, spreading, monolayer growth, and soft agar colony formation of transfected CHO cells [36]. Transfection also stimulates PIP2 hydrolysis, Ca^{2+} mobilization, arachidonate acid release, ERK1/2 and p38 MAPK phosphorylation, and stress fiber formation while inhibiting cell proliferation [37]. The potential role of *KiSS-1* in prostate cancer is also currently under investigation.

The remaining MSGs mentioned above have been characterized in the context of the Dunning rat prostate cancer model. Of these, data to this point indicates that at least two – *KAI-1* and *CD44* – suppress metastasis at an early stage of the metastatic cascade. Preliminary data for the as of yet unidentified MSG activities on

Table 1. Chromosomal regions that suppress prostate cancer metastases *in vivo* as identified by microcell-mediated chromosomal transfer

Chromosomal location	Tumor types	Cell line tested (species of origin)	*In vitro* phenotype*	*In vivo* phenotype
2p25–22	Prostate [25]	AT6.1 (rat)	↓ Invasion	↓ Spontaneous mets
7q21–22 and/or 7q31.2–32	Prostate [26]	AT6.3 (rat)	ND	↓ Spontaneous mets ↓ Experimental mets
8p21–p12	Prostate [27,28]	AT6.2 (rat)	↓ Invasion	↓ Spontaneous mets
10cen–10q23	Prostate [29]	AT6.3 (rat)	ND	↓ Spontaneous mets
12qcen–q13 and/or 12q24–ter	Prostate [30]	AT6.1 (rat)	ND	↓ Spontaneous mets No micrometastases observed at the experimental endpoint
16q24.2	Prostate [31]	AT6.1 (rat)	ND	↓ Spontaneous mets
20p11.23–12	Prostate [32]	AT6.1 (rat)	↓ Invasion	↓ Spontaneous mets ↓ Experimental mets

ND = not determined, mets = metastases.
*Invasion was measured by migration through Matrigel.

other chromosomes (Table 1) suggests that many of these genes may also act at an early stage. Positional cloning efforts to identify the MSGs encoded by these chromosomes are underway.

3.3. KAI-1

KAI-1 was, notably, the first prostate cancer MSG identified functionally using MMCT [38]. Mapped to 11p11.2 [39], *KAI-1* reduces the invasiveness of AT6.1 cells and has since been implicated in the progression of a number of other human cancers. When transfected into MDA-MB-231 cells, which normally express *KAI-1* at low levels, *KAI-1* significantly suppresses *in vitro* invasion and clonogenicity in soft agar [40]. In response to PMA, a phorbol ester, activating protein kinase C has been shown to induce expression of *KAI-1* in metastatic cells [41] that otherwise down-regulate *KAI-1*. Nerve growth factor has also been demonstrated to induce re-expression of *KAI-1* in DU145 and PC-3 cells [42]. Etoposide, a topoisomerase II inhibitor, is further believed to activate expression of *KAI-1* in these and other cell lines via p53 and c-Jun [43]. Treatment of cells with PMA, nerve growth factor, or etoposide reduced invasiveness in all cases. When examined in clinical samples, down-regulation of *KAI-1* has been found to be coincident with advanced lung, breast, and prostate cancers [44–46]. Epigenetic regulation studies have not indicated a mechanism of *KAI-1* down-regulation [47]. Current evidence for loss of heterozygosity (LOH) at the *KAI-1* locus in human samples suggests LOH or allelic imbalance may occur in only a subset of cases. In Japan, 7 of 10 metastatic samples exhibited loss [48], but samples from American patients did not show any loss in 12 lymph node metastases [49]. The discovery of a microsatellite marker more tightly linked to the *KAI-1* locus than previously used markers may permit a better overall assessment of LOH in human disease [50].

3.4. CD44

Another MSG identified at the same time as *KAI-1* and mapped to the same region of chromosome 11 is *CD44*. There is a broad literature documenting the potential functions of *CD44* in the metastatic ability of various cell and tissue types [51,52]. In any case, *CD44* encodes an integral membrane glycoprotein that acts as a receptor for hyaluronic acid and osteopontin and influences cellular adhesion [53], perhaps through its binding to the protein merlin [52]. DNA hypermethylation has been implicated in the down-regulation of CD44 [54], and down-regulation of CD44 and its v6 isoform correlates with higher tumor grade in clinical samples [53,55,56].

The remaining prostate cancer MSG identified appears to regulate growth at the secondary site, late in the metastatic cascade.

3.5. MKK4

We have recently reported the identification of *MKK4* as a MSG on human chromosome 17 that suppresses the metastatic ability of AT6.1 Dunning rat prostate cancer cells. At the experimental endpoint, the number of overt surface metastases observed in the lungs from mice with *MKK4*-expressing tumors was reduced 15 to 30-fold compared to lungs from mice bearing parental AT6.1 tumors [57]. At first glance, this suppression could have been due to the inhibition of any step within the metastatic cascade. However, *in vivo* experiments did not suggest a decrease in the number or viability of tumor cells colonizing the lung, leading us to hypothesize that metastatic suppression was occurring in the lung itself. AT6.1 cells expressing MKK4 were therefore transduced with a β-galactosidase reporter gene construct and tested in spontaneous metastasis assays. These studies revealed blue-staining microscopic metastases in numbers comparable to the numbers of macroscopic metastases observed with control AT6.1 cells. Furthermore, no evidence was found to suggest an anti-angiogenic mechanism in our model. Taken together, our *in vivo* data suggest that *MKK4*-suppressed cells escape from the primary tumor, but are growth inhibited at the secondary site [58].

Evaluation of the expression of components of the *MKK4* signaling cascade showed a loss or down-regulation of expression of *MKK4* or c-Jun, a downstream mediator of *MKK4*, in six of eight human prostate cancer cell lines [59]. *MKK4* expression was next assessed during the development of clinical prostate cancer by immunohistochemical study. Normal prostate tissue expressed high levels of *MKK4* only in the epithelial compartment. Neoplastic tissue showed a direct, inverse relationship between *MKK4* expression and Gleason pattern [59]. These results demonstrate that *MKK4* is consistently down-regulated during prostate cancer progression and support a role for dysregulation of its signaling cascade in clinical disease. LOH analysis of *MKK4* revealed allelic loss in

31% (5 of 16) of metastatic prostate cancer lesions that was not associated with coding region mutations [59].

4. Conclusions

The metastatic cascade is comprised of a number of specific steps that tumor cells must complete in order to form a metastasis at a secondary site. These include escape from the primary tumor, invasion into the surrounding tissue and intravasation, survival in the circulation, arrest and/or extravasation at a secondary site, and progressive growth at the secondary site. Suppression of metastasis may therefore in principle occur at any point in this cascade, and MSG studies have revealed that these genes can indeed act both early and late in the cascade.

To our surprise, MSG products appear to have a role controlling the progressive growth of cancer cells at the secondary site, prior to the need for angiogenesis. The data reviewed here indicate that, even though cells may be able to travel through the circulation, simply reaching the secondary site is insufficient for metastasis formation. Cells may extravasate and remain dormant or die upon reaching the secondary site, or they may be unable to grow beyond the size of a microscopic focus.

While differential display techniques have identified a number of genes associated with metastasis or suppression of the metastatic phenotype, additional functional *in vivo* assays are needed to determine whether this association is causative or correlative. The coupling of MMCT with *in vivo* assays is one approach that has enabled the functional identification of the majority of known MSGs. MMCT continues to prove its utility with the discovery of additional MSG activities on various chromosomes.

5. Key unanswered questions

What molecular and cellular mechanisms govern the growth of disseminated tumor cells at a secondary site? This is one question we must ask after considering the data presented here. Metastasis suppression can no longer be thought of as occurring only at the site of a primary tumor. Instead, each step of the metastatic cascade must now be taken into account, particularly the lodging and subsequent growth of disseminated cells into clinically significant metastases. While the literature often views organ-specificity as a result of preferential 'homing' of cancer cells to an organ,

a growing body of work shows that disseminated cells are likely to be present in multiple organs [5,60,61]. This data points to an important role for the microenvironment in permitting the survival and growth of only certain cancer cell types.

As translational researchers, our goals are to improve the ability of pathologists to distinguish unambiguously malignant from indolent lesions and to help clinicians differentiate between tumors that are highly likely to metastasize from those that are not. The practical question therefore becomes, how can we use MSGs, or the pathways they regulate, to improve patient management? The initial challenge of simply identifying MSGs is largely behind us, due to the immense amount of genetic information that has become readily available. Now the challenge is to identify those genes that are functionally relevant to the acquisition of metastatic ability. The realization of this goal will depend upon the use of well-characterized *in vivo* animal models in conjunction with clinical correlative studies. We must here emphasize that *in vitro* models do not accurately reflect *in vivo* metastasis [62], and that none of the MSGs described in this review could have been identified by traditional *in vitro* assays.

References

1. Poste G, Fidler IJ: The pathogenesis of cancer metastasis. Nature 283: 139–146, 1980
2. MacDonald NJ, Steeg PS: Molecular basis of tumour metastasis. Cancer Surv 16: 175–199, 1993
3. Welch DR, Rinker-Schaeffer CW: What defines a useful marker of metastasis in human cancer? J Natl Cancer Inst 91: 1351–1353, 1999
4. Yoshida BA, Sokoloff MM, Welch DR, Rinker-Schaeffer CW: Metastasis-suppressor genes: A review and perspective on an emerging field. J Natl Cancer Inst 92: 1717–1730, 2000
5. Fidler IJ: Critical factors in the biology of human cancer metastasis: Twenty-eighth G.H.A. Clowes memorial award lecture. Cancer Res 50: 6130–6138, 1990
6. Chambers AF: The metastatic process: Basic research and clinical implications. Oncol Res 11: 161–168, 1999
7. Melchior SW, Corey E, Ellis WJ, Ross AA, Layton TJ, Oswin MM, Lange PH, Vessella RL: Early tumor cell dissemination in patients with clinically localized carcinoma of the prostate. Clin Cancer Res 3: 249–256, 1997
8. Christiano AP, Yoshida BA, Dubauskas Z, Sokoloff M, Rinker-Schaeffer CW: Development of markers of prostate cancer metastasis: Review and perspective. Urol Oncol 5: 217–223, 2000
9. Wood DP Jr, Banerjee M: Presence of circulating prostate cells in the bone marrow of patients undergoing radical

148

prostatectomy is predictive of disease-free survival. J Clin Oncol 15: 3451–3457, 1997

10. Yang M, Jiang P, Sun FX, Hasegawa S, Baranov E, Chishima T, Shimada H, Moossa AR, Hoffman RM: A fluorescent orthotopic bone metastasis model of human prostate cancer. Cancer Res 59: 781–786, 1999

11. Al-Mehdi AB, Tozawa K, Fisher AB, Shientag L, Lee A, Muschel RJ: Intravascular origin of metastasis from the proliferation of endothelium-attached tumor cells: A new model of metastasis. Nat Med 6: 100–102, 2000

12. Cameron MD, Schmidt EE, Kerkvliet N, Nadkarni KV, Morris VL, Groom AC, Chambers AF, MacDonald IC: Temporal progression of metastasis in lung: Cell survival, dormancy, and location dependence of metastatic inefficiency. Cancer Res 60: 2541–2546, 2000

13. Freije JMP, MacDonald NJ, Steeg PS: Differential gene expression in tumor metastasis: Nm23. In: Gunthert U, Shlag PM, Birchmeier W (eds) Attempts to Understand Metastasis Formation II: Regulatory Factors. Springer-Verlag, Berlin, 1996, pp 215–232

14. Lee HY, Lee H: Inhibitory activity of nm23-H1 on invasion and colonization of human prostate carcinoma cells is not mediated by its NDP kinase activity. Cancer Lett 145: 93–99, 1999

15. Stravodimos K, Constantinides C, Manousakas T, Pavlaki C, Pantazopoulos D, Giannopoulos A, Dimopoulos C: Immunohistochemical expression of transforming growth factor beta 1 and nm-23H1 antioncogene in prostate cancer: Divergent correlation with clinicopathological parameters. Anticancer Res 20: 3823–3828, 2000

16. Nelson PS, Han D, Rochon Y, Corthals GF, Lin B, Monson A, Nguyen V, Franza BR, Plymate SR, Aebersold R, Hood L: Comprehensive analyses of prostate gene expression: Convergence of expressed sequence tag databases, transcript profiling and proteomics. Electrophoresis 21: 1823–1831, 2000

17. Otsuki Y, Tanaka M, Yoshii S, Kawazoe N, Nakaya K, Sugimura H: Tumor metastasis suppressor nm23H1 regulates Rac1 GTPase by interaction with Tiam1. Proc Natl Acad Sci USA 98: 4385–4390, 2001

18. Ohkura N, Kishi M, Tsukada T, Yamaguchi K: Menin, a gene product responsible for multiple endocrine neoplasia type 1, interacts with the putative tumor metastasis suppressor nm23. Biochem Biophys Res Commun 282: 1206–1210, 2001

19. Zou Z, Gao C, Nagaich AK, Connell T, Saito S, Moul JW, Seth P, Appella E, Srivistava S: p53 regulates the expression of the tumor suppressor gene maspin. J Biol Chem 275: 6051–6054, 2000

20. Machtens S, Serth J, Bokemeyer C, Bathke W, Minssen A, Koomannsberger C, Hartmann J, Knuchel R, Kondo M, Jonas U, Kuczyk M: Expression of the p53 and maspin protein in primary prostate cancer: Correlation with clinical features. Int J Cancer 95: 337–342, 2001

21. McGowen R, Biliran H Jr, Sager R, Sheng S: The surface of prostate carcinoma DU145 cells mediates the inhibition of urokinase-type plasminogen activator by maspin. Cancer Res 60: 4771–4778, 2000

22. Kirschmann DA, Lininger RA, Gardner LMG, Seftor EA, Odero VA, Ainsztein AM, Earnshaw WC, Wallrath LL, Hendrix MJC: Down-regulation of HP1Hs alpha expression is associated with the metastatic phenotype in breast cancer. Cancer Res 60: 3359–3363, 2000

23. Fujita H, Okada F, Hamada J, Hosokawa M, Moriuchi T, Koya RC, Kuzumaki N: Gelsolin functions as a metastasis suppressor in B16-BL6 mouse melanoma cells and requirement of the carboxyl-terminus for its effect. Int J Cancer 93: 773–780, 2001

24. Ichikawa T, Ichikawa Y, Isaacs JT: Genetic factors and suppression of metastatic ability of prostatic cancer. Cancer Res 51: 3788–3792, 1991

25. Mashimo T, Goodarzi G, Watabe M, Cuthbert AP, Newbold RF, Pai SK, Hirota S, Hosobe S, Miura K, Bandyopadhyay S, Gross SC, Watabe K: Localization of a novel tumor metastasis suppressor region on the short arm of human chromosome 2. Genes Chromosomes Cancer 28: 285–293, 2000

26. Nihei N, Ohta S, Kuramochi H, Kugoh H, Oshimura M, Barrett JC, Isaacs JT, Igarashi T, Ito H, Masai M, Ichikawa Y, Ichikawa T: Metastasis-suppressor gene(s) for rat prostate cancer on the long arm of human chromosome 7. Genes Chromosomes Cancer 24: 1–8, 1999

27. Nihei N, Ichikawa T, Kawana Y, Kuramochi H, Kugoh H, Oshimura M, Hayata I, Shimazaki J, Ito H: Mapping of metastasis-suppressor gene(s) for rat prostate cancer on the short arm of human chromosome 8 by irradiated microcell-mediated chromosome transfer. Genes Chromosomes Cancer 17: 260–268, 1996

28. Kuramochi H, Ichikawa T, Nihei N, Kawana Y, Suzuki H, Schalken JA, Takeichi M, Nagafuchi A, Ito H, Shimazaki J: Suppression of invasive ability of highly metastatic rat prostate cancer by introduction of human chromosome 8. Prostate 31: 14–20, 1997

29. Nihei N, Ichikawa T, Kawana Y, Kuramochi H, Kugo H, Oshimura M, Killary AM, Rinker-Schaeffer CW, Barrett JC, Isaacs JT: Localization of metastasis suppressor gene(s) for rat prostatic cancer to the long arm of human chromosome 10. Genes Chromosomes Cancer 14: 112–119, 1995

30. Luu HH, Zagaja GP, Dubauskas Z, Chen SL, Smith RC, Watabe K, Ichikawa Y, Ichikawa T, Davis EM, Le Beau MM, Rinker-Schaeffer CW: Identification of a novel metastasis-suppressor region on human chromosome 12. Cancer Res 58: 3561–3565, 1998

31. Mashimo T, Watabe M, Cuthbert AP, Newbold RF, Rinker-Schaeffer CW, Helfer E, Watabe K: Human chromosome 16 suppresses metastasis but not tumorigenesis in rat prostatic tumor cells. Cancer Res 58: 4572–4576, 1998

32. Goodarzi G, Mashimo T, Watabe M, Cuthbert AP, Newbold RF, Pai SK, Hirota S, Hosobe S, Miura K, Bandyopadhyay S, Gross SC, Balaji KC, Watabe K: Identification of tumor metastasis suppressor region on the short arm of chromosome 20. Genes Chromosomes Cancer 32: 33–42, 2001

33. Seraj MJ, Samant RS, Verderame MF, Welch DR: Functional evidence for a novel human breast carcinoma metastasis suppressor, BRMS1, encoded at chromosome 11q13. Cancer Res 60: 2764–2769, 2000

34. Saunders MM, Seraj MJ, Li Z, Zhou Z, Winter CR, Welch DR, Donahue HJ: Breast cancer metastatic potential correlates with a breakdown in homospecific and heterospecific gap junctional intercellular communication. Cancer Res 61: 1765–1767, 2001

35. Ohtaki T, Shintani Y, Honda S, Matsumoto H, Hori A, Kanehashi K, Terao Y, Kumano S, Takatsu Y, Masuda Y, Ishibashi Y, Watanabe T, Asada M, Yamada T, Suenaga M, Kitada C, Usuki S, Kurokawa T, Onda H, Nishimura O, Fujino M: Metastasis-suppressor gene *KiSS-1* encodes peptide ligand of a G-protein-coupled receptor. Nature 411: 613–616, 2001

36. Hori A, Honda S, Asada M, Ohtaki T, Oda K, Watanabe T, Shintani Y, Yamada T, Suenaga M, Kitada C, Onda H, Kurokawa T, Nishimura O, Fujino M: Metastin suppresses the motility and growth of CHO cells transfected with its receptor. Biochem Biophys Res Commun 286: 958–963, 2001

37. Kotani M, Detheux M, Vandenbogaerde A, Communi D, Vanderwinden JM, Le Poul E, Brezillon S, Tyldesley R, Suarez-Huerta N, Vandeput F, Blanpain C, Schiffmann SN, Vassart G, Parmentier M: The metastasis-suppressor gene *KiSS-1* encodes kisspeptins, the natural ligands of the orphan G protein-coupled receptor GPR54. J Biol Chem 276: 34631–34636, 2001

38. Ichikawa T, Ichikawa Y, Dong J, Hawkins AL, Griffin CA, Isaacs WB, Oshimura M, Barrett JC, Isaacs JT: Localization of metastasis-suppressor gene(s) for prostatic cancer to the short arm of human chromosome 11. Cancer Res 52: 3486–3490, 1992

39. Dong JT, Lamb PW, Rinker-Schaeffer CW, Vukanovic J, Ichikawa T, Isaacs JT, Barrett JC: KAI1, a metastasis-suppressor gene for prostate cancer on human chromosome 11p11.2. Science 268: 884–886, 1995

40. Yang X, Wei LL, Tang C, Slack R, Mueller S, Lippman ME: Overexpression of KAI1 suppresses *in vitro* invasiveness and *in vivo* metastasis in breast cancer cells. Cancer Res 61: 5284–5288, 2001

41. Akita H, Iizuka A, Hashimoto Y, Kohri K, Ikeda K, Nakanishi M: Induction of KAI-1 expression in metastatic cancer cells by phorbol esters. Cancer Lett 153: 79–83, 2000

42. Sigala S, Faraoni I, Botticini D, Paez-Pereda M, Missale C, Bonmassar E, Spano P: Suppression of telomerase, reexpression of KAI1, and abrogation of tumorigenicity by nerve growth factor in prostate cancer cell lines. Clin Cancer Res 5: 1211–1218, 1999

43. Mashimo T, Bandyopadhyay S, Goodarzi G, Watabe M, Pai SK, Gross SC, Watabe K: Activation of the tumor metastasis-suppressor gene, KAI1, by etoposide is mediated by p53 and c-Jun genes. Biochem Biophys Res Commun 274: 370–376, 2000

44. Tagawa K, Arihiro K, Takeshima Y, Hiyama E, Yamasaki M, Inai K: Down-regulation of KAI1 messenger RNA expression is not associated with loss of heterozygosity of the KAI1 gene region in lung adenocarcinoma. Jpn J Cancer Res 90: 970–976, 1999

45. Yang X, Wei L, Tang C, Slack R, Montgomery E, Lippman M: KAI1 protein is down-regulated during the pro-gression of human breast cancer. Clin Cancer Res 6: 3424–3429, 2000

46. Bouras T, Frauman AG: Expression of the prostate cancer metastasis suppressor gene KAI1 in primary prostate cancers: A biphasic relationship with tumor grade. J Pathol 188: 382–388, 1999

47. Sekita N, Suzuki H, Ichikawa T, Kito H, Akakura K, Igarashi T, Nakayama T, Watanabe M, Shiraishi T, Toyota M, Yoshie O, Ito H: Epigenetic regulation of the KAI-1 metastasis-suppressor gene in human prostate cancer cell lines. Jpn J Cancer Res 92: 947–951, 2001

48. Kawana Y, Komiya A, Ueda T, Nihei N, Kuramochi H, Suzuki H, Yatani R, Imai T, Dong JT, Imai T, Yoshie O, Barrett JC, Isaacs JT, Shimazaki J, Ito H, Ichikawa T: Location of KAI1 on the short arm of human chromosome 11 and frequency of allelic loss in advanced human prostate cancer. Prostate 32: 205–213, 1997

49. Dong JT, Suzuki H, Pin SS, Bova GS, Schalken JA, Isaacs WB, Barrett JC, Isaacs JT: Down-regulation of the KAI1 metastasis-suppressor gene during the progression of human prostatic cancer infrequently involves gene mutation or allelic loss. Cancer Res 56: 4387–4390, 1996

50. Maraj BH, Leek JP, Carr IM, Markham AF: Identification of a novel microsatellite marker tightly linked to the KAI-1 gene for predicting prostate cancer progression. Eur Urol 37: 228–233, 2000

51. Bajorath J: Molecular organization, structural features, and ligand binding characteristics of CD44, a highly variable cell surface glycoprotein with multiple functions. Proteins 39: 103–111, 2000

52. Herrlich P, Morrison H, Sleeman J, Orian-Rousseau V, Konig H, Weg-Remers S, Ponta H: CD44 acts both as a growth- and invasiveness-promoting molecule and as a tumor-suppressing cofactor. Ann NY Acad Sci 910: 106–118, 2000

53. Braun S, Pantel K, Muller P, Janni W, Hepp F, Kentenich CR, Gastroph S, Wischnik A, Dimpfl T, Kindermann G, Riethmuller G, Schlimok G: Cytokeratin-positive cells in the bone marrow and survival of patients with stage I, II, or III breast cancer. N Engl J Med 342: 525–533, 2000

54. Lou W, Krill D, Dhir R, Becich MJ, Dong JT, Frierson HF Jr, Isaacs WB, Isaacs JT, Gao AC: Methylation of the CD44 metastasis-suppressor gene in human prostate cancer. Cancer Res 59: 2329–2331, 1999

55. Aaltomaa S, Lipponen P, Ala-Opas M, Kosma VM: Expression and prognostic value of CD44 standard and variant v3 and v6 isoforms in prostate cancer. Eur Urol 39: 138–144, 2001

56. Noordzij MA, van Steenbrugge GJ, Schroder FH, Van der Kwast TH: Decreased expression of CD44 in metastatic prostate cancer. Int J Cancer 84: 478–483, 1999

57. Chekmareva MA, Hollowell CM, Smith RC, Davis EM, LeBeau MM, Rinker-Schaeffer CW: Localization of prostate cancer metastasis-suppressor activity on human chromosome 17. Prostate 33: 271–280, 1997

58. Chekmareva MA, Kadkhodaian MM, Hollowell CM, Kim H, Yoshida BA, Luu HH, Stadler WM, Rinker-Schaeffer CW: Chromosome 17-mediated dormancy

150

of AT6.1 prostate cancer micrometastases. Cancer Res 58: 4963–4969, 1998

59. Kim HL, Griend DJ, Yang X, Benson DA, Dubauskas Z, Yoshida BA, Chekmareva MA, Ichikawa Y, Sokoloff MH, Zhan P, Karrison T, Lin A, Stadler WM, Ichikawa T, Rubin MA, Rinker-Schaeffer CW: Mitogen-activated protein kinase kinase 4 metastasis-suppressor gene expression is inversely related to histological pattern in advancing human prostatic cancers. Cancer Res 61: 2833–2837, 2001

60. Radinsky R, Fidler IJ: Regulation of tumor cell growth at organ-specific metastases. *In vivo* 6: 325–331, 1992

61. Fidler IJ: Critical determinants of melanoma metastasis. J Investig Dermatol Symp Proc 1: 203–208, 1996

62. Welch DR: Technical considerations for studying cancer metastasis *in vivo*. Clin Exp Metastasis 15: 272–306, 1997

Address for offprints: C.W. Rinker-Schaeffer, The University of Chicago Urology Research Laboratory, Pennsylvania State College of Medicine, PA, USA; *Tel:* 313 993 8197; *Fax:* 313 993 4112; *e-mail:* crinker@surgerybsd.uchicago.edu

The urokinase-type plasminogen activator system in prostate cancer metastasis

Shijie Sheng
Department of Pathology, Wayne State University School of Medicine, Detroit, MI, USA

Key words: gene expression, proteolysis, extracellular matrix, tumor growth, invasion, metastasis

Abstract

Accumulated clinical and experimental evidence indicates that the urokinase-type plasminogen activator (uPA) and its regulators are causatively involved in the metastatic phenotype of many types of cancers. In the past couple of decades, investigation on the role of the uPA system in human prostate cancer (PC) has been intensified and has yielded valuable insights. This review summarizes recent advances made in several areas regarding the clinical relevance, the function and the molecular mechanisms of the uPA system in PC metastasis. A current consensus suggests that the uPA system promotes PC metastasis by mediating pericellular plasminogen activation. Towards the development of therapeutic strategies that specifically target uPA-mediated PC metastasis, several remaining issues are discussed.

Introduction

Localized pericellular proteolysis has been recognized as a critical mechanism for extracellualar matrix (ECM) remodeling, cell–matrix interaction and the generation of biologically active molecules that mediate diverse cellular functions including cell proliferation, adhesion, invasion and tumor metastasis. Urokinase-type plasminogen activator (uPA), a membrane-associated serine protease, has been implicated in human prostate cancer (PC) [1–3]. Recent advances in several areas suggest that the pericellular uPA system may serve as a useful molecular marker to predict a poor prognosis of PC [1–3], and may be a therapeutic target for PC intervention. uPA catalyzes the extracellular proteolytic conversion of zymogen plasminogen to active plasmin. The localized pericellular uPA activity is facilitated by cell surface-anchored uPA receptor, uPAR [4,5], and can be specifically inhibited by several plasminogen activator inhibitors (PAI) [6]. Overwhelming evidence in the literature demonstrates that the cell surface-associated uPA/uPAR complex is causatively involved in tumor invasion and metastasis of many types of cancers by exerting multifaceted functions via either direct or indirect interactions with

integrins, endocytosis receptors, and growth factors (see review [6]). Thus, the task to effectively block the uPA-mediated tumor invasion and metastasis without causing adverse side effects appears rather challenging. This review is intended to put into perspective the clinical relevance, the function and the regulation of the uPA system in human PC, and help to identify remaining critical issues that hamper the development of therapeutic strategies that target uPA-mediated PC metastasis.

The key components of the uPA system

uPA is a 54-kDa serine protease. The primary substrate of uPA is plasminogen [7]. uPA catalyzes the cleavage of the zymogen plasminogen to plasmin. Plasmin is a serine protease with a relatively broad substrate specificity. The major biological function of plasmin is to cleave fibrin polymers of the clot in thrombolysis [8,9], and to degrade several key ECM components [10,11]. *In vitro* evidence suggests that plasmin can also activate other zymogen proteases such as matrix metalloproteinases [12]. In addition to plasminogen, uPA also catalyzes the activation of two plasminogen homologues, hepatocyte growth factor/scatter

M.L. Cher, K.V. Honn and A. Raz (eds.), Prostate Cancer: New Horizons in Research and Treatment, 151–160.
© 2002 *Kluwer Academic Publishers.*

factor (HGF/SF) [13] and macrophage-stimulating protein (MSP) [14], by a proteolytic cleavage similar to that in plasminogen activation. A recent *in vitro* study showed that in the presence of free sulfhydryl donors (FSDs), uPA also converts plasminogen to an alternatively cleaved product angiostatin [15], which has been shown to inhibit tumor-induced angiogenesis [16,17].

uPA is initially secreted as a single chain zymogen, pro-uPA, without plasminogen-activating activity. Pro-uPA is bound to the cell surface-anchored uPAR and is cleaved, primarily by plasmin, at the peptide bond K158–I159 into an active two-chain molecule [8,9,18]. The mature uPA protein is a disulfide bond-linked heterodimer containing an A chain (the N-terminal fragment) that binds to uPAR and the catalytic B-chain (the C-terminal fragment). uPAR, lacking an intracellular domain, is attached to the cell membrane by a glycosyl phosphatidyl inositol (GPI) [4,5]. Accumulated evidence demonstrates that uPAR not only facilitates the proteolytic activation of uPA, but also directly interacts with (and is, perhaps, regulated by) the integrin receptors of ECM proteins, ECM components, as well as proteins on adjacent cells [10,19,20]. The binding of uPAR to its ligand uPA, thus, is thought to allow for both spatial and temporal regulation of uPA activity.

Several serine protease inhibitors (serpins) including plasminogen activator inhibitor type-1 (PAI-1), plasminogen activator inhibitor type-2 (PAI-2) and maspin have been shown to neutralize the proteolytic activity of uPA. PAI-1 and PAI-2 inhibit the uPAR-bound uPA more efficiently than soluble uPA [21–23]. Interestingly, the novel serpin maspin only inhibits the cell surface-associated uPA, but not the soluble uPA [24]. *In vitro* biochemical evidence further suggests that these serpins inhibit uPA by docking their reactive site loop (RSL) into the catalytic domain of uPA, and forming a stable uPA/serpin complex [25]. The interaction between uPA and serpin inhibitors may be regulated by serpin cofactors such as heparin [26,27]. PAI-1 has been shown to regulate the integrin-mediated cell adhesion to vitronectin by directly binding to vitronectin in an uPA-independent manner [28,29].

The clinical relevance of uPA in human prostate cancer

In PC patients, the elevation of either uPA or uPAR, or both, in serum could be used as a predictor of poor prognosis. The serum levels of uPA and uPAR are moderately elevated in individuals with benign prostate hyperplasia (BPH) [3], and significantly elevated in patients with PC [2,3,30]. The elevated serum levels of uPA and uPAR correlate with the serum level of prostate specific antigen (PSA) and the development of PC metastasis [1,31], and inversely correlate with the overall survival rate among PC patients [1,3]. Consistently, the density of uPA and uPAR in tumor tissues are significantly higher than in prostate tissues from healthy individuals [1]. Interestingly, the elevated uPA/uPAR expression is, in some cases, accompanied by an up-regulation of PAI-1 in high-grade PC patients [32]. The correlation between the uPA level/activity and the metastatic potential of PC has been observed also with prostate tumor tissues in short-term cultures *in vitro* [33]. In addition, elevated uPA appears to correlate with increased activation of type-2 and type-9 matrix metalloproteinases (MMP-2 and MMP-9) [34–36].

Similar differential expression patterns of uPA and uPAR have been observed in established human PC cell lines of different invasive and metastatic potentials [37], as well as in animal models for PC. Among three commonly used PC cell lines (PC3, DU145, and LNCaP), PC3 cells initially derived from a PC bone metastasis express uPA at the highest level and have the highest net plasminogen activation activity. PC3 cells also express tissue-type plasminogen activator (tPA), PAI-1 and PAI-2. DU145 cells, established from a brain metastasis, express uPA at a moderate level, and do not express tPA [38,39]. The only androgen-sensitve cell line LNCaP expresses little or no uPA in the presence of dihydrotestosterone (DHT) [39,40]. uPAR is expressed in all these cell lines [38,39]. To date, the role of tPA in PC metastasis remains unclear. When cell lines originating from the Dunning rat R-3327 prostate tumor were analyzed for their production of uPA, MMPs, as well as their capacities to mediate ECM degradation, only uPA-mediated ECM-degradation correlated with their known metastatic potentials [34].

The molecular mechanisms underlying the up-regulation of uPA and uPAR in PC appear to be complex. The elevated uPA and uPAR expression may result from accumulated genetic changes in PC cells such as gene amplification as evident in some high-grade PC tissues and in the highly invasive and metastastic PC3 cell line [41]. In addition, elevated uPA expression in PC tissues and cultured PC cell lines has been shown to correlate with up-regulated ets family paralogues Fli and Elf-1, and in some cases, with c-Fos and C-Jun activity [42,43]. Thus, the differential expression of uPA may also result from the evolving epigenetic stimulations during PC progression. In fact, numerous paracrine growth factors have been shown to activate the transcription of uPA and lead to elevated pericellular uPA activity, including androgen [44–46], interleukins [47], thrombin [48], bombesin [49], lipopolysaccharide [40], IGF [50], EGF [44], and TGF-β [44]. In the case of TGF-β, latent form TGF-β derived from osteoblasts has been shown to undergo proteolytic activation by PC cell-associated uPA. The active TGF-β, in turn, may stimulate the overexpression of both uPA and PAI-1, resulting in a net increase in pericellular plasminogen activation, increased activation of MMP-9, and increased tumor cell invasion of matrigel [51,52]. Interestingly, when cultured on fibronectin substratum, LNCaP cells express uPA at a reduced level as compared to control cells that are cultured on regular plastic culture dishes [40]. This result suggests that the signaling events that regulate the expression of the uPA system may be further modulated by the extracellular matrix components encountered by the tumor cells during PC progression.

It is of particular importance to note that in contrast to PAI-1, which is sometimes up-regulated in invasive PC cells [32], the expression of maspin inversely correlates with PC progression [53]. Both clinical evidence and *in vitro* studies on maspin promoter activity suggest that maspin expression in normal prostate epithelial cells may be directly activated by the wild-type tumor suppressor p53 [53,54], or suppressed by a hormone-responsive element [55]. It is likely that the down-regulation of maspin expression may result from the loss of either the hormone sensitivity, or the activity of wild type p53.

uPA promotes prostate cancer metastasis

Consistent with the differential expression patterns of the components in the uPA system in PC, accumulated experimental evidence further supports the development of PC intervention strategies that specifically target the uPA system. In cell culture, the capacities of three human PC cell lines (LNCaP, DU145, and PC3) to invade matrigel correspond to their abilities to activate plasminogen [39]. Growth factor EGF and bombesin (a potent inducer of signal transduction pathways) stimulate the expression of uPA, and stimulate the activation of MMP-2 and MMP-9 in PC cells [49]. In response to bombesin treatment, DU145 and PC3 cells

exhibited a stimulated cell proliferation rate and elevated invasive potential. These effects of bombesin can be neutralized either by a uPA-neutralizing antibody or by p-aminobenzamidine, a synthetic serine protease inhibitor [49].

It has been recognized that the uPA system also affects prostate tumor growth. PAI-1 variants inhibit the growth of DU145 and LNCaP xenografts in SCID mice [56]. In cell culture, the proliferation of LNCaP cells that express little or no endogenous uPA can be significantly stimulated by exogenously added uPA [39]. The mechanism underlying this growth stimulatory effect of uPA is not clear. Based on a cell cycle analysis, it seems unlikely that the uPA system directly regulates the cell cycle machinery [57]. On the other hand, a recent report suggests that PAI-1 may protect PC cells from induced apoptosis [58]. Little is known about whether the anti-apoptotic effect of PAI-1 depends on its association with the cell surface-anchored uPA/uPAR complex.

The role of the uPA system in tumor invasion and metastasis has been reproduced in the experimental Dunning rat PC model. When injected subcutaneously into Copenhagen rats, Dunning Mat LyLu PC cells developed skeletal metastasis that led to hind limb paralysis [59]. In this model, uPA-overexpressing cells derived from Mat LyLu cells exhibited increased skeletal metastasis, while parallel Mat LyLu-derived transfectant cells that expressed the uPA antisense cDNA developed skeletal metastasis at a significantly slower pace. When Copenhagen rats were infused with a synthetic uPA inhibitor, B-428, the Dunning rat PC implants were inhibited in primary tumor growth and in metastasis to lymph nodes and lungs [60]. Consistently, constitutive expression of an uPA-mutant that binds to uPAR but does not activate plasminogen in Mat LyLu-derived stable transfectant cells inhibits tumor xenograft growth and tumor-induced angiogenesis in Copenhagen rats [61].

Specific inhibition of the cell surface-associated uPA may be achieved by blocking the interaction of uPA to uPAR. PC3 cells transfected with the cDNA of a mutant uPA which binds to uPAR but lacks enzymatic activity were markedly inhibited in their capacity to mediate pericellular uPA activity *in vitro*, and their metastatic potential *in vivo* [62]. On the other hand, specific enzymatic inhibitors of uPA have been used successfully to block uPA-mediated PC invasion and metastasis. Overexpression of PAI-1 limits the PC cell-mediated pericellular accumulation of plasmin as well as the activation of MMP-2 and MMP-9 [39]. Specific neutralizing antibody against uPA A-chain that blocks the interaction between uPA and uPAR inhibits the growth of uPA-producing PC3 cells and DU145 cells [39]. Alpha-emitting radiation therapy using Tb-149 or Bi-213 conjugated to PAI-2 has been shown to specifically target PC cells with high cytotoxicity *in vitro* [63]. As compared to mock control cells, several PAI-1 overexpressing clonal cell lines derived from PC3 by stable transfection developed significantly smaller tumors when injected subcutaneously into nude mice. These PAI-1 expressing PC3 transfectants also developed significantly less neovascularization and micrometastases to the lung and liver [32]. Purified recombinant PAI-1 and small molecular weight uPA inhibitors such as p-aminobenzamidine and amiloride have also been shown to inhibit the growth of DU145 and LNCaP tumor xenografts in SCID mice [56,64].

Recently, purified mouse maspin was shown to inhibit the growth and neovascularization of LNCaP xenograft in nude mice [65]. It is interesting to note that although *in vitro* evidence demonstrates a critical role of maspin reactive site (RSL) in inhibiting tumor cell-mediated uPA activity, a truncation mutant of maspin lacking the RSL sequence was active in inhibiting tumor induced angiogenesis *in vivo* [65]. It is not clear, however, whether the RSL-independent tumor suppressive activity of maspin was also independent of the cell surface-associated uPA/uPAR complex. On the other hand, both purified recombinant maspin and endogenously expressed maspin inhibited the motility and invasion of PC cell lines in cell culture [66]. The dual inhibitory effect of maspin on PC cell motility and invasion seems to support the hypothesis that maspin targets the cell surface-associated uPA/uPAR complex. Research on the uPA system in other types of cells suggests that the uPA/uPAR complex may exert a dual stimulatory effect on cell motility and invasion by concertedly degrading ECM and regulating the integrin-mediated signal transduction pathways [10,67–73]. Although it is yet to be tested whether the uPA/uPAR complex interacts with the focal adhesion complex in PC cells, it has been shown that the binding of uPA to uPAR on the surface of LNCaP cells lead to the tyrosine phosphorylation of two proteins involved in $\alpha 5\beta 1$ integrin-mediated signaling: focal adhesion kinase (FAK) and the crk-associated substrate p130 (Cas) [67].

Epigenetic down-regulation of uPA expression in PC cells can also effectively block the uPA-mediated invasive phenotypes. Studies of Xing and Rabbani showed

that overexpression of wildtype androgen receptor (AR) in PC3 cells restored the androgen responsiveness in these cells. Treatment of these AR-expressing PC3 cells with DHT led to a dose-dependent decrease in the production of the uPA messenger RNA and uPA protein, resulting in decreased invasive potential *in vitro*, and decreased tumor metastasis in nude mice [74]. The down-regulation of uPA in DU145 cells that resulted from retinoic acid treatment correlated with decreased cell-mediated ECM degradation (specifically fibronectin and laminin) and significantly reduced tumor invasion of matrigel [75–77]. In addition, synthetic retinoid N-(4-hydroxyphenyl) retinamide simultaneously stimulated PAI-1 expression and repressed uPA expression in PC cells and inhibited cellular adhesion, motility, and cell-mediated ECM-degradation [75,78–80].

The uPA system may stimulate multiple invasive steps of PC metastasis. Endogenous PAI-1 and maspin have been shown to inhibit PC-induced angiogenesis *in vivo* [64,65]. Purified recombinant PAI-1 also inhibits PC-induced experimental angiogenesis [56]. The anti-angiogenic effect of prostate tumor-associated macrophage was thought to be due, in part, to their ability to secrete granulocyte-macrophage colony-stimulating factor (GM-CSF) which, in turn, up-regulates the expression of PAI-2 [81]. Interestingly, an *in vitro* study showed that uPA and FSDs (such as N-acetyl-L-cysteine, D-penicillamine, captopril, L-cysteine, or reduced glutathione) secreted by PC3 cells were sufficient to convert plasminogen to angiostatin [15], a potent naturally occurring inhibitor of angiogenesis [16,17]. The PC3 cell-associated uPA system has been implicated in the proteolytic activation of osteoblasts-derived latent TGF-β [35,52]. The activated TGF-β may subsequently stimulate the overexpression of uPA and PAI-1 in PC3 cells, enhance the net pericellular activation of plasminogen and MMP-9, and promote the survival of PC cells in bone environment [35,52,82,83]. Thus, the uPA system may also promote organ-specific metastasis of PC to bone.

Remaining issues and future directions

Taken together, both clinical and experimental evidence indicate that the cell-associated uPA/uPAR system plays a key role in PC invasion and metastasis. Overexpression of uPA and uPAR leads to accelerated prostate tumor growth, invasion, angiogenesis, and metastasis. In contrast, inhibition of the uPA system either by manipulating gene expression or by uPA-blocking agents inhibits PC invasion and metastasis both in cell culture and in animal models. In light of the future development of anti-metastasis strategies that specifically target the uPA system, the following issues remain to be addressed.

The imbalance between uPA and its inhibitors may underlie the tumor promoting activity of uPA. Thus, restoring the biological balance between uPA and its inhibitors should be a pharmacological goal in combating PC metastasis without inflicting adverse side effects on normal tissue function. It is not surprising that the uPAR-bound uPA, capable of turning on a powerful pericellular proteolytic cascade, can be efficiently neutralized by multiple serpin inhibitors such as PAI-1, PAI-2, and maspin. However, achieving a quantitative balance between uPA and its inhibitors may not be sufficient. The inhibition of uPA activity by different serpins may lead to differential cellular responses to tumor–host interactions. To this end, it is important to note that the metastatic phenotype of many types of cancer does not correlate with an imbalance between uPA and PAI-1. In fact, PAI-1 is often found up-regulated along with uPA and uPAR [84–86]. The uPA detected in serum exists in the uPA/PAI-1 complex [87,88]. Furthermore, overexpression of PAI-1, at least in some experimental systems, inhibits tumor cell apoptosis [58] and has been shown to be essential for angiogenesis in a murine mammary carcinoma model [89] and in a murine fibrosarcoma model [90]. PAI-2 [38,91,92] and maspin [53,93–96], on the other hand, have been shown to be down-regulated in many types of cancers including PC, and play a tumor suppressive role. It is possible that a switch of the uPA cognate inhibitor from the tumor suppressive type (e.g. PAI-2 and maspin) to the tumor promoting type (e.g. PAI-1) may lead to a qualitative imbalance between uPA and its inhibitors, and may represent a gain of function at critical steps of PC progression. Thus, it is important to delineate the specific mode of uPA inhibition that blocks PC metastasis. To achieve this goal, detailed biological, biochemical, and pharmacological properties of these natural uPA inhibitors in PC progression should be compared by a systematic approach both *in vitro* and in animal models.

Since uPAR facilitates the activation of uPA on the cell surface, it is an appealing idea to block uPA-mediated pericellular proteolysis by disrupting the interaction between uPA and uPAR. However, it is important to bear in mind that uPAR also plays a critical role for uPA inhibition by serpins. The complete inhibition of uPA/uPAR on the cell surface may ultimately depend on an efficient internalization mechanism that quenches the cell surface uPA activity. Accumulated evidence demonstrates that endocytosis receptor α2-MR/LRP (alpha2-macroglobulin receptor/low density lipoprotein receptor-related protein) mediates the internalization of the uPAR/uPA/PAI-1 complex [97–100]. Biliran et al. have shown that endogenous maspin also induces an LRP-mediated internalization of uPA and uPAR in DU145 cells [101]. A uPAR associated protein uPARAP, a member of the macrophage mannose receptor protein family, has been recently identified as an additional receptor for the cell-associated uPA/uPAR complex [102]. uPARAP is a constitutively recycling internalization receptor. *In vitro* studies suggest that uPARAP forms a ternary complex with pro-uPA and uPAR on the cell surface in all tissues undergoing primary ossification, and may function as a mediator of the uPA/uPAR internalization [102]. Thus, uPAR appears to play a biphasic role in regulating the proteolytic activity of cell surface-associate uPA. On the one hand, uPAR facilitates the proteolytic activation of pro-uPA to active uPA. On the other hand, uPAR is a critical component of the uPA internalization complex that ultimately quenches the cell surface uPA activity. In fact, it has been shown that PAI-1, in some cases, inhibits uPA-induced chemotaxis by stimulating the internalization of the cell surface-associated uPA/uPAR complex [100]. The internalization of the uPA complex represents an additional dimension of uPA regulation and raises the need to explore uPA inhibitors that antagonize the activity of uPAR-bound uPA, but do not interfere with subsequent uPA/uPAR internalization.

The evidence obtained so far from PC research leads to a consensus that the uPA system promotes tumor growth, invasion, and metastasis by degrading extracellular matrix. Furthermore, the uPA-mediated pericellular proteolysis depends on its cell surface-anchored receptor uPAR. Increasing evidence generated from studies using other experimental systems shows that uPAR is a multifunctional protein. In invasive carcinoma cells, the uPA/uPAR complex is localized in caveolae [68,103], and this may further enhance pericellular plasminogen activation at the leading edge of an invading cell. At the leading edge of the invasive cells, uPAR may directly interact with integrins

156

and promote integrin-mediated signal transduction [10,68–73]. Although it is not clear whether the N-terminal domain of uPA exists as a natural product, *in vitro* studies have shown that this domain alone binds to uPAR to induce proteolysis-independent signaling events [69,70], and promotes tumor cell motility and invasion [70,104–106]. Consistently, a recent report showed that uPA stimulated cell migration of DU145 cells by a mechanism that requires FAK [107]. It is intriguing to hypothesize that the localization of uPA to cell surface anchored uPAR provides a versatile mechanism to facilitate ECM degradation in response to the evolving cell–matrix interaction at key steps of tumor invasion and metastasis. Thus, to specifically block tumor-promoting uPA activity, more extensive studies are needed to obtain critical insights into how cell–matrix interactions at each step of PC metastasis (i.e. local invasion, angiogenesis, and organ-specific metastasis) differentially regulate the activity of the uPA/uPAR complex. In the meantime, it is critical to understand how PC cells of different genetic background and signaling transduction capacities utilize the uPA/uPAR system. For example, it needs to be clarified whether hormone sensitive and hormone refractory PCs differ in terms of the expression, the activity, as well as the regulation of the pericellular uPA system.

Concluding remarks

The uPA system has been implicated in promoting the metastasis of many types of cancers. Clinical evidence also indicates that up-regulation of uPA along with uPAR correlates with an aggressive phenotype and poor prognosis of human PC. As summarized in this review, the role of the uPA system in PC is promotion of tumor metastasis primarily by facilitating pericellular plasminogen activation and, subsequently, ECM degradation. Despite the exciting leads obtained in the past decade, the investigation of the uPA system in PC progression is yet in its early stage and several critical issues need to be systematically addressed. Nonetheless, the accumulated evidence supports the development of PC intervention strategies that specifically target the uPA system.

References

1. Miyake H, Hara I, Yamanaka K, Arakawa S, Kamidono S: Elevation of urokinase-type plasminogen activator and its receptor densities as new predictors of disease progression and prognosis in men with prostate cancer. Int J Oncol 14: 535–541, 1999
2. Miyake H, Hara I, Yamanaka K, Gohji K, Arakawa S, Kamidono S: Elevation of serum levels of urokinase-type plasminogen activator and its receptor is associated with disease progression and prognosis in patients with prostate cancer. Prostate 39: 123–129, 1999
3. McCabe NP, Angwafo FF III, Zaher A, Selman SH, Kouinche A, Jankun J: Expression of soluble urokinase plasminogen activator receptor may be related to outcome in prostate cancer patients. Oncol Rep 7: 879–882, 2000
4. Roldan AL, Cubellis MV, Masucci MT, Behrendt N, Lund LR, Dano K, Appella E, Blasi F: Cloning and expression of the receptor for human urokinase plasminogen activator, a central molecule in cell surface, plasmin dependent proteolysis. EMBO J 9, 1990
5. Ploug M, Kjalke M, Ronne E, Weidle U, Hoyer-Hansen G, Dano K: Localization of the disulfide bonds in the NH2-terminal domain of the cellular receptor for human urokinase-type plasminogen activator. A domain structure belonging to a novel superfamily of glycolipid-anchored membrane proteins. J Biol Chem 268: 17539–17546, 1993
6. Andreasen PA, Kjoller L, Christensen L, Duffy MJ: The urokinase-type plasminogen activator system in cancer metastasis: a review. Int J Cancer 72: 1–22, 1997
7. Rickli EE: The activation mechanism of human plasminogen. Thromb Diath Haemorrh 34: 386–395, 1975
8. Robison AK, Collen D: Activation of the fibrinolytic system. Cardiol Clin 5: 13–19, 1987
9. Gurewich V: Fibrinolysis: an unfinished agenda. Blood Coagul Fibrinolysis 11: 401–408, 2000
10. Rabbani SA, Mazar AP: The role of the plasminogen activation system in angiogenesis and metastasis. Surg Oncol Clin N Am 10: 393–415, 2001
11. Pepper MS: Role of the matrix metalloproteinase and plasminogen activator-plasmin systems in angiogenesis. Arterioscler Thromb Vasc Biol 21: 1104–1117, 2001
12. Legrand C, Polette M, Tournier JM, de Bentzmann S, Huet E, Monteau M, Birembaut P: uPA/plasmin system-mediated MMP-9 activation is implicated in bronchial epithelial cell migration. Exp Cell Res 264: 326–336, 2001
13. Naldini L, Tamagnone L, Vigna E, Sachs M, Hartmann G, Birchmeier W, Daikuhara Y, Tsubouchi H, Blasi F, Comoglio PM: Extracellular proteolytic cleavage by urokinase is required for activation of hepatocyte growth factor/scatter factor. EMBO J 11: 4825–4833, 1992
14. Miyazawa K, Wang Y, Minoshima S, Shimizu N, Kitamura N: Structural organization and chromosomal localization of the human hepatocyte growth factor activator gene – phylogenetic and functional relationship with blood coagulation factor XII, urokinase, and tissue-type plasminogen activator. Eur J Biochem 258: 355–361, 1998
15. Gately S, Twardowski P, Stack MS, Cundiff DL, Grella D, Castellino FJ, Enghild J, Kwaan HC, Lee F, Kramer RA, Volpert O, Bouck N, Soff GA: The mechanism of cancer-mediated conversion of plasminogen to the angiogenesis inhibitor angiostatin. Proc Natl Acad Sci USA 94: 10868–10872, 1997

16. O'Reilly MS: Angiostatin: an endogenous inhibitor of angiogenesis and of tumor growth. EXS 79: 273–294, 1997

17. Soff GA: Angiostatin and angiostatin-related proteins. Cancer Metastasis Rev 19: 97–107, 2000

18. Rijken DC: Plasminogen activators and plasminogen activator inhibitors: biochemical aspects. Baillieres Clin Haematol 8: 291–312, 1995

19. Ossowski L, Aguirre-Ghiso JA: Urokinase receptor and integrin partnership: coordination of signaling for cell adhesion, migration and growth. Curr Opin Cell Biol 12: 613–620, 2000

20. Preissner KT, Kanse SM, May AE: Urokinase receptor: a molecular organizer in cellular communication. Curr Opin Cell Biol 12: 621–628, 2000

21. Schwartz BS, Espana F: Two distinct urokinase-serpin interactions regulate the initiation of cell surface-associated plasminogen activation. J Biol Chem 274: 15278–15283, 1999

22. Ellis V, Wun TC, Behrendt N, Ronne E, Dano K: Inhibition of receptor-bound urokinase by plasminogen-activator inhibitors. J Biol Chem 265: 9904–9908, 1990

23. Schwartz BS: Differential inhibition of soluble and cell surface receptor-bound single-chain urokinase by plasminogen activator inhibitor type 2. A potential regulatory mechanism. J Biol Chem 269: 8319–8323, 1994

24. McGowen R, Biliran H Jr, Sager R, Sheng S: The surface of prostate carcinoma DU145 cells mediates the inhibition of urokinase-type plasminogen activator by maspin. Cancer Res 60: 4771–4778, 2000

25. Yamamoto M, Sawaya R, Mohanam S, Rao VH, Bruner JM, Nicolson GL, Ohshima K, Rao JS: Activities, localizations, and roles of serine proteases and their inhibitors in human brain tumor progression. J Neuro-Oncol 22: 139–151, 1994

26. Engh RA, Huber R, Bode W, Schulze AJ: Divining the serpin inhibition mechanism: a suicide substrate 'springe'? Trends Biotechnol 13: 503–510, 1995

27. Pratt CW, Church FC: General features of the heparin-binding serpins antithrombin, heparin cofactor II and protein C inhibitor. Blood Coagul Fibrinolysis 4: 479–490, 1993

28. Salonen EM, Vaheri A, Pollanen J, Stephens R, Andreasen P, Mayer M, Dano K, Gailit J, Ruoslahti E: Interaction of plasminogen activator inhibitor (PAI-1) with vitronectin. J Biol Chem 264: 6339–6343, 1989

29. Deng G, Royle G, Seiffert D, Loskutoff DJ: The PAI-1/vitronectin interaction: two cats in a bag? Thromb Haemost 74: 66–70, 1995

30. Van Veldhuizen PJ, Sadasivan R, Cherian R, Wyatt A: Urokinase-type plasminogen activator expression in human prostate carcinomas. Am J Med Sci 312: 8–11, 1996

31. Kirchheimer JC, Pfluger H, Ritschl P, Hienert G, Binder BR: Plasminogen activator activity in bone metastases of prostatic carcinomas as compared to primary tumors. Invasion Metastasis 5: 344–355, 1985

32. Soff GA, Sanderowitz J, Gately S, Verrusio E, Weiss I, Brem S, Kwaan HC: Expression of plasminogen activator inhibitor type 1 by human prostate carcinoma cells inhibits primary tumor growth, tumor-associated angiogenesis, and metastasis to lung and liver in an athymic mouse model. J Clin Invest 96: 2593–2600, 1995

33. Festuccia C, Vincentini C, di Pasquale AB, Aceto G, Zazzeroni F, Miano L, Bologna M: Plasminogen activator activities in short-term tissue cultures of benign prostatic hyperplasia and prostatic carcinoma. Oncol Res 7: 131–138, 1995

34. Quax PH, de Bart AC, Schalken JA, Verheijen JH: Plasminogen activator and matrix metalloproteinase production and extracellular matrix degradation by rat prostate cancer cells *in vitro*: correlation with metastatic behavior *in vivo*. Prostate 32: 196–204, 1997

35. Festuccia C, Giunciuglio D, Guerra F, Villanova I, Angelucci A, Manduca P, Teti A, Albini A, Bologna M: Osteoblasts modulate secretion of urokinase-type plasminogen activator (uPA) and matrix metalloproteinase-9 (MMP-9) in human prostate cancer cells promoting migration and matrigel invasion. Oncol Res 11: 17–31, 1999

36. Rabbani SA: Metalloproteases and urokinase in angiogenesis and tumor progression. *In Vivo* 12: 135–142, 1998

37. Hollas W, Hoosein N, Chung LW, Mazar A, Henkin J, Kariko K, Barnathan ES, Boyd D: Expression of urokinase and its receptor in invasive and non-invasive prostate cancer cell lines. Thromb Haemost 68: 662–666, 1992

38. Lyon PB, See WA, Xu Y, Cohen MB: Diversity and modulation of plasminogen activator activity in human prostate carcinoma cell lines. Prostate 27: 179–186, 1995

39. Festuccia C, Dolo V, Guerra F, Violini S, Muzi P, Pavan A, Bologna M: Plasminogen activator system modulates invasive capacity and proliferation in prostatic tumor cells. Clin Exp Metastasis 16: 513–528, 1998

40. Pentyala SN, Whyard TC, Waltzer WC, Meek AG, Hod Y: Androgen induction of urokinase gene expression in LNCaP cells is dependent on their interaction with the extracellular matrix. Cancer Lett 130: 121–126, 1998

41. Helenius MA, Saramaki OR, Linja MJ, Tammela TL, Visakorpi T: Amplification of urokinase gene in prostate cancer. Cancer Res 61: 5340–5344, 2001

42. Gavrilov D, Kenzior O, Evans M, Calaluce R, Folk WR: Expression of urokinase plasminogen activator and receptor in conjunction with the ets family and AP-1 complex transcription factors in high grade prostate cancers. Eur J Cancer 37: 1033–1040, 2001

43. D'Orazio D, Besser D, Marksitzer R, Kunz C, Hume DA, Kiefer B, Nagamine Y: Cooperation of two PEA3/AP1 sites in uPA gene induction by TPA and FGF-2. Gene 201: 179–187, 1997

44. Desruisseau S, Ghazarossian-Ragni E, Chinot O, Martin PM: Divergent effect of TGFbeta1 on growth and proteolytic modulation of human prostatic-cancer cell lines. Int J Cancer 66: 796–801, 1996

45. Wilson MJ, Ludowese C, Sinha AA, Estensen RD: Effects of castration on plasminogen activator activities and plasminogen activator inhibitor type 1 in the rat ventral prostate. Prostate 28: 239–250, 1996

46. Xing RH, Rabbani SA: Regulation of urokinase production by androgens in human prostate cancer cells: effect on tumor growth and metastases *in vivo*. Endocrinology 140, 1999

158

47. Ohta S, Niiya K, Sakuragawa N, Fuse H: Induction of urokinase-type plasminogen activator by lipopolysaccharide in PC-3 human prostatic cancer cells. Thromb Res 97: 343–347, 2000

48. Yoshida E, Verrusio EN, Mihara H, Oh D, Kwaan HC: Enhancement of the expression of urokinase-type plasminogen activator from PC-3 human prostate cancer cells by thrombin. Cancer Res 54: 3300–3304, 1994

49. Festuccia C, Guerra F, D'Ascenzo S, Giunciuglio D, Albini A, Bologna M: In vitro regulation of pericellular proteolysis in prostatic tumor cells treated with bombesin. Int J Cancer 75: 418–431, 1998

50. Angelloz-Nicoud P, Binoux M: Autocrine regulation of cell proliferation by the insulin-like growth factor (IGF) and IGF binding protein-3 protease system in a human prostate carcinoma cell line (PC-3). Endocrinology 136: 5485–5492, 1995

51. Festuccia C, Angelucci A, Gravina GL, Villanova I, Teti A, Albini A, Bologna M, Abini A: Osteoblast-derived TGF-beta1 modulates matrix degrading protease expression and activity in prostate cancer cells. Int J Cancer 85: 407–415, 2000

52. Festuccia C, Bologna M, Gravina GL, Guerra F, Angelucci A, Villanova I, Millimaggi D, Teti A: Osteoblast conditioned media contain TGF-beta1 and modulate the migration of prostate tumor cells and their interactions with extracellular matrix components. Int J Cancer 81: 395–403, 1999

53. Machtens S, Serth J, Bokemeyer C, Bathke W, Minssen A, Kollmannsberger C, Hartmann J, Knuchel R, Kondo M, Jonas U, Kuczyk M: Expression of the p53 and Maspin protein in primary prostate cancer: correlation with clinical features. Int J Cancer 95: 337–342, 2001

54. Zou Z, Gao C, Nagaich AK, Connell T, Saito S, Moul JW, Seth P, Appella E, Srivastava S: p53 regulates the expression of the tumor suppressor gene maspin. J Biol Chem 275: 6051–6054, 2000

55. Zhang M, Magit D, Sager R: Expression of maspin in prostate cells is regulated by a positive ets element and a negative hormonal responsive element site recognized by androgen receptor. Proc Natl Acad Sci USA 94: 5673–5678, 1997

56. Jankun J, Keck RW, Skrzypczak-Jankun E, Swiercz R: Inhibitors of urokinase reduce size of prostate cancer xenografts in severe combined immunodeficient mice. Cancer Res 57: 559–563, 1997

57. Plas E, Carroll VA, Jilch R, Simak R, Mihaly J, Melchior S, Thuroff JW, Binder BR, Pfluger H: Variations of components of the plasminogen activation system with the cell cycle in benign prostate tissue and prostate cancer. Cytometry 46: 184–189, 2001

58. Kwaan HC, Wang J, Svoboda K, Declerck PJ: Plasminogen activator inhibitor 1 may promote tumour growth through inhibition of apoptosis. Br J Cancer 82: 1702–1708, 2000

59. Achbarou A, Kaiser S, Tremblay G, Ste-Marie LG, Brodt P, Goltzman D, Rabbani SA: Urokinase overproduction results in increased skeletal metastasis by prostate cancer cells in vivo. Cancer Res 54: 2372–2377, 1994

60. Rabbani SA, Harakidas P, Davidson DJ, Henkin J, Mazar AP: Prevention of prostate-cancer metastasis in vivo by a novel synthetic inhibitor of urokinase-type plasminogen activator (uPA). Int J Cancer 63: 840–845, 1995

61. Evans CP, Elfman F, Parangi S, Conn M, Cunha G, Shuman MA: Inhibition of prostate cancer neovascularization and growth by urokinase-plasminogen activator receptor blockade. Cancer Res 57: 3594–3599, 1997

62. Crowley CW, Cohen RL, Lucas BK, Liu G, Shuman MA, Levinson AD: Prevention of metastasis by inhibition of the urokinase receptor. Proc Natl Acad Sci USA 90: 5021–5025, 1993

63. Allen BJ, Rizvi S, Li Y, Tian Z, Ranson M: In vitro and preclinical targeted alpha therapy for melanoma, breast, prostate and colorectal cancers. Crit Rev Oncol Hematol 39: 139–146, 2001

64. Swiercz R, Keck RW, Skrzypczak-Jankun E, Selman SH, Jankun J: Recombinant PAI-1 inhibits angiogenesis and reduces size of LNCaP prostate cancer xenografts in SCID mice. Oncol Rep 8: 463–470, 2001

65. Zhang M, Volpert O, Shi YH, Bouck N: Maspin is an angiogenesis inhibito. Nat Med 6: 196–199, 2000

66. Sheng S, Carey J, Seftor EA, Dias L, Hendrix MJ, Sager R: Maspin acts at the cell membrane to inhibit invasion and motility of mammary and prostatic cancer cells. Proc Natl Acad Sci USA 93: 11669–11674, 1996

67. Yebra M, Goretzki L, Pfeifer M, Mueller BM: Urokinase-type plasminogen activator binding to its receptor stimulates tumor cell migration by enhancing integrin-mediated signal transduction. Exp Cell Res 250: 231–240, 1999

68. Koshelnick Y, Ehart M, Hufnagl P, Heinrich PC, Binder BR: Urokinase receptor is associated with the components of the JAK1/STAT1 signaling pathway and leads to activation of this pathway upon receptor clustering in the human kidney epithelial tumor cell line TCL-598. J Biol Chem 272: 28563–28567, 1997

69. Dumler I, Kopmann A, Weis A, Mayboroda OA, Wagner K, Gulba DC, Haller H: Urokinase activates the Jak/Stat signal transduction pathway in human vascular endothelial cells. Arterioscler Thromb Vasc Biol 19: 290–297, 1999

70. Nguyen DH, Hussaini IM, Gonias SL: Binding of urokinase-type plasminogen activator to its receptor in MCF-7 cells activates extracellular signal-regulated kinase 1 and 2 which is required for increased cellular motility. J Biol Chem 273: 8502–8507, 1998

71. Wei Y, Yang X, Liu Q, Wilkins JA, Chapman HA: A role for caveolin and the urokinase receptor in integrin-mediated adhesion and signaling. J Cell Biol 144: 1285–1294, 1999

72. Nguyen DH, Catling AD, Webb DJ, Sankovic M, Walker LA, Somlyo AV, Weber MJ, Gonias SL: Myosin light chain kinase functions downstream of Ras/ERK to promote migration of urokinase-type plasminogen activator-stimulated cells in an integrin-selective manner. J Cell Biol 146: 149–164, 1999

73. Degryse B, Orlando S, Resnati M, Rabbani SA, Blasi F: Urokinase/urokinase receptor and vitronectin/alpha(v)beta(3) integrin induce chemotaxis and

cytoskeleton reorganization through different signaling pathways. Oncogene 20: 2032–2043, 2001

74. Xing RH, Rabbani SA: Regulation of urokinase production by androgens in human prostate cancer cells: effect on tumor growth and metastases *in vivo*. Endocrinology 140: 4056–4064, 1999

75. Webber MM, Bello-DeOcampo D, Quader S, Deocampo ND, Metcalfe WS, Sharp RM: Modulation of the malignant phenotype of human prostate cancer cells by N-(4-hydroxyphenyl)retinamide (4-HPR). Clin Exp Metastasis 17: 255–263, 1999

76. Webber MM, Waghray A: Urokinase-mediated extracellular matrix degradation by human prostatic carcinoma cells and its inhibition by retinoic acid. Clin Cancer Res 1: 755–761, 1995

77. Waghray A, Webber MM: Retinoic acid modulates extracellular urokinase-type plasminogen activator activity in DU-145 human prostatic carcinoma cells. Clin Cancer Res 1: 747–753, 1995

78. Kim JH, Tanabe T, Chodak GW, Rukstalis DB: *In vitro* anti-invasive effects of N-(4-hydroxyphenyl)-retinamide on human prostatic adenocarcinoma. Anticancer Res 15: 1429–1434, 1995

79. Tanabe T: Effects of N-(4-hydroxyphenyl) retinamide on urokinase-type plasminogen activator and plasminogen activator inhibitor-1 in prostate adenocarcinoma cell lines. Hiroshima J Med Sci 49: 67–72, 2000

80. Igawa M, Tanabe T, Chodak GW, Rukstalis DB: N-(4-hydroxyphenyl) retinamide induces cell cycle specific growth inhibition in PC3 cells. Prostate 24: 299–305, 1994

81. Joseph IB, Isaacs JT: Macrophage role in the anti-prostate cancer response to one class of antiangiogenic agents. J Natl Cancer Inst 90: 1648–1653, 1998

82. Festuccia C, Teti A, Bianco P, Guerra F, Vicentini C, Tennina R, Villanova I, Sciortino G, Bologna M: Human prostatic tumor cells in culture produce growth and differentiation factors active on osteoblasts: a new biological and clinical parameter for prostatic carcinoma. Oncol Res 9: 419–431, 1997

83. Goltzman D: Mechanisms of the development of osteoblastic metastases. Cancer 80: 1581–1587, 1997

84. Konecny G, Untch M, Arboleda J, Wilson C, Kahlert S, Boettcher B, Felber M, Beryt M, Lude S, Hepp H, Slamon D, Pegram M: Her-2/neu and urokinase-type plasminogen activator and its inhibitor in breast cancer. Clin Cancer Res 7: 2448–2457, 2001

85. Konecny G, Untch M, Pihan A, Kimmig R, Gropp M, Stieber P, Hepp H, Slamon D, Pegram M: Association of urokinase-type plasminogen activator and its inhibitor with disease progression and prognosis in ovarian cancer. Clin Cancer Res 7: 1743–1749, 2001

86. Miseljic S, Galandiuk S, Myers SD, Wittliff JL: Expression of urokinase-type plasminogen activator and plasminogen activator inhibitor in colon disease. J Clin Lab Anal 9: 413–417, 1995

87. Pedersen AN, Christensen IJ, Stephens RW, Briand P, Mouridsen HT, Dano K, Brunner N: The complex between urokinase and its type-1 inhibitor in primary breast cancer: relation to survival. Cancer Res 60: 6927–6934, 2000

88. Pedersen AN, Hoyer-Hansen G, Brunner N, Clark GM, Larsen B, Poulsen HS, Dano K, Stephens RW: The complex between urokinase plasminogen activator and its type-1 inhibitor in breast cancer extracts quantitated by ELISA. J Immunol Methods 203: 55–65, 1997

89. Bajou K, Noel A, Gerard RD, Masson V, Brunner N, Holst-Hansen C, Skobe M, Fusenig NE, Carmeliet P, Collen D, Foidart JM: Absence of host plasminogen activator inhibitor 1 prevents cancer invasion and vascularization. Nat Med 4: 923–928, 1998

90. Gutierrez LS, Schulman A, Brito-Robinson T, Noria F, Ploplis VA, Castellino FJ: Tumor development is retarded in mice lacking the gene for urokinase-type plasminogen activator or its inhibitor, plasminogen activator inhibitor-1. Cancer Res 60: 5839–5847, 2000

91. Stephens RW, Brunner N, Janicke F, Schmitt M: The urokinase plasminogen activator system as a target for prognostic studies in breast cancer. Breast Cancer Res Treat 52: 99–111, 1998

92. Chambers SK, Ivins CM, Carcangiu ML: Expression of plasminogen activator inhibitor-2 in epithelial ovarian cancer: a favorable prognostic factor related to the actions of CSF-1. Int J Cancer 74: 571–575, 1997

93. Zou Z, Anisowicz A, Hendrix MJ, Thor A, Neveu M, Sheng S, Rafidi K, Seftor E, Sager R: Maspin, a serpin with tumor-suppressing activity in human mammary epithelial cells. Science 263: 526–529, 1994

94. Reddy KB, McGowen R, Schuger L, Visscher D, Sheng S: Maspin expression inversely correlates with breast tumor progression in MMTV/TGF-alpha transgenic mouse model. Oncogene 20: 6538–6543, 2001

95. Xia W, Lau YK, Hu MC, Li L, Johnston DA, Sheng Sj, El-Naggar A, Hung MC: High tumoral maspin expression is associated with improved survival of patients with oral squamous cell carcinoma. Oncogene 19: 2398–2403, 2000

96. Martin KJ, Kritzman BM, Price LM, Koh B, Kwan CP, Zhang X, Mackay A, O'Hare MJ, Kaelin CM, Mutter GL, Pardee AB, Sager R: Linking gene expression patterns to therapeutic groups in breast cancer. Cancer Res 60: 2232–2238, 2000.

97. Nykjaer A, Petersen CM, Moller B, Jensen PH, Moestrup SK, Holtet TL, Etzerodt M, Thogersen HC, Munch M, Andreasen PA: Purified alpha 2-macroglobulin receptor/LDL receptor-related protein binds urokinase plasminogen activator inhibitor type-1 complex. Evidence that the alpha 2-macroglobulin receptor mediates cellular degradation of urokinase receptor-bound complexes. J Biol Chem 267: 14543–14546, 1992

98. Kounnas MZ, Henkin J, Argraves WS, Strickland DK: Low density lipoprotein receptor-related protein/alpha 2-macroglobulin receptor mediates cellular uptake of pro-urokinase. J Biol Chem 268: 21862–21867, 1993

99. Zhang L, Strickland DK, Cines DB, Higazi AA: Regulation of single chain urokinase binding, internalization, and degradation by a plasminogen activator inhibitor 1-derived peptide. J Biol Chem 272: 27053–27057, 1997

160

100. Degryse B, Sier CF, Resnati M, Conese M, Blasi F: PAI-1 inhibits urokinase-induced chemotaxis by internalizing the urokinase receptor. FEBS Lett 505: 249–254, 2001

101. Biliran H Jr, Sheng S: Pleiotrophic Inhibition of Pericellular Urokinase-type Plasminogen Activator System by Endogenous Tumor Suppressive Maspin. Cancer Res (in press), 2001

102. Engelholm LH, Nielsen BS, Dano K, Behrendt N: The urokinase receptor associated protein (uPARAP/endo180): a novel internalization receptor connected to the plasminogen activation system. Trends Cardiovasc Med 11: 7–13, 2001

103. Stahl A, Mueller BM: The urokinase-type plasminogen activator receptor, a GPI-linked protein, is localized in caveolae. J Cell Biol 129: 335–344, 1995

104. Lu H, Mabilat C, Yeh P, Guitton JD, Li H, Pouchelet M, Shoevaert D, Legrand Y, Soria J, Soria C: Blockage of urokinase receptor reduces in vitro the motility and the deformability of endothelial cells. FEBS Lett 380: 21–24, 1996

105. Masucci MT, Pedersen N, Blasi F: A soluble, ligand binding mutant of the human urokinase plasminogen activator receptor. J Biol Chem 266: 8655–8658, 1991

106. Kobayashi H, Ohi H, Shinohara H, Sugimura M, Fujii T, Terao T, Schmitt M, Goretzki L, Chucholowski N, Janicke F: Saturation of tumour cell surface receptors for urokinase-type plasminogen activator by amino-terminal fragment and subsequent effect on reconstituted basement membranes invasion. Br J Cancer 67: 537–544, 1993

107. Slack JK, Adams RB, Rovin JD, Bissonette EA, Stoker CE, Parsons JT: Alterations in the focal adhesion kinase/Src signal transduction pathway correlate with increased migratory capacity of prostate carcinoma cells. Oncogene 20: 1152–1163, 2001

Address for offprints: Shijie Sheng, Department of Pathology, Wayne State University School of Medicine, 540 East Canfield Avenue, Detroit, MI 48201, USA; *Tel:* 313-993-8197; *Fax:* 313-993-4112; *e-mail:* ssheng@med.wayne.edu

Angiogenesis in prostate cancer: Biology and therapeutic opportunities

Brian Nicholson, Greg Schaefer and Dan Theodorescu
Department of Urology, University of Virginia, Charlottesville, VA, USA

Key words: angiogenesis, antiangiogenic, therapy, VEGF, prostate, cancer

Abstract

Tumor growth is limited in size without the incorporation of new blood vessels. Tumor cells release soluble factors (angiogenic factors) that induce neovascularization and allow subsequent growth beyond 2–3 mm in diameter meeting the need for cellular uptake of oxygen and nutrients. This process is referred to as the 'angiogenic switch' and indicates the acquisition of an angiogenic phenotype. Tumor angiogenesis requires an imbalance between proangiogenic and antiangiogenic factors with formation of new vessels being a highly regulated process. In this review we discuss the mediators of angiogenesis, the strategies for manipulating angiogenic factors, and possible therapeutic applications with a special emphasis on prostate cancer.

Introduction

Tumors are, 'hot, and red, and bloody' according to Dr. Judah Folkman, and it was with this observation that the field of angiogenesis began [1]. Decades of research led to a general recognition that tumor progression is critically dependent upon the tumor's ability to 'recruit (its) own private blood supply' [2]. Initially, the scientific establishment was slow to embrace this concept. Folkman suggests that the difficulties in understanding this hypothesis occurred because investigators relied too heavily upon data from histologic specimens, as opposed to identifying what occurs in the intact living organism. The field of cancer research still confronts the problem of translating *in vitro* experimentation into relevant tools for addressing the true biology of tumor growth.

Folkman's insight arose from experimentation performed after the United States Navy drafted him into service in 1960 [3]. The Navy asked Folkman et al. to develop a blood substitute that could be 'freeze-dried' like coffee and reconstituted with salt water. He and Dr. Frederick Becker developed a crude circulatory system, and found that a rabbit thyroid could survive within their system. Tumor cells placed into the system grew initially, but became quiescent after some time. When the thyroid-tumors were reinjected into the donor animal, they were startled to find that the cells had not in fact died – but rather the tumors resumed growth and also developed significant vascularization.

In 1973, Folkman published results showing that injection of human tumor cells into the rabbit cornea induced angiogenesis [4]. Surprisingly, another group showed that insertion of uric acid had a similar effect in this system which led Folkman to demonstrate that macrophage invasion, in response to the irritant led to vascularization. This example illustrates how administered agents or endogenous factors may regulate angiogenesis in either a direct or indirect fashion, or both. Conversely, it is important to identify whether therapeutic inhibitors of angiogenesis act directly, by recruiting secondary factors that subsequently regulate the angiogenic process, or whether they have a direct cytostatic or cytotoxic effect. Investigators often struggle to demonstrate that treatments actually act at the level of angiogenesis, rather than by tumor ablation via apoptosis or necrosis. Indeed, some effectors may inhibit angiogenesis and concomitantly suppress tumor growth. Additionally, because antiangiogenic therapy is often cytostatic, combination therapies with cytotoxic chemotherapies are being tested (which are showing some effectiveness in preclinical trials) and arguments exist on the proper endpoint for these studies.

M.L. Cher, K.V. Honn and A. Raz (eds.), Prostate Cancer: New Horizons in Research and Treatment, 161–183.
© 2002 *Kluwer Academic Publishers.*

Cancer angiogenesis

Tumor growth is limited in size without the incorporation of new blood vessels [5]. Cellular uptake of oxygen and nutrients occurs by diffusion in small avascular tumors, but tumor cells release soluble factors (angiogenic factors) that induce neovascularization and allow subsequent growth beyond 2–3 mm [6]. This process is referred to as the 'angiogenic switch' indicating the acquisition of an angiogenic phenotype [7]. Some reports indicate that tumor growth originating in vascular tissues may also co-opt existing blood vessels prior to the induction of tumor neovascularization [8]. Furthermore, some evidence suggests that developing tumors can use homeostatic mechanisms to their advantage to promote angiogenesis [9].

Angiogenesis, is a critical step for both continuous tumor growth and metastatic development [10]. It is a dynamic process of multiple, sequential, and integrated steps: degradation of the basement membrane surrounding capillaries, endothelial migration into the extracellular matrix (ECM) towards angiogenic stimuli, proliferation of endothelial cells, organization of endothelial cells into cylindrical structures, and capillary differentiation and fusion into a tubular network of new blood vessels [11]. Angiogenesis in tumors occurs due to an imbalance between proangiogenic and antiangiogenic factors (Table 1) [12]. Tumor cells may overexpress constitutive angiogenic factors or may respond to external stimuli, which

leads to changes in regulation concerning angiogenic factors.

Tumor cell migration into the circulatory system is directly related to the surface area of vessels within the tumor [13]. Phenotypically, newly formed vessels can be quite different from mature vessels as can tumor vasculature from vessels in normal tissues. For instance, vascular endothelial growth factor (VEGF) receptors are up-regulated in newly formed blood vessels [14], and elevated levels of staining by antibodies to the integrins $\alpha V\beta 3$ and $\alpha V\beta 5$ are found in tumor vessels when compared to normal vessels [15]. Further evidence is the heterogeneity of the ability of tumor endothelium to bind specific peptide sequences [16]. Interestingly, prostate-specific membrane antigen (PSMA) has been found to be present in tumor-associated neovasculature, including tumors from a non-prostatic origin, yet not in benign tissue vasculature [17].

Endothelia from different tissues are phenotypically distinct, and may respond differently to various regulators of angiogenesis [16]. Differential regulation of angiogenesis is tissue specific and is regulated by expression of cytokines and growth factors within the tissue microenvironment [18]. In addition, interactions between tumors and adjacent tissues with the surrounding ECM are particularly relevant in angiogenesis. These principles are exemplified by mouse models where human xenografts exhibit enhanced tumorigenesis, angiogenesis, and metastatic potential when grown in an orthotopic location, as opposed to heterotopically implanted tumor cells [19,20].

Table 1. Angiogenic factors in prostate cancer

	Proangiogenic	Antiangiogenic
Endogenous factors	Matrix metalloproteinases (MMPs)	Tissue inhibitor of metalloproteinase 1 (TIMP-1)
	Vascular endothelial growth factor (VEGF)	
	Basic fibroblast growth factor 2 (bFGF-2)	Interleukin-10 (IL-10)
	Fibroblast growth factor 4 (FGF-4)	Angiostatin
	Transforming growth factor β_1 (TGF-β_1)	Endostatin
	Interleukin 8 (IL-8)	
	Interleukin 6 (IL-6)	Prostate specific antigen (PSA)
	Interleukin 1β (IL-1β)	
	Cyclooxygenase 2 (COX-2)	Interferon (IFN)
	Nitric oxide (NO)	
	Tumor necrosis factor (TNF)	
	Insulin growth factor 1 (IGF-I)	
Pharmaceutical agents		Neutralizing antibodies
		MMP inhibitors
		Fumagillin analogue
		Linomide
		Carboxyamido-triazole

Assessing angiogenesis in the prostate: Microvessel density

Staining tissue with specific antiendothelial antibodies and subsequently counting the vessels under the microscope with a grid allows quantitation of small vessels immunohistochemically. Since the description of the endothelial cell–cell adhesion molecule PECAM-1 [21] and subsequent identification of the molecule in solid tumor cell lines, including the prostate cancer cell lines DU145 and PPC-1, anti-PECAM-1 [22] antibodies have been used to visualize microvessels in tumor specimens. Additional antibodies used in microvessel density (MVD) analysis include anti-Factor VIII-related antigen, anti-von Willebrand Factor (vWF), anti-CD34, and others [23]. An early study of MVD in specimens from 74 invasive prostate cancers, 29 of whom had metastatic disease, showed a significant correlation with cancers from patients with metastasis having nearly a 2-fold increase in MVD over cancers from patients with locally invasive disease. MVD also increased with Gleason score, but only in the poorly differentiated tumors [24]. Another study demonstrated increases in MVD between clinically localized prostate cancers and locally invasive or metastatic tumors. These authors also report that prostatic intraepithelial neoplasia in acini and ductules had increased microvascularity relative to benign epithelium in 18 of 25 tumors [25].

The MVD assay is somewhat subjective, as it relies upon the observer's eye to first find a 'hot spot' designated as the area with the greatest MVD, and then count the vessels. A recent study looked at the reproducibility of MVD quantitation by a single observer performing three repeated measurements on 60 specimens. They found that MVD counts were similar, with a reliability coefficient of 0.82. This same group evaluated 100 randomly selected radical prostatectomy specimens to evaluate the usefulness of MVD as a prognostic marker. Thirteen cases were excluded and the median follow-up time was 36 months. MVD using immunostaining with anti-PECAM-1 antibody in these 87 cases was not associated with Gleason sum, tumor stage, surgical margin status, or seminal vesicle invasion. MVD was also not associated with prostate specific antigen failure in the 20 (23%) patients who had a biochemical relapse during the 36-month median follow-up time [26].

A long-term study evaluated radical prostatectomy specimens from 42 patients who were not treated with adjuvant hormonal therapy, and who were followed until death. Pathologic specimens from these patients were immunohistochemically stained for p53, retinoblastoma, chromogranin A, and MVD assays were performed. Multivariate analysis revealed that p53 and retinoblastoma had the greatest prognostic importance regarding disease-specific survival and chromogranin A and MVD values were of no additional significance when p53 and retinoblastoma were assessed [27]. Contrasting these findings, many groups are finding that increased MVD does have some prognostic value in prostate cancer. One study evaluated both the mean and the maximal MVD in 64 consecutive radical prostatectomy specimens. Immunostaining against vWF and analysis by both a univariate and a multivariate method demonstrated that the maximal MVD, in contrast to the mean MVD, was significantly associated with survival in prostate cancer patients [28]. Another group reported on MVD by anti-Factor VIII-related antigen in 221 prostate needle biopsies from patients managed by watchful waiting. The median length of follow-up was 15 years and MVD was statistically significantly correlated with clinical stage ($p < 0.0001$) and histopathological grade ($p < 0.0001$). The authors also performed a multivariate analysis demonstrating that MVD was a significant predictor of disease-specific survival in the entire cancer population ($p = 0.0004$), as well as in the clinically localized cancer population ($p < 0.0001$) [29].

Bostwick et al. [30] reported on a multi-institutional study to determine the predictive power of an enhancement of MVD analysis in combination with Gleason score and serum prostatic specific antigen (PSA) to predict extraprostatic extension. This group evaluated randomly selected prostate needle biopsy specimens from 186 patients as well as matched samples from radical prostatectomy specimens. They used an automated digital image analysis system to measure microvessel morphology and to calculate the optimized microvessel density (OMVD) in the biopsy samples. Prediction of extraprostatic extension was increased significantly when OMVD analysis was added to Gleason score and pre-operative serum PSA concentration. Prediction by OMVD did not extend to outcome in patients with margin-free organ-confined prostate cancer with Gleason sums of 6–9.

Specimens from 147 radical prostatectomies were stained with an antibody against Factor VIII-related antigen using the OMVD method. Mean follow-up was 6 years with 58 patients demonstrating clinical or biochemical relapse; 12 patients died during this period but only one of these from prostate cancer. OMVD was not found to be significantly associated with DNA ploidy, Gleason grade, unilateral or bilateral disease, nor to pre-operative PSA. Similarly, OMVD was not a significant univariate or multivariate predictor of clinical or biochemical recurrence [31]. Contrasting this report is a study looking at the differences between anti-PECAM-1 and anti-CD34 MVD assays and their relationship to prostate specific antigen biochemical failure in 102 patients that underwent radical prostatectomy without adjuvant hormonal therapy. They found that the average MVD determined by CD31 staining was significantly lower than that obtained by CD34 staining. Using Kaplan–Meier analysis, anti-CD34 and anti-CD31 MVDs were associated strongly with PSA recurrence on a univariate level. However, only anti-CD34 MVD was an independent predictor of PSA failure [32]. It appears that the disparate results of the use of MVD as a prognostic indicator may be related to the different antibodies used.

Angiogenic mechanisms in prostate cancer

Although there are many factors have been shown to contribute to the angiogenic process, we have focused on those which have some association with prostate cancer angiogenesis. However, those that currently do not, may in the future be related to this tumor type.

Tumor suppressor genes

Although there exist reports linking up-regulation of VEGF to mutations of the tumor suppressor gene p53, in many different cancers, the only report to date on prostate cancer concludes that although VEGF expression correlated with tumor grade, stage, and clinical outcome, it was independent of p53 expression [33]. Inactivation of the tumor suppressor PTEN, however, has been detected in a minority of clinically localized prostate cancers, is common in metastatic disease, and is associated with increased angiogenesis in these tumors [34]. Interestingly, enhanced angiogenesis in this study did not rely on reduction of thrombospondin 1 expression as had previously been reported in gliomas cells *in vitro* [35].

Stromal-epithelial interactions and hypoxia-induced angiogenesis

The interactions between prostate cancer and the surrounding stroma have long been appreciated [36].

Stromal fibroblasts, co-inoculated with the human prostate cancer cell line PC-3, in three-dimensional culture are required for angiogenesis [37]. Additionally, normal human prostate epithelial cells have been shown to express a variety of cytokines with angiogenic and/or endothelial cell-activating properties [38]. Prostate cancer cells have also been shown to express angiogenic factors, most notably VEGF and interleukin-8 (IL-8) [39]. Further evidence is seen in endothelial cell cultures that are stimulated by the addition of conditioned medium or grown in co-culture with prostate cancer cells [40].

Hypoxia is known to induce expression of the hypoxia-inducible factor-1 (HIF-1) [41], which has been shown to increase growth rate and metastatic ability in prostate cancer cells independent of the oxygen tension in the cellular environment [42]. Furthermore, one immunohistochemical study found that HIF-1 protein levels are higher, relative to normal tissue, in 13 of 19 tumor types, including prostate cancer [43]. A recent report demonstrates that hypoxia can up-regulate expression of VEGF in prostate cancer *in vitro* [44]. Zhong et al. [45] have linked the signal transduction pathway from receptor tyrosine kinases to phosphatidylinositol 3-kinase (PI3K), AKT (protein kinase B), and its effector FKBP-rapamycin-associated protein (FRAP), which occurs via autocrine stimulation or inactivation of the tumor suppressor, and VEGF-induced angiogenesis in prostate cancer. Growth factor- and mitogen-induced secretion of VEGF, the product of a known HIF-1 target gene, was inhibited by LY294002 and rapamycin, inhibitors of PI3K and FRAP, respectively, in an *in vitro* prostate cancer system. Cyclooxygenase-2 (COX-2), an inducible enzyme that catalyzes the formation of prostaglandins from arachidonic acid, has been demonstrated to be induced by hypoxia. The up-regulation of VEGF in PC-3ML human prostate cancer cells is accompanied by a persistent induction of COX-2 mRNA and protein and is significantly suppressed following exposure to NS398, a selective COX-2 inhibitor [46].

Androgen and macrophage regulation

Androgens are involved in regulating the blood flow *in vivo* in both the normal rat ventral prostate and in the Dunning tumor rat model [47,48]. Castration, one form of antiandrogen therapy that is widely utilized in patients with advanced prostate cancer, has been shown to inhibit VEGF expression and induce apoptosis of endothelial cells preceding the apoptosis of tumor cells in an *in vivo* model [49]. Chemical castration 7–28 days prior to radical prostatectomy, results in tremendous recruitment of inflammatory cells, as well as induction of apoptosis, in the resected histologic specimens. Tumor-associated macrophages (TAMs), one such inflammatory cell, play an important role in tumor angiogenesis [50], and reduced infiltration of TAMs has been associated with prostate cancer progression [51]. TAMs have the capability to influence each phase of the angiogenic process, such as alterations of the local ECM, induction of endothelial cells to migrate or proliferate, and inhibition of vascular growth with formation of differentiated capillaries [52]. Other studies have demonstrated that castration inhibited prostate tumor VEGF production, but had no effect on other angiogenic factors [53].

Proteinases acting on the extracellular matrix

Two families of proteinases, plasminogen activators (PAs) and matrix metalloproteinases (MMPs), are implicated in the degradation of the basement membrane [54]. Urokinase type plasminogen activator (uPA), a PA family proteinase, and its receptor (uPAR) are expressed in aggressive human prostate cancer cell lines DU145 and PC-3 and are absent in the less aggressive LNCaP cell line [55]. Furthermore, blocking the uPA receptor inhibits tumor growth and neovascularization in prostate cancer cells [56]. *In vitro*, the primary human prostate cancer cell line 1013L was found to express no uPA, while DU145, a cell line derived from a metastatic lesion, expressed high levels of uPA. Using a Xenograft mouse model, 1013L tumor homogenates had hardly detectable levels of uPA, that is, 300-fold lower than were found in the invasive prostate xenograft DU145 [57]. The human prostate carcinoma cells PC-3, DU145, and LNCaP also express enzymatic activity converting plasminogen to the endogenous inhibitor of angiogenesis angiostatin [58]. It has been demonstrated that basic fibroblast growth factor (bFGF), besides stimulating uPA production by vascular endothelial cells, also increases the production of receptors, which modulates their capacity to focalize this enzyme on the cell surface [59].

The type IV collagenases MMP-9 and MMP-2 are also involved in basement membrane degradation [60]. Radical prostatectomy specimens from 40 patients were examined using rapid colorimetric *in situ* hybridization technique to evaluate the expression level of E-cadherin and MMPs types 2 and 9. While E-cadherin stained in a more central region of the tumor, both MMPs predominately stained at the leading edges of the tumor. Decreased expression of E-cadherin, as well as increased expression of MMP-2 and MMP-9 was significantly associated with the Gleason score of the tumors. The authors also found that irrespective of serum PSA level or Gleason score, the ratio between expression of MMPs and E-cadherin at the invasive edge of tumors exhibited the strongest association with non-organ-confined prostate cancer. Perhaps E-cadherin and MMPs expression levels could be useful to delineate organ-confined and non-organ-confined disease [61]. MMP-9 and MMP-2 have both been demonstrated to be regulated by transforming growth factor beta 1 (TGF-β_1) in prostate cancer cell lines [62]. MMP-2 and TGF-β_1 expression were both demonstrated to be directly related to the angiogenic and metastatic phenotype in the aggressive PC-3ML cell line. Inhibition of this phenotype was effected by IL-10, which has been shown to induce the tissue inhibitor of metalloproteinase-1 (TIMP-1) [63]. Further studies linked TGF-β_1 and IL-10 regulation and demonstrated that TGF-β_1 transfected cells had greater metastatic growth and that these tumors stained poorly for IL-10 [64].

Vascular endothelial growth factor

VEGF, otherwise known as vascular permeability factor, was first described by Senger et al. in 1983 [65]. The gene encoding VEGF resides on chromosome 6p21.3 with a coding region that spans approximately 14,000 bases. The human VEGF gene contains eight exons and at least six isoforms of the protein are found secondary to alternative splicing of the mRNA. All six spliced mRNAs are homologous in exons 1–5 and in exon 8, but differ due to variation in exons 6 and 7. The resulting isoforms are named VEGF plus the amino acid content of the protein: $VEGF_{121}$, $VEGF_{145}$, $VEGF_{165}$, $VEGF_{183}$, $VEGF_{189}$, and $VEGF_{206}$ [66]. VEGF isoforms are secreted as homodimers of the cysteine-knot superfamily and show greatest similarity to the platelet-derived growth factor (PDGF) family [67]. VEGF binds three tyrosine kinase receptors; exon 3 codes for three acidic residues that binds the fms-like tyrosine kinase-3 receptor (Flt-1 or VEGFR-1), while three basic amino acid residues encoded in exon 4 bind the kinase insert domain-containing receptor/fetal liver kinase 1 (KDR/Flk-1 or VEGFR-2) [68,69]. Flt-4 (VEGFR-3) is related to VEGFR-1 and VEGFR-2 but is only found in embryonic lymphatic endothelium [70].

Three isoforms of VEGF (VEGF$_{121}$, VEGF$_{165}$, and VEGF$_{189}$) are preferentially expressed in VEGF-producing cells [71]. VEGF$_{165}$ has a moderate affinity for heparin via a heparin-binding domain, while VEGF$_{121}$ lacks the heparin-binding region [72]. Therefore, while VEGF$_{121}$ is freely secreted, VEGF$_{165}$ remains mostly associated with cells and the ECM, likely due to interactions with heparan sulfate proteoglycans (HSPGs) [73]. Similarly, VEGF$_{189}$ and VEGF$_{206}$ have additional heparin-binding domains and are completely sequestered to the ECM and cell surface [74]. It has been demonstrated that recombinant VEGF$_{189}$ and VEGF$_{206}$ were unable to stimulate endothelial cell proliferation, while recombinant VEGF$_{121}$ and VEGF$_{165}$ did induce endothelial proliferation [75]. More recently, VEGF$_{189}$ has been shown to exert its biological effects by stimulating the FGF pathway [76]. Additional growth factors belonging to the VEGF family, which share common receptors with VEGF have been discovered. The discovery of placenta growth factor (PlGF) [77] was followed by the recent discovery of four additional growth factors belonging to the VEGF family (VEGF B–E) [78–81].

During angiogenesis, endothelial cells are switched from a resting state to one of rapid growth by diffusible factors secreted by tumor cells [11]. VEGF was the first selective angiogenic growth factor to be purified, and is still a preeminent molecule in this area [82]. Many human tumor biopsies exhibit enhanced expression of VEGF mRNAs by malignant cells and VEGF receptor mRNAs in adjacent endothelial cells. Abrogation of VEGF function with monoclonal anti-VEGF antibodies results in complete suppression of prostate cancer induced angiogenesis and prevents tumor growth beyond the initial prevascular growth phase [83]. Immunohistochemical (IHC) studies [84] have demonstrated that in human prostate cancer tissues, the cancer cells stained positively for VEGF and this correlated with MVD. On the other hand, benign prostatic hyperplasia (BPH) and normal prostate cells displayed little VEGF staining and vascularity [39]. Finally, increased VEGF expression [85] has been related to neuroendocrine differentiation in prostate cancer, a known poor prognostic factor for survival [86]. Taken together, these data suggest that the prostate tumor growth advantage conferred by VEGF

expression appears to be a consequence of stimulation of angiogenesis.

VEGF expression is mediated by a plethora of external factors such as hypoxia, growth factors and cytokines. Regulation of VEGF can occur at transcriptional [87], post transcriptional [88], and translational levels [89]. Cytokines, growth factors, and gonadotropins that do not stimulate angiogenesis directly can modulate angiogenesis by modulating VEGF expression in specific cell types, and thus exert an indirect angiogenic or antiangiogenic effect [18]. Factors that can potentiate VEGF production include fibroblast growth factor 2 (FGF-2) [90], fibroblast growth factor 4 (FGF-4) [91], PDGF [92], tumor necrosis factor (TNF) [93], transforming growth factor β (TGF-β) [94], insulin growth factor 1 (IGF-I) [95], interleukin 1β (IL-1β) [96], and IL-6 [97]. Reciprocal regulation between VEGF and the small molecule nitric oxide (NO) exists; NO up-regulates VEGF and the production of VEGF in turn up-regulates NO, indicating that a positive feedback loop exists between these two factors [98]. In addition, NO contributes to the blood vessel-permeabilizing effects of VEGF and to VEGF-stimulated vasodilatation. NO synthetase-2 has recently been reported to have an elevated expression by immunohistochemistry in both prostate cancer and prostatic intraepithelial neoplasia as compared to normal prostate tissue, albeit in a small study [99].

While the soluble factors and other stimuli mentioned above are known to induce VEGF transcription, the exact signaling intermediates used in this process are less well defined. Recently, several papers have shed some light on this issue and have implicated the Ras, Raf, and Src gene products as VEGF signaling intermediates [100]. Overexpression of activated forms of these genes, is associated with marked elevation of both VEGF mRNA and secreted functional protein levels [101]. Tumorigenic VEGF expression is critical for Ras-mediated tumorigenesis, and the loss of tumorigenic expression causes dramatic decreases in vascular density and permeability and increases in tumor cell apoptosis [102]. While Ras, Raf, and Src activating mutations are unusual in human prostate cancer, this does not in any way detract from their possible role as a major signaling molecules whose circuits can be corrupted in prostate cancer [103]. Thus, any factor that stimulates Ras, Raf, and Src mediated signaling pathways may contribute to the growth of a solid tumor by a direct effect on tumor cell proliferation and indirectly, by facilitating tumor angiogenesis via the induction of

VEGF. Additionally, VEGF transcription can also be regulated by cell surface contacts mediated by either cell–cell or cell–ECM interactions. A novel regulatory pathway mediating this effect was shown to involve focal adhesion kinase (FAK), Src, phosphatidylinositol 3 kinase (PI3K), Raf, and MAPK kinase (MEK) in a Ras-independent manner. This third major avenue of VEGF regulation may serve to explain a number of fundamental issues in prostate cancer biology such as the organ tropism of prostate cancer metastasis [104].

Devising a novel 'confrontation culture' system, using small clusters of both embryonic stem cells and the human prostate cancer line DU145, Wartenberg et al. [105] were able to demonstrate 'vascularization' of prostate spheroids mediated by the stem cells. In the confrontation culture, protein levels of VEGF and HIF-1 rose until approximately the same day that vascularization became evident. When vascularization became clearly visible, levels of both proteins had fallen to approximately 20–30% of their day 3 peak levels. VEGF and the platelet endothelial cell adhesion molecule (PECAM) staining were most pronounced at the point where the embryoid body contacted the DU145 tumor spheroid. Interestingly, while the authors found that the partial pressure of oxygen in the vascularized spheroid was lower than that in the avascular spheroid, evidence of central necrosis disappeared when vascularization was present. The authors therefore suggest that central necrosis in the avascular spheroid may not be exclusively due to the hypoxic conditions at the tumor center.

A transgenic adenocarcinoma of the mouse prostate (TRAMP mouse) was developed by insertion of the SV40 T antigen gene under a prostate-specific promoter into the germ line of mice. Heterozygous animals develop well-differentiated prostate tumors from between 10 and 16 weeks, and progression to both poorly differentiated primary prostatic tumors and metastatic lesions occur at 18–24 weeks. In this model system the temporal and spatial expression patterns of PECAM, HIF-1, VEGF, and the cognate receptors VEGFR-1 and VEGFR-2 were characterized. IHC and *in situ* analyses of prostate tissue specimens identified a distinct early angiogenic switch consistent with the expression of PECAM-1, HIF-1, and VEGFR-1 and the recruitment of new vasculature to lesions representative of high-grade prostatic intra epithelial neoplasia (PIN) HIF-1 expression localized to the nucleus correlating with and possibly preceding VEGF expression. Furthermore, expression of the VEGF-165 isoform was not seen in normal prostate, high-

grade PIN, or moderately to well differentiated prostate adenocarcinoma, but was found in poorly differentiated prostate cancers. The authors further demonstrated a distinct late angiogenic switch consistent with decreased expression of VEGFR-1, increased expression of VEGFR-2, and the transition from a differentiated adenocarcinoma to a more poorly differentiated state [106].

Studies have evaluated the expression of VEGF in LNCaP, which does not exhibit a metastatic phenotype, and two of its derivatives: LNCaP-Pro5 (slightly metastatic) and LNCaP-LN3 (highly metastatic) after orthotopic implantation into athymic nude mice. *In vitro*, VEGF production by LNCaP-LN3 was significantly higher than those of both LNCaP and LNCaP-Pro5 cells. *In vivo*, LNCaP-LN3 tumors exhibited higher levels of VEGF mRNA and protein as well as VEGFR-2 protein and had higher MVD than either LNCaP tumors or LNCaP-Pro5 tumors. The authors conclude that metastatic human prostate cancer cells exhibited enhanced VEGF production and tumor vascularity compared with prostate cancer cells of lower metastatic potential [107]. Two other prostate cancer cell lines were evaluated for VEGF expression by enzyme-linked immunosorbent assay (ELISA) by yet another group. Orthotopic implantation of PC-3M (highly metastatic) and DU145 (poorly metastatic) was performed in nude mice. They found that angiogenesis was much more evident in PC-3M tumors as compared with DU145 tumors, but ELISA-determined VEGF levels were approximately 3-fold higher in both DU145 cell tumors, and in the conditioned media of DU145 cells. To characterize this apparent contradiction, they then detected VEGF isoforms by Western blotting in both solid tumor extracts, and in culture medium conditioned by the same cell lines. Western blotting showed that PC-3M tumors, but not conditioned media, contained VEGF isoforms not identified by an ELISA antibody raised against the VEGF$_{165}$ isoform. Other isoforms of VEGF may therefore be predominate in PC-3M cells [108].

Finally, one study sought to determine whether tumor overexpression of VEGF is causally related to organ specific tumor growth in bone using a prostate cancer xenograft model. Transfection of the LNCaP derivative C4-2, which is modestly tumorigenic and metastasizes preferentially to bone, with a full-length cDNA encoding VEGF$_{165}$, did not seem to affect *in vitro* cell growth. Although such overexpression did affect tumorigenicity and *in vivo* tumor growth rates when cells were inoculated subcutaneously, no such effect was observed when cells were inoculated orthotopically or into intrafemoral sites. These results suggest that the biological impact of prostate tumor VEGF overexpression is organ/site specific, leading to the speculation that it may play a part in the observed organ tropism of metastatic spread [109].

Basic fibroblast growth factor (bFGF)

The gene for bFGF is located at 4q25–q27, while the protein consists of 155 amino acids. Dimerization occurs when bound to the tyrosine kinase FGF receptor 1 (flg) that requires bFGF binding to cell surface HSPGs. The rabbit corneal model has been used to demonstrate a dose-dependent induction of angiogenesis in response to bFGF [110]. VEGF and bFGF have been shown to be synergistic for induction of angiogenesis. Microvascular endothelial cells grown on the surface of three-dimensional collagen gels were stimulated with VEGF and/or bFGF and induces the cells to invade the underlying matrix and to form capillary-like tubules; bFGF was found to be twice as potent, at equimolar concentrations, as VEGF for stimulating angiogenesis. VEGF and bFGF together, induced an *in vitro* angiogenic response that was far greater than additive, and which occurred with greater rapidity than the response to either cytokine alone [111]. Comparisons in bFGF and its receptor (flg) expression were performed on prostate cancer cell lines. Androgen-sensitive and nonmetastatic LNCaP cells did not produce measurable amounts of bFGF, expressed small but measurable amounts of FGF receptor mRNA, and did respond to exogenous bFGF. Androgen-independent, but moderately metastatic DU145 cells did produce measurable amounts of biologically active bFGF, expressed large amounts of FGF receptor mRNA, and responded to exogenous bFGF. While the androgen-independent and highly metastatic PC-3 cells also produced measurable amounts of bFGF, but did not demonstrate a growth response to exogenous bFGF even though large amounts of FGF receptor mRNA were expressed [112]. Another study utilized co-culture of LNCaP cells with bFGF-dependent human adrenal carcinoma SW-13 cell line as target cells. They found that LNCaP cells stimulated SW-13 cell growth, that this stimulation was magnified in androgen-treated LNCaP cells, that specific anti-bFGF antibodies inhibited the LNCaP stimulated growth of SW-13 cells, and that no proliferation of SW-13 cells occurred in the absence of LNCaP cells. These

data suggest that androgen may regulate bFGF secretion by LNCaP cells *in vitro* [113]. Orthotopic tumors from PC-3M and DU145 cells were evaluated by ELISA for bFGF levels and the more aggressive PC-3M cell line, which was more angiogenic, displayed greater staining than the less aggressive DU145 cell line [108].

Studies evaluating the usefulness of measuring urinary and serum VEGF and bFGF levels have shown no correlation with prognosis and have been found to be less useful than serum PSA measurements [114,115]. Reverse transcription polymerase chain reaction (RT-PCR) with primer sets for FGF-3, FGF-4, and FGF-6 was performed on 26 prostate cancer RNA samples. As opposed to normal prostate RNA, in which these FGF factors are not amplified, 14 of 26 samples expressed FGF-6 while no amplification of either FGF-3 or FGF-4 was detected. Further analysis by ELISA with a specific antibody against FGF-6 showed an absence of the factor in normal prostate, but was elevated in 4 of 9 PIN lesions and in 15 of 24 prostate cancers. IHC analysis with anti-FGF-6 antibody revealed weak staining of prostatic basal cells in normal prostate, but was markedly elevated in PIN lesions. In the prostate cancers, the majority of cases revealed expression of FGF-6 in the prostate cancer cells, in two cases, expression was present in prostatic stromal cells. The authors then found that exogenous FGF-6 was able to stimulate proliferation of primary prostatic epithelial and stromal cells, immortalized prostatic epithelial cells, and prostate cancer cell lines in tissue culture. They conclude that FGF-6 is increased in PIN lesions and prostate cancer and can promote the proliferation of the transformed prostatic epithelial cells via paracrine and autocrine mechanisms [116].

Transforming growth factor beta 1

TGF-β is a known inhibitor of the growth of epithelial cells, in a cytostatic manner, but may stimulate the growth of stromal cells, such as fibroblasts. Indeed the growth of prostate cancer cells *in vitro* are also inhibited by TGF-β_1 under restrictive conditions, however this inhibition may be overcome with the addition of growth factors or in the presence of ECM components [117]. Prostate cancer cells *in vivo* do secrete TGF-β_1 but seem to acquire resistance to this inhibition as they progress to more aggressive phenotypes. Overproduction of TGF-β_1 and loss of TGF-β receptor type II expression has been shown to be associated with poor clinical outcome in prostate cancer and

TGF-β_1 expression correlated with tumor vascularity, tumor grade, and metastasis [118]. Therefore, resistance to TGF-β_1 growth inhibition as well as TGF-β_1 stimulated angiogenesis and metastasis may explain this apparent paradox. IHC studies have localized TGF-β_1, to intracellular and extracellular locations, in prostate cancer as well as benign prostatic hypertrophy. Extracellular and epithelial cell staining were found to be more extensive in prostate cancer versus benign prostatic hypertrophy samples, and conversely, staining was more extensive intracellularly and in stromal cells in benign prostatic hypertrophy when compared to prostate cancer [119]. Similar results were shown by a group comparing prostate tissue from local and metastatic prostate cancers with the additional finding of increased intracellular staining in patients with lymph node involvement when compared to patients with localized disease [120].

A mechanism for prostate cancer to escape the inhibitory regulation by TGF-β_1 was proposed by IHC studies on 2 of the 3 receptors for this factor. TGF-β type I and type II receptors were localized to epithelial cells in 8 specimens of benign prostatic hypertrophy, but in 32 specimens of prostate cancer loss of staining in 4 samples for type II receptor and in 8 samples in type I receptors was found [121]. These data were corroborated in another study that also noted decreasing expression of type II receptors significantly related to increasing histological grade of tumors [122]. Evaluation of TGF-β receptors in primary tumors and lymph node metastases displayed weak IHC staining as compared to normal prostate and lack of staining for both type I and type II receptors in 25% and 45% of samples, respectively. Further analysis of mRNA by RT-PCR and Northern blotting revealed decreased expression of both type I and type II receptors secondary to down-regulation of gene transcription [123]. The expression of TGF-β_1 in several rat prostate adenocarcinoma models was also evaluated by Northern blotting. TGF-β_1 mRNA levels were demonstrated to be much higher in rat prostate adenocarcinomas (Dunning R3327 Mat-LyLu, AT2, G, HI, and H sublines) than in normal prostate. Additionally, TGF-β_1 mRNA levels were found to be unchanged 2 weeks after castration [124].

Interleukin 8

IL-8 has been shown to be a macrophage-derived mediator of angiogenesis. It is a promoter of angiogenesis in the rat cornea model and is a chemotactic and mitogenic factor for human endothelial cells from the umbilical vein [125]. IL-8 expression in normal human prostate epithelial cells has been demonstrated by RT-PCR, as well as in conditioned media by ELISA [38]. Ferrer et al. [39,84] compared VEGF expression with that of IL-8 in human prostate cancer cells. *Ex vivo* IHC staining of human prostate cancer specimens, benign prostatic hypertrophy, and normal prostate tissues showed that adenocarcinoma cells stained positively for VEGF (20 of 25 slides) and IL-8 (25 of 25 slides), while benign prostatic hypertrophy and normal prostate cells displayed little staining for either angiogenesis factor. IL-8 was present throughout the cytoplasm of cancer cells and no difference in staining pattern between tumors of different Gleason grade was noted. Additionally, DU145 cells grown in culture were stimulated with cytokines showed induction of both VEGF and IL-8. Interestingly, cytokine stimulation of DU145 cells resulted in differential stimulation, whereby TNF was the predominantly induced VEGF and IL-1 was the predominant inducer of IL-8 [39]. Another *in vitro* study on the highly metastatic human PC-3M-LN4 prostate cancer cell lines measured IL-8 mRNA by Northern blot and colorimetric *in situ* hybridization techniques. Highly metastatic cell lines constitutively and uniformly expressed higher levels of IL-8 when compared to parenteral PC-3M cells or poorly metastatic cell lines. The authors also showed that prostate cancer cells implanted subcutaneously expressed less IL-8 mRNA than cells implanted orthotopically, indicating that the expression of these genes was dependent on the organ environment [126].

A different group performed studies on the highly metastatic PC-3M-LN4 cell line, which overexpresses IL-8 and the poorly metastatic PC-3P cell line that expresses relatively low amounts of IL-8. They transfected PC-3P cells with the full-length sense IL-8 cDNA, whereas PC-3M-LN4 cells were transfected with the full-sequence antisense IL-8 cDNA. *In vitro*, sense-transfected PC-3P cells overexpressed IL-8 mRNA and protein, which resulted in up-regulation of MMP-9 mRNA, and collagenase activity, resulting in increased invasion through Matrigel. Antisense IL-8 cDNA transfection of the PC-3M-LN4 cells greatly reduced IL-8 and MMP-9 expression, collagenase activity, and invasion. After orthotopic implantation into athymic nude mice, the sense-transfected PC-3P cells were highly tumorigenic and metastatic, and displayed significantly increased neovascularity and IL-8 expression, when compared with either PC-3P cells or controls [127].

Cyclooxygenase-2

Cyclooxygenase is involved in hypoxia-induced angiogenesis through interactions with VEGF, as previously mentioned; however, some evidence exists to suggest that inhibition of this factor may also induce apoptosis in prostate cancer cells, although this relationship with angiogenesis is undefined [128]. IHC staining of 30 samples of benign prostatic hypertrophy and 82 samples of prostate cancer revealed that for both benign prostatic hypertrophy and prostate cancer, COX-1 expression was primarily in the fibromuscular stroma, with variable weak cytoplasmic expression in glandular neoplastic epithelial cells. In contrast, COX-2 expression differed markedly between benign prostatic hypertrophy and cancer; in benign prostatic hypertrophy membranous expression of COX-2 in luminal glandular cells was found, but without stromal expression. In cancer, the stromal expression of COX-2 was unaltered, but expression by tumor cells was significantly greater with a change in the staining pattern from membranous to cytoplasmic. Additionally, COX-2 expression was significantly higher in poorly differentiated than in well-differentiated tumors. Immunoblotting confirmed these results as four times greater expression of COX-2 in cancer than in benign prostatic hypertrophy was demonstrated [129].

Antiangiogenic mechanisms and therapy in prostate cancer

The rationale behind interrupting angiogenesis is based on tumors' requirement of this process for proliferation and metastasis. Three basic strategies are used to inhibit tumor angiogenesis with the goals of preventing further growth of tumors or perhaps inducing tumor regression and diminishing or eliminating the ability of a tumor to metastasize. Although antiangiogenesis therapy has long been considered merely antiproliferative, a study using the antiangiogenic molecule angiostatin, which inhibits endothelial cell response to angiogenic therapy, was able to cause regression in three human and three murine primary carcinomas in mice, without apparent toxicity. The human carcinomas regressed to microscopic dormant foci in which tumor cell proliferation was balanced by apoptosis, a state termed dormancy,

in the presence of blocked angiogenesis [130]. It may therefore be possible to cause tumor regression with prolonged antiangiogenic therapy. Therapeutic strategies include inhibiting the release of proangiogenic molecules by tumor cells or cells surrounding tumors, inhibiting the angiogenic stimulating action of these molecules, and inhibiting the endothelial cell response to proangiogenic molecules. Another approach would be delivery or induction of endogenous antiangiogenic molecules. Furthermore, therapies may either target the tumor or supporting cells directly, or may target the endothelial cells. Modulating the endothelial cells has the advantages of easy drug delivery from an intravenous route and decreased likelihood of endothelial cell alterations which may lead to resistance to the therapy.

Matrix metalloproteinase inhibitors

The tissue inhibitors of MMPs are secreted by epithelial cells and are in part stimulated by IL-6 and IL-10 [131]. Levels of MMPs and TIMPs secreted by epithelial cultures of normal, benign, and malignant prostate were compared in an early study. Analysis of conditioned media showed both normal and prostate cancer tissues grown in culture secreted latent and active forms of both MMP-2 and MMP-9. Normal juvenile and adult prostates secreted significant amounts of free TIMPs, but they were either markedly reduced or not detectable in conditioned media from neoplastic tissues [132]. IHC staining of fetal and normal prostate tissues, benign prostatic hyperplasia and prostate cancer showed TIMP-1 and TIMP-2 were expressed at elevated levels in the stroma of Gleason sum 5 tissues, while in higher Gleason sum tissues (8–10), TIMP-1 and TIMP-2 were not expressed. Furthermore, TIMP-1 and TIMP-2 expression was high in organ-confined specimens, somewhat lower in specimens with capsular penetration, and low or negative in samples with positive surgical margins or seminal vesicle involvement and lymph node metastases [133]. Cocultures of prostate cancer cells derived from primary and metastatic tumors with primary or immortalized stromal cells showed enhanced levels of pro-MMP-9 and reduced levels of TIMP-1 and TIMP-2. Enhanced expression of pro-MMP-9 occurred in prostate cancer cells and the TIMPs were down-regulated in stromal cells. Furthermore, induction of pro-MMP-9 and reduction of TIMP expression did not require cell–cell contact and were mediated by a soluble factor(s) present in the conditioned medium of the effector cell [134].

IL-10 treatment of PC-3ML cell tumors in the severe combined immunodeficiency (SCID) mouse model was an effective inhibitor of spinal metastasis and increased tumor-free survival rates. IL-10 treatment of the PC-3 ML cells and the SCID mice reduced the number of spinal metastases from 70% seen in the natural progression of the model to 5% of the mice. Additionally, following discontinuation of IL-10 treatment after 30 days, the mice remained tumor-free and mouse survival rates increased dramatically, from less than 30% in untreated mice to about 85% in IL-10-treated mice. To further delineate the mechanism behind these findings, the authors measured expression of MMPs and TIMPs by ELISA in IL-10 treated PC-3ML cells. IL-10 treatment of the PC-3 ML cells down-regulated MMP-2 and MMP-9 while up-regulating TIMP-1, but not TIMP-2, expression. IL-10-treated mice exhibited similar changes in MMP-2, MMP-9, and TIMP-1 expression. Lastly, IL-10 receptor antibodies blocked the IL-10 effects on PC-3ML cells [135]. Alendronate, a potent bisphosphonate compound has been shown to inhibit TGF-β_1 induced MMP-2 secretion in PC-3ML cells, while TIMP-2 secretion was unaffected. The relative imbalance between the molar stoichiometry of TIMP-2 to MMP-2 resulted in decreased collagen solubilization [136].

Several well tolerated, orally active MMP inhibitors (MMPIs) have been generated that demonstrate efficacy in mouse cancer models. Marimastat (BB-2516) was the first MMPI to have entered clinical trials in the field of oncology and has completed phase I [137] and phase II trials in prostate and colon cancer patients. Marimastat was generally well tolerated in phase I trials and phase II trials used serum PSA as a marker in patients with prostate cancer. The authors reported a 58% response rate (no increase in serum PSA over the course of the study plus partial response defined as 0–25% increase in serum PSA per 4 weeks) using doses of greater than 50 mg twice daily [138]. Another MMPI batimastat (BB-94) was demonstrated to inhibit invasion of DU145 cells in Matrigel and in a murine diaphragm invasion assay [139]. Another in vitro study looked at the effect of batimastat on Mat-LyLu cancer cells and went on to describe its in vivo effect on tumor growth in the orthotopic cancer R3327 Dunning tumor rat model. Significant inhibition of tumor cell proliferation in vitro occurred and after orthotopic cell inoculation, tumors grew to mean weights of almost one-half the weight of the control group [140]. Other MMPIs

have been developed, are in various stages of preclinical and clinical trials, and include Bay 12-9566 and prinomastat (Ag3340).

Overexpression of uPA by the rat prostate-cancer cell line Dunning R3227, Mat-LyLu, results in increased tumor metastasis to several sites. Histological examination of skeletal lesions has shown them to be primarily osteoblastic. A selective inhibitor of uPA enzymatic activity, 4-iodo benzo(b)thiophene-2-carboxamidine (B-428) was used in this model resulted in a marked decrease in primary tumor volume and weight as well as in the development of tumor metastases when compared with controls [141]. In a similar study, a mutant recombinant murine uPA, that retains receptor binding but not proteolytic activity, was made by polymerase chain reaction mutagenesis and transfected into the highly metastatic rat Dunning Mat-LyLu prostate cancer cell line. A clone stably expressing uPA was injected into Copenhagen rats and tumors found in these animals were significantly smaller with fewer metastases than in control animals. Additionally, mean MVD in transfected tumors was 4-fold lower than that in animals with tumors derived from the control tumor cell line [56]. These studies demonstrate that uPA-specific inhibitors can decrease primary tumor volume and invasiveness as well as metastasis in a model of prostate cancer. To determine the effect bone cells have on prostate cancer cell expression of basement membrane degrading proteins, serum-free conditioned medium harvested from osteoblast cultures was used to stimulate the in vitro chemotaxis of prostate cancer cells and invasion of a reconstituted basement membrane (Matrigel). This enhanced invasive activity was due to osteoblast cell conditioned media stimulated secretion of uPA and matrix MMP-9. Additionally, inhibition of these matrix-degrading proteases by neutralizing antibodies or by inhibitors of their catalytic activity reduced Matrigel invasion. Thus demonstrating that factors produced during osteogenesis by bone cells stimulates prostate cancer cell chemotaxis and matrix proteases expression, thus representing potential targets for alternative therapies deterring the progression of prostate cancer metastasis to bone [142].

The work of Stearns et al. [63] has demonstrated that antibodies to MMP-2 and MMP-9 inhibit induction of microvessel formation in vitro. MMP-9 expression is partly inhibited by anti-alpha-2-integrin antibody, a major collagen I receptor [134]. Since MMPs are involved primarily in the initial stages of angiogenesis, therapies against these molecules would probably best be used early in cancer development or metastasis.

Angiostatin

Angiostatin is a circulating inhibitor of angiogenesis, first discovered in the presence of a murine Lewis lung tumor. A mouse corneal neovascularization model stimulated by a bFGF pellet detected circulating inhibitors of angiogenesis generated by PC-3 human prostate carcinoma grown in immunodeficient mice. These mice demonstrated significant inhibition of angiogenesis in the cornea, significant inhibition of vessel length, clock-hours of neovascularization, and vessel density [143]. A mechanism behind angiostatin generation in human prostate carcinoma cell lines (PC-3, DU145, and LNCaP) was found in the expression of serine protease enzymatic activity that can generate bioactive angiostatin from purified human plasminogen or plasmin [58]. Endogenous molecules sufficient for angiostatin generation were later identified as uPA and free sulfhydryl donors (FSDs) in PC-3 cells. Furthermore, in a defined cell-free system, plasminogen activators such as uPA, tissue-type plasminogen activator (tPA), or streptokinases, in combination with one of a series of free sulfhydryl groups (N-acetyl-L-cysteine, D-penicillamine, captopril, L-cysteine, or reduced glutathione) generate angiostatin from plasminogen.

Cell-free derived angiostatin inhibited angiogenesis *in vitro* and *in vivo* and suppressed the growth of Lewis lung carcinoma metastases [144]. Interestingly, the serine protease PSA is able to convert plasminogen to biologically active angiostatin-like fragments. In an *in vitro* morphogenesis assay was then performed and the purified angiostatin-like fragments inhibited proliferation and tubular formation of human umbilical vein endothelial cells with the same efficacy as angiostatin [145]. Incubating plasminogen with conditioned media from prostate cancer cells resulted in purification of procathepsin D, a lysosomal proenzyme, which when converted to pseudocathepsin D generated two angiostatic peptides shown to inhibit angiogenesis both *in vitro* and *in vivo* [146].

Endostatin

Endostatin was discovered as an angiogenesis inhibitor produced by hemangioendothelioma, and was determined to be a 20 kDa C-terminal fragment of collagen XVIII. Endostatin was demonstrated to specifically inhibit endothelial proliferation and was found to be a potent inhibitor of angiogenesis and tumor growth. Primary tumors treated with endostatin were regressed to dormant microscopic lesions similar, to those found in the aforementioned angiostatin treated tumors [130], with immunohistochemistry revealing high proliferation balanced by apoptosis in tumor cells and blocked angiogenesis without apparent toxicity [147].

A transgenic mouse model developed by insertion of an SV40 early-region transforming sequence under the regulatory control of a rat prostatic steroid-binding promoter was used to evaluate the effects of endostatin treatment on spontaneous prostate cancer tumorigenesis. The SV40 Tag functionally inactivates p53 and Rb through the direct binding to these proteins and appears to interfere with cell cycle regulation. Adenomas develop in about one-third of animals between 6 and 8 months of age and approximately 40% of male mice develop invasive prostate adenocarcinomas by 9 months of age. Mouse endostatin expressed in yeast was administered to mice 7 weeks prior to the expected visibility of tumors. While the authors do not report a decrease in tumor burden as seen with mammary adenocarcinomas in transgenic females with this model, they did demonstrate prolonged survival time for an additional 74 days for males [148]. In human patients with prostate cancer, a single nucleotide polymorphism (D104N) may have impaired the function of endostatin in 13 men heterozygous for the polymorphism D104N and 13 men homozygous for the allele men diagnosed with prostate cancer. Serum ELISA analysis demonstrated endostatin levels were similar both in carriers and non-carriers of this mutation. The results of statistical analysis predict that individual heterozygous for N104 have a 2.5 times greater chance of developing prostate cancer when compared with men containing two wild-type endostatin alleles. Based on sequence comparison and structural modeling, this polymorphism in endostatin may inhibit the ability to interact with other molecules [149].

Prostate specific antigen

PSA (also known as kallikrein-3 (KLK-3)) translation is regulated by androgen and there are two androgen response elements (AREs) in the 5′ untranslated region of the mRNA. Antiangiogenic property of PSA was described by looking at the administration of PSA to bovine endothelial cells and human endothelial cell lines (HUVEC and HMVEC-d) and subsequent stimulation with FGF-2 or VEGF. PSA was demonstrated to be antiproliferative *in vitro*, in a dose-dependent manner, in all three cell lines with and IC_{50} (concentration at which inhibition was 50%) ranging from $0.6\,\mu M$ to $4.0\,\mu M$ after stimulation with FGF-2. However, PC-3 cells were not inhibited by PSA *in vitro*, nor were the murine melanoma cells (B16BL6). HUVEC cells treated with PSA and stimulated with VEGF showed an IC_{50} of $4\,\mu M$ versus an IC_{50} of $1.2\,\mu M$ in FGF-2 stimulated cells in wound-migration assays. Similarly, Boyden chamber assays found PSA ($5\,\mu M$) to inhibit FGF-2 stimulated HUVEC invasion by 77%, while PSA (300 nM to $3\,\mu M$) inhibited tube formation of HUVEC in Matrigel, in a dose-dependent manner, by approximately 50%. The authors state that on a molar basis, PSA inhibition on both endothelial cell proliferation and migration was 5- to 10-fold less potent than angiostatin and endostatin (no data given). PSA was then administered to mice at $9\,\mu M$ for 11 consecutive days, after intravenous inoculation of B16BL6 melanoma cells, to assess its ability to inhibit the formation of lung colonies; PSA treatment resulted in a 40% reduction in the mean number of lung tumor nodules in this model [150]. These authors then expressed a recombinant human PSA in the yeast *Pichia pastoris* and compared its activity with that of PSA purified from seminal plasma in a modified Boyden chamber migration assay. They found that this assay was more sensitive to the inhibitory effects of PSA and demonstrated that concentrations in the 100 nM range, for both forms of PSA, resulted in 50% inhibition of endothelial cell migration [151].

Interferons

Interferons (IFNs) have been used to modulate the immune regulation in many cancers but may also have effects on angiogenesis in carcinomas. The antiviral activity of IFNs led to their discovery, but later data revealed that they also control cell growth and differentiation, inhibit expression of oncogenes, and activate T lymphocytes, natural killer cells, and macrophages [152]. IFNs have been extensively studied in clinical trials and have been shown to be effective against many vascular tumors. Some reports have suggested that this effect is due to inhibition of angiogenesis [153].

An *in vitro* study evaluated the effect of purified human fibroblast IFN-β and recombinant IFN-α on cell proliferation in PC-3 and DU145 cells. Both cell lines responded to the antiproliferative action of IFN, IFN-β being more effective than IFN-α. PC-3 cells were more sensitive than the DU145 cell line, showing 95% inhibition of cell proliferation at the highest concentration of IFN-β [154]. A human renal carcinoma cell metastatic line (SN12PM6) was established in culture from a lung metastasis and SN12PM6-resistant cells were selected *in vitro* for resistance to the antiproliferative effects of IFN-α or IFN-β. IFN-α and IFN-β, but not IFN-γ, down-regulated the expression of bFGF at the mRNA and protein levels by a mechanism independent of their antiproliferative effects. The withdrawal of IFN-α or IFN-β from the medium permitted SN12PM6-resistant cells to resume production of bFGF. Additionally, the incubation of human prostate carcinoma cells with non-cytostatic concentrations of IFN-α or IFN-β also produced down-regulation of bFGF production [155]. Therefore, the inhibitory action of IFN-α and IFN-β on angiogenesis may act indirectly through down-regulation of bFGF.

Orthotopic and subcutaneous implantation of PC-3M human prostate cancer cells, engineered to constitutively produce murine IFN-β, and PC-3M-P and PC-3M-Neo cells *in vivo* in nude mice demonstrated antiproliferative effects of IFN-β. PC-3M-P and PC-3M-Neo cells produced rapidly growing tumors and regional lymph node metastases, whereas PC-3M-IFN-β cells did not. PC-3M-IFN-β also suppressed the tumorigenicity of bystander non-transduced prostate cancer cells, and IHC staining revealed that tumors were homogeneously infiltrated by macrophages. Furthermore, MVD assays showed that control tumors contained more blood vessels than PC-3M-IFN-β tumors. The authors suggest that suppression of tumorigenicity and metastasis of PC-3M-IFN-β cells is due to inhibition of angiogenesis and activation of host effector cells [156]. Small clinical trials have only shown limited effectiveness IFN-β in patients with advanced hormone refractory prostate cancer [157].

Anti-vascular endothelial growth factor antibodies

A neutralizing anti-VEGF antibody (A4.6.1) was evaluated for effects on the growth and angiogenic activity of spheroids of the human prostatic cell line DU145 implanted subcutaneously in nude mice. Tumor cells were prelabeled with a fluorescent vital dye (CMTMR), which allowed measurement of size of the implanted tumor spheroids throughout a 2-week observation period and FITC-dextran was used for plasma enhancement to visualize angiogenic activity. Tumors of control animals induced angiogenesis with high vascular density, whereas in animals treated with the anti-VEGF antibody, there was complete inhibition of angiogenesis of the micro tumors and complete inhibition of tumor growth after the initial prevascular angiogenesis independent growth phase [83]. A similar study examined the effect of inhibiting VEGF on primary tumor growth and metastases in an *in vivo* model of established metastatic prostate cancer. Using luciferase as a reporter, DU145 cells, which were found to secrete VEGF, and DU145-luciferase were injected subcutaneously and consistently formed tumors in severe combined immunodeficient mice. After 6 weeks, luciferase assays were performed in whole lung lysates and showed significant activity, consistent with the presence of micrometastasis. Twice weekly treatment with antibody A4.6.1 not only suppressed primary tumor growth, but inhibited metastatic dissemination to the lungs. When treatment was delayed until the primary tumors were well established, further growth was still inhibited, as was the progression of metastatic disease [158]. A study on glioma cells has shown that overexpression of transfected anti-sense-VEGF cDNA led to decreased expression of VEGF *in vitro* and tumor growth *in vivo* was greatly reduced [159]. A strategy utilizing anti-sense-VEGF cDNA with gene therapy may therefore be plausible and might possibly translate to prostate cancer.

Anti-interleukin 6 antibodies

A recent report demonstrates that anti-IL-6 monoclonal antibodies, with or without concurrent etoposide, caused tumor regression and apoptosis. Xenografts of the human prostate cancer cell line PC-3, which produces IL-6, were established in nude mice and tumors were measured over a 4-week treatment period. Tumor volume and terminal deoxynucleotidyl transferase (TdT)-mediated dUTP-biotin nick end-labeling (TUNEL) assay was performed. Anti-IL-6 antibody, with or without etoposide, induced a 60% tumor regression compared to initial tumor size in addition to apoptosis. Furthermore, etoposide alone did not induce tumor regression or apoptosis in this animal model, and no synergy was demonstrated between anti-IL-6

antibody and etoposide [160]. Although MVD and angiogenesis were not evaluated in this report, given the association of IL-6 induction of VEGF and angiogenesis [97] reduction of angiogenesis may be one mechanism underlying the observed tumor effects.

Fumagillin analogue TNP-470

Despite many pharmacological studies, the current knowledge of TNP-470's molecular mode of action is limited. A previous study has shown that TNP-470 exerts biphasic growth inhibition; reversible cytostatic activity toward endothelial cells is observed at low doses (complete growth inhibition at 0.75 nM), but cytotoxic effects are observed at higher concentrations (75 μM) for all cell types tested [161]. The cytostatic inhibition is thought to be responsible for its antiangiogenic effect, because the serum concentration of TNP-470 in rats after systemic administration was much lower than that required for cytotoxic inhibition. In addition, incorporation of thymidine, but not uridine and leucine, in HUVEC is inhibited by TNP-470 treatment, suggesting specific inhibition of DNA synthesis. At the molecular level, TNP-470 does not inhibit early G_1 mitogenic events, such as cellular protein tyrosyl phosphorylation or the expression of immediate early genes [162]. However, TNP-470 potently inhibits the activation of CDK2 and CDC2 as well as retinoblastoma protein phosphorylation, although not through direct kinase inhibition [162].

TNP-470 potently inhibits the tumor growth of hormone-independent prostate cancer PC-3 cell xenografts *in vivo* with maximum inhibition of 96%. Combination therapy with cisplatin and TNP-470 showed an additive antiproliferative effect against PC-3 cells. *In vitro* studies demonstrate PC-3 cells are considerably insensitive to TNP-470 in monolayer cultures (50% inhibitory concentration at 5 μg/ml), whereas TNP-470 did inhibit the anchorage-independent growth of PC-3 (50% inhibitory concentration at 50 pg/ml) [163]. It is important to note that one group demonstrated that induction of TNP-470 therapy increased the secretion of PSA up to 1.5-fold irrespective of tumoricidal effects [164] which may erroneously suggest tumor progression unless clinicians are aware of this paradoxical effect.

Phase I dose escalation trial of alternate-day intravenous TNP-470 therapy in 33 patients with metastatic and androgen-independent prostate cancer has been completed. The dose-limiting toxic effect was a characteristic neuropsychiatric symptom complex (anesthesia, gait disturbance, and agitation) that resolved upon cessation of therapy. No definite antitumor activity of TNP-470 was observed; however, transient stimulation of the serum PSA concentration occurred in some of the patients treated [165].

Thalidomide

Thalidomide was marketed in Europe as a sedative, but was withdrawn 30 years ago because it has potent teratogenic effects that cause stunted limb growth (dysmelia) in humans. *In vitro* data suggested that thalidomide has antiangiogenic activity induced by bFGF in a rabbit cornea assay [166]. A report on a randomized phase II study of thalidomide in patients with androgen-independent prostate cancer has recently been released. A total of 63 patients were enrolled in the study; 50 patients were on the low-dose arm and received a dose of 200 mg/day, while 13 patients were on the high-dose arm and received an initial dose of 200 mg/day that escalated to 1200 mg/day. A serum PSA level decline of greater than or equal to 50% was noted in 18% of patients on the low-dose arm, but in none of the patients on the high-dose arm. Also, a total of 27% of all patients had a decline in PSA of greater than or equal to 40%, often associated with an improvement of clinical symptoms. Only 4 patients were maintained for greater than 150 days and the most prevalent complications were constipation, fatigue, and neurological disorders. The authors note that the decline in PSA in these patients may be particularly important as pre-clinical studies showed thalidomide increasing PSA levels [167].

Calcium channel blocker carboxyamido-triazole

Phase II clinical trial of the antiproliferative, antimetastatic, and antiangiogenic agent carboxyamido-triazole (CAI) was evaluated with 15 patients with stage D2 androgen-independent prostate cancer with soft tissue metastases. Because CAI previously had been shown to decrease PSA secretion *in vitro*, this marker was not used. Fourteen of 15 patients were evaluable for response and all of these 14 patients demonstrated progressive disease at approximately 2 months. Twelve patients progressed by computed tomography and/or bone scan at 2 months, whereas 2 patients demonstrated clinical progression at 1.5 and 2 months. One patient was removed from study at 6 weeks due to grade II peripheral neuropathy lasting >1 month. No clinical responses were noted, but a 28% decrease in serum VEGF concentration was observed. CAI does not possess clinical activity in patients with androgen-independent prostate cancer and soft tissue metastases [168].

Linomide

Linomide (N-phenylmethyl-1, 2-dihydro-4-hydroxyl-1-methyl-2-oxo-quinoline-3-carboxamide) is a quinoline 3-carboxamide which previously has been demonstrated to modulate immune response and produce antitumor effects when given *in vivo*. Five distinct Dunning R3327 rat prostatic cancer subline models were treated daily with intraperitoneal injections of linomide and demonstrated a reproducible antitumor effect against all of the prostatic cancers tested, regardless of their growth rate, degree of morphologic differentiation, metastatic ability, or androgen responsiveness. This antitumor effect was observed only *in vivo*, not *in vitro*, and was cytotoxic to prostatic cancer cells. This cytotoxic response resulted in the retardation of the growth rate of both primary prostatic cancers and in metastatic lesions. Interestingly, the authors found that growth retardation due to linomide was reversible, and continuous daily treatment was required for maximal antitumor response. Additionally, the antitumor effects of linomide were demonstrated in prostatic cancer-bearing athymic nude rats. These data suggest that the antitumor effects of linomide against rat prostatic cancers may involve both immune and non-immune host mechanisms, including perhaps angiogenesis [169].

This group recognized evidence that linomide treatment has antiangiogenic activity, namely the observation that prostatic cancers from linomide treated rats have more focal necrosis than size matched tumors from untreated rats. They then demonstrated that linomide has dose dependent, antiangiogenic activity in the rat using a Matrigel-based quantitative *in vivo* angiogenic assay [170]. In another series of experiments, linomide was unable to inhibit either basal or hypoxia-induced secretion of VEGF in human prostate cancer cells [53]. Linomide also has no effect on secreted bFGF levels. Castration inhibited tumor VEGF but had no effect on bFGF levels in both the androgen-responsive PC-82 and A-2 human prostatic cancers when grown in severe combined immunodeficient mice. When given in combination, castration potentiated the inhibition of tumor growth induced by linomide alone. This potentiation is not due to a further inhibition in tumor VEGF levels induced by castration. Although both castration and linomide inhibit angiogenesis, the former accomplishes it by inhibiting VEGF secretion, whereas the latter has multiple effects at several steps in the angiogenic process other than VEGF secretion. Based on their different but complementary mechanisms of action, simultaneous combination of androgen ablation with linomide enhances the antiprostatic cancer efficacy compared to either monotherapies alone and appears to warrant testing in humans.

National Cancer Institute trials database

There are several trials using antiangiogenic strategies in prostate cancer listed in the National Cancer Institute database (Table 2). This database can be found at *http://cancernet.nci.nih.gov/trialsrch.shtml.* This page is updated on a regular basis, and is intended as an overview of some of the current trials of anti-angiogenesis agents. However, it is not a comprehensive summary of all of the clinical trials ongoing with drugs that inhibit angiogenesis with additional trials, and additional sponsors, not represented.

Table 2. Current clinical trials of angiogenesis related therapies in prostate cancer

Search criteria (http://cancernet.nci.nih.gov/trialsrch.shtml)			
Date search	November 2001	NIH Clinical Center only	no
Cancer	prostate	Version of results	health professional
Type of trial	all types	Stage of cancer	all stages
Accrual in trial	open or closed	Modality	antiangiogenesis therapy
State	all states	Phase of trial	all phases
Country	all countries	Sponsor of trial	all

Title of clinical trial	Protocol ID number(s)
Trials closed to accrual	
Phase I study of carboxyamido-triazole for refractory cancers	NCI-92-C-0054P
	NCI-T91-0170N
	NCI-MB-281
Phase I study of SU006668 in patients with advanced solid tumors	UCLA-0004061
	NCI-G01-2010
	SUGEN-SU6668.004
Phase II randomized study of CT-2584 in patients with hormone refractory, metastatic adenocarcinoma of the prostate	CTI-1038
	CPMC-IRB-8781
Phase II randomized study of oral thalidomide in patients with hormone refractory adenocarcinoma of the Prostate	NCI-95-C-0178L
	NCI-T95-0038N
	NCI-CPB-372
Phase II study of oral carboxyamido-triazole in patients with androgren-independent prostate cancer	NCI-97-C-0059C
	NCI-T96-0053
Phase III randomized study of low molecular weight heparin (dalteparin) plus standard therapy versus standard therapy alone in patients with advanced cancer	NCCTG-979251
	NCI-P98-0139
Phase III randomized study of MMPI AG3340 in combination with mitoxantrone and prednisone in patients with hormone refractory prostate cancer	AG-3340-009
Trials open to accrual	
Phase I study of SU5416 with standard androgen ablation and radiotherapy in patients with intermediate or advanced-stage prostate cancer	UCCRC-NCI-4390
	NCI-4390
Phase II randomized study of dexamethasone with or without SU5416 in patients with hormone refractory prostate cancer	UCCRC-10428
	NCI-49
	UCCRC-NCI-49
Phase II randomized study of docetaxel with or without thalidomide in patients with androgen-independent metastatic prostate cancer	NCI-00-C-0033
Phase II study of bevacizumab, estramustine, and docetaxel in patients with hormone refractory metastatic prostate cancer	CLB-90006
Phase III randomized study of oral thalidomide versus placebo in patients with androgen-dependent stage IV nonmetastatic prostate cancer following limited hormonal ablation	NCI-00-C-0080
	NCI-T99-0053

Key unanswered questions

A provocative strategy is the targeting of endothelial cells themselves with the use of immunoconjugates that selectively occlude the vasculature of solid tumors [171]. Attacking microvessels could offer advantages over challenging tumors themselves. First, tumor dependence on a blood supply could lead to tremendous apoptotic response upon local interruption of the tumor vasculature. Second, the tumor vascular endothelium is in direct contact with the bloodstream, facilitating the delivery of endothelial cell toxic molecules. Third, lack of tumor vascular endothelial cell transformation suggests that they are unlikely to acquire mutations that render them resistant to therapy. One study has looked at the use of human tissue factor to tumor vascular endothelium in a mouse model. Tissue factor is the major initiating receptor for the blood coagulation cascades and assembly of cell surface tissue factor with factor VII/VIIa generates the functional tissue factor–factor VIIa complex. This complex rapidly activates the serine protease zymogen factors IX and X by limited proteolysis, leading to the formation of thrombin and, ultimately, a blood clot. The investigators used a recombinant form of tissue factor that contains only the cell surface domain of the protein. This truncated tissue factor contains factor X-activating activity that is about five orders of magnitude less than that of native transmembrane tissue factor in an appropriate phospholipid membrane environment. By using an antibody to target this truncated form of tissue factor to tumor vascular endothelium, it was brought into proximity with a cell surface and recovered in part its native function resulting in locally initiated thrombosis. Such an antibody-truncated tissue factor conjugate could selectively thrombose tumor vasculature [172].

Another group demonstrated that a single intravascular injection of a cyclic peptide or monoclonal antibody antagonist of integrin $\alpha V\beta 3$ disrupts ongoing angiogenesis in the chick chorioallantoic membrane (CAM) assay and leading to the rapid regression of human tumors transplanted onto the CAM. The authors state that induction of angiogenesis by a tumor or cytokine promotes vascular cell entry into the cell cycle and results in expression of integrin $\alpha V\beta 3$. After angiogenesis is initiated, antagonists of this integrin induce apoptosis of the proliferative angiogenic vascular cells, leaving preexisting quiescent blood vessels unaffected [15].

Conclusion

Angiogenesis has clearly been demonstrated to be a vital requirement for prostate cancer to proliferate locally and to metastasize. This makes antiangiogenic therapy particularly attractive as an antitumor modality. There are a myriad of targets as the regulation of tumor angiogenesis involves numerous molecules both on the proangiogenic and antiangiogenic sides of the balance. Finally, differences in protein expression between newly formed tumor vessels and more mature vessels offer an additional avenue for future antiangiogenic drug discovery.

References

1. Linde N: NOVA: Cancer warrior. In: Linde N (ed.) NOVA, PBS, Alexandria, Virginia, 2001
2. Gimbrone MA, Jr., Leapman SB, Cotran RS, Folkman J: Tumor dormancy *in vivo* by prevention of neovascularization. J Exp Med 136(2): 261–276, 1972
3. Ezzell C: Starving tumors of their lifeblood. Sci Am 279(4): 33–34, 1998
4. Gimbrone MA, Jr., Leapman SB, Cotran RS, Folkman J: Tumor angiogenesis: Iris neovascularization at a distance from experimental intraocular tumors. J Natl Cancer Inst 50(1): 219–228, 1973
5. Folkman J: The role of angiogenesis in tumor growth. Semin Cancer Biol 3(2): 65–71, 1992
6. Folkman J, Klagsbrun M: Angiogenic factors. Science 235(4787): 442–447, 1987
7. Hanahan D, Folkman J: Patterns and emerging mechanisms of the angiogenic switch during tumorigenesis. Cell 86(3): 353–364, 1996
8. Holash J, Maisonpierre PC, Compton D, Boland P, Alexander CR, Zagzag D, Yancopoulos GD, Wiegand SJ: Vessel cooption, regression, and growth in tumors mediated by angiopoietins and VEGF. Science 284(5422): 1994–1998, 1999
9. Fidler IJ: Modulation of the organ microenvironment for treatment of cancer metastasis. J Natl Cancer Inst 87(21): 1588–1592, 1995
10. Fidler IJ, Ellis LM: The implications of angiogenesis for the biology and therapy of cancer metastasis. Cell 79(2): 185–188, 1994
11. Folkman J, Watson K, Ingber D, Hanahan D: Induction of angiogenesis during the transition from hyperplasia to neoplasia. Nature 339(6219): 58–61, 1989
12. Liotta LA, Steeg PS, Stetler-Stevenson WG: Cancer metastasis and angiogenesis: An imbalance of positive and negative regulation. Cell 64(2): 327–336, 1991
13. Liotta LA, Saidel MG, Kleinerman J: The significance of hematogenous tumor cell clumps in the metastatic process. Cancer Res 36(3): 889–894, 1976

178

14. Feng D, Nagy JA, Brekken RA, Pettersson A, Manseau EJ, Pyne K, Mulligan R, Thorpe PE, Dvorak HF, Dvorak AM: Ultrastructural localization of the vascular permeability factor/vascular endothelial growth factor (VPF/VEGF) receptor-2 (FLK-1, KDR) in normal mouse kidney and in the hyperpermeable vessels induced by VPF/VEGF-expressing tumors and adenoviral vectors. J Histochem Cytochem 48(4): 545–556, 2000

15. Brooks PC, Montgomery AM, Rosenfeld M, Reisfeld R A, Hu T, Klier G, Cheresh DA: Integrin alpha v beta 3 antagonists promote tumor regression by inducing apoptosis of angiogenic blood vessels. Cell 79(7): 1157–1164, 1994

16. Pasqualini R, Ruoslahti E: Organ targeting in vivo using phage display peptide libraries. Nature 380(6572): 364–366, 1996

17. Chang SS, O'Keefe DS, Bacich DJ, Reuter VE, Heston WD, Gaudin PB: Prostate-specific membrane antigen is produced in tumor-associated neovasculature. Clin Cancer Res 5(10): 2674–2681, 1999

18. Fidler IJ: Angiogenic heterogeneity: Regulation of neoplastic angiogenesis by the organ microenvironment. J Natl Cancer Inst 93(14): 1040–1041, 2001

19. Naito S, von Eschenbach AC, Giavazzi R, Fidler IJ: Growth and metastasis of tumor cells isolated from a human renal cell carcinoma implanted into different organs of nude mice. Cancer Res 46(8): 4109–4115, 1986

20. Fidler IJ, Naito S, Pathak S: Orthotopic implantation is essential for the selection, growth and metastasis of human renal cell cancer in nude mice (corrected). Cancer Metastasis Rev 9(2): 149–165, 1990

21. Albelda SM, Muller WA, Buck CA, Newman PJ: Molecular and cellular properties of PECAM-1 (endo-CAM/CD31): A novel vascular cell–cell adhesion molecule. J Cell Biol 114(5): 1059–1068, 1991

22. Tang DG, Chen YQ, Newman PJ, Shi L, Gao X, Diglio CA, Honn KV: Identification of PECAM-1 in solid tumor cells and its potential involvement in tumor cell adhesion to endothelium. J Biol Chem 268(30): 22883–22894, 1993

23. Brawer MK, Bigler SA, Deering RE: Quantitative morphometric analysis of the microcirculation in prostate carcinoma. J Cell Biochem 16H(Suppl): 62–64, 1992

24. Weidner N, Carroll PR, Flax J, Blumenfeld W, Folkman J: Tumor angiogenesis correlates with metastasis in invasive prostate carcinoma. Am J Pathol 143(2): 401–409, 1993

25. Brawer MK, Deering RE, Brown M, Preston SD, Bigler SA: Predictors of pathologic stage in prostatic carcinoma. The role of neovascularity. Cancer 73(3): 678–687, 1994

26. Rubin MA, Buyyounouski M, Bagiella E, Sharir S, Neugut A, Benson M, de la Taille A, Katz AE, Olsson CA, Ennis RD: Microvessel density in prostate cancer: Lack of correlation with tumor grade, pathologic stage, and clinical outcome. Urology 53(3): 542–547, 1999

27. Krupski T, Petroni GR, Frierson HF, Jr., Theodorescu JU: Microvessel density, p53, retinoblastoma, and chromogranin A immunohistochemistry as predictors of disease-specific survival following radical prostatectomy for carcinoma of the prostate. Urology 55(5): 743–749, 2000

28. Offersen BV, Borre M, Overgaard J: Immunohistochemical determination of tumor angiogenesis measured by the maximal microvessel density in human prostate cancer. APMIS 106(4): 463–469, 1998

29. Borre M, Offersen BV, Nerstrom B, Overgaard J: Microvessel density predicts survival in prostate cancer patients subjected to watchful waiting. Br J Cancer 78(7): 940–944, 1998

30. Bostwick DG, Wheeler TM, Blute M, Barrett DM, MacLennan GT, Sebo TJ, Scardino PT, Humphrey PA, Hudson MA, Fradet Y, Miller GJ, Crawford ED, Blumenstein BA, Mahran HE, Miles BJ: Optimized microvessel density analysis improves prediction of cancer stage from prostate needle biopsies. Urology 48(1): 47–57, 1996

31. Gettman MT, Bergstralh EJ, Blute M, Zincke H, Bostwick DG: Prediction of patient outcome in pathologic stage T2 adenocarcinoma of the prostate: Lack of significance for microvessel density analysis. Urology 51(1): 79–85, 1998

32. de la Taille A, Katz AE, Bagiella E, Buttyan R, Sharir S, Olsson CA, Burchardt T, Ennis RD, Rubin MA: Microvessel density as a predictor of PSA recurrence after radical prostatectomy. A comparison of CD34 and CD31. Am J Clin Pathol 113(4): 555–562, 2000

33. Strohmeyer D, Rossing C, Bauerfeind A, Kaufmann O, Schlechte H, Bartsch G, Loening S: Vascular endothelial growth factor and its correlation with angiogenesis and p53 expression in prostate cancer. Prostate 45(3): 216–224, 2000

34. Giri D, Ittmann M: Inactivation of the PTEN tumor suppressor gene is associated with increased angiogenesis in clinically localized prostate carcinoma. Hum Pathol 30(4): 419–424, 1999

35. Wen S, Stolarov J, Myers MP, Su JD, Wigler MH, Tonks NK, Durden DL: PTEN controls tumor-induced angiogenesis. Proc Natl Acad Sci USA 98(8): 4622–4627, 2001

36. Camps JL, Chang SM, Hsu TC, Freeman MR, Hong SJ, Zhau HE, von Eschenbach AC, Chung LW: Fibroblast-mediated acceleration of human epithelial tumor growth in vivo. Proc Natl Acad Sci USA 87(1): 75–79, 1990

37. Janvier R, Sourla A, Koutsilieris M, Doillon CJ: Stromal fibroblasts are required for PC-3 human prostate cancer cells to produce capillary-like formation of endothelial cells in a three-dimensional co-culture system. Anticancer Res 17(3A): 1551–1557, 1997

38. Campbell CL, Savarese DM, Quesenberry PJ, Savarese TM: Expression of multiple angiogenic cytokines in cultured normal human prostate epithelial cells: Predominance of vascular endothelial growth factor. Int J Cancer 80(6): 868–874, 1999

39. Ferrer FA, Miller LJ, Andrawis RI, Kurtzman SH, Albertsen PC, Laudone VP, Kreutzer DL: Angiogenesis and prostate cancer: In vivo and in vitro expression of angiogenesis factors by prostate cancer cells. Urology 51(1): 161–167, 1998

40. Hepburn PJ, Griffiths K, Harper ME: Angiogenic factors expressed by human prostatic cell lines: Effect on endothelial cell growth in vitro. Prostate 33(2): 123–132, 1997

41. Semenza GL, Wang GL: A nuclear factor induced by hypoxia via de novo protein synthesis binds to the human erythropoietin gene enhancer at a site required for transcriptional activation. Mol Cell Biol 12(12): 5447–5454, 1992

42. Zhong H, Agani F, Baccala AA, Laughner E, Rioseco-Camacho N, Isaacs WB, Simons JW, Semenza GL: Increased expression of hypoxia inducible factor-1alpha in rat and human prostate cancer. Cancer Res 58(23): 5280–5284, 1998

43. Zhong H, De Marzo AM, Laughner E, Lim M, Hilton DA, Zagzag D, Buechler P, Isaacs WB, Semenza GL, Simons JW: Overexpression of hypoxia-inducible factor 1alpha in common human cancers and their metastases. Cancer Res 59(22): 5830–5835, 1999

44. Cvetkovic D, Movsas B, Dicker AP, Hanlon AL, Greenberg RE, Chapman JD, Hanks GE, Tricoli JV: Increased hypoxia correlates with increased expression of the angiogenesis marker vascular endothelial growth factor in human prostate cancer. Urology 57(4): 821–825, 2001

45. Zhong H, Chiles K, Feldser D, Laughner E, Hanrahan C, Georgescu MM, Simons JW, Semenza GL: Modulation of hypoxia-inducible factor 1alpha expression by the epidermal growth factor/phosphatidylinositol 3-kinase/PTEN/AKT/FRAP pathway in human prostate cancer cells: Implications for tumor angiogenesis and therapeutics. Cancer Res 60(6): 1541–1545, 2000

46. Liu XH, Kirschenbaum A, Yao S, Stearns ME, Holland JF, Claffey K, Levine AC: Upregulation of vascular endothelial growth factor by cobalt chloride-simulated hypoxia is mediated by persistent induction of cyclooxygenase-2 in a metastatic human prostate cancer cell line. Clin Exp Metastasis 17(8): 687–694, 1999

47. Lekas E, Johansson M, Widmark A, Bergh A, Damber JE: Decrement of blood flow precedes the involution of the ventral prostate in the rat after castration. Urol Res 25(5): 309–314, 1997

48. Hartley-Asp B, Vukanovic J, Joseph IB, Strandgarden K, Polacek J, Isaacs JT: Anti-angiogenic treatment with linomide as adjuvant to surgical castration in experimental prostate cancer. J Urol 158(3 Pt 1): 902–907, 1997

49. Jain RK, Safabakhsh N, Sckell A, Chen Y, Jiang P, Benjamin L, Yuan F, Keshet E: Endothelial cell death, angiogenesis, and microvascular function after castration in an androgen-dependent tumor: Role of vascular endothelial growth factor. Proc Natl Acad Sci USA 95(18): 10820–10825, 1998

50. Lissbrant IF, Stattin P, Wikstrom P, Damber JE, Egevad L, Bergh A: Tumor associated macrophages in human prostate cancer: Relation to clinicopathological variables and survival. Int J Oncol 17(3): 445–451, 2000

51. Shimura S, Yang G, Ebara S, Wheeler TM, Frolov A, Thompson TC: Reduced infiltration of tumor-associated macrophages in human prostate cancer: Association with cancer progression. Cancer Res 60(20): 5857–5861, 2000

52. Sunderkotter C, Steinbrink K, Goebeler M, Bhardwaj R, Sorg C: Macrophages and angiogenesis. J Leukoc Biol 55(3): 410–422, 1994

53. Joseph IB, Isaacs JT: Potentiation of the antiangiogenic ability of linomide by androgen ablation involves downregulation of vascular endothelial growth factor in human androgen-responsive prostatic cancers. Cancer Res 57(6): 1054–1057, 1997

54. Rabbani SA: Metalloproteases and urokinase in angiogenesis and tumor progression. In Vivo 12(1): 135–142, 1998

55. Hoosein NM, Boyd DD, Hollas WJ, Mazar A, Henkin J, Chung LW: Involvement of urokinase and its receptor in the invasiveness of human prostatic carcinoma cell lines. Cancer Commun 3(8): 255–264, 1991

56. Evans CP, Elfman F, Parangi S, Conn M, Cunha G, Shuman MA: Inhibition of prostate cancer neovascularization and growth by urokinase-plasminogen activator receptor blockade. Cancer Res 57(16): 3594–3599, 1997

57. Billstrom A, Lecander I, Dagnaes-Hansen F, Dahllof B, Stenram U, Hartley-Asp B: Differential expression of uPA in an aggressive (DU 145) and a nonaggressive (1013L) human prostate cancer xenograft. Prostate 26(2): 94–104, 1995

58. Gately S, Twardowski P, Stack MS, Patrick M, Boggio L, Cundiff DL, Schnaper HW, Madison L, Volpert O, Bouck N, Enghild J, Kwaan HC, Soff GA: Human prostate carcinoma cells express enzymatic activity that converts human plasminogen to the angiogenesis inhibitor, angiostatin. Cancer Res 56(21): 4887–4890, 1996

59. Mignatti P, Mazzieri R, Rifkin DB: Expression of the urokinase receptor in vascular endothelial cells is stimulated by basic fibroblast growth factor. J Cell Biol 113(5): 1193–1201, 1991

60. Nagakawa O, Murakami K, Yamaura T, Fujiuchi Y, Murata J, Fuse H, Saiki I: Expression of membrane-type 1 matrix metalloproteinase (MT1-MMP) on prostate cancer cell lines. Cancer Lett 155(2): 173–179, 2000

61. Kuniyasu H, Troncoso P, Johnston D, Bucana CD, Tahara E, Fidler IJ, Pettaway CA: Relative expression of type IV collagenase, E-cadherin, and vascular endothelial growth factor/vascular permeability factor in prostatectomy specimens distinguishes organ-confined from pathologically advanced prostate cancers. Clin Cancer Res 6(6): 2295–2308, 2000

62. Sehgal I, Thompson TC: Novel regulation of type IV collagenase (matrix metalloproteinase-9 and -2) activities by transforming growth factor-beta1 in human prostate cancer cell lines. Mol Biol Cell 10(2): 407–416, 1999

63. Stearns ME, Rhim J, Wang M: Interleukin 10 (IL-10) inhibition of primary human prostate cell-induced angiogenesis: IL-10 stimulation of tissue inhibitor of metalloproteinase-1 and inhibition of matrix metalloproteinase-(MMP)-2/MMP-9 secretion. Clin Cancer Res 5(1): 189–196, 1999

64. Stearns ME, Garcia FU, Fudge K, Rhim J, Wang M: Role of interleukin 10 and transforming growth factor beta1 in the angiogenesis and metastasis of human prostate primary tumor lines from orthotopic implants in severe combined immunodeficiency mice. Clin Cancer Res 5(3): 711–720, 1999

65. Senger DR, Galli SJ, Dvorak AM, Perruzzi CA, Harvey VS, Dvorak HF: Tumor cells secrete a vascular permeability factor that promotes accumulation of ascites fluid. Science 219(4587): 983–985, 1983

66. Robinson CJ, Stringer SE: The splice variants of vascular endothelial growth factor (VEGF) and their receptors. J Cell Sci 114(Pt 5): 853–865, 2001

180

67. Muller YA, Christinger HW, Keyt BA, de Vos AM: The crystal structure of vascular endothelial growth factor (VEGF) refined to 1.93 A resolution: Multiple copy flexibility and receptor binding. Structure 5(10): 1325–1338, 1997

68. Mustonen T, Alitalo K: Endothelial receptor tyrosine kinases involved in angiogenesis. J Cell Biol 129(4): 895–898, 1995

69. Keyt BA, Nguyen HV, Berleau LT, Duarte CM, Park J, Chen H, Ferrara N: Identification of vascular endothelial growth factor determinants for binding KDR and FLT-1 receptors. Generation of receptor-selective VEGF variants by site-directed mutagenesis. J Biol Chem 271(10): 5638–5646, 1996

70. Kaipainen A, Korhonen J, Mustonen T, van Hinsbergh VW, Fang GH, Dumont D, Breitman M, Alitalo K: Expression of the fms-like tyrosine kinase 4 gene becomes restricted to lymphatic endothelium during development. Proc Natl Acad Sci USA 92(8): 3566–3570, 1995

71. Nicosia RF. What is the role of vascular endothelial growth factor-related molecules in tumor angiogenesis? Am J Pathol 153(1): 11–16, 1998

72. Fairbrother WJ, Champe MA, Christinger HW, Keyt BA, Starovasnik MA: Solution structure of the heparin-binding domain of vascular endothelial growth factor. Structure 6(5): 637–648, 1998

73. Houck KA, Leung DW, Rowland AM, Winer J, Ferrara N: Dual regulation of vascular endothelial growth factor bioavailability by genetic and proteolytic mechanisms. J Biol Chem 267(36): 26031–26037, 1992

74. Park JE, Keller GA, Ferrara N: The vascular endothelial growth factor (VEGF) isoforms: Differential deposition into the subepithelial extracellular matrix and bioactivity of extracellular matrix-bound VEGF. Mol Biol Cell 4(12): 1317–1326, 1993

75. Houck KA, Ferrara N, Winer J, Cachianes G, Li B, Leung DW: The vascular endothelial growth factor family: Identification of a fourth molecular species and characterization of alternative splicing of RNA. Mol Endocrinol 5(12): 1806–1814, 1991

76. Jonca F, Ortega N, Gleizes PE, Bertrand N, Plouet J: Cell release of bioactive fibroblast growth factor 2 by exon 6-encoded sequence of vascular endothelial growth factor. J Biol Chem 272(39): 24203–24209, 1997

77. Maglione D, Guerriero V, Viglietto G, Delli-Bovi P, Persico MG: Isolation of a human placenta cDNA coding for a protein related to the vascular permeability factor. Proc Natl Acad Sci USA 88(20): 9267–9271, 1991

78. Paavonen K, Horelli-Kuitunen N, Chilov D, Kukk E, Pennanen S, Kallioniemi OP, Pajusola K, Olofsson B, Eriksson U, Joukov V, Palotie A, Alitalo K: Novel human vascular endothelial growth factor genes VEGF-B and VEGF-C localize to chromosomes 11q13 and 4q34, respectively. Circulation 93(6): 1079–1082, 1996

79. Joukov V, Pajusola K, Kaipainen A, Chilov D, Lahtinen I, Kukk E, Saksela O, Kalkkinen N, Alitalo K: A novel vascular endothelial growth factor, VEGF-C, is a ligand for the Flt4 (VEGFR-3) and KDR (VEGFR-2) receptor tyrosine kinases. EMBO J 15(2): 290–298, 1996

80. Yamada Y, Nezu J, Shimane M, Hirata Y: Molecular cloning of a novel vascular endothelial growth factor, VEGF-D. Genomics 42(3): 483–488, 1997

81. Ogawa S, Oku A, Sawano A, Yamaguchi S, Yazaki Y, Shibuya M: A novel type of vascular endothelial growth factor, VEGF-E (NZ-7 VEGF), preferentially utilizes KDR/Flk-1 receptor and carries a potent mitotic activity without heparin-binding domain. J Biol Chem 273(47): 31273–31282, 1998

82. Senger DR, Perruzzi CA, Feder J, Dvorak HF: A highly conserved vascular permeability factor secreted by a variety of human and rodent tumor cell lines. Cancer Res 46(11): 5629–5632, 1986

83. Borgstrom P, Bourdon MA, Hillan KJ, Sriramarao P, Ferrara N: Neutralizing anti-vascular endothelial growth factor antibody completely inhibits angiogenesis and growth of human prostate carcinoma micro tumors in vivo. Prostate 35(1): 1–10, 1998

84. Ferrer FA, Miller LJ Andrawis RI, Kurtzman SH, Albertsen PC, Laudone VP, Kreutzer DL: Vascular endothelial growth factor (VEGF) expression in human prostate cancer: In situ and in vitro expression of VEGF by human prostate cancer cells. J Urol 157(6): 2329–2333, 1997

85. Harper ME, Glynne-Jones E, Goddard L, Thurston VJ, Griffiths K: Vascular endothelial growth factor (VEGF) expression in prostatic tumours and its relationship to neuroendocrine cells. Br J Cancer 74(6): 910–916, 1996

86. Noordzij MA, van der Kwast TH, van Steenbrugge GJ, Hop WJ, Schroder FH: The prognostic influence of neuroendocrine cells in prostate cancer: Results of a long-term follow-up study with patients treated by radical prostatectomy. Int J Cancer 62(3): 252–258, 1995

87. Mazure NM, Chen EY, Yeh P, Laderoute KR, Giaccia AJ: Oncogenic transformation and hypoxia synergistically act to modulate vascular endothelial growth factor expression. Cancer Res 56(15): 3436–3440, 1996

88. Levy AP, Levy NS, Goldberg MA: Post-transcriptional regulation of vascular endothelial growth factor by hypoxia. J Biol Chem 271(5): 2746–2753, 1996

89. Akiri G, Nahari D, Finkelstein Y, Le SY, Elroy-Stein O, Levi BZ: Regulation of vascular endothelial growth factor (VEGF) expression is mediated by internal initiation of translation and alternative initiation of transcription. Oncogene 17(2): 227–236, 1998

90. Seghezzi G, Patel S, Ren CJ, Gualandris A, Pintucci G, Robbins ES, Shapiro RL, Galloway AC, Rifkin DB, Mignatti P: Fibroblast growth factor-2 (FGF-2) induces vascular endothelial growth factor (VEGF) expression in the endothelial cells of forming capillaries: An autocrine mechanism contributing to angiogenesis. J Cell Biol 141(7): 1659–1673, 1998

91. Deroanne CF, Hajitou A, Calberg-Bacq CM, Nusgens BV, Lapiere CM: Angiogenesis by fibroblast growth factor 4 is mediated through an autocrine up-regulation of vascular endothelial growth factor expression. Cancer Res 57(24): 5590–5597, 1997

92. Finkenzeller G, Marme D, Weich HA, Hug H: Platelet-derived growth factor-induced transcription of the vascular

endothelial growth factor gene is mediated by protein kinase C. Cancer Res 52(17): 4821–4823, 1992

93. Giraudo E, Primo L, Audero E, Gerber HP, Koolwijk P, Soker S, Klagsbrun M, Ferrara N, Bussolino F: Tumor necrosis factor-alpha regulates expression of vascular endothelial growth factor receptor-2 and of its co-receptor neuropilin-1 in human vascular endothelial cells. J Biol Chem 273(34): 22128–22135, 1998

94. Pertovaara L, Kaipainen A, Mustonen T, Orpana A, Ferrara N, Saksela O, Alitalo K: Vascular endothelial growth factor is induced in response to transforming growth factor-beta in fibroblastic and epithelial cells. J Biol Chem 269(9): 6271–6274, 1994

95. Warren RS, Yuan, H, Matli MR, Ferrara N, Donner DB: Induction of vascular endothelial growth factor by insulin-like growth factor 1 in colorectal carcinoma. J Biol Chem 271(46): 29483–29488, 1996

96. Li J, Perrella MA, Tsai JC, Yet SF, Hsieh CM, Yoshizumi M, Patterson C, Endege WO, Zhou F, Lee ME: Induction of vascular endothelial growth factor gene expression by interleukin-1 beta in rat aortic smooth muscle cells. J Biol Chem 270(1): 308–312, 1995

97. Cohen T, Nahari D, Cerem LW, Neufeld G, Levi BZ: Interleukin 6 induces the expression of vascular endothelial growth factor. J Biol Chem 271(2): 736–741, 1996

98. Dembinska-Kiec A, Dulak J, Partyka L, Huk I, Mailnski T: VEGF-nitric oxide reciprocal regulation. Nat Med 3(11): 1177, 1997

99. Uotila P, Valve E, Martikainen P, Nevalainen M, Nurmi M, Harkonen P: Increased expression of cyclooxygenase-2 and nitric oxide synthase-2 in human prostate cancer. Urol Res 29(1): 23–28, 2001

100. Rak J, Mitsuhashi Y, Sheehan C, Tamir A, Viloria-Petit A, Filmus J, Mansour SJ, Ahn NG, Kerbel RS: Oncogenes and tumor angiogenesis: Differential modes of vascular endothelial growth factor up-regulation in ras-transformed epithelial cells and fibroblasts. Cancer Res 60(2): 490–498, 2000

101. Grugel S, Finkenzeller G, Weindel K, Barleon B, Marme D: Both v-Ha-Ras and v-Raf stimulate expression of the vascular endothelial growth factor in NIH 3T3 cells. J Biol Chem 270(43): 25915–25919, 1995

102. Grunstein J, Roberts WG, Mathieu-Costello O, Hanahan D, Johnson RS: Tumor-derived expression of vascular endothelial growth factor is a critical factor in tumor expansion and vascular function. Cancer Res 59(7): 1592–1598, 1999

103. Konishi N, Hiasa Y, Tsuzuki T, Tao M, Enomoto T, Miller GJ: Comparison of ras activation in prostate carcinoma in Japanese and American men. Prostate 30(1): 53–57, 1997

104. Sheta EA, Harding MA, Conaway MR, Theodorescu D: Focal adhesion kinase, Rap1, and transcriptional induction of vascular endothelial growth factor. J Natl Cancer Inst 92(13): 1065–1073, 2000

105. Wartenberg M, Donmez F, Ling FC, Acker H, Hescheler J, Sauer H: Tumor-induced angiogenesis studied in confrontation cultures of multicellular tumor spheroids and embryoid bodies grown from pluripotent embryonic stem cells. FASEB J 15(6): 995–1005, 2001

106. Huss WJ, Hanrahan CF, Barrios RJ, Simons JW, Greenberg NM: Angiogenesis and prostate cancer: Identification of a molecular progression switch. Cancer Res 61(6): 2736–2743, 2001

107. Balbay MD, Pettaway CA, Kuniyasu H, Inoue K, Ramirez E, Li E, Fidler IJ, Dinney CP: Highly metastatic human prostate cancer growing within the prostate of athymic mice overexpresses vascular endothelial growth factor. Clin Cancer Res 5(4): 783–789, 1999

108. Connolly JM, Rose DP: Angiogenesis in two human prostate cancer cell lines with differing metastatic potential when growing as solid tumors in nude mice. J Urol 160(3 Pt 1): 932–936, 1998

109. Krupski T, Harding MA, Herce ME, Gulding KM, Stoler MH, Theodorescu D: The role of vascular endothelial growth factor in the tissue specific in vivo growth of prostate cancer cells. Growth Factors 18(4): 287–302, 2001

110. Gaudric A, N'Guyen T, Moenner M, Glacet-Bernard A, Barritault D: Quantification of angiogenesis due to basic fibroblast growth factor in a modified rabbit corneal model. Ophthalmic Res 24(3): 181–188, 1992

111. Pepper MS, Ferrara N, Orci L, Montesano R: Potent synergism between vascular endothelial growth factor and basic fibroblast growth factor in the induction of angiogenesis in vitro. Biochem Biophys Res Commun 189(2): 824–831, 1992

112. Nakamoto T, Chang CS, Li AK, Chodak GW: Basic fibroblast growth factor in human prostate cancer cells. Cancer Res 52(3): 571–577, 1992

113. Zuck B, Goepfert C, Nedlin-Chittka A, Sohrt K, Voigt KD, Knabbe C: Regulation of fibroblast growth factor-like protein(s) in the androgen-responsive human prostate carcinoma cell line LNCaP. J Steroid Biochem Mol Biol 41(3–8): 659–663, 1992

114. Bok RA, Halabi S, Fei DT, Rodriquez CR, Hayes DF, Vogelzang NJ, Kantoff P, Shuman MA, Small EJ: Vascular endothelial growth factor and basic fibroblast growth factor urine levels as predictors of outcome in hormone-refractory prostate cancer patients: A cancer and leukemia group B study. Cancer Res 61(6): 2533–2536, 2001

115. Walsh K, Sherwood RA, Dew TK, Mulvin D: Angiogenic peptides in prostatic disease. BJU Int 84(9): 1081–1083, 1999

116. Ropiquet F, Giri D, Kwabi-Addo B, Mansukhani A, Ittmann M: Increased expression of fibroblast growth factor 6 in human prostatic intraepithelial neoplasia and prostate cancer. Cancer Res 60(15): 4245–4250, 2000

117. Morton DM, Barrack ER: Modulation of transforming growth factor beta 1 effects on prostate cancer cell proliferation by growth factors and extracellular matrix. Cancer Res 55(12): 2596–2602, 1995

118. Wikstrom P, Stattin P, Franck-Lissbrant I, Damber JE, Bergh A: Transforming growth factor beta1 is associated with angiogenesis, metastasis, and poor clinical outcome in prostate cancer. Prostate 37(1): 19–29, 1998

119. Truong LD, Kadmon D, McCune BK, Flanders KC, Scardino PT, Thompson TC: Association of transforming growth factor-beta 1 with prostate cancer: An immunohistochemical study. Hum Pathol 24(1): 4–9, 1993

182

120. Eastham JA, Truong LD, Rogers E, Kattan M, Flanders KC, Scardino PT, Thompson TC: Transforming growth factor-beta 1: Comparative immunohistochemical localization in human primary and metastatic prostate cancer. Lab Inves 73(5): 628–635, 1995

121. Kim IY, Ahn HJ, Zelner DJ, Shaw JW, Lang S, Kato M, Oefelein MG, Miyazono K, Nemeth JA, Kozlowski JM, Lee C: Loss of expression of transforming growth factor beta type I and type II receptors correlates with tumor grade in human prostate cancer tissues. Clin Cancer Res 2(8): 1255–1261, 1996

122. Williams RH, Stapleton AM, Yang G, Truong LD, Rogers E, Timme TL, Wheeler TM, Scardino PT, Thompson TC: Reduced levels of transforming growth factor beta receptor type II in human prostate cancer: An immunohistochemical study. Clin Cancer Res 2(4): 635–640, 1996

123. Guo Y, Jacobs SC, Kyprianou N: Down-regulation of protein and mRNA expression for transforming growth factor-beta (TGF-beta1) type I and type II receptors in human prostate cancer. Int J Cancer 71(4): 573–579, 1997

124. Steiner MS, Zhou ZZ, Tonb DC, Barrack ER: Expression of transforming growth factor-beta 1 in prostate cancer. Endocrinology 135(5): 2240–2247, 1994

125. Koch AE, Polverini PJ, Kunkel SL, Harlow LA, DiPietro LA, Elner VM, Elner SG, Strieter RM: Interleukin-8 as a macrophage-derived mediator of angiogenesis. Science 258(5089): 1798–1801, 1992

126. Greene GF, Kitadai Y, Pettaway CA, von Eschenbach AC, Bucana CD, Fidler IJ: Correlation of metastasis-related gene expression with metastatic potential in human prostate carcinoma cells implanted in nude mice using an *in situ* messenger RNA hybridization technique. Am J Pathol 150(5): 1571–1582, 1997

127. Inoue K, Slaton JW, Eve BY, Kim SJ, Perrotte P, Balbay MD, Yano S, Bar-Eli M, Radinsky R, Pettaway CA: Interleukin 8 expression regulates tumorigenicity and metastases in androgen-independent prostate cancer. Clin Cancer Res 6(5): 2104–2119, 2000

128. Hsu AL, Ching TT, Wang DS, Song X, Rangnekar VM, Chen CS: The cyclooxygenase-2 inhibitor celecoxib induces apoptosis by blocking Akt activation in human prostate cancer cells independently of Bcl-2. J Biol Chem 275(15): 11397–11403, 2000

129. Madaan S, Abel PD, Chaudhary KS, Hewitt R, Stott M A, Stamp GW, Lalani EN: Cytoplasmic induction and over-expression of cyclooxygenase-2 in human prostate cancer: Implications for prevention and treatment. BJU Int 86(6): 736–741, 2000

130. O'Reilly MS, Holmgren L, Chen C, Folkman J: Angiostatin induces and sustains dormancy of human primary tumors in mice. Nat Med 2(6): 689–692, 1996

131. Stearns M, Wang M, Stearns ME: Cytokine (IL-10, IL-6) induction of tissue inhibitor of metalloproteinase 1 in primary human prostate tumor cell lines. Oncol Res 7(3–4): 173–181, 1995

132. Lokeshwar BL, Selzer MG, Block NL, Gunja-Smith Z: Secretion of matrix metalloproteinases and their inhibitors (tissue inhibitor of metalloproteinases) by human prostate in explant cultures: Reduced tissue inhibitor of metalloproteinase secretion by malignant tissues. Cancer Res 53(19): 4493–4498, 1993

133. Wood M, Fudge K, Mohler JL, Frost AR, Garcia F, Wang M, Stearns ME: *In situ* hybridization studies of metalloproteinases 2 and 9 and TIMP-1 and TIMP-2 expression in human prostate cancer. Clin Exp Metastasis 15(3): 246–258, 1997

134. Dong Z, Nemeth JA, Cher ML, Palmer KC, Bright RC, Fridman R: Differential regulation of matrix metalloproteinase-9, tissue inhibitor of metalloproteinase-1 (TIMP-1) and TIMP-2 expression in co-cultures of prostate cancer and stromal cells. Int J Cancer 93(4): 507–515, 2001

135. Stearns ME, Fudge K, Garcia F, Wang M: IL-10 inhibition of human prostate PC-3 ML cell metastases in SCID mice: IL-10 stimulation of TIMP-1 and inhibition of MMP-2/MMP-9 expression. Invasion Metastasis 17(2): 62–74, 1997

136. Stearns ME: Alendronate blocks TGF-beta1 stimulated collagen 1 degradation by human prostate PC-3 ML cells. Clin Exp Metastasis 16(4): 332–339, 1998

137. Nemunaitis J, Poole C, Primrose J, Rosemurgy A, Malfetano J, Brown P, Berrington A, Cornish A, Lynch K, Rasmussen H, Kerr D, Cox D, Millar A: Combined analysis of studies of the effects of the matrix metalloproteinase inhibitor marimastat on serum tumor markers in advanced cancer: Selection of a biologically active and tolerable dose for longer-term studies. Clin Cancer Res 4(5): 1101–1109, 1998

138. Steward WP: Marimastat (BB2516): Current status of development. Cancer Chemother Pharmacol 43(Suppl): S56–S60, 1999

139. Knox JD, Bretton L, Lynch T, Bowden GT, Nagle RB: Synthetic matrix metalloproteinase inhibitor, BB-94, inhibits the invasion of neoplastic human prostate cells in a mouse model. Prostate 35(4): 248–254, 1998

140. Lein M, Jung K, Le DK, Hasan T, Ortel B, Borchert D, Winkelmann B, Schnorr D, Loenings SA: Synthetic inhibitor of matrix metalloproteinases (batimastat) reduces prostate cancer growth in an orthotopic rat model. Prostate 43(2): 77–82, 2000

141. Rabbani SA, Harakidas P, Davidson DJ, Henkin J, Mazar AP: Prevention of prostate-cancer metastasis *in vivo* by a novel synthetic inhibitor of urokinase-type plasminogen activator (uPA). Int J Cancer 63(6): 840–845, 1995

142. Festuccia C, Giunciuglio D, Guerra F, Villanova I, Angelucci A, Manduca P, Teti A, Albini A, Bologna M: Osteoblasts modulate secretion of urokinase-type plasminogen activator (uPA) and matrix metalloproteinase-9 (MMP-9) in human prostate cancer cells promoting migration and matrigel invasion. Oncol Res 11(1): 17–31, 1999

143. Chen C, Parangi S, Tolentino MJ, Folkman J: A strategy to discover circulating angiogenesis inhibitors generated by human tumors. Cancer Res 55(19): 4230–4233, 1995

144. Gately S, Twardowski P, Stack MS, Cundiff DL, Grella D, Castellino FJ, Enghild J, Kwaan HC, Lee F, Kramer RA, Volpert O, Bouck N, Soff GA: The mechanism of cancer-mediated conversion of plasminogen to the angiogenesis inhibitor angiostatin. Proc Natl Acad Sci USA 94(20): 10868–10872, 1997

145. Heidtmann HH, Nettelbeck DM, Mingels A, Jager R, Welker HG, Kontermann RE: Generation of

angiostatin-like fragments from plasminogen by prostate-specific antigen. Br J Cancer 81(8): 1269–1273, 1999

146. Morikawa W, Yamamoto K, Ishikawa S, Takemoto S, Ono M, Fukushi J, Naito S, Nozaki C, Iwanaga S, Kuwano M: Angiostatin generation by cathepsin D secreted by human prostate carcinoma cells. J Biol Chem 275(49): 38912–38920, 2000

147. O'Reilly MS, Boehm T, Shing Y, Fukai N, Vasios G, Lane WS, Flynn E, Birkhead JR, Olsen BR, Folkman J: Endostatin: An endogenous inhibitor of angiogenesis and tumor growth. Cell 88(2): 277–285, 1997

148. Yokoyama Y, Green JE, Sukhatme VP, Ramakrishnan S: Effect of endostatin on spontaneous tumorigenesis of mammary adenocarcinoma in a transgenic mouse model. Cancer Res 60(16): 4362–4365, 2000

149. Iughetti P, Suzuki O, Godoi PH, Ferreira Alves VA, Sertie AL, Zorick T, Soares F, Camargo A, Moreira ES, di Loreto C, Moreira-Filho CA, Simpson A, Oliva G, Passos-Bueno MR: A polymorphism in endostatin, an angiogenesis inhibitor, predisposes for the development of prostatic adenocarcinoma. Cancer Res 61(20): 7375–7378, 2001

150. Fortier AH, Nelson BJ, Grella DK, Holaday JW: Antiangiogenic activity of prostate-specific antigen. J Natl Cancer Inst 91(19): 1635–1640, 1999

151. Fortier AH, Grella DK, Nelson BJ, Holaday JW: RESPONSE: re: Antiangiogenic activity of prostate-specific antigen. J Natl Cancer Inst 92(4): 345A–346, 2000

152. Krown SE: Interferons in malignancy: Biological products or biological response modifiers? J Natl Cancer Inst 80(5): 306–309, 1988

153. Dinney CP, Bielenberg DR, Perrotte P, Reich R, Eve BY, Bucana CD, Fidler IJ: Inhibition of basic fibroblast growth factor expression, angiogenesis, and growth of human bladder carcinoma in mice by systemic interferon-alpha administration. Cancer Res 58(4): 808–814, 1998

154. Sica G, Fabbroni L, Castagnetta L, Cacciatore M, Pavone-Macaluso M: Antiproliferative effect of interferons on human prostate carcinoma cell lines. Urol Res 17(2): 111–115, 1989

155. Singh RK, Gutman M, Bucana CD, Sanchez R, Llansa N, Fidler IJ: Interferons alpha and beta down-regulate the expression of basic fibroblast growth factor in human carcinomas. Proc Natl Acad Sci USA 92(10): 4562–4566, 1995

156. Dong Z, Greene G, Pettaway C, Dinney CP, Eue I, Lu W, Bucana CD, Balbay MD, Bielenberg D, Fidler IJ: Suppression of angiogenesis, tumorigenicity, and metastasis by human prostate cancer cells engineered to produce interferon-beta. Cancer Res 59(4): 872–879, 1999

157. Bulbul MA, Huben RP, Murphy GP: Interferon-beta treatment of metastatic prostate cancer. J Surg Oncol 33(4): 231–233, 1986

158. Melnyk O, Zimmerman M, Kim KJ, Shuman M: Neutralizing anti-vascular endothelial growth factor antibody inhibits further growth of established prostate cancer and metastases in a pre-clinical model. J Urol 161(3): 960–963, 1999

159. Saleh M, Stacker SA, Wilks AF: Inhibition of growth of C6 glioma cells *in vivo* by expression of antisense vascular endothelial growth factor sequence. Cancer Res 56(2): 393–401, 1996

160. Smith PC, Keller ET: Anti-interleukin-6 monoclonal antibody induces regression of human prostate cancer xenografts in nude mice. Prostate 48(1): 47–53, 2001

161. Kusaka M, Sudo K, Matsutani E, Kozai Y, Marui S, Fujita T, Ingber D, Folkman J: Cytostatic inhibition of endothelial cell growth by the angiogenesis inhibitor TNP-470 (AGM-1470). Br J Cancer 69(2): 212–216, 1994

162. Abe J, Zhou W, Takuwa N, Taguchi J, Kurokawa K, Kumada M, Takuwa Y: A fumagillin derivative angiogenesis inhibitor, AGM-1470, inhibits activation of cyclin-dependent kinases and phosphorylation of retinoblastoma gene product but not protein tyrosyl phosphorylation or protooncogene expression in vascular endothelial cells. Cancer Res 54(13): 3407–3412, 1994

163. Yamaoka M, Yamamoto T, Ikeyama S, Sudo K, Fujita T: Angiogenesis inhibitor TNP-470 (AGM-1470) potently inhibits the tumor growth of hormone-independent human breast and prostate carcinoma cell lines. Cancer Res 53(21): 5233–5236, 1993

164. Horti J, Dixon SC, Logothetis CJ, Guo Y, Reed E, Figg WD: Increased transcriptional activity of prostate-specific antigen in the presence of TNP-470, an angiogenesis inhibitor. Br J Cancer 79(9–10): 1588–1593, 1999

165. Logothetis CJ, Wu KK, Finn LD, Daliani D, Figg W, Ghaddar H, Gutterman JU: Phase I trial of the angiogenesis inhibitor TNP-470 for progressive androgen-independent prostate cancer. Clin Cancer Res 7(5): 1198–1203, 2001

166. D'Amato RJ, Loughnan MS, Flynn E, Folkman J: Thalidomide is an inhibitor of angiogenesis. Proc Natl Acad Sci USA 91(9): 4082–4085, 1994

167. Figg WD, Dahut W, Duray P, Hamilton M, Tompkins A, Steinberg SM, Jones E, Premkumar A, Linehan WM, Floeter MK, Chen CC, Dixon S, Kohler DR, Kruger EA, Gubish E, Pluda JM, Reed E: A randomized phase II trial of thalidomide, an angiogenesis inhibitor, in patients with androgen-independent prostate cancer. Clin Cancer Res 7(7): 1888–1893, 2001

168. Bauer KS, Figg WD, Hamilton JM, Jones EC, Premkumar A, Steinberg SM, Dyer V, Linehan WM, Pluda JM, Reed E: A pharmacokinetically guided Phase II study of carboxyamido-triazole in androgen-independent prostate cancer. Clin Cancer Res 5(9): 2324–2329, 1999

169. Ichikawa T, Lamb JC, Christensson PI, Hartley-Asp B, Isaacs JT: The antitumor effects of the quinoline-3-carboxamide linomide on Dunning R-3327 rat prostatic cancers. Cancer Res 52(11): 3022–3028, 1992

170. Vukanovic J, Passaniti A, Hirata T, Traystman RJ, Hartley-Asp B, Isaacs JT: Antiangiogenic effects of the quinoline-3-carboxamide linomide. Cancer Res 53(8): 1833–1837, 1993

171. Ruoslahti E: Targeting tumor vasculature with homing peptides from phage display. Semin Cancer Biol 10(6): 435–442, 2000

172. Huang X, Molema G, King S, Watkins L, Edgington TS, Thorpe PE: Tumor infarction in mice by antibody-directed targeting of tissue factor to tumor vasculature. Science 275(5299): 547–550, 1997

Address for offprints: Dan Theodorescu, Department of Urology, Health Sciences System, University of Virginia, P.O. Box 800422, Charlottesville, VA 22908-0422, USA; *e-mail:* dt9d@virginia.edu

Integrins and prostate cancer metastases

Mara Fornaro, Thomas Manes and Lucia R. Languino
Department of Pathology, Yale University School of Medicine, New Haven, CT, USA

Key words: integrin, adhesion, migration, survival, proliferation, signaling

Abstract

Integrins have emerged as modulators of a variety of cellular functions. They have been implicated in cell migration, survival, normal and aberrant cellular growth, differentiation, gene expression, and modulation of intracellular signal transduction pathways.

In this review article, the structural and functional characteristics of integrins, their expression and their potential role in prostate cancer metastases will be discussed.

1. Introduction

Integrins are crucial regulators of differentiation, growth, survival, migration and invasion. Thus, they can control the events that characterize the phenotype of a malignant tumor: lack of differentiation, abnormal growth and increased survival, local invasion and infiltration of surrounding normal tissues, and finally, metastatic spread.

In prostate cancer, tumor cells have a markedly different surrounding matrix than normal cells; thus, changes in the integrin profile may be functionally relevant and contribute to metastasis establishment and growth (as discussed below in 4).

The altered integrin and extracellular matrix (ECM) repertoire in metastatic prostate cancer is likely to affect predominantly cell migration. The mechanisms that control cell migration have been shown *in vitro* to be mediated by integrin-activated signaling molecules, such as focal adhesion kinase (FAK), phosphatidylinositol 3-kinase (PI 3-kinase), and members of the extracellular signal-regulated kinase 1 and 2/mitogen-activated protein (ERK1 and 2/MAP) kinase family. Thus, it is predicted that the study of alterations of these signaling pathways controled by integrins will contribute to the understanding of the mechanisms that support metastasis establishment and growth *in vivo* in prostate cancer (as discussed below in 5).

Due to space constraints, studies performed using prostate cancer cell lines *in vitro* will not be discussed in this review.

2. The integrin family of adhesion receptors

Adhesive contacts between cells and ECM components play a crucial role in organ development, abnormal tissue growth, tumor progression and metastatic spread. These interactions are mediated by *integrins*, the most widely distributed gene superfamily of adhesion receptors, expressed by all mammalian cells [1]. Integrins can also mediate cell–cell interactions, although the ability to mediate cell–cell contact is restricted to a few members of the family ($\alpha_L\beta_2$, $\alpha_M\beta_2$, $\alpha_X\beta_2$, $\alpha_D\beta_2$, $\alpha_4\beta_1$, and $\alpha_4\beta_7$) [1].

2.1. α and β subunits

Integrins are structurally organized into heterodimeric transmembrane complexes, variously assembled through the non-covalent association between an α and a β subunit [1]. So far, 18 α subunits, 8 β subunits, and 24 complexes have been identified and their expression and function characterized in various cell types. The integrin family is divided into subfamilies that share the β subunit [2]. Each β subunit associates with one to twelve α subunits and each α can associate with more than one β subunit. Functional specificity is determined by the specific associated subunits and by the cell type that expresses the heterodimeric complex (Table 1).

Integrins are expressed as constitutively active or inactive receptors for ECM ligands. Their functional state is cell type-dependent as well as ligand-dependent [3,4]. These different functional states might

M.L. Cher, K.V. Honn and A. Raz (eds.), Prostate Cancer: New Horizons in Research and Treatment, 185–195.
© 2002 *Kluwer Academic Publishers.*

186

Table 1. The integrin family

Subunit		Ligand
$\beta_{1(A)}$	α_1	Laminin, Collagen
	α_2	Laminin, Collagen
	α_{3A}, α_{3B}	Laminin, Collagen, Fibronectin, Entactin
	α_4	Fibronectin, VCAM1
	α_5	Fibronectin, L1
	$\alpha_{6A}, \alpha_{6B}, \alpha_{6X1}, \alpha_{6X2}$	Laminin
	$\alpha_{7A}, \alpha_{7B}, \alpha_{7X1}, \alpha_{7X1X2}$	Laminin
	α_8	Fibronectin, Tenascin, Vitronectin, Osteopontin
	α_9	Tenascin
	α_{10}	Collagen
	α_{11}	Collagen
	α_v	Fibronectin, Osteopontin, TGFβ-LAP
$\beta_{1B}, \beta_{1C}, \beta_{1C-2}, \beta_{1D}$		
β_2	α_L	ICAM1, ICAM2, ICAM3, ICAM4
	α_M	iC3b, Fibrinogen, Factor X, ICAM1, ICAM2, ICAM4
	α_X	iC3b, Fibrinogen
	α_D	ICAM3
β_{3A}	$\alpha_{IIb}, \alpha_{IIbalt}$	Fibrinogen, Fibronectin, von Willebrand Factor, Vitronectin, Thrombospondin, Disintegrin, Osteopontin
	α_v	Vitronectin, Fibrinogen, Fibronectin, von Willebrand Factor, Thrombospondin, Disintegrin, L1, MMP2, Osteopontin
β_{3B}, β_{3C}		
β_{4A}	α_{6A}, α_{6B}	Laminin-5
$\beta_{4B}, \beta_{4C}, \beta_{4D}$		
β_{5A}	α_v	Vitronectin, Osteopontin, TGFβ-LAP
β_{5B}		
β_6	α_v	Fibronectin, Tenascin, Vitronectin, TGFβ-LAP
β_7	α_4	Fibronectin, VCAM, MAdCAM1
	α_{IEL}	
β_8	α_v	Vitronectin, Fibronectin, Laminin, TGFβ- LAP

be crucial in modulating integrin-mediated functions *in vivo*.

2.2. Integrin cytoplasmic domains

Recent experimental evidence obtained with recombinant deletion mutants and chimeric forms of integrin α and β cytoplasmic domains has demonstrated that cytoplasmic tails modulate receptor distribution, receptor surface expression, ligand binding affinity of the extracellular domain, cell adhesion, and cell spreading [5,6]. Therefore, structural differences in the primary sequences of the integrin intracellular domains are predicted to determine the specificity of a variety of integrin-mediated events. In support of this hypothesis, mutations, and deletions in the integrin cytoplasmic domain have been found in the β_3 and β_4 integrin subgroups in, respectively, Glanzmann's thrombasthenia [7] and junctional epidermolysis bullosa [8], thus pointing to the cytoplasmic domain as a key player in determining crucial cellular responses *in vivo*.

Alternatively spliced forms of the α ($\alpha_3, \alpha_6, \alpha_7$) and β ($\beta_1, \beta_3, \beta_4, \beta_5$) integrin cytoplasmic domains have been identified (for review see [5] and [6]) thus adding further complexity to the regulatory pathways mediated by integrins. It is well established that the cytoplasmic domain of the β_1 subunit is required for integrins to modulate many cellular functions as well as to trigger signaling events which result in protein phosphorylation and interactions with intracellular proteins [6]. Five different β_1 isoforms containing alternatively spliced cytoplasmic domains have been identified ($\beta_{1A}, \beta_{1B}, \beta_{1C}, \beta_{1C-2}$, and β_{1D}) and have been shown to differentially affect receptor localization, cell proliferation, cell adhesion and migration, interactions with intracellular proteins and, ultimately, phosphorylation and activation of signaling molecules [6].

The expression of integrin variants is tissue and cell-type specific [6]. A selective expression has been shown for the β_{1C} integrin subunit, an inhibitor of cell proliferation [6], in hematopoietic cells, platelets, activated endothelial cells, and epithelial cells of liver, kidney, lung, breast as well as prostate [6,9–12]. The β_{1B} isoform has been found to be restricted to skin and liver, while the β_{1D} subunit has been detected in striated muscle, where it replaces the common β_{1A} isoform. Similar to β_1 variants, a differential distribution of the variant forms $\beta_{3A}, \beta_{3B}, \alpha_{3A}, \alpha_{3B}, \alpha_{6A}, \alpha_{6B}, \alpha_{7A}$, and α_{7B} in relationship to their wild type counterparts has also been described using protein and mRNA analysis [6]. The functional differences described for these variants suggest that modulation of splicing patterns of β_1 mRNA may provide an accessory mechanism to regulate signaling pathways initiated by integrins [13–15].

3. Integrin modulation of cellular functions

By interacting with the ECM and, inside the cell, with the cytoskeleton, integrins transfer signals from the extracellular environment to intracellular compartments and control many cellular functions, such as migration, survival, proliferation, differentiation, and gene expression [16–18]. These signals are initiated after integrin engagement with natural ligands or surrogate antibody ligands and include increases in cytosolic free $[Ca^{2+}]_i$, tyrosine phosphorylation, elevation of intracellular pH, and stimulated transcription and translation of immediate and early inflammatory genes [18]. Integrins can act synergistically with growth factors in modulating cellular functions [18]. Overall, the published studies show that such modulation of cellular functions is mediated by adhesion- and spreading-dependent events as well as by integrin expression. A series of excellent reviews are available on these topics [19–22].

It is worth mentioning that p27^{kip1} levels are regulated in response to integrin expression and engagement and are regulated in prostate cancer. Cell adhesion to the ECM is required for cell cycle progression and proliferation in different cell types [16]. Loss of cell anchorage to the ECM has been shown to up-regulate the expression of cyclin kinase inhibitors (CKIs) such as p27^{kip1}, while at the same time decreasing the levels of cyclin D1 and A [16]. Engagement of β_1 integrins has been shown to regulate the cell cycle machinery by modulating p27^{kip1} protein levels in either a positive or a negative fashion depending upon the cellular context [9,23,24]. p27^{kip1} is a CKI that controls cell cycle progression by associating with cyclin D-, E-, and A-cdk complexes. p27^{kip1} is highly expressed in non-proliferative, quiescent cells and its levels are increased by growth-inhibitory signals. Furthermore, its forced overexpression is sufficient to inhibit cell proliferation. The pathophysiological relevance of p27^{kip1} regulated expression is suggested by recent studies showing that in prostate cancer, as well as in several types of cancer, loss of p27^{kip1} is an adverse prognostic factor that correlates with poor patient survival [25–29]. Some reports have also shown that low p27^{kip1} expression correlates with lymph node metastasis [30–32]. Previous data from our laboratory have shown that β_{1C} integrin is down-regulated in prostate cancer and that forced expression of β_{1C} in vitro is accompanied by an increase in p27^{kip1} levels [9]. Moreover, in vivo β_{1C} integrin and p27^{kip1} expressions are concurrently down-regulated in neoplastic prostate epithelial cells, thus describing for the first time, an in vivo correlation of expression of integrins and a cell cycle inhibitor [9]. The results highlight the role of β_{1C} as an upstream regulator of p27^{kip1}. Since in vivo down-regulation of β_{1C} is likely to occur at an earlier stage than p27^{kip1}'s loss in the pathogenesis of prostate cancer, we expect β_{1C} to be a sensitive prognostic indicator of potentially high clinical value to predict therapy and patient survival.

4. Integrin expression in prostate cancer

Integrin expression in normal prostate and various prostate cancer specimens has been investigated by several laboratories, most typically by using immunohistochemical techniques (Table 2). With one exception (LM609 antibody that recognizes the $\alpha_v\beta_3$ integrin), the antibodies recognize epitopes on single integrin subunits. In order to extract information regarding the changes in functional integrin heterodimers, the findings must therefore be interpreted based on what is known about the association of integrin subunits.

Dramatic changes seen in integrin levels are those of β_{1C}, β_3, β_4 and a truncated version of α_{IIb}, which lacks the transmembrane and cytoplasmic domains. β_{1C} is expressed in benign glandular epithelial cells, but is markedly down-regulated in adenocarcinomas, regardless of the histological grade [9,12,33,34]. In contrast, β_3 is undetectable in normal prostate, but is expressed in adenocarcinoma and metastatic lesions [35] (Jain, Zheng and Languino, unpublished). β_3 is known to associate with α_v and α_{IIb}. However, even though the levels of α_v have been shown to be decreased in carcinoma compared to normal or benign prostate [36], $\alpha_v\beta_3$ is known to be present on primary prostate adenocarcinoma cells as a functional vitronectin receptor [35]. The truncated α_{IIb} integrin contains a unique sequence at its carboxy terminus, which enabled its detection in adenocarcinoma cells [37]. This epitope was not detected in normal prostate [37]. The integrin studied most intensively is $\alpha_6\beta_4$. β_4, paired with α_6 in hemidesmosomal structures at the interface of normal glandular basal cells and basal lamina, disappears as cells in prostatic

Table 2. Altered expression of integrins in prostate cancer

Integrin	Sample	Method	Altered expression	Reference
β_1	Tissue	IHC	Up-regulated and redistributed with progression	Knox et al. (1994); Murant et al. (1997)
β_{1C}	Tissue	IHC, immunoblot	Down-regulated in adenocarcinoma, expressed in benign epithelium	Fornaro et al. (1996, 1998, 1999); Perlino et al. (2000)
β_3	Freshly isolated cells from tissue and primary cultures, tissue	FACS analysis, immunoblot, IHC	Expressed in adenocarcinoma and metastatic lesions, not in normal cells	Zheng et al. (1999); #Jain et al. unpublished
β_4	Tissue	IHC	Down-regulated in carcinoma	Nagle et al. (1995); Allen et al. (1998); Davis et al. (2001)
α_2	Tissue	IHC	Down-regulated in carcinoma, up-regulated in metastases	Nagle et al. (1994); Bonkhoff et al. (1993)
α_3	Tissue	IHC	Down-regulated in carcinoma	Nagle et al. (1994)
α_4	Tissue	IHC	Down-regulated in carcinoma	Nagle et al. (1994)
α_5	Tissue	IHC	Down-regulated in carcinoma	Nagle et al. (1994)
α_6	Tissue	IHC, TEM	Polarized distribution in benign, less polarized in HGPIN, not polarized in lymph node metastases; hemidesmosomal $\alpha 6$ absent in carcinoma cells; up-regulated in metastases	Bonkhoff et al. (1993); Knox et al. (1994); Nagle et al. (1995)
α_v	Tissue	IHC	Down-regulated in carcinoma	Nagle et al. (1994)
α_{IIb} (truncated)	Tissue	IHC	Expressed in adenocarcinoma, not in normal tissue	Trikha et al. (1998)

IHC: immunohistochemistry; TEM: transmission electron microscopy; FACS: fluorescence activated cell sorting; HGPIN: high grade prostatic intraepithelial neoplasia; #Jain, Zheng and Languino, unpublished results.

intraepithelial neoplasia (PIN) lesions become transformed, and is absent in carcinoma cells [36,38–40]. The expression of α_6, however, is still maintained in prostatic neoplasms, but its distribution becomes more disperse and its density at sites of contact with the basement membrane diminishes with increasing histologic grade [41,42]. Since the only other integrin that α_6 is known to associate with is β_1, this re-distribution of α_6 probably represents the $\alpha_6\beta_1$ integrin. In addition, α_6 is up-regulated in lymph node metastases compared to primary lesions [41]. Most other α integrins, that is, α_2, α_3, α_4, α_5 and, as mentioned above, α_v, have been reported to be down-regulated in adenocarcinoma [36,38]. In one study, increased staining for α_2 was found in lymph node metastases compared to primary lesions [41]. While not distinguishing between the four known different isoforms of β_1, Murant et al. [43] report a slight increase in expression levels of β_1 with increasing Gleason grade. Taken with the reduction of the aforementioned α integrins, this would therefore represent a shift in β_1 heterodimer composition with the

progression of prostate cancer. However, it should be noted that some of the α integrin subunits that heterodimerize with β_1, that is, α_1, α_7, α_8, and α_9, have not yet been investigated.

The expression of integrins in normal prostate and prostate cancer has also been investigated at the mRNA level. Indirectly, a massive effort is represented by the Cancer Genome Anatomy Project (CGAP). At the CGAP web site, libraries prepared from many different samples, ranging from normal tissue to metastatic lesions, can be compared. However, not much information regarding integrins is yet available. Even so, integrin protein levels cannot be inferred from mRNA levels. This has been documented in two recent studies. In an investigation of β_1 variant gene expression in normal and neoplastic prostate, Perlino et al. [12] showed that β_{1C} mRNA levels were down-regulated in neoplastic specimens, in agreement with β_{1C} protein levels, but total β_1 mRNA was also down-regulated, in contrast to total β_1 protein levels. Recently, Hao et al. [44] showed that the mRNA of β_4 was at least at the same level in malignant as compared to normal tissue, which is unexpected given the well-documented decrease in β_4 protein levels. These recent findings indicate that the control of integrin expression in the progression of prostate cancer is complex and deserves further investigations.

5. Signaling pathways activated by integrins: Molecular alterations in prostate cancer

Integrins are likely involved in cancer initiation and/or progression because of their ability not only to mediate interactions with ECM proteins, but also to regulate multiple intracellular signaling molecules that are necessary for cell motility, cell survival and proliferation [1,21]. The mechanisms of signaling that occur proximal to the membrane are poorly known; integrin clustering or association with members of the transmembrane 4 superfamily might be ways to trigger proliferation signals and, consequently, regulate tumor invasion and growth [45].

This section focuses on gene products that have been shown to be involved in signaling events mediated by integrins that affect cell motility and whose expression levels and activity are altered in prostate cancer. The best characterized pathways activated by integrins are the FAK, the PI 3-kinase and the Ras/MAP kinase pathways (Figure 1 and Table 3). Other molecules that are regulated by integrins but have not been implicated in cell migration, such as the tumor suppressors p53 and Rb, cyclins D and A, and the cyclin kinase inhibitor p21[cip1] have been shown to be frequently mutated and/or overexpressed in prostate cancer. An overview of the most frequent alterations of these molecules in prostate cancer can be found in recent excellent reviews [46,47] and elsewhere in this issue.

5.1. FAK

FAK is a non-receptor protein tyrosine kinase that has been shown to co-localize with integrins at focal contact sites [48]. FAK becomes tyrosine phosphorylated in response to integrin engagement and other stimuli [48–50]. FAK inhibition induces apoptosis and overexpression of FAK prevents apoptosis induced either in absence of ECM survival signals or in response to other

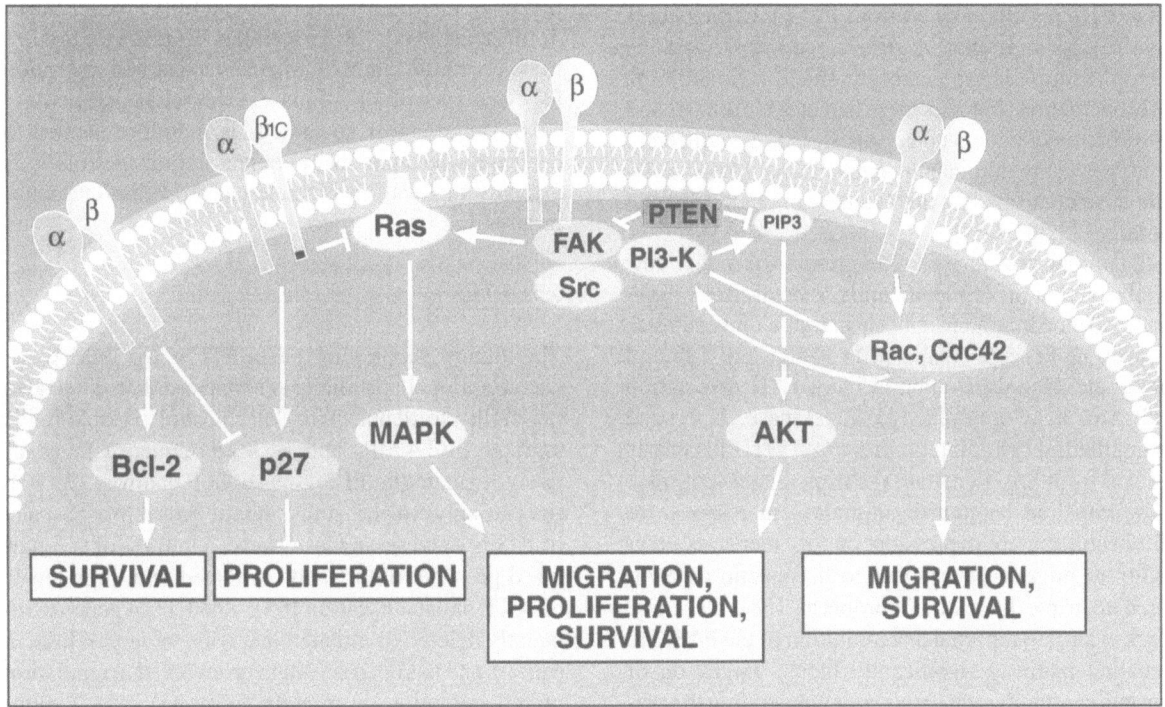

Figure 1. Signaling pathways activated by integrins and altered in prostate cancer. Schematic drawing showing the signal transduction pathways activated by integrins that control cell migration, survival and proliferation; these pathways are altered in prostate cancer. PIP3, phosphatidylinositol (3,4,5) triphosphate.

Table 3. Integrin signaling pathways that control cell migration and are altered in prostate cancer

Signaling molecule	Regulation by integrins	Alteration
FAK	Kinase activity	Up-regulation
AKT	Kinase activity	Increased kinase activity/phosphorylation
PTEN	Nd	Deletions/point mutations/down-regulation
Ras	GTPase activity	Low frequency point mutations
MAP kinase	Kinase activity	Up-regulation and increased kinase activity/phosphorylation

Nd, not determined.
Up-regulation, refers to protein levels.
Down-regulation, refers to protein levels.

stimuli [50]. Several studies have suggested a role for FAK in controling cell migration in response to integrin engagement or to growth factors [50]. Direct evidence on the role of FAK *in vivo* in regulating cell migration has been obtained with the generation of FAK null mice. Ablation of the FAK gene results in embryonic lethality at day 8.0–8.5 due to severe mesodermal defects [51]. Cells derived from these embryos show a decreased migration *in vitro* as compared to cells derived from wild type embryos [51,52]. In addition, FAK overexpression in chinese hamster fibroblasts and perturbation of endogenous FAK signaling in different cell types using dominant negative forms of the molecule have confirmed its involvement in controling cell motility [35,50,53,54].

In normal prostate, FAK expression is either low or absent but it is significantly increased in high-grade adenocarcinomas and in invasive and metastatic prostate cancers compared to benign prostate and low grade adenocarcinoma [55,56]. FAK association with Src, a cytoplasmic tyrosine kinase, is crucial for regulating cell migration *in vitro* [57]. Fibroblasts derived from Src, Fyn, and Yes triple knock-out mice show impaired haptotactic migration in response to fibronectin and re-expression of Src increases their ability to migrate in response to fibronectin as compared to triple knock-out fibroblasts [58]. Recently, Slack et al. [59] reported that inhibition of the FAK/Src signaling pathway significantly blocks migration of prostate carcinoma cells *in vitro*, demonstrating the crucial role exerted by these molecules in the regulation of prostate cell motility. However, analysis of Src gene alterations, protein expression and activity in prostate cancer tissues has not been performed.

5.2. *PI 3-kinase/AKT*

In addition to stimulating FAK, integrins can also activate the PI 3-kinase pathway [60]. PI 3-kinases comprise a family of lipid kinases activated by a wide variety of extracellular stimuli. The lipid products of PI 3-kinases, specifically phosphatidylinositol(3,4)biphosphate [$PI(3,4)P_2$] and (3,4,5)triphosphate [$PI(3,4,5)P_3$], affect cell proliferation, survival, differentiation, and migration by targeting specific signaling molecules such as the serine/threonine protein kinase B, also known as AKT [61–63]. Integrin-mediated adhesion to the ECM stimulates the production of $PI(3,4)P_2$ and $PI(3,4,5)P_3$ [64,65], the association of the p85 PI 3-kinase subunit with FAK [66] and AKT activation [64,65]. AKT plays an important role in transducing survival signals in response to several growth factors and to integrin engagement [64,67]. Recent studies have shown a significant increase in AKT kinase activity and phosphorylation associated with prostate cancer progression; specifically, the highest levels of phosphorylated AKT correlated with high Gleason grade, tumor stage III/IV and invasive cancer [68,69]. Several studies have reported that integrins control cancer cell motility through the PI 3-kinase pathway [70] which has been shown *in vitro* to be crucial for human prostate cancer cell migration [4]. Analysis of PI 3-kinase expression and activity on prostate cancer specimens is therefore needed to determine the clinicopathological significance of the PI 3-kinase pathway in prostate cancer initiation and/or progression.

5.3. *PTEN*

The tumor suppressor gene PTEN (or MMAC-1) encodes a dual specificity phosphatase but it has also the ability to dephosphorylate inositol phospholipids such as $PI(3,4,5)P_3$ and as a consequence to negatively regulate the PI 3-kinase/AKT pathway [71,72]. Interestingly, in the study mentioned above absence of PTEN expression was observed in 60% of the analyzed prostate tumors and correlated with high levels of AKT phosphorylation [68]. The PTEN gene is frequently deleted or mutated in a wide variety of human cancers and has been shown to be involved in regulation of cell migration on integrin substrates [72]. Tamura et al. [73] have shown that FAK is one of the PTEN substrates. PTEN inhibits cell migration and invasion by dephosphorylating FAK and the adapter protein Shc, thereby antagonizing integrin-triggered signaling

[72]. The PTEN gene was located at 10q23.3 [74,75]. Loss of heterozygosity (LOH) in the region 10q23.3 is present in 29–42% of clinically localized prostate cancers [76,77]. Similarly, LOH at 10q23 is present in more than 50% of metastatic prostate tumors [76–78]. PTEN is also frequently mutated or deleted in prostate cancer and prostate cancer cell lines [74,76,78,79]. PTEN is expressed at the protein level in secretory epithelia in normal adult prostate and loss of PTEN protein expression in primary prostate cancers correlates with high Gleason grade and advanced pathological stage [80]. It is, thus, conceivable that reduced PTEN expression levels might result in increased prostate cancer cell migration in vivo.

5.4. Ras/MAP kinase

Ras proteins belong to a large family of GTPases which function as signal transducers by cycling from an active GTP-bound form to an inactive GDP-bound form and activated Ras stimulates numerous signaling cascades such as the ERK1 and 2/MAP kinase pathway [81]. The Ras/MAP kinase pathway plays a pivotal role in modulating gene expression, cell cycle progression, survival and motility [82,83]. Integrin clustering has been shown to stimulate Ras GTP-loading [65,84–87] and to activate specific effectors of the Ras/MAP kinase signaling cascade [88,89] which results in increased cell proliferation, cell cycle progression and survival [90]. Some integrins exert a negative effect on the Ras/MAP kinase pathway which leads to cell cycle arrest and differentiation [91] and inhibition of cell proliferation [15]. There is evidence that cell motility is controled by integrins via a signaling cascade involving Shc and MEK1 and the MAP kinases ERK1 and 2, respectively [92,93]. Sustained activation of the Ras/MAP kinase pathway can also prevent apoptosis triggered by loss of cell–ECM contacts [94–96]. Recently it has been reported that migration and survival mechanisms promoted by integrin engagement are coordinately regulated through activation of pathways that involve ERK activity [97]. The activity and expression levels of MAP kinase are significantly higher in primary prostatic adenocarcinoma and in metastatic lesions than the levels detected in benign prostate [98–100]. Increased MAP kinase activation correlates with high Gleason score and tumor stage [98]. Since Ras mutations are uncommon in prostate cancer [46], chronic stimulation of the Ras/MAP kinase pathway is most likely achieved by alterations in the levels of upstream regulators such as integrins, growth factors and growth factor receptors during prostate cancer initiation and/or progression. Several studies suggest that integrin engagement activates members of the Rho-family of small GTPases [20,70]. Specifically, Rho, Rac, and Cdc42 have been shown to be required for cell motility [20,70]. However, analysis of Rho-family of small GTPases' gene alterations, protein expression or activity in prostate cancer tissues has not been performed.

5.5. Bcl-2

The Bcl-2 protein is a proto-oncogene that promotes cell survival [101] and is a member of a large family that consists of pro-apoptotic and pro-survival factors [102]. The Bcl-2 gene is activated by chromosomal translocation in the majority of non-Hodgkin's lymphomas and is also up-regulated in many solid tumors, indicating that it might contribute to resistance to apoptosis in response to chemotherapeutic agents and radiation therapy [102]. Adhesion to fibronectin through $\alpha_5\beta_1$ and $\alpha_v\beta_1$ and to vitronectin through $\alpha_v\beta_3$ integrins was shown to up-regulate Bcl-2 transcription and protein levels and resulted in protection from apoptosis induced by serum deprivation [103,104].

Bcl-2 protein levels are low or absent in normal prostate and Bcl-2 expression is restricted to basal cells [105]. In prostate carcinoma Bcl-2 is up-regulated and its expression correlates with hormone-refractory disease [46,105] and with poor survival [46]. Analysis of metastatic lesions obtained from prostate cancer patients after hormone treatment (hormone-refractory tumors) stained positive for Bcl-2 [106]. There is evidence for a role for Bcl-2 in promoting cancer cell motility and invasion. Overexpression of Bcl-2 increases migration and metastatic potential of breast cancer cells [107] and therefore its involvement in prostate cell migration deserves to be investigated.

6. Conclusions

This review highlights the current knowledge of the alterations that occur in prostate cancer and in prostate cancer metastases and that involve integrins and integrin-activated pathways. Although the specific functions of integrins, their ligands and their modulators in prostate cancer are not completely understood, recent publications outlining their expression pave the way for future investigations describing the role of integrin isoforms and of integrin signaling in prostate cancer cell invasion, metastatic establishment and growth.

Future research will focus on functional correlates, combining general knowledge of integrins and integrin signaling with an increasing appreciation for the role of the ECM in prostate cancer progression.

Since a single 'metastasis gene' has not been found, it is expected that multiple genetic alterations have to occur at the same time to make a cell 'metastatic'. Therefore, in addition to the disregulated expression of either integrins or integrin-activated pathways in prostate cancer, alterations of other molecules that control cell adhesion or increase either proteolysis of ECM or migration may have an important role in disease progression and metastatic spread. Among others, KAI-1, a 'prostate cancer metastasis suppressor gene' described elsewhere in details in this issue, deserves further consideration for its ability to inhibit cell migration and potentially affect integrin–ligand binding. Similarly, changes in integrin affinity, avidity, or activation state are likely to control cell–ECM interaction; additional investigations on these topics will help understanding the role of integrins in prostate cancer metastases.

Acknowledgements

This work was supported by grants from the National Institutes of Health: grants R29 CA-71870 and RO1 CA-89720 (to L.R.L.), and from the Army PCRP grant DAMD17-98-1-8506 (to L.R.L. and M.F.) and DK-07556T32 training grant (to T.M.). We thank Ms. N. Bennett for expert assistance in preparing the manuscript.

References

1. Hynes RO: Cell adhesion: Old and new questions. Trends Cell Biol 9: M33–M37, 1999
2. Ruoslahti E: Integrins as signaling molecules and targets for tumor therapy. Kidney Int 51: 1413–1417, 1997
3. Byzova TV, Rabbani R, D'Souza SE, Plow EF: Role of integrin $\alpha v \beta 3$ in vascular biology. Thromb Haemost 80: 726–734, 1998
4. Zheng DQ, Woodard AS, Tallini G, Languino LR: Substrate specificity of $\alpha v \beta 3$ integrin-mediated cell migration and PI 3-kinase/AKT pathway activation. J Biol Chem 275: 24565–24574, 2000
5. Hemler ME, Weitzman JB, Pasqualini R, Kawaguchi S, Kassner PD, Berdichevsky FB: Structure, biochemical properties, and biological functions of integrin cytoplasmic domains. In: Takada Y (ed) Integrins: The Biological Problems. CRC Press Inc., Boca Raton, 1995, pp 1–35
6. Fornaro M, Languino LR: Alternatively spliced variants: A new view of the integrin cytoplasmic domain. Matrix Biol 16: 185–193, 1997
7. Williams MJ, Hughes PE, O'Toole TE, Ginsberg MH: The inner world of cell adhesion: Integrin cytoplasmic domains. Trends Cell Biol 4: 109–112, 1994
8. Vidal F, Aberdam D, Miquel C, Christiano AM, Pulkkinen L, Uitto J, Ortonne J-P, Meneguzzi G: Integrin $\beta 4$ mutations associated with junctional epidermolysis bullosa with pyloric atresia. Nat Genet 10: 229–234, 1995
9. Fornaro M, Tallini G, Zheng DQ, Flanagan WM, Manzotti M, Languino LR: p27kip1 acts as a downstream effector of and is coexpressed with the β_{1C} integrin in prostatic adenocarcinoma. J Clin Invest 103: 321–329, 1999
10. Patriarca C, Alfano RM, Sonnenberg A, Graziani D, Cassani B, de Melker A, Colombo P, Languino LR, Fornaro M, Warren WH, Coggi G, Gould VE: Integrin laminin receptor profile of pulmonary squamous cell and adenocarcinomas. Hum Pathol 29: 1208–1215, 1998
11. Manzotti M, Dell'Orto P, Maisonneuve P, Fornaro M, Languino LR, Viale G: Down-regulation of β_{1C} integrin in breast carcinomas correlates with high proliferative fraction, high histological grade, and larger size. Am J Pathol 156: 169–174, 2000
12. Perlino E, Lovecchio M, Vacca RA, Fornaro M, Moro L, Ditonno P, Battaglia M, Selvaggi FP, Mastropasqua MG, Bufo P, Languino LR: Regulation of mRNA and protein levels of β_1 integrin variants in human prostate carcinoma. Am J Pathol 157: 1727–1734, 2000
13. Belkin AM, Retta SF, Pletjushkina OY, Balzac F, Silengo L, Fassler R, Koteliansky VE, Burridge K, Tarone G: Muscle $\beta 1D$ integrin reinforces the cytoskeleton-matrix link: Modulation of integrin adhesive function by alternative splicing. J Cell Biol 139: 1583–1595, 1997
14. Retta SF, Balzac F, Ferraris P, Belkin AM, Fassler R, Humphries MJ, De Leo G, Silengo L, Tarone G: $\beta 1$-integrin cytoplasmic subdomains involved in dominant negative function. Mol Biol Cell 9: 715–731, 1998
15. Fornaro M, Steger CA, Bennett AM, Wu JJ, Languino LR: Differential role of β_{1C} and β_{1A} integrin cytoplasmic variants in modulating focal adhesion kinase, protein kinase B/AKT, and Ras/Mitogen-activated protein kinase pathways. Mol Biol Cell 11: 2235–2249, 2000
16. Bottazzi ME, Assoian RK: The extracellular matrix and mitogenic growth factors control G1 phase cyclins and cyclin-dependent kinase inhibitors. Trends Cell Biol 7: 348–352, 1997
17. Frisch SM, Ruoslahti E: Integrins and anoikis. Curr Opin Cell Biol 9: 701–706, 1997
18. Schwartz MA, Schaller MD, Ginsberg MH: Integrins: Emerging paradigms of signal transduction. Annu Rev Cell Dev Bio 11: 549–599, 1995
19. Holly SP, Larson MK, Parise LV: Multiple roles of integrins in cell motility. Exp Cell Res 261: 69–74, 2000
20. Parise LV, Lee J, Juliano RL: New aspects of integrin signaling in cancer. Semin Cancer Biol 10: 407–414, 2000
21. Ruoslahti E, Reed JC: Anchorage dependence, integrins and apoptosis. Cell 77: 477–478, 1994

22. Assoian RK, Schwartz MA: Coordinate signaling by integrins and receptor tyrosine kinases in the regulation of G_1 phase cell-cycle progression. Curr Opin Genet Dev 11: 48–53, 2001

23. Henriet P, Zhong ZD, Brooks PC, Weinberg KI, DeClerck YA: Contact with fibrillar collagen inhibits melanoma cell proliferation by up-regulating p27KIP1. Proc Natl Acad Sci USA 97: 10026–10031, 2000

24. Qiang YW, Kitagawa M, Higashi M, Ishii G, Morimoto C, Harigaya K: Activation of mitogen-activated protein kinase through $\alpha 5\beta 1$ integrin is required for cell cycle progression of B progenitor cell line, Reh, on human marrow stromal cells. Exp Hematol 28: 1147–1157, 2000

25. Tsihlias J, Kapusta LR, DeBoer G, Morava-Protzner I, Zbieranowski I, Bhattacharya N, Catzavelos GC, Koltz LH, Slingerland M: Loss of cyclin-dependent kinase inhibitor p27Kip1 is a novel prognostic factor in localized human prostate adenocarcinoma. Cancer Res 58: 542–548, 1998

26. Yang RM, Naitoh J, Murphy M, Wang HJ, Phillipson J, deKernion JB, Loda M, Reiter RE: Low P27 expression predicts poor disease-free survival in patients with prostate cancer. J Urol 159: 941–945, 1998

27. Catzavelos C, Bhattacharya N, Ung YC, Wilson JA, Roncari L, Sandhu C, Shaw P, Yeger H, Morava-Protzner I, Kapusta L, Franssen E, Pritchard KI, Slingerland JM: Decreased levels of the cell-cycle inhibitor p27Kip1 protein: Prognostic implications in primary breast cancer. Nat Med 3: 227–230, 1997

28. Porter PL, Malone KE, Heagerty PJ, Alexander GM, Gatti LA, Firpo EJ, Daling JR, Roberts JM: Expression of cell-cycle regulators p27Kip1 and cyclin E, alone and in combination, correlate with survival in young breast cancer patients. Nat Med 3: 222–226, 1997

29. Loda M, Cukor B, Tam SW, Lavin P, Fiorentino M, Draetta GF, Jessup JM, Pagano M: Increased proteasome-dependent degradation of the cyclin-dependent kinase inhibitor p27 in aggressive colorectal carcinomas. Nat Med 3: 231–234, 1997

30. Cheville J, Lloyd R, Sebo T, Cheng L, Erickson L, Bostwick D, Lohse C, Wollan P: Expression of p27kip1 in prostatic adenocarcinoma. Mod Pathol 11: 324–328, 1998

31. Erdamar S, Yang G, Harper JW, Lu X, Kattan MW, Thompson TC, Wheeler TM: Levels of expression of p27KIP1 protein in human prostate and prostate cancer: An immunohistochemical analysis. Mod Pathol 12: 751–755, 1999

32. Fernandez PL, Arce Y, Farre X, Martinez A, Nadal A, Rey MJ, Peiro N, Campo E, Cardesa A: Expression of p27/Kip1 is down-regulated in human prostate carcinoma progression. J Pathol 187: 563–566, 1999

33. Fornaro M, Tallini G, Bofetiado CJM, Bosari S, Languino LR: Down-regulation of β_{1C} integrin, an inhibitor of cell proliferation, in prostate carcinoma. Am J Pathol 149: 765–773, 1996

34. Fornaro M, Manzotti M, Tallini G, Slear AE, Bosari S, Ruoslahti E, Languino LR: β_{1C} integrin in epithelial cells correlates with a nonproliferative phenotype: Forced expression of β_{1C} inhibits prostate epithelial cell proliferation. Am J Pathol 153: 1079–1087, 1998

35. Zheng DQ, Woodard AS, Fornaro M, Tallini G, Languino LR: Prostatic carcinoma cell migration via $\alpha_v\beta_3$ integrin is modulated by a focal adhesion kinase pathway. Cancer Res 59: 1655–1664, 1999

36. Nagle RB, Knox JD, Wolf C, Bowden GT, Cress AE: Adhesion molecules, extracellular matrix, and proteases in prostate carcinoma. J Cell Biochem (19 Suppl): 232–237, 1994

37. Trikha M, Cai Y, Grignon D, Honn KV: Identification of a novel truncated αIIb integrin. Cancer Res 58: 4771–4775, 1998

38. Nagle RB, Hao J, Knox JD, Dalkin BL, Clark V, Cress AE: Expression of hemidesmosomal and extracellular matrix proteins by normal and malignant human prostate tissue. Am J Pathol 146: 1498–1507, 1995

39. Allen MV, Smith GJ, Juliano R, Maygarden SJ, Mohler JL: Downregulation of the β_4 integrin subunit in prostatic carcinoma and prostatic intraepithelial neoplasia. Hum Pathol 29: 311–318, 1998

40. Davis TL, Cress AE, Dalkin BL, Nagle RB: Unique expression pattern of the $\alpha 6\beta 4$ integrin and laminin-5 in human prostate carcinoma. Prostate 46: 240–248, 2001

41. Bonkhoff H, Stein U, Remberger K: Differential expression of $\alpha 6$ and $\alpha 2$ very late antigen integrins in the normal, hyperplastic, and neoplastic prostate: Simultaneous demonstration of cell surface receptors and their extracellular ligands. Hum Pathol 24: 243–248, 1993

42. Bonkhoff H: Analytical molecular pathology of epithelial-stromal interactions in the normal and neoplastic prostate. Analyt Quant Cytol Histol 20: 437–442, 1998

43. Murant SJ, Handley J, Stower M, Reid N, Cussenot O, Maitland NJ: Coordinated changes in expression of cell adhesion molecules in prostate cancer. Eur J Cancer 33: 263–271, 1997

44. Hao J, Jackson L, Calaluce R, McDaniel K, Dalkin BL, Nagle RB: Investigation into the mechanism of the loss of laminin 5 ($\alpha 3\beta 3\gamma 2$) expression in prostate cancer. Am J Pathol 158: 1129–1135, 2001

45. Hemler M, Mannion B, Berditchevski F: Association of TM4SF proteins with integrins: Relevance to cancer. Biochim Biophys Acta 1287: 67–71, 1996

46. Augustus M, Moul JW, Srivastava S: The Molecular Phenotype of the Malignant Prostate, IOS Press, Washington DC, 1999

47. Burton JL, Oakley N, Anderson JB: Recent advances in the histopathology and molecular biology of prostate cancer. BJU Int 85: 87–94, 2000

48. Guan JL, Trevithick JE, Hynes RO: Fibronectin/integrin interaction induces tyrosine phosphorylation of a 120 kDa protein. Cell Regul 2: 951, 1991

49. Kornberg L, Earp H, Turner C, Prockop C, Juliano R: Signal transduction by integrins: Increased protein tyrosine phosphorylation caused by clustering in β_1 integrins. Proc Natl Acad Sci USA 88: 8392–8396, 1991

50. Schaller MD: Biochemical signals and biological responses elicited by the focal adhesion kinase. Biochim Biophys Acta 1540: 1–21, 2001

51. Ilic D, Furuta Y, Kanazawa S, Takeda N, Sobue K, Nakatsuji N, Nomura S, Fujimoto J, Okada M,

Yamamoto T, Aizawa S: Reduced cell motility and enhanced focal adhesion contact formation in cells from FAK-deficient mice. Nature 377: 539–543, 1995

52. Ilic D, Kanazawa S, Furuta Y, Yamamoto T, Aizawa S: Impairment of mobility in endodermal cells by FAK deficiency. Exp Cell Res 222: 298–303, 1996

53. Cary LA, Chang JF, Guan J-L: Stimulation of cell migration by overexpression of focal adhesion kinase and its association with Src and Fyn J Cell Sci 109: 1787–1794, 1996

54. Gilmore A, Romer H: Inhibition of focal adhesion kinase (FAK) signaling in focal adhesions decreases cell motility and proliferation. Mol Biol Cell 7: 1209–1224, 1996

55. Tremblay L, Hauck W, Aprikian AG, Begin LR, Chapdelaine A, Chevalier S: Focal adhesion kinase pp^{125FAK} expression, activation and association with paxillin and p^{50CSK} in human metastatic prostate carcinoma. Int J Cancer 68: 164–171, 1996

56. Stanzione R, Picascia A, Chieffi P, Imbimbo C, Palmieri A, Mirone V, Staibano S, Franco R, De Rosa G, Schlessinger J, Tramontano D: Variations of proline-rich kinase Pyk2 expression correlate with prostate cancer progression. Lab Invest 81: 51–59, 2001

57. Sieg DJ, Hauck CR, Schlaepfer DD: Required role of focal adhesion kinase (FAK) for integrin-stimulated cell migration. J Cell Sci 112: 2677–2691, 1999

58. Klinghoffer RA, Sachsenmaier C, Cooper JA, Soriano P: Src family kinases are required for integrin but not PDGFR signal transduction. EMBO J 18: 2459–2471, 1999

59. Slack JK, Adams RB, Rovin JD, Bissonette EA, Stoker CE, Parsons JT: Alterations in the focal adhesion kinase/Src signal transduction pathway correlate with increased migratory capacity of prostate carcinoma cells. Oncogene 20: 1152–1163, 2001

60. Keely P, Parise L, Juliano R: Integrins and GTPases in tumor cell growth, motility and invasion. Trends Cell Biol 8: 101–106, 1998

61. Rameh LE, Cantley LC: The role of phosphoinositide 3-kinase lipid products in cell function. J Biol Chem 274: 8347–8350, 1999

62. Jiang BH, Aoki M, Zheng JZ, Li J, Vogt PK: Myogenic signaling of phosphatidylinositol 3-kinase requires the serine-threonine kinase Akt/protein kinase B. Proc Natl Acad Sci USA 96: 2077–2081, 1999

63. Morales-Ruiz M, Fulton D, Sowa G, Languino LR, Fujio Y, Walsh K, Sessa WC: Vascular endothelial growth factor-stimulated actin reorganization and migration of endothelial cells is regulated via the serine/threonine kinase Akt. Circ Res 86: 892–896, 2000

64. Khwaja A, Rodriguez-Viciana P, Wennstrom S, Warne PH, Downward J: Matrix adhesion and Ras transformation both activate a phosphoinositide 3-OH kinase and protein kinase B/Akt cellular survival pathway. EMBO J 16: 2783–2793, 1997

65. King WG, Mattaliano MD, Chan TO, Tsichlis PN, Brugge JS: Phosphatidylinositol 3-kinase is required for integrin-stimulated AKT and Raf-1/mitogen-activated protein kinase pathway activation. Mol Cell Biol 17: 4406–4418, 1997

66. Chen H-C, Guan J-L: Association of focal adhesion kinase with its potential substrate phosphatidylinositol 3-kinase. Proc Natl Acad Sci USA 91: 10148–10152, 1994

67. Downward J: Mechanisms and consequences of activation of protein kinase B/Akt. Curr Opin Cell Biol 10: 262–267, 1998

68. Sun M, Wang G, Paciga JE, Feldman RI, Yuan ZQ, Ma XL, Shelley SA, Jove R, Tsichlis PN, Nicosia SV, Cheng JQ: AKT1/PKBalpha kinase is frequently elevated in human cancers and its constitutive activation is required for oncogenic transformation in NIH3T3 cells. Am J Pathol 159: 431–437, 2001

69. Paweletz CP, Charboneau L, Bichsel VE, Simone NL, Chen T, Gillespie JW, Emmert-Buck MR, Roth MJ, Petricoin IE, Liotta LA: Reverse phase protein microarrays which capture disease progression show activation of pro-survival pathways at the cancer invasion front. Oncogene 20: 1981–1989, 2001

70. Mercurio AM, Rabinovitz I, Shaw LM: The $\alpha6\beta4$ integrin and epithelial cell migration. Curr Opin Cell Biol 13: 541–545, 2001

71. Maehama T, Dixon JE: PTEN: A tumour suppressor that functions as a phospholipid phosphatase. Trends Cell Biol 9: 125–128, 1999

72. Tamura M, Gu J, Tran H, Yamada KM: PTEN gene and integrin signaling in cancer. J Natl Cancer Inst 91: 1820–1828, 1999

73. Tamura M, Gu J, Matsumoto K, Aota S, Parsons R, Yamada KM: Inhibition of cell migration, spreading and focal adhesions by tumor suppressor PTEN. Science 280: 1614–1617, 1998

74. Li J, Yen C, Liaw D, Podsypanina K, Bose S, Wang SI, Puc J, Miliaresis C, Rodgers L, McCombie R, Bigner SH, Giovanella BC, Ittmann M, Tycko B, Hibshoosh H, Wigler MH, Parsons R: *PTEN*, a putative protein tyrosine phosphatase gene mutated in human brain, breast, and prostate cancer. Science 275: 1943–1947, 1997

75. Steck PA, Pershouse MA, Jasser SA, Yung WK, Lin H, Ligon AH, Langford LA, Baumgard ML, Hattier T, Davis T, Frye C, Hu R, Swedlund B, Teng DH, Tavtigian SV: Identification of a candidate tumour suppressor gene, MMAC1, at chromosome 10q23.3 that is mutated in multiple advanced cancers. Nat Genet 15: 356–362, 1997

76. Cairns P, Okami K, Halachmi S, Halachmi N, Esteller M, Herman JG, Jen J, Isaacs WB, Bova GS, Sidransky D: Frequent inactivation of *PTEN/MMAC1* in primary prostate cancer. Cancer Res 57: 4997–5000, 1997

77. Suzuki H, Freije D, Nusskern DR, Okami K, Cairns P, Sidransky D, Isaacs WB, Bova GS: Interfocal heterogeneity of PTEN/MMAC1 gene alterations in multiple metastatic prostate cancer tissues. Cancer Res 58: 204–209, 1998

78. Teng DH, Hu R, Lin H, Davis T, Iliev D, Frye C, Swedlund B, Hansen KL, Vinson VL, Gumpper KL, Ellis L, El-Naggar A, Frazier M, Jasser S, Langford LA, Lee J, Mills GB, Pershouse MA, Pollack RE, Tornos C, Troncoso P, Yung WK, Fujii G, Berson A, Steck PA, et al.: MMAC1/PTEN mutations in primary tumor specimens and tumor cell lines. Cancer Res 57: 5221–5225, 1997

195

79. Vlietstra RJ, van Alewijk DCJG, Hermans KGL, van Steenbrugge GJ, Trapman J: Frequent inactivation of *PTEN* in prostate cancer cell lines and xenografts. Cancer Res 58: 2720–2723, 1998

80. McMenamin ME, Soung P, Perera S, Kaplan I, Loda M, Sellers WR: Loss of PTEN expression in paraffin-embedded primary prostate cancer correlates with high Gleason score and advanced stage. Cancer Res 59: 4291–4296, 1999

81. Campbell SL, Khosravi-Far R, Rossman KL, Clark GJ, Der CJ: Increasing complexity of Ras signaling. Oncogene 17: 1395–1413, 1998

82. Robinson MJ, Cobb MH: Mitogen-activated protein kinase pathways. Curr Opin Cell Biol 9: 180–186, 1997

83. Chang L, Karin M: Mammalian MAP kinase signalling cascades. Nature 410: 37–40, 2001

84. Clark E, Hynes R: Ras activation is necesary for integrin-mediated activation of extracellular signal-regulated kinase 2 and cytosolic phospholipase A_2 but not for cytoskeletal organization. J Biol Chem 271: 14814–14818, 1996

85. Wary KK, Mainiero F, Isakoff SJ, Marcantonio EE, Giancotti FG: The adaptor protein Shc couples a class of integrins to the control of cell cycle progression. Cell 87: 733–743, 1996

86. Mainiero F, Murgia C, Wary KK, Curatola AM, Pepe A, Blumemberg M, Westwick JK, Der CJ, Giancotti FG: The coupling of $\alpha_6\beta_4$ integrin to Ras-MAP kinase pathways mediated by Shc controls keratinocyte proliferation. EMBO J 16: 2365–2375, 1997

87. Miranti CK, Ohno S, Brugge JS: Protein kinase C regulates integrin-induced activation of the extracellular regulated kinase pathway upstream of Shc. J Biol Chem 274: 10571–10581, 1999

88. Schlaepfer DD, Hunter T: Integrin signalling and tyrosine phosphorylation: Just the FAKs? Trends Cell Biol 8: 151–157, 1998

89. Howe A, Aplin AE, Alahari SK, Juliano RL: Integrin signaling and cell growth control. Curr Opin Cell Biol 10: 220–231, 1998

90. Schwartz MA, Assoian RK: Integrins and cell proliferation: Regulation of cyclin-dependent kinases via cytoplasmic signaling pathways. J Cell Sci 114: 2553–2560, 2001

91. Sastry SK, Lakonishok M, Wu S, Truong TQ, Huttenlocher A, Turner CE, Horwitz AF: Quantitative changes in integrin and focal adhesion signaling regulate myoblast cell cycle withdrawal. J Cell Biol 144: 1295–1309, 1999

92. Gu J, Tamura M, Pankov R, Danen EH, Takino T, Matsumoto K, Yamada KM: Shc and FAK differentially regulate cell motility and directionality modulated by PTEN. J Cell Biol 146: 389–403, 1999

93. Cheresh DA, Leng J, Klemke RL: Regulation of cell contraction and membrane ruffling by distinct signals in migratory cells. J Cell Biol 146: 1107–1116, 1999

94. Frisch SM, Screaton RA: Anoikis mechanisms. Curr Opin Cell Biol 13: 555–562, 2001

95. Le Gall M, Chambard JC, Breittmayer JP, Grall D, Pouyssegur J, Van Obberghen-Schilling E: The p42/p44 MAP kinase pathway prevents apoptosis induced by anchorage and serum removal. Mol Biol Cell 11: 1103–1112, 2000

96. Rosen K, Rak J, Leung T, Dean NM, Kerbel RS, Filmus J: Activated Ras prevents downregulation of Bcl-X(L) triggered by detachment from the extracellular matrix. A mechanism of Ras-induced resistance to anoikis in intestinal epithelial cells. J Cell Biol 149: 447–456, 2000

97. Cho SY, Klemke RL: Extracellular-regulated kinase activation and CAS/Crk coupling regulate cell migration and suppress apoptosis during invasion of the extracellular matrix. J Cell Biol 149: 223–236, 2000

98. Gioeli D, Mandell JW, Petroni GR, Frierson HF Jr, Weber MJ: Activation of mitogen-activated protein kinase associated with prostate cancer progression. Cancer Res 59: 279–284, 1999

99. Magi-Galluzzi C, Mishra R, Fiorentino M, Montironi R, Yao H, Capodieci P, Wishnow K, Kaplan I, Stork PJ, Loda M: Mitogen-activated protein kinase phosphatase 1 is overexpressed in prostate cancers and is inversely related to apoptosis. Lab Invest 76: 37–51, 1997

100. Price DT, Rocca GD, Guo C, Ballo MS, Schwinn DA, Luttrell LM: Activation of extracellular signal-regulated kinase in human prostate cancer. J Urol 162: 1537–1542, 1999

101. Vaux DL, Cory S, Adams JM: Bcl-2 gene promotes haemopoietic cell survival and cooperates with c-myc to immortalize pre-B cells. Nature 335: 440–442, 1988

102. Reed JC: Mechanisms of apoptosis. Am J Pathol 157: 1415–1430, 2000

103. Zhang Z, Vuori K, Reed JC, Ruoslahti E: The $\alpha_5\beta_1$ integrin supports survival of cells on fibronectin and up-regulates Bcl-2 expression. Proc Natl Acad Sci USA 92: 6161–6165, 1995

104. Matter ML, Ruoslahti E: A signaling pathway from the $\alpha5\beta1$ and $\alpha V\beta3$ integrins that elevates bcl-2 transcription. J Biol Chem 276: 27757–27763, 2001

105. Bruckheimer EM, Gjertsen BT, McDonnell TJ: Implications of cell death regulation in the pathogenesis and treatment of prostate cancer. Semin Oncol 26: 382–398, 1999

106. Colombel M, Symmans F, Gil S, O'Toole KM, Chopin D, Benson M, Olsson CA, Korsmeyer S, Buttyan R: Detection of the apoptosis-suppressing oncoprotein bcl-2 in hormone-refractory human prostate cancers. Am J Pathol 143: 390–400, 1993

107. Del Bufalo D, Biroccio A, Leonetti C, Zupi G: Bcl-2 overexpression enhances the metastatic potential of a human breast cancer line. FASEB J 11: 947–953, 1997

108. Knox JD, Cress AE, Clark V, Manriquez L, Affinito Kit-Sahn, Dalkin BL, Nagle RB: Differential expression of extracellular matrix molecules and the α_6-integrins in the normal and neoplastic prostate. Am J Pathol 145: 167–174, 1994

Address for offprints: Lucia R. Languino, Department of Pathology, Yale University School of Medicine, P.O. Box 208023, 310 Cedar Street, New Haven, CT 06520, USA; *Tel:* (203) 737-1454; *Fax:* (203) 737-1455; *e-mail:* lucia.languino@yale.edu

Prostate carcinoma skeletal metastases: Cross-talk between tumor and bone

Evan T. Keller[1], Jian Zhang[1], Carlton R. Cooper[2], Peter C. Smith[1], Laurie K. McCauley[3],
Kenneth J. Pienta[2] and Russell S. Taichman[3]
[1]Unit for Laboratory Animal Medicine, [2]Department of Surgery, [3]Department of
Periodontics/Prevention/Geriatrics, University of Michigan, Ann Arbor, MI, USA

Key words: prostatic neoplasms, skeletal metastases, bone morphogenetic protein, parathyroid hormone-related
protein, stromal-derived factor, matrix metalloproteinase

Abstract

The majority of men with progressive prostate cancer develop metastases with the skeleton being the most prevalent
metastatic site. Unlike many other tumors that metastasize to bone and form osteolytic lesions, prostate carcinomas
form osteoblastic lesions. However, histological evaluation of these lesions reveals the presence of underlying osteoclastic activity. These lesions are painful, resulting in diminished quality of life of the patient. There is emerging
evidence that prostate carcinomas establish and thrive in the skeleton due to cross-talk between the bone microenvironment and tumor cells. Bone provides chemotactic factors, adhesion factors, and growth factors that allow the
prostate carcinoma cells to target and proliferate in the skeleton. The prostate carcinoma cells reciprocate through
production of osteoblastic and osteolytic factors that modulate bone remodeling. The prostate carcinoma-induced
osteolysis promotes release of the many growth factors within the bone extracellular matrix thus further enhancing the progression of the metastases. This review focuses on the interaction between the bone and the prostate
carcinoma cells that allow for development and progression of prostate carcinoma skeletal metastases.

1. Introduction

Prostate carcinoma is the most frequently diagnosed
cancer in men and the second leading cause of cancer
death among men in the United States [1]. The most
common site of prostate carcinoma metastasis is the
bone with skeletal metastases identified at autopsy in
up to 90% of patients dying from prostate carcinoma
[2–4]. Skeletal metastasis results in significant complications that diminish the quality of life in affected
patients. These complications include bone pain,
impaired mobility, pathological fracture, spinal cord
compression and symptomatic hypercalcemia [5–7].
Despite advances in the diagnosis and management
of prostate carcinoma, advanced disease with skeletal metastasis remains incurable. Current therapeutic
modalities are mostly palliative, and include hormonal
therapy, pharmacological management of bone pain,
radiotherapy for pain and spinal cord compression [8],
various chemotherapy regimens, and the use of bisphosphonates to inhibit osteoclast activity [9]. In spite of
the severe complications of prostate carcinoma skeletal

metastasis, there have not been many advances in the
therapeutic arena to prevent or diminish these lesions.
It is critical that a solid understanding of the pathophysiology of prostate carcinoma skeletal metastatic
process is developed to provide the basis for creating
strategies to prevent or diminish their occurrence and
associated complications. A preponderance of evidence suggests that establishment and progression of
prostate carcinoma bone metastases is dependent on
interaction between the bone microenvironment and
the prostate carcinoma cell through both soluble and
cell-membrane bound bioactive factors. In this review,
we will summarize some of the cross-talk mechanisms
between bone and prostate carcinoma.

2. The effects of bone on prostate carcinoma metastasis

In agreement with the 'seed and soil' theory of metastases espoused by Paget [10], the predilection of
prostate carcinoma to establish metastases in bone as

M.L. Cher, K.V. Honn and A. Raz (eds.), Prostate Cancer: New Horizons in Research and Treatment, 197–213.
© 2002 Kluwer Academic Publishers.

198

opposed to other organs suggests that the bone microenvironment offers a fertile soil for prostate carcinoma growth. Prior to interacting on the bone cells and bone matrix, the prostate carcinoma cells must enter the bone compartment. This is accomplished by several general mechanisms that include chemotaxis from the circulation, attachment to bone endothelium, extravasation, and invasion. The bone microenvironment is a complicated mixture of mineralized and non-mineralized bone matrix and endothelial, hematopoietic, immune, and bone marrow stromal cells. Each of these components of the bone microenvironment may contribute to the establishment of prostate carcinoma metastases through provision of chemotactic, angiogenic, adhesion and growth factors.

2.1. Chemotaxis

When prostate carcinoma cells are injected adjacent to adult human bone implanted in SCID mice, the prostate carcinoma cells to migrate to adult human bone [11]. This observation provides evidence that bone provides chemotactic factors for prostate carcinoma cells. This is further supported by the observation that bone undergoing active resorption facilitated adhesion [12] and chemotaxis [13,14] of tumor cells to bone compared to non-resorbing bone. Collagen products appear to be one component of bone that induces tumor chemotaxis [15]. The factors through which bone induces chemotaxis are not clear. However, low glycosylated osteonectin was found to be an active chemotaxic factor in crude bone extracts that promoted chemotaxis of human prostate epithelial cells and increased the invasive ability of human prostate carcinoma cells [16]. In contrast with this observation, purified fibronectin, but not crude bone extracts induced migration of the prostate carcinoma DU-145 cell line [17]. Cell line specificity may account for these differences. Epidermal growth factor induced migration of the TSU-pr1 prostate carcinoma cell line [18]. Since EGF is present in medullary bone, this observation suggests that it may act as a chemotactic factor for bone metastases. Finally, the Rho-kinase inhibitor, Y-27632, inhibited *in vitro* chemotactic migration to bone marrow fibroblast conditioned media and metastatic growth in immune-compromised mice of highly invasive human prostatic cancer (PC3) cells [19]. This observation suggests that modulation of kinase activity may prove fruitful in inhibition of skeletal metastasis.

In addition to the above substances, which typically are not considered chemotactic factors, prostate carcinoma cells may commandeer the normal leukocyte bone marrow homing mechanism using the chemokine pathway [20]. Chemokines are classified based upon the relative position of cysteine residues near the NH2-terminus into four major families: CC,CXC,C,CX$_3$C (as reviewed in [21]). Chemokines activate receptors that are members of the large family of seven-transmembrane G protein–coupled proteins. In addition to the role that chemokines have in cell migration, they play significant roles in normal development, inflammation, atherosclerosis and angiogenesis. The rapidly increasing knowledge of chemokines has begun to impact many aspects of tumor biology including modulation of proliferation, angiogenesis and immune response to tumor (as reviewed in [22]).

An important role for chemokines may be to regulate metastatic behavior. Localization in tissues and migration to target organs are essential steps in the pathobiology of metastasis which strongly support the analogy to hematopoietic cell homing. In this context, the CXC chemokine stromal-derived factor (SDF-1; CXCL12) and its receptor, CXCR4 appear to be critical molecular determinants for these events [23,24]. This has been substantiated in gene knockout investigations [25,26] and by the demonstration that level of CXCR4 expression correlates with the ability of human hematopoietic progenitors to engraft into nude mice [26]. In the bone marrow, SDF-1 is constitutively produced by osteoblasts, fibroblasts and endothelial cells [27]. However, not all vascular endothelial cells express SDF-1, suggesting that organ-specific expression SDF-1 may account for the selectivity of metastases to target certain organs [28].

Several lines of evidence suggest that SDF-1 contributes to the pathogenesis of prostate carcinoma metastases. Inhibition of chemokines diminished *in vitro* proliferation of PC-3 cells [29] and anti-CXCR2 antibody inhibited IL-8-stimulated migration of PC-3 cells *in vitro* [30]. These studies suggest that chemokines contribute to prostate metastatic pathophysiology. This possibility is reinforced by the observation that CXCR4 is expressed in normal prostate tissues, albeit at low levels [31], as well as several neoplasms that invade the marrow (e.g., breast cancers, Burkitt's lymphoma, leukemias) [31–33]. Furthermore, several prostate carcinoma cell lines express CXCR4 mRNA, and SDF-1 increased migration of these cells *in vitro* [34]. It was recently demonstrated that normal breast tissues express little CXCR4, whereas breast neoplasms express high levels of CXCR4 [35,36], and antibody to CXCR4 blocked the metastatic spread of the tumors to the bone in an experimental metastasis model [35]. Taken together, these data suggest that SDF-1 and CXCR4 are likely critical regulators of prostate carcinoma metastasis to bone.

2.2. Attachment to endothelium

Cell adhesion plays a vital role in cancer metastasis. In fact, the ability of cancer cells to adhere to organ-specific cells and components may be a critical regulator of their metastatic pattern. A cancer cell in the circulation initially interacts with the organ's microvascular endothelium and subsequently the organ's extracellular matrix (ECM) components [37,38]. Cell adhesion molecules (CAMs) expressed on both the cancer and endothelial cells mediate these interactions. CAMs expressed on the endothelial cells are regulated by an organ's microenvironment, which results in CAM expression specific to each organ [39]. The organ-specific composition of ECM proteins such as laminin, fibronectin, and vitronectin that are recognized by CAMs expressed on cancer cells contribute significantly to organ-specific metastasis [40,41].

It has been proposed that prostate carcinoma metastasis to bone is mediated, in part, by preferential adhesion to bone marrow endothelium as opposed to endothelium from other sites [42,43]. Two studies demonstrated that prostate carcinoma cells adhered preferentially to immortalized human bone marrow endothelial (HBME) cells as compared to human umbilical vein endothelial cells (HUVEC), immortalized human aortic endothelial cells (HAEC-I), and immortalized human dermal microvascular endothelial cells (HDMVEC) [42,44]. This observation was confirmed in another study that demonstrated preferential adhesion of PC-3 cells to HBME cells as compared to HUVECs and lung endothelial cells, Hs888Lu [45]. Interestingly, this adhesion was enhanced when HBME cells were grown on bone ECM components [44]. The PC-3 cell line was used as a model for prostate carcinoma in these studies because it was derived from a bone metastasis. To determine the CAMs involved in prostate carcinoma (PC)–HBME interaction, galactose-rich-modified citrus pectin (MCP) and several antibodies to known CAMs expressed on HBME cell monolayers, were used in adhesion assays. MCP was used because it was reported to interfere with interactions mediated by carbohydrate-binding proteins such as galectins [46]. The data demonstrated that MCP and antibodies to galectin-3, vascular cell adhesion molecule (VCAM), CD11a

(alpha-L), CD18 (beta-2), and leukocyte functional antigen-1 (LFA-1) pectin, reduced PC-3 cell adhesion to HBME cell monolayers [42]. This observation suggests that carbohydrate-binding proteins, VCAM, alpha-L, beta-2, and LFA-1 may be partially involved in prostate carcinoma cell adhesion to HBME cells. Beta-1 integrins expressed on HUVEC were demonstrated to mediate PC-3 cell adhesion to this endothelial cell line [47]. Surprisingly, the beta-1 integrins expressed on HBME cells were not involved in PC-3 cell adhesion to HBME cell monolayers [48]; however, beta-1 integrins, expressed on PC-3 cells, did mediate its interaction with HBME cell monolayers [45]. Hyaluronan and galactosyl receptor, a cell surface C-type lectin expressed on PC-3 cells, were also shown to mediate PC–HBME interaction [49,50].

The ability of metastatic prostate cells to adhere to the bone matrix may also contribute to prostate carcinoma frequent metastasis to bone matrix [51,52]. Kostenuik demonstrated that PC-3 cells adhered to the collagen type I in the bone matrix. This adhesion was mediated by $\alpha2\beta1$ expressed on PC-3 cells and was upregulated by transforming growth factor-β (TGF-β), a major bone-derived cytokine [53]. Festuccia and colleagues [52] showed that osteoblast-conditioned media containing TGF-β, modulated the PC-3 interaction with ECM proteins, including collagen type I. These results provide evidence that TGF-β, present in the bone marrow, can influence prostate carcinoma cell adhesion to the bone matrix by modulating surface expression of selected integrins.

2.3. Growth factors

The calcified bone matrix is replete with putative prostate carcinoma growth factors including insulin-like growth factors (IGF), bone morphogenetic proteins (BMP), fibroblast growth factors (FGF) and transforming growth factor (TGF)-beta, which are released upon resorption of bone [54,55]. Furthermore, experimental evidence that resorption of calcified bone matrix promotes tumor growth was suggested by the observation that conditioned media for bone cultures undergoing resorption stimulated cancer cell growth of a variety of tumor cell lines [56]. Taken together, these data suggest that inhibiting bone resorption will diminish cancer growth by decreasing growth factors availability in the bone microenvironment.

Several purified factors from bone matrix have been demonstrated to stimulate prostate carcinoma cell growth in vitro [57–59]. For example, IGF-I and IGF-II are important mediators of prostate carcinoma growth (as reviewed in [60,61]). Prostate carcinoma cells have IGF receptors [62] and proliferate in response to IGF [57]. Transfection of LNCaP cells with FGF-8 expression vector induced an increased growth rate, higher soft agar clonogenic efficiency, enhanced *in vitro* invasion, and increased *in vivo* tumorigenesis [58]. The source of these growth factors is diverse. For example, osteoblast-derived factors influence prostate carcinoma growth, adhesion, and motility [16,17,63]. Additionally, bone marrow stromal cells, as opposed to non-skeletal fibroblasts, induced prostate carcinoma cell growth *in vitro* and *in vivo* [64–66]. As research continues on the extracellular matrix of bone, it is very likely that additional prostate carcinoma growth factors will be discovered.

3. The effect of prostate carcinoma on the bone: Osteoblastic

3.1. Prostate skeletal metastases are mixed osteoblastic and osteolytic lesions

Once in the bone, prostate carcinoma tumors have pathobiology that appears to be somewhat unique to cancer skeletal metastases. Specifically, prostate carcinoma skeletal metastases are most often characterized as osteoblastic (i.e., increased mineral density at the site of the lesion) as opposed to osteolytic. Other tumors, such as breast cancer, can form osteoblastic lesions; however, these occur less frequently [67,68]. In spite of the radiographic osteoblastic appearance it is clear from histological evidence that prostate carcinoma metastases form a heterogeneous mixture of osteolytic and osteoblastic lesions although osteoblastic lesions predominate [69–72]. Sites of prostate carcinoma bone metastases are often demonstrated to have increases in osteoid surface, osteoid volume, mineralization rates [73,74]. Recent evidence shows that osteoblastic metastases form on trabecular bone at sites of previous osteoclastic resorption, and that such resorption may be required for subsequent osteoblastic bone formation [75,76]. Clinical evidence demonstrates increased systemic markers of both bone production and bone resorption in prostate carcinoma patients [77,78] in addition to bone histomorphometric findings of increased indices of bone resorption [71]. These findings suggest that prostate carcinoma induces bone production through an overall increase in bone remodeling, which in the non-pathologic state

is a balance between osteoclastic resorption of bone and osteoblast-mediated replacement of resorbed bone (as reviewed in [79–81]). In the case of prostate carcinoma, it appears the induction of osteoblast-mediated mineralization outweighs the increase in osteoclast resorption resulting in overall formation of osteoblastic lesions. The osteoblastic lesions result in overall weakening of the bone for the following reasons; mature, healthy bone is formed of lamellar bone, which allows for tight packing of collagen bundles and optimum bone strength. In contrast, prostate carcinoma induces production of *woven* bone, which is composed of loosely packed, randomly oriented collagen bundles that produce bone with suboptimal strength [82,83]. Thus, the combination of underlying osteolysis and production of weak bone leads to a predisposition to fracture. The mechanisms through which prostate carcinoma cells promote bone mineralization remain poorly understood.

3.2. A variety of factors may contribute to prostate carcinoma-mediated bone mineralization

Prostate carcinoma produces osteoblastic factors that mediate their effect through activation of the osteoblast transcription factor Cbfa1 in the osteoblast precursor [84]. This suggests that induction of osteosclerosis occurs through normal osteoblast differentiation pathways. In addition to this observation, the prostate carcinoma cell itself demonstrates increased expression of Cbfa1 an the ability to mineralize *in vitro*, suggesting that it directly contributes to osteosclerosis [85]. Many factors that have direct or indirect osteogenic properties have been implicated in prostate carcinoma's osteogenic activity (Table 1) (as reviewed in [86, 87–89]). Although, initially identified as a nondefined osteoblastic activity from prostate carcinoma cells *in vitro* [90], many specific factors have been

Table 1. Osteogenic factors produced by cancer cells

Factor	Reference
Bone morphogenetic proteins (BMP)	[93,169]
Endothelin-1 (ET-1)	[94,136]
Insulin-like growth factors (IGF)	[231,232].
Interleukin-1 and -6	[233,234]
Osteoprotegerin (OPG)	[100,101]
Parathyroid hormone-related peptide (PTHrP)	[96,97]
Transforming growth factor-β (TFG-β)	[99]
Urinary plasminogen activator (urokinase)	[235]

identified that may promote osteoblastic lesions. Some of these factors, such as bone morphogenetic proteins (BMP) [91–93] and enodothlin-1 (ET-1) [94] may directly stimulate differentiation of osteoblast precursors to mature mineral-producing osteoblasts [95] or induce osteoblast protein production [93]. Other factors such as parathyroid hormone-related protein (PTHrP) may work through inhibition of osteoblast apoptosis [96,97]. Additionally, there are proteins that may work indirectly to enhance bone production, such as the serine proteases, prostate specific antigen (PSA) and urinary plasminogen activator (uPA), which can activate latent forms of osteogenic proteins, such as transforming growth factor-β (TFG-β) [98,99]. Finally, some molecules, such as osteoprotegerin (OPG) [100–102] and ET-1 (in a dual role with its osteoblast-stimulating activity) [103] can enhance osteosclerosis through inhibiting osteoclastogenesis. Other tumor types, such as osteosarcoma, are also known to produce a variety of osteoblastic factors [104–106]. With such a large number of factors, it is difficult to determine which the key factor is, and most likely several of these osteogenic factors work in concert to produce maximal bone production.

3.2.1. Parathyroid hormone related protein (PTHrP)
PTHrP was originally identified as a tumor-derived factor responsible for humoral hypercalcemia of malignancy (HHM). It has limited homology with the endocrine hormone, parathyroid hormone, sharing 7 of the first 13 N-terminal amino acids, but otherwise is dissimilar and immunologically distinct [107]. PTH AND PTHrP bind to the same receptor (the PTH-1 receptor) and evoke the same biological activity due to similarities in their steric configurations at the region of 25–34 amino acids. Patients with solid tumors and hypercalcemia have increased serum PTHrP in 80% of the cases, emphasizing the impact of this peptide to increase bone resorption and renal tubular resorption of calcium [107]. Subsequent to its characterization in HHM, PTHrP was found to be produced by many normal tissues including, epithelium, lactating mammary gland, and cartilage where it has an autocrine, paracrine, or intracrine role [107]. PTHrP plays a critical role in the development of the skeleton as evidenced by its lethality upon gene ablation and the severe skeletal chondrodysplasia found in these animals [108]. These studies have led to the conclusion that PTHrP in cartilage functions to accelerate the growth of cartilage cells and to oppose their progression to a terminally differentiated cell [109].

Many features of PTHrP make it an attractive candidate for influencing prostate carcinoma growth. PTHrP is produced by normal prostate epithelial cells, from which prostate carcinoma arises, and PTHrP is found in the seminal fluid [87,110]. PTHrP has been immunohistochemically identified in prostate carcinoma tissue in patients with clinically localized disease [111], is found in higher levels in prostate intraepithelial neoplasia than in normal prostate epithelium, is found in higher levels in prostate carcinoma than in benign prostatic hyperplasia [112,113], and is found in human metastatic lesions in bone [114]. There is also evidence that PTHrP can regulate malignant tumor growth in an autocrine manner in human renal cell carcinoma [115], enhance breast cancer metastasis to bone [116,117], and act as an autocrine growth factor for prostate carcinoma cells *in vitro* [118]. Recent evidence indicates that expression of nuclear-targeted PTHrP can protect prostate and other cells from apoptosis [114,119], bind RNA [120], and act as a mitogen [121,122]. PTHrP production by primary prostatic tumors is associated with increased tumor size and rate of growth in an animal model [114] suggesting that PTHrP acts in autocrine or intracrine mechanisms to promote tumor growth. In contrast, in this same model and in an intracardiac injection model of prostate carcinoma, PTHrP was not associated with an increase in metastatic potential [83,114]. This suggests that PTHrP is not important in the process of metastasis to bone but once in the bone microenvironment where target cells with receptors are present (osteoblasts); it may play a critical role in the bone response to prostate carcinoma. Of particular interest to prostate carcinoma, PSA has been shown to cleave PTHrP leading to an inactivation of the PTHrP-stimulation of cAMP which is a key pathway for the actions of PTHrP in bone [123]. More recent studies indicate that in colon cancer cells, PTHrP enhances adhesion of cells to type I collagen but not fibronectin or laminin [124]. All these data suggest that PTHrP has a critical role in the local bone microenvironment of metastatic prostate carcinoma; but what this precise role is has yet to be determined.

3.2.2. Endothelin-1
ET-1 is a member of the ET family which is composed of ET-1, -2, and -3. The ET family members are synthesized as a 203 amino acid precursor peptide that is cleaved to a 21 amino acid peptide with the same two characteristic disulfide bridges [125]. Initially

identified as a potent vasoconstrictor, ET-1 interacts with cell surface ET_A and ET_B receptors to induce a variety of responses including modulation of cell growth and fetal development (as reviewed in [125]). ETs are found in a variety of tissues including vascular endothelium, parathyroid gland, mammary tissue, and macrophages [125].

The role of ET-1 in bone remodeling is controversial. For example, in the murine osteoblast precursor cell, MC3T3-E1, E1 inhibits differentiation, reduces both alkaline phosphatase activity and osteocalcin expression and diminishes *in vitro* mineralization suggesting that ET-1 will diminish bone production [126,127]. In contrast, ET-1 has been shown to inhibit bone resorption [128], induce collagen synthesis [129] and osteopontin and alkaline phosphatase production [130,131] in a variety of osteoblastic cell lines. The conflicting results may be due to differences in cell lines, particularly with regards to ET receptor expression. Although these *in vitro* data are in apparent conflict, the *in vivo* data support that ET-1 promotes bone formation [132]. Specifically, administration of an ET_A receptor antagonist in mice resulted in reduced bone mass [132].

ET-1 is secreted by normal prostate epithelial cells into the ejaculate [133–135] and is now considered a putative mediator of prostate carcinoma pathophysiology (as reviewed in [136]). The ectopic expression of ET-1 in the bone metastatic site by prostate carcinoma cells may enable ET-1 to influence the bone remodeling process locally. This is supported by the report that para-tibial injection of an amniotic cell line overexpressing ET-1 induced new bone formation in the tibiae of mice, which was diminished by blockade of ET_A receptor [137]. Additionally, administration of an ETA receptor antagonist diminished breast cancer-induced bone production in a murine model [138]. Furthermore, co-incubating the androgen-independent prostate carcinoma cell lines DU-145 and PC-3, but not the androgen-responsive cell line LNCaP, with bone slices induced ET-1 expression from the prostate carcinoma cells [103]. The DU-145 and PC-3 cell lines also induced osteoclastogenic activity that was blocked by anti-human ET-1 antibody. Taken together, these reports suggest that ET-1 may contribute to prostate carcinoma metastases-induced osteoblastic lesions. In apparent conflict with these models, is the observation that serum ET-1 levels are elevated in people with Paget's disease, which is characterized by low bone mineral density secondary to increased osteoclastic activity [139].

3.2.3. Bone morphogenetic proteins

BMPs are members of the transforming growth factor (TFG)-β superfamily. More than 30 BMPs have been identified to date [140]. While originally discovered because of their ability to induce new bone formation, BMPs are now recognized to perform many functions, particularly in the role of development, such as apoptosis, differentiation, proliferation and morphogenesis (as reviewed in [141–143]). BMPs are synthesized as large precursor molecules that undergo proteolytic cleavage to release the mature protein, which form active hetero- or homodimers [144,145]. BMPs bind to receptors (BMPR-IA and -IB) and a BMP type II receptor (BMPR-II), which induces Smad phosphorylation [146] resulting in modulation of gene regulation. Target genes of BMPs include osteoblast proteins such as OPG [147] and the osteoblast-specific transcription factor Cbfa-1 [148,149]. Several proteins that antagonize BMP action have been identified. For example, noggin and gremlin inhibit BMP-2, -4 and -7 by binding to them [150–152]. Furthermore, the BMPs themselves regulate their own inhibitors in an apparent negative feedback mechanism [153,154].

Many *in vitro* studies have demonstrated that BMPs induce osteogenic differentiation including the ability of BMP-7 (also called osteogenic protein-1; OP-1) to induce osteogenic differentiation of newborn rat calvarial cells and rat osteosarcoma cells [155–157]. The BMPs' osteogenic properties appear to be specific to the differentiation stage of the target cells. Specifically, BMPs can induced uncommitted stem cells [155,158,159] and myoblasts [160] to express osteoblast parameters such as alkaline phosphatase or osteocalcin expression [79,161]; whereas, BMPs do not stimulate mature osteoblasts or fibroblasts [158,162–164] to increase expression of these proteins. Examination of genetically modified mice provides further evidence of the importance of BMP in bone development. The *bmp7* homozygous null condition in mice is a postnatal lethal mutation and is associated with, in addition to renal and ocular abnormalities, retarded skeletal ossification [165]. In contrast, *bmp6* null mice are viable and fertile, and the skeletal elements of newborn and adult mutants are indistinguishable from wildtype [166]. However, careful examination of skeletogenesis in late gestation embryos reveals a consistent delay in ossification strictly confined to the developing sternum. Finally, mice with mutations of the *bmp5* gene have skeletal abnormalities and inefficient fracture repair [167]. Taken together, these data provide evidence that BMPs are important regulators of the osteogenesis. Thus, dysregulation of their expression in the bone microenvironment would most likely impact bone remodeling.

A few studies have examined the expression of BMPs in normal and neoplastic prostate tissues. Using Northern analysis, Harris et al. [92] examined BMP-2, -3, -4 and -6 mRNA expression in human normal prostate and prostate carcinoma cell lines. They found that normal human prostate predominantly expressed BMP-4. The androgen-dependent non-metastatic LNCaP human prostate carcinoma cell line produced very low to undetectable levels of BMPs. Whereas, the aggressive androgen-independent PC-3 cell line expressed very high levels of BMP-3 and slightly lower levels of BMP-2, -4 and -6 compared to normal cells, but much higher than LNCaP cells. In support of these results, Weber et al. [168], using PCR analysis, identified 16 (73%) of 22 prostate carcinoma samples that were positive for BMP-7 mRNA compared to eight (57%) of 14 normal prostate tissue samples. In another PCR based analysis, Bentley et al. [169], found that several BMPs were expressed in both benign and malignant prostate tissue and in the PC3 and DU145 prostate carcinoma cell lines. BMP-6 expression was detected in the prostate tissue of over 50% of patients with clinically defined metastatic prostate adenocarcinoma, but was not detected in non-metastatic or benign prostate samples. In another study focused on BMP-6 mRNA and protein expression, Barnes et al. [170] observed that BMP-6 was produced by normal and neoplastic human prostate (radical prostatectomy specimens and human carcinoma cell lines DU145 and PC3). However, BMP-6 mRNA and protein expression was higher in prostate carcinoma as compared with adjacent normal prostate, with higher-grade tumors (Gleason score of 6 or more) having greater BMP-6 immunostaining than the lower-grade tumors (Gleason score of 4 or less). These results were consistent with a later study by Hamdy et al. [171], who reported that BMP-6 mRNA expression was detected exclusively in malignant epithelial cells in 20 of 21 patients (95%) with metastases, in 2 of 11 patients (18%) with localized cancer, and undetectable in 8 benign samples. In addition to BMP, there have been several reports that prostate carcinoma expresses BMP receptors. It appears that as prostate carcinoma progress, the cells down-regulate their own expression of BMP receptors [172,173], which may be a protective mechanism as it has been demonstrated that BMP-2 can inhibit prostate

carcinoma cell proliferation [174]. Taken together, these observations demonstrate that prostate carcinoma cells produce increasing levels of BMPs as they progress to a more aggressive phenotype and suggest that the up-regulation of BMP expression in prostate carcinoma cells localized in the bone is a critical component of the mechanism of development of osteoblastic lesions at prostate carcinoma metastatic sites.

4. The effect of prostate carcinoma on the bone: Osteolytic

Although the osteoblastic component of prostate carcinoma metastases has received attention, limited research has been performed on the osteoclastic aspect of prostate carcinoma. Similar to the reports for breast cancer bone metastases [175,176], several lines of evidence suggest that resorption of bone is an important mediator of prostate carcinoma bone metastases. For example, administration of bisphosphonates, inhibitors of osteoclast activity, to patients with prostate carcinoma bone metastases relieves bone pain and lowers systemic indices of bone resorption [177–179]. Furthermore, administration of osteoclast inhibitors such as OPG or bisphosphonates prevents tumor establishment or diminished tumor burden in animal models [76,180–182]. It is not clear if bisphosphonates have a direct antitumor effect [183–185] or inhibit tumor growth through its ability to diminish osteoclast activity [186,187]. In some instances, it may be a combination of activities. As described above, in addition to serum levels of bone resorption markers being elevated in men with prostate carcinoma skeletal metastases, the lesions usually are demonstrated to have histological evidence of osteoclast activity. Thus, osteoclast activity may play an important role in development and progression of prostate carcinoma metastases. Prostate carcinoma cells secrete a variety of factors that may promote bone lysis, such as interleukin-6 (as reviewed in [188]) and PTHrP. However, it appears that these factors mediate their osteolytic effects through induction of a key pro-osteoclastogenic molecule, receptor activator of NFκB ligand (RANKL).

4.1. Receptor activator of NFkB ligand-OPG axis

A member of the tumor necrosis factor family, RANKL is initially expressed as a membrane anchored molecule; however, a small fraction of RANKL is released through proteolytic cleavage from the cell surface as a soluble 245 amino acid homotrimeric molecule (sRANKL) [189]. Both soluble and membrane bound RANKL promote osteoclast formation and activation by binding to RANK on the osteoclast precursor membrane [189–193].

In addition to RANKL and RANK, another key modulator of osteoclastogenesis is osteoprotegerin (OPG)(also known as osteoclastogenesis inhibitory factor-OCIF) [102,194]. OPG serves as a decoy receptor that binds RANKL and thus blocks its ability to bind to RANK and induce osteoclastogenesis. In contrast to RANKL and RANK, whose expression is mainly restricted at low levels to the skeletal and immune systems, OPG is expressed in a variety of tissues, such as liver, lung, heart, kidney, stomach, intestines, skin and calvaria in mice and lung, heart, kidney and placenta in human [102,195–201]. In bone, OPG is mainly produced by osteoblastic lineage cells and its expression increases as the cells become more differentiated [199,202,203]. Administration of recombinant OPG to normal rodents resulted in increased bone mass [102,196] and completely prevented ovariectomy-induced bone loss without apparent adverse skeletal and extraskeletal side effects [102]. In fact, based on this activity, the balance ratio of RANKL to OPG appears to be very important in controlling the overall activity (i.e., lysis vs no lysis) that will be observed [204–206].

A number of reports have shown that osteoclastic bone resorptive lesions are important to the development of bone metastases in several cancer types including breast cancer, lung cancer and prostate carcinoma [207]. These cancers may induce osteoclast activity through secretion of IL-1α, PTHrP or PGE2 [208,209]. However, tumor-mediated osteolysis occurs indirectly through expression of molecules, such as PTHrP, that induce RANKL in osteoblasts [210,211]. This contrasts with the observations that giant cell tumors directly promote osteoclast activity via RANKL [212] and our observation that prostate carcinoma cells directly induce osteoclastogenesis through RANKL [76]. Another factor that may play a role in tumor-induced osteoclastogenesis is human macrophage inflammatory protein-1α (hMIP-1α), which has been shown to be produced by myeloma cells [213]. Because of the osteoclastic activity induced by many cancers, antiresorptive approaches such as administration of bisphosphonates or anti-PTHrP neutralizing antibody have been reported in breast cancer animal models to be able to block the tumor expansion in bone [214,215].

Furthermore, OPG has been recently shown to inhibit primary bone sarcoma-induced osteolysis and tumor-induced bone pain, but not tumor burden in mice [100]. However, OPG not only blocked osteolytic bone metastasis induced by human neuroblastoma NB-19 cells [216], but also reduced tumor burden in that model. In addition to OPG, a soluble form of RANK (sRANK) has been shown to inhibit myeloma-induced lytic lesions in murine models [217].

4.2. Matrix metalloproteinases

Matrix metalloproteinases (MMPs) are family of enzymes whose primary function is to degrade the extracellular matrix. MMPs contribute to metastatic invasion, including destruction of bone [218]. Prostate carcinomas and their cell lines express a large number of MMPs [219–226]. The initial functional data in prostate carcinoma bone metastasis that suggested bone remodeling is modulated through MMPs was provided by in vitro studies. Specifically, blocking MMP activity with 1,10-phenanthroline, a MMP inhibitor, diminished bone matrix degradation induced by PC-3 cells in vitro [227,228]. The importance of MMPs in bone metastasis has been further confirmed in vivo. An MMP inhibitor, batimistat, has been shown to inhibit development bone resorption in vitro and in vivo in murine models of breast [229] and prostate carcinoma [230]. The mechanism through which prostate carcinoma-produced MMPs induce bone resorption is not clear; however, it appears to involve induction of osteoclastogenesis as inhibition of MMPs reduced the number of osteoclasts associated with prostate tumor growth in human bone implants in mice [230].

5. Conclusions

A model summarizing the cross-talk between prostate carcinoma and the bone microenvironment that leads to development and progression of prostate carcinoma skeletal metastases is presented in Figure 1. The bone contributes many aspects of the metastatic cascade including chemotaxis, endothelial attachment, invasion and tumor proliferation. Once in the bone microenvironment, the prostate carcinoma cells modulate bone remodeling which favors tumor progression. The presence of many different active factors produced by both the bone and the prostate carcinoma cells that appear to contribute to the pathobiology of skeletal metastases

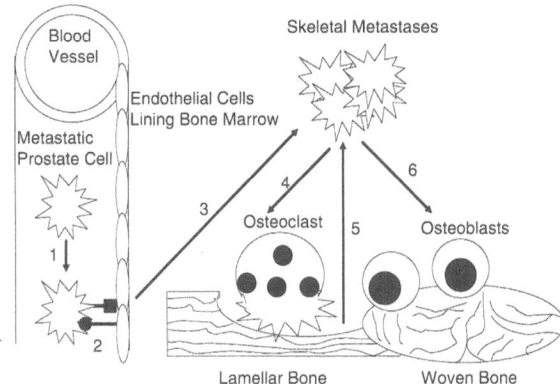

Figure 1. Model of cross-talk between prostate carcinoma cells and the bone microenvironment. The bone produces chemotactic factors that attract prostate carcinoma cells to migrate (1) through the vascular system towards the skeleton. The bone marrow endothelia displays adhesion molecules that complement those expressed by the prostate carcinoma cell, resulting in attachment of the cell (2). The prostate carcinoma cell extravasates and invades into the skeletal extracellular tissue (3), at which point it releases factors that stimulate osteoclastogenesis (4). The subsequent bone resorption is accompanied by release of growth factors that stimulate prostate carcinoma proliferation (5). The progressing prostate carcinoma releases factors that promote osteoblast production and inhibit osteoblast apoptosis (6) resulting in production of woven bone and the characteristic osteosclerotic lesion. This process continues in a cyclical fashion with continued induction of osteoclastic activity, carcinoma cell proliferation and bone production.

suggests that defining the mechanisms of prostate carcinoma skeletal metastases will be challenging. Continued research on how these interactions occur may lead to identification of targets to interrupt this crosstalk and prevent the establishment or progression of prostate cancer skeletal metastases.

Acknowledgements

This work was supported by USAMRMC Prostate carcinoma Research Program Grant # DAMD17-00-1-053, National Institutes of Health Grants SPORE 1 P50 CA69568 and T32 RR07008.

References

1. Landis SH, Murray T, Bolden S, Wingo PA: Cancer statistics, 1999. CA Cancer J Clin 49: 8–31, 1999
2. Abrams H, Spiro R, Goldstein N: Metastases in carcinoma. Cancer 3: 74–85, 1950
3. Bubendorf L, Schopfer A, Wagner U, Sauter G, Moch H, Willi N, Gasser TC, Mihatsch MJ: Metastatic patterns of prostate cancer: an autopsy study of 1,589 patients. Hum Pathol 31: 578–583, 2000
4. Rana A, Chisholm GD, Khan M, Sekharjit SS, Merrick MV, Elton RA: Patterns of bone metastasis and their prognostic significance in patients with carcinoma of the prostate. Br J Urol 72: 933–936, 1993
5. Galasko CS: Skeletal metastases. Clin Orthop 1986: 18–30, 1986
6. Coleman RE: Skeletal complications of malignancy. Cancer 80: 1588–1594, 1997
7. Moul JW, Lipo DR: Prostate cancer in the late 1990s: Hormone refractory disease options. Urol Nurs 19: 125–131; quiz 132–123, 1999
8. Szostak MJ, Kyprianou N: Radiation-induced apoptosis: predictive and therapeutic significance in radiotherapy of prostate cancer (review). Oncol Rep 7: 699–706, 2000
9. Papapoulos SE, Hamdy NA, van der Pluijm G: Bisphosphonates in the management of prostate carcinoma metastatic to the skeleton. Cancer 88: 3047–3053, 2000
10. Paget S: The distribution of secondary growth in cancer of the breast. Lancet 1: 571–573, 1829
11. Tsingotjidou AS, Zotalis G, Jackson KR, Sawyers C, Puzas JE, Hicks DG, Reiter R, Lieberman JR: Development of an animal model for prostate cancer cell metastasis to adult human bone. Anticancer Res 21: 971–978, 2001
12. Magro C, Orr FW, Manishen WJ, Sivananthan K, Mokashi SS: Adhesion, chemotaxis, and aggregation of Walker carcinosarcoma cells in response to products of resorbing bone. J Natl Cancer Inst 74: 829–838, 1985
13. Orr W, Varani J, Gondex MK, Ward PA, Mundy GR: Chemotactic responses of tumor cells to products of resorbing bone. Science 203: 176–179, 1979
14. Orr FW, Varani J, Gondek MD, Ward PA, Mundy GR: Partial characterization of a bone-derived chemotactic factor for tumor cells. Am J Pathol 99: 43–52, 1980
15. Wass JA, Varani J, Piontek GE, Ward PA, Orr FW: Responses of normal and malignant cells to collagen, collagen-derived peptides and the C5-related tumor cell chemotactic peptide. Cell Differ 10: 329–332, 1981
16. Jacob K, Webber M, Benayahu D, Kleinman HK: Osteonectin promotes prostate cancer cell migration and invasion: a possible mechanism for metastasis to bone. Cancer Res 59: 4453–4457, 1999
17. Hullinger TG, McCauley LK, DeJoode ML, Somerman MJ: Effect of bone proteins on human prostate cancer cell lines *in vitro*. Prostate 36: 14–22, 1998
18. Rajan R, Vanderslice R, Kapur S, Lynch J, Thompson R, Djakiew D: Epidermal growth factor (EGF) promotes chemomigration of a human prostate tumor cell line, and EGF immunoreactive proteins are present at sites of metastasis in the stroma of lymph nodes and medullary bone. Prostate 28: 1–9, 1996
19. Somlyo AV, Bradshaw D, Ramos S, Murphy C, Myers CE, Somlyo AP: Rho-kinase inhibitor retards migration and *in vivo* dissemination of human prostate cancer cells. Biochem Biophys Res Commun 269: 652–659, 2000
20. Baggiolini M: Chemokines and leukocyte traffic. Nature 392: 565–568, 1998

206

21. Rossi D, Zlotnik A: The biology of chemokines and their receptors. Annu Rev Immunol 18: 217–242, 2000

22. Strieter RM: Chemokines: Not just leukocyte chemoattractants in the promotion of cancer. Nat Immunol 2: 285–286, 2001

23. Aiuti A, Tavian M, Cipponi A, Ficara F, Zappone E, Hoxie J, Peault B, Bordignon C: Expression of CXCR4, the receptor for stromal cell-derived factor-1 on fetal and adult human lympho-hematopoietic progenitors. Eur J Immunol 29: 1823–1831, 1999

24. Kim CH, Broxmeyer HE: SLC/exodus2/6Ckine/TCA4 induces chemotaxis of hematopoietic progenitor cells: Differential activity of ligands of CCR7, CXCR3, or CXCR4 in chemotaxis vs. suppression of progenitor proliferation. J Leukoc Biol 66: 455–461, 1999

25. Nagasawa T, Hirota S, Tachibana K, Takakura N, Nishikawa S, Kitamura Y, Yoshida N, Kikutani H, Kishimoto T: Defects of B-cell lymphopoiesis and bone-marrow myelopoiesis in mice lacking the CXC chemokine PBSF/SDF-1. Nature 382: 635–638, 1996

26. Peled A, Petit I, Kollet O, Magid M, Ponomaryov T, Byk T, Nagler A, Ben-Hur H, Many A, Shultz L, Lider O, Alon R, Zipori D, Lapidot T: Dependence of human stem cell engraftment and repopulation of NOD/SCID mice on CXCR4. Science 283: 845–848, 1999

27. Ponomaryov T, Peled A, Petit I, Taichman RS, Habler L, Sandbank J, Arenzana-Seisdedos F, Magerus A, Caruz A, Fujii N, Nagler A, Lahav M, Szyper-Kravitz M, Zipori D, Lapidot T: Induction of the chemokine stromal-derived factor-1 following DNA damage improves human stem cell function. J Clin Invest 106: 1331–1339, 2000

28. Imai K, Kobayashi M, Wang J, Shinobu N, Yoshida H, Hamada J, Shindo M, Higashino F, Tanaka J, Asaka M, Hosokawa M: Selective secretion of chemoattractants for haemopoietic progenitor cells by bone marrow endothelial cells: a possible role in homing of haemopoietic progenitor cells to bone marrow. Br J Haematol 106: 905–911, 1999

29. Moore BB, Arenberg DA, Stoy K, Morgan T, Addison CL, Morris SB, Glass M, Wilke C, Xue YY, Sitterding S, Kunkel SL, Burdick MD, Strieter RM: Distinct CXC chemokines mediate tumorigenicity of prostate cancer cells. Am J Pathol 154: 1503–1512, 1999

30. Reiland J, Furcht LT, McCarthy JB: CXC-chemokines stimulate invasion and chemotaxis in prostate carcinoma cells through the CXCR2 receptor. Prostate 41: 78–88, 1999

31. Gupta SK, Pillarisetti K: Cutting edge: CXCR4-Lo: Molecular cloning and functional expression of a novel human CXCR4 splice variant. J Immunol 163: 2368–2372, 1999

32. Sehgal A, Ricks S, Boynton AL, Warrick J, Murphy GP: Molecular characterization of CXCR-4: A potential brain tumor-associated gene. J Surg Oncol 69: 239–248, 1998

33. Mohle R, Failenschmid C, Bautz F, Kanz L: Overexpression of the chemokine receptor CXCR4 in B cell chronic lymphocytic leukemia is associated with increased functional response to stromal cell-derived factor-1 (SDF-1). Leukemia 13: 1954–1959, 1999

34. Taichman R, McCauley L, Taichman N: Use of the SDF-1/CXCR4 pathway in prostate cancer metastasis to bone. Blood 96: 571a, 2000

35. Muller C, Homey B, Sato H, Ge N, Catron D, Buchanan M, McClanahan T, Murphy E, Yuan W, Wagners S, Barrera J, Mohar A, Verastegui E, Zlotnik A: Involvement of chemokine receptors in breast cancer metastasis. Nature 410: 50–56, 2001

36. Liotta LA: An attractive force in metastasis. Nature 410: 24–25, 2001

37. Miyasaka M: Cancer metastasis and adhesion molecules. Clin Orthop 312: 10–18, 1995

38. Orr FW, Wang HH, Lafrenie RM, Scherbarth S, Nance DM: Interactions between cancer cells and the endothelium in metastasis. J Pathol 190: 310–329, 2000

39. Pauli BU, Augustin-Voss HG, El-Sabban ME, Johnson RC, Hammer DA: Organ-preference of metastasis. Cancer and Metastasis Rev 9: 175–189, 1990

40. Deroock IB, Pennington ME, Sroka TC, Lam KS, Bowden GT, Bair EL, Cress AE: Synthetic peptides inhibit adhesion of human tumor cells to extracellular matrix proteins. Cancer Res 61: 3308–3313, 2001

41. vanderPluijm G, Vloedgraven H, Papapoulos S, Lowik C, Grzesik W, Kerr J, Robey PG: Attachment characteristics and involvement of integrins in adhesion of breast cancer cell lines to extracellular bone matrix components. Lab Inves 77: 665–675, 1997

42. Lehr JE, Pienta KJ: Preferential adhesion of prostate cancer cells to a human bone marrow endothelial cell line (see comments). J Natl Cancer Inst 90: 118–123, 1998

43. Cooper CR, Pienta KJ: Cell adhesion and chemotaxis in prostate cancer metastasis to bone: a minireview. Prostate Canc Prostatic Dis 3: 6–12, 2000

44. Cooper CR, Mclean L, Walsh M, Taylor J, Hayasaka S, Bhatia J, Pienta KJ: Preferential adhesion to prostate cancer cells to bone is mediated by binding to bone marrow endothelial cells as compared to extracellular matrix components in vitro. Clin Cancer Res 6: 4839–4847, 2000

45. Scott LJ, Clarke NW, George NJ, Shanks JH, Testa NG, Lang SH: Interactions of human prostatic epithelial cells with bone marrow endothelium: binding and invasion. Br J Cancer 84: 1417–1423, 2001

46. Pienta KJ, Naik H, Akhtar A, Yamazaki K, Replogle TS, Lehr J, Donat TL, Tait L, Hogan V, Raz A: Inhibition of spontaneous metastasis in a rat prostate cancer model by oral administration of modified citrus pectin. J Natl Cancer Inst 87: 348–353, 1995

47. Romanov VI, Goligorsky MS: RGD-recognizing integrins mediate interactions of human prostate carcinoma cells with endothelial cells in vitro. Prostate 39: 108–118, 1999

48. Cooper CR, McLean L, Mucci NR, Poncza P, Pienta KJ: Prostate cancer cell adhesion to quiescent endothelial cells is not mediated by beta-1 integrin subunit. Anticancer Res 20: 4159–4162, 2000

49. Simpson MA, Reiland J, Burger SR, Furch LT, Spice AP, Theodore R. Oegema J, McCarthy JB: Hyaluronan synthase elevation in metastatic prostate carcinoma cells correlates with hyaluronan surface retention, a prerequisite for

rapid adhesion to bone marrow endothelial cells. J Biol Chem 276: 17949–17957, 2001

50. Kierszenbaum AL, Rivkin E, Chang PL, Tres LL, Olsson CA: Galactosyl receptor, a cell surface C-type lectin of normal and tumoral prostate epithelial cells with binding affinity to endothelial cells. Prostate 43: 175–183, 2000

51. Kostenuik PJ, Sanchez-Sweatman O, Orr FW, Singh G: Bone cell matrix promotes the adhesion of human prostatic carcinoma cells via the alpha 2 beta 1 integrin. Clin Exp Metastasis 14: 19–26, 1996

52. Festuccia C, Bologna M, Gravina GL, Guerra F, Angelucci A, Villonava I, Millimaggi D, Teti A: Osteoblast conditioned media contained TGF-beta1 and modulat the migration of prostate tumor cells and their interactions with extracellular matrix components. Int J Cancer 81: 395–403, 1999

53. Kostenuik PJ, Singh G, Orr FW: Transforming growth factor-beta upregulates the integrin-mediated adhesion of human prostatic carcinoma cells to type I collagen. Clin Exp Metastasis 15: 41–52, 1997

54. Martinez J, Fuentes M, Cambiazo V, Santibanez JF: Bone extracellular matrix stimulates invasiveness of estrogen-responsive human mammary MCF-7 cells. Int J Cancer 83: 278–282, 1999

55. Linkhart TA, Mohan S, Baylink DJ: Growth factors for bone growth and repair: IGF, TGF beta and BMP. Bone 19: 1S–12S, 1996

56. Manishen WJ, Sivananthan K, Orr FW: Resorbing bone stimulates tumor cell growth. A role for the host microenvironment in bone metastasis. Am J Pathol 123: 39–45, 1986

57. Ritchie CK, Andrews LR, Thomas KG, Tindall DJ, Fitzpatrick LA: The effects of growth factors associated with osteoblasts on prostate carcinoma proliferation and chemotaxis: Implications for the development of metastatic disease. Endocrinology 138: 1145–1150, 1997

58. Song Z, Powell WC, Kasahara N, van Bokhoven A, Miller GJ, Roy-Burman P: The effect of fibroblast growth factor 8, isoform b, on the biology of prostate carcinoma cells and their interaction with stromal cells. Cancer Res 60: 6730–6736, 2000

59. Desruisseau S, Ghazarossian-Ragni E, Chinot O, Martin PM: Divergent effect of TGFbeta1 on growth and proteolytic modulation of human prostatic-cancer cell lines. Int J Cancer 66: 796–801, 1996

60. Djavan B, Waldert M, Seitz C, Marberger M: Insulin-like growth factors and prostate cancer. World J Urol 19: 225–233, 2001

61. Peehl DM, Cohen P, Rosenfeld RG: The insulin-like growth factor system in the prostate. World J Urol 13: 306–311, 1995

62. Cohen P, Peehl DM, Lamson G, Rosenfeld RG: Insulin-like growth factors (IGFs), IGF receptors, and IGF-binding proteins in primary cultures of prostate epithelial cells. J Clin Endocrinol Metab 73: 401–407, 1991

63. Festuccia C, Giunciuglio D, Guerra F, Villanova I, Angelucci A, Manduca P, Teti A, Albini A, Bologna M: Osteoblasts modulate secretion of urokinase-type plasminogen activator (uPA) and matrix metalloproteinase-9 (MMP-9) in human prostate cancer cells promoting migration and matrigel invasion. Oncol Res 11: 17–31, 1999

64. Lang SH, Clarke NW, George NJ, Allen TD, Testa NG: Interaction of prostate epithelial cells from benign and malignant tumor tissue with bone-marrow stroma. Prostate 34: 203–213, 1998

65. Gleave ME, Hsieh JT, von Eschenbach AC, Chung LW: Prostate and bone fibroblasts induce human prostate cancer growth in vivo: Implications for bidirectional tumor-stromal cell interaction in prostate carcinoma growth and metastasis. J Urol 147: 1151–1159, 1992

66. Gleave M, Hsieh JT, Gao CA, von Eschenbach AC, Chung LW: Acceleration of human prostate cancer growth in vivo by factors produced by prostate and bone fibroblasts. Cancer Res 51: 3753–3761, 1991

67. Yamashita K, Aoki Y, Hiroshima K: Metastatic epidural bony tumor causing spinal cord compression: A case report. Clin Orthop 1996: 231–235, 1996

68. Munk PL, Poon PY, O'Connell JX, Janzen D, Coupland D, Kwong JS, Gelmon K, Worsley D: Osteoblastic metastases from breast carcinoma with false-negative bone scan. Skeletal Radiol 26: 434–437, 1997

69. Berruti A, Piovesan A, Torta M, Raucci CA, Gorzegno G, Paccotti P, Dogliotti L, Angeli A: Biochemical evaluation of bone turnover in cancer patients with bone metastases: Relationship with radiograph appearances and disease extension. Br J Cancer 73: 1581–1587, 1996

70. Vinholes J, Coleman R, Eastell R: Effects of bone metastases on bone metabolism: Implications for diagnosis, imaging and assessment of response to cancer treatment. Cancer Treat Rev 22: 289–331, 1996

71. Urwin GH, Percival RC, Harris S, Beneton MN, Williams JL, Kanis JA: Generalised increase in bone resorption in carcinoma of the prostate. Br J Urol 57: 721–723, 1985

72. Roudier M, Sherrard D, True L, Ott-Ralp S, Meligro C, MBerrie M, Soo C, Felise D, Quinn JE, Vessella R: Heterogenous bone histomorphometric patterns in metastatic prostate cancer. J Bone Miner Res 15S1: S567, 2000

73. Clarke NW, McClure J, George NJ: Osteoblast function and osteomalacia in metastatic prostate cancer. Eur Urol 24: 286–290, 1993

74. Charhon SA, Chapuy MC, Delvin EE, Valentin-Opran A, Edouard CM, Meunier PJ: Histomorphometric analysis of sclerotic bone metastases from prostatic carcinoma special reference to osteomalacia. Cancer 51: 918–924, 1983

75. Carlin BI, Andriole GL: The natural history, skeletal complications, and management of bone metastases in patients with prostate carcinoma. Cancer 88: 2989–2994, 2000

76. Zhang J, Dai J, Qi Y, Lin DL, Smith P, Strayhorn C, Mizokami A, Fu Z, Westman J, Keller ET: Osteoprotegerin inhibits prostate cancer-induced osteoclastogenesis and prevents prostate tumor growth in the bone. J Clin Invest 107: 1235–1244, 2001

77. Maeda H, Koizumi M, Yoshimura K, Yamauchi T, Kawai T, Ogata E: Correlation between bone metabolic markers and bone scan in prostatic cancer. J Urol 157: 539–543, 1997

208

78. Demers LM, Costa L, Lipton A: Biochemical markers and skeletal metastases. Cancer 88: 2919–2926, 2000
79. Karsenty G: Bone formation and factors affecting this process. Matrix Biol 19: 85–89, 2000
80. Parfitt AM: The mechanism of coupling: A role for the vasculature. Bone 26: 319–323, 2000
81. Boyce BF, Hughes DE, Wright KR, Xing L, Dai A: Recent advances in bone biology provide insight into the pathogenesis of bone diseases. Lab Invest 79: 83–94, 1999
82. Rosol TJ: Pathogenesis of bone metastases: Role of tumor-related proteins. J Bone Miner Res 15: 844–850, 2000
83. Blomme EA, Dougherty KM, Pienta KJ, Capen CC, Rosol TJ, McCauley LK: Skeletal metastasis of prostate adenocarcinoma in rats: Morphometric analysis and role of parathyroid hormone-related protein. Prostate 39: 187–197, 1999
84. Yang J, Fizazi K, Peleg S, Sikes CR, Raymond AK, Jamal N, Hu M, Olive M, Martinez LA, Wood CG, Logothetis CJ, Karsenty G, Navone NM: Prostate cancer cells induce osteoblast differentiation through a Cbfa1-dependent pathway. Cancer Res 61: 5652–5659, 2001
85. Lin DL, Tarnowski CP, Zhang J, Dai J, Rohn E, Patel AH, Morris MD, Keller ET: Bone metastatic LNCaP-derivative C4-2B prostate cancer cell line mineralizes *in vitro*. Prostate 47: 212–221, 2001
86. Boyce BF, Yoneda T, Guise TA: Factors regulating the growth of metastatic cancer in bone. Endocr Relat Cancer 6: 333–347, 1999
87. Deftos LJ: Prostate carcinoma: Production of bioactive factors. Cancer 88: 3002–3008, 2000
88. Yoneda T: Cellular and molecular mechanisms of breast and prostate cancer metastasis to bone. Eur J Cancer 34: 240–245, 1998
89. Goltzman D, Bolivar I, Rabbani SA: Studies on the pathogenesis of osteoblastic metastases by prostate cancer. Adv Exp Med Biol 324: 165–171, 1992
90. Koutsilieris M, Rabbani SA, Goltzman D: Selective osteoblast mitogens can be extracted from prostatic tissue. Prostate 9: 109–115, 1986
91. Autzen P, Robson CN, Bjartell A, Malcolm AJ, Johnson MI, Neal DE, Hamdy FC: Bone morphogenetic protein 6 in skeletal metastases from prostate cancer and other common human malignancies. Br J Cancer 78: 1219–1223, 1998
92. Harris SE, Harris MA, Mahy P, Wozney J, Feng JQ, Mundy GR: Expression of bone morphogenetic protein messenger RNAs by normal rat and human prostate and prostate cancer cells. Prostate 24: 204–211, 1994
93. Hullinger TG, Taichman RS, Linseman DA, Somerman MJ: Secretory products from PC-3 and MCF-7 tumor cell lines upregulate osteopontin in MC3T3-E1 cells. J Cell Biochem 78: 607–616, 2000
94. Nelson JB, Hedican SP, George DJ, Reddi AH, Piantadosi S, Eisenberger MA, Simons JW: Identification of endothelin-1 in the pathophysiology of metastatic adenocarcinoma of the prostate. Nat Med 1: 944–949, 1995
95. Kimura G, Sugisaki Y, Masugi Y, Nakazawa N: Calcification in human osteoblasts cultured in medium conditioned by the prostatic cancer cell line PC-3 and prostatic acid phosphatase. Urol Int 48: 25–30, 1992
96. Karaplis AC, Vautour L: Parathyroid hormone-related peptide and the parathyroid hormone/parathyroid hormone-related peptide receptor in skeletal development. Curr Opin Nephrol Hypertens 6: 308–313, 1997
97. Cornish J, Callon KE, Lin C, Xiao C, Moseley JM, Reid IR: Stimulation of osteoblast proliferation by C-terminal fragments of parathyroid hormone-related protein. J Bone Miner Res 14: 915–922, 1999
98. Rabbani SA, Gladu J, Mazar AP, Henkin J, Goltzman D: Induction in human osteoblastic cells (SaOS2) of the early response genes fos, jun, and myc by the amino terminal fragment (ATF) of urokinase. J Cell Physiol 172: 137–145, 1997
99. Killian CS, Corral DA, Kawinski E, Constantine RI: Mitogenic response of osteoblast cells to prostate-specific antigen suggests an activation of latent TGF-beta and a proteolytic modulation of cell adhesion receptors. Biochem Biophys Res Commun 192: 940–947, 1993
100. Honore P, Luger NM, Sabino MA, Schwei MJ, Rogers SD, Mach DB, O'Keefe PF, Ramnaraine ML, Clohisy DR, Mantyh PW: Osteoprotegerin blocks bone cancer-induced skeletal destruction, skeletal pain and pain-related neurochemical reorganization of the spinal cord. Nat Med 6: 521–528, 2000
101. Guise TA: Molecular mechanisms of osteolytic bone metastases. Cancer 88: 2892–2898, 2000
102. Simonet WS, Lacey DL, Dunstan CR, Kelley M, Chang MS, Luthy R, Nguyen HQ, Wooden S, Bennett L, Boone T, Shimamoto G, DeRose M, Elliott R, Colombero A, Tan HL, Trail G, Sullivan J, Davy E, Bucay N, Renshaw-Gegg L, Hughes TM, Hill D, Pattison W, Campbell P, Boyle WJ: Osteoprotegerin: A novel secreted protein involved in the regulation of bone density. Cell 89: 309–319, 1997
103. Chiao JW, Moonga BS, Yang YM, Kancherla R, Mittelman A, Wu-Wong JR, Ahmed T: Endothelin-1 from prostate cancer cells is enhanced by bone contact which blocks osteoclastic bone resorption. Br J Cancer 83: 360–365, 2000
104. Laitinen M, Marttinen A, Aho AJ, Lindholm TS: Bone morphogenetic protein in bone neoplasms: Comparison of different detection methods. Eur Surg Res 30: 168–174, 1998
105. Raval P, Hsu HH, Schneider DJ, Sarras MP Jr., Masuhara K, Bonewald LF, Anderson HC: Expression of bone morphogenetic proteins by osteoinductive and non-osteoinductive human osteosarcoma cells. J Dent Res 75: 1518–1523, 1996
106. Wlosarski K, Reddi AH: Tumor cells stimulate *in vivo* periosteal bone formation. Bone Miner 2: 185–192, 1987
107. Strewler GJ: The physiology of parathyroid hormone-related protein. N Engl J Med 342: 177–185, 2000
108. Lanske B, Amling M, Neff L, Guiducci J, Baron R, Kronenberg HM: Ablation of the PTHrP gene or the PTH/PTHrP receptor gene leads to distinct abnormalities in bone development. J Clin Invest 104: 399–407, 1999
109. Amizuka N, Henderson JE, White JH, Karaplis AC, Goltzman D, Sasaki T, Ozawa H: Recent studies on the biological action of parathyroid hormone (PTH)-related

peptide (PTHrP) and PTH/PTHrP receptor in cartilage and bone. Histol Histopathol 15: 957–970, 2000

110. Iwamura M, Abrahamsson PA, Schoen S, Cockett AT, Deftos LJ: Immunoreactive parathyroid hormone-related protein is present in human seminal plasma and is of prostate origin. J Androl 15: 410–414, 1994

111. Iwamura M, di Sant'Agnese PA, Wu G, Benning CM, Cockett AT, Deftos LJ, Abrahamsson PA: Immunohistochemical localization of parathyroid hormone-related protein in human prostate cancer. Cancer Res 53: 1724–1726, 1993

112. Asadi F, Farraj M, Sharifi R, Malakouti S, Antar S, Kukreja S: Enhanced expression of parathyroid hormone-related protein in prostate cancer as compared with benign prostatic hyperplasia. Hum Pathol 27: 1319–1323, 1996

113. Iwamura M, Gershagen S, Lapets O, Moynes R, Abrahamsson PA, Cockett AT, Deftos LJ, di Sant'Agnese PA: Immunohistochemical localization of parathyroid hormone-related protein in prostatic intra-epithelial neoplasia. Hum Pathol 26: 797–801, 1995

114. Dougherty KM, Blomme EA, Koh AJ, Henderson JE, Pienta KJ, Rosol TJ, McCauley LK: Parathyroid hormone-related protein as a growth regulator of prostate carcinoma. Cancer Res 59: 6015–6022, 1999

115. Burton PB, Moniz C, Knight DE: Parathyroid hormone related peptide can function as an autocrine growth factor in human renal cell carcinoma. Biochem Biophys Res Commun 167: 1134–1138, 1990

116. Bouizar Z, Spyratos F, De vernejoul MC: The parathyroid hormone-related protein (PTHrP) gene: use of downstream TATA promotor and PTHrP 1-139 coding pathways in primary breast cancers vary with the occurrence of bone metastasis. J Bone Miner Res 14: 406–414, 1999

117. Yin JJ, Selander K, Chirgwin JM, Dallas M, Grubbs BG, Wieser R, Massague J, Mundy GR, Guise TA: TGF-beta signaling blockade inhibits PTHrP secretion by breast cancer cells and bone metastases development. J Clin Invest 103: 197–206, 1999

118. Iwamura M, Abrahamsson PA, Foss KA, Wu G, Cockett AT, Deftos LJ: Parathyroid hormone-related protein: a potential autocrine growth regulator in human prostate cancer cell lines. Urology 43: 675–679, 1994

119. Henderson JE, Amizuka N, Warshawsky H, Biasotto D, Lanske BM, Goltzman D, Karaplis AC: Nucleolar localization of parathyroid hormone-related peptide enhances survival of chondrocytes under conditions that promote apoptotic cell death. Mol Cell Biol 15: 4064–4075, 1995

120. Aarts MM, Levy D, He B, Stregger S, Chen T, Richard S, Henderson JE: Parathyroid hormone-related protein interacts with RNA. J Biol Chem 274: 4832–4838, 1999

121. Ye Y, Falzon M, Seitz PK, Cooper CW: Overexpression of parathyroid hormone-related protein promotes cell growth in the rat intestinal cell line IEC-6. Regul Pept 99: 169–174, 2001

122. Massfelder T, Dann P, Wu TL, Vasavada R, Helwig JJ, Stewart AF: Opposing mitogenic and anti-mitogenic actions of parathyroid hormone-related protein in vascular smooth muscle cells: a critical role for nuclear targeting. Proc Natl Acad Sci USA 94: 13630–13635, 1997

123. Cramer SD, Chen Z, Peehl DM: Prostate specific antigen cleaves parathyroid hormone-related protein in the PTH-like domain: Inactivation of PTHrP-stimulated cAMP accumulation in mouse osteoblasts. J Urol 156: 526–531, 1996

124. Ye Y, Seitz PK, Cooper CW: Parathyroid hormone-related protein overexpression in the human colon cancer cell line HT-29 enhances adhesion of the cells to collagen type I. Regul Pept 101: 19–23, 2001

125. Stjernquist M: Endothelins–vasoactive peptides and growth factors. Cell Tissue Res 292: 1–9, 1998

126. Takuwa Y, Ohue Y, Takuwa N, Yamashita K: Endothelin-1 activates phospholipase C and mobilizes Ca^{2+} from extra- and intracellular pools in osteoblastic cells. Am J Physiol 257: E797–803, 1989

127. Hiruma Y, Inoue A, Shiohama A, Otsuka E, Hirose S, Yamaguchi A, Hagiwara H: Endothelins inhibit the mineralization of osteoblastic MC3T3-E1 cells through the A-type endothelin receptor. Am J Physiol 275: R1099–1105, 1998

128. Zaidi M, Alam AS, Bax BE, Shankar VS, Bax CM, Gill JS, Pazianas M, Huang CL, Sahinoglu T, Moonga BS, et al.: Role of the endothelial cell in osteoclast control: New perspectives. Bone 14: 97–102, 1993

129. Tatrai A, Foster S, Lakatos P, Shankar G, Stern PH: Endothelin-1 actions on resorption, collagen and noncollagen protein synthesis, and phosphatidylinositol turnover in bone organ cultures. Endocrinology 131: 603–607, 1992

130. Shioide M, Noda M: Endothelin modulates osteopontin and osteocalcin messenger ribonucleic acid expression in rat osteoblastic osteosarcoma cells. J Cell Biochem 53: 176–180, 1993

131. Kasperk CH, Borcsok I, Schairer HU, Schneider U, Nawroth PP, Niethard FU, Ziegler R: Endothelin-1 is a potent regulator of human bone cell metabolism in vitro. Calcif Tissue Int 60: 368–374, 1997

132. Tsukahara H, Hori C, Hiraoka M, Yamamoto K, Ishii Y, Mayumi M: Endothelin subtype A receptor antagonist induces osteopenia in growing rats. Metabolism 47: 1403–1407, 1998

133. Langenstroer P, Tang R, Shapiro E, Divish B, Opgenorth T, Lepor H: Endothelin-1 in the human prostate: Tissue levels, source of production and isometric tension studies. J Urol 150: 495–499, 1993

134. Walden PD, Ittmann M, Monaco ME, Lepor H: Endothelin-1 production and agonist activities in cultured prostate-derived cells: Implications for regulation of endothelin bioactivity and bioavailability in prostatic hyperplasia. Prostate 34: 241–250, 1998

135. Casey ML, Byrd W, MacDonald PC: Massive amounts of immunoreactive endothelin in human seminal fluid. J Clin Endocrinol Metab 74: 223–225, 1992

136. Nelson JB, Carducci MA: The role of endothelin-1 and endothelin receptor antagonists in prostate cancer. BJU Int 85(Suppl 2): 45–48, 2000

137. Nelson JB, Nguyen SH, Wu-Wong JR, Opgenorth TJ, Dixon DB, Chung LW, Inoue N: New bone formation in an osteoblastic tumor model is increased by endothelin-1

overexpression and decreased by endothelin A receptor blockade. Urology 53: 1063–1069, 1999

138. Yin J, Grubbs B, Cui Y, Weu-Wong J, Wessale J, Padley R, Guise T: Endothelin A receptor blockade inhibits osteoblastic metastases. J Bone Miner Res 15: S201, 2000

139. Tarquini R, Perfetto F, Tarquini B: Endothelin-1 and Paget's bone disease: Is there a link? Calcif Tissue Int 63: 118–120, 1998

140. Ducy P, Karsenty G: The family of bone morphogenetic proteins. Kidney Int 57: 2207–2214, 2000

141. Reddi AH: Bone morphogenetic proteins: An unconventional approach to isolation of first mammalian morphogens. Cytokine Growth Factor Rev 8: 11–20, 1997

142. Hogan BL: Bone morphogenetic proteins in development. Curr Opin Genet Dev 6: 432–438, 1996

143. Hall BK, Miyake T: All for one and one for all: condensations and the initiation of skeletal development. Bioessays 22: 138–147, 2000

144. Wozney JM: The bone morphogenetic protein family and osteogenesis. Mol Reprod Dev 32: 160–167, 1992

145. Suzuki A, Kaneko E, Maeda J, Ueno N: Mesoderm induction by BMP-4 and -7 heterodimers. Biochem Biophys Res Commun 232: 153–156, 1997

146. Wrana JL: Regulation of Smad activity. Cell 100: 189–192, 2000

147. Wan M, Shi X, Feng X, Cao X: Transcriptional mechanisms of bone morphogenetic protein induced osteoprotegrin gene expression. J Biol Chem 276: 10119–10125, 2001

148. Tsuji K, Ito Y, Noda M: Expression of the PEBP2alphaA/AML3/CBFA1 gene is regulated by BMP4/7 heterodimer and its overexpression suppresses type I collagen and osteocalcin gene expression in osteoblastic and nonosteoblastic mesenchymal cells. Bone 22: 87–92, 1998

149. Gori F, Thomas T, Hicok KC, Spelsberg TC, Riggs BL: Differentiation of human marrow stromal precursor cells: Bone morphogenetic protein-2 increases OSF2/CBFA1, enhances osteoblast commitment, and inhibits late adipocyte maturation. J Bone Miner Res 14: 1522–1535, 1999

150. Abe E, Yamamoto M, Taguchi Y, Lecka-Czernik B, O'Brien CA, Economides AN, Stahl N, Jilka RL, Manolagas SC: Essential requirement of BMPs-2/4 for both osteoblast and osteoclast formation in murine bone marrow cultures from adult mice: antagonism by noggin. J Bone Miner Res 15: 663–673, 2000

151. Zimmerman LB, De Jesus-Escobar JM, Harland RM: The Spemann organizer signal noggin binds and inactivates bone morphogenetic protein 4. Cell 86: 599–606, 1996

152. Merino R, Rodriguez-Leon J, Macias D, Ganan Y, Economides AN, Hurle JM: The BMP antagonist Gremlin regulates outgrowth, chondrogenesis and programmed cell death in the developing limb. Development 126: 5515–5522, 1999

153. Nifuji A, Noda M: Coordinated expression of noggin and bone morphogenetic proteins (BMPs) during early skeletogenesis and induction of noggin expression by BMP-7. J Bone Miner Res 14: 2057–2066, 1999

154. Nifuji A, Kellermann O, Noda M: Noggin expression in a mesodermal pluripotent cell line C1 and its regulation by BMP. J Cell Biochem 73: 437–444, 1999

155. Li IW, Cheifetz S, McCulloch CA, Sampath KT, Sodek J: Effects of osteogenic protein-1 (OP-1, BMP-7) on bone matrix protein expression by fetal rat calvarial cells are differentiation stage specific. J Cell Physiol 169: 115–125, 1996

156. Asahina I, Sampath TK, Nishimura I, Hauschka PV: Human osteogenic protein-1 induces both chondroblastic and osteoblastic differentiation of osteoprogenitor cells derived from newborn rat calvaria. J Cell Biol 123: 921–933, 1993

157. Maliakal JC, Asahina I, Hauschka PV, Sampath TK: Osteogenic protein-1 (BMP-7) inhibits cell proliferation and stimulates the expression of markers characteristic of osteoblast phenotype in rat osteosarcoma (17/2.8) cells. Growth Factors 11: 227–234, 1994

158. Yamaguchi A, Ishizuya T, Kintou N, Wada Y, Katagiri T, Wozney JM, Rosen V, Yoshiki S: Effects of BMP-2, BMP-4, and BMP-6 on osteoblastic differentiation of bone marrow-derived stromal cell lines, ST2 and MC3T3-G2/PA6. Biochem Biophys Res Commun 220: 366–371, 1996

159. Katagiri T, Yamaguchi A, Ikeda T, Yoshiki S, Wozney JM, Rosen V, Wang EA, Tanaka H, Omura S, Suda T: The non-osteogenic mouse pluripotent cell line, C3H10T1/2, is induced to differentiate into osteoblastic cells by recombinant human bone morphogenetic protein-2. Biochem Biophys Res Commun 172: 295–299, 1990

160. Katagiri T, Akiyama S, Namiki M, Komaki M, Yamaguchi A, Rosen V, Wozney JM, Fujisawa-Sehara A, Suda T: Bone morphogenetic protein-2 inhibits terminal differentiation of myogenic cells by suppressing the transcriptional activity of MyoD and myogenin. Exp Cell Res 230: 342–351, 1997

161. Ducy P, Schinke T, Karsenty G: The osteoblast: A sophisticated fibroblast under central surveillance. Science 289: 1501–1504, 2000

162. Knutsen R, Wergedal JE, Sampath TK, Baylink DJ, Mohan S: Osteogenic protein-1 stimulates proliferation and differentiation of human bone cells in vitro. Biochem Biophys Res Commun 194: 1352–1358, 1993

163. Kim KJ, Itoh T, Kotake S: Effects of recombinant human bone morphogenetic protein-2 on human bone marrow cells cultured with various biomaterials. J Biomed Mater Res 35: 279–285, 1997

164. Groeneveld EH, Burger EH: Bone morphogenetic proteins in human bone regeneration. Eur J Endocrinol 142: 9–21, 2000

165. Jena N, Martin-Seisdedos C, McCue P, Croce CM: BMP7 null mutation in mice: Developmental defects in skeleton, kidney, and eye. Exp Cell Res 230: 28–37, 1997

166. Solloway MJ, Dudley AT, Bikoff EK, Lyons KM, Hogan BL, Robertson EJ: Mice lacking Bmp6 function. Dev Genet 22: 321–339, 1998

167. Kingsley DM, Bland AE, Grubber JM, Marker PC, Russell LB, Copeland NG, Jenkins NA: The mouse short ear skeletal morphogenesis locus is associated with defects

in a bone morphogenetic member of the TGF beta super-family. Cell 71: 399–410, 1992

168. Weber KL, Bolander ME, Rock MG, Pritchard D, Sarkar G: Evidence for the upregulation of osteogenic protein-1 mRNA expression in musculoskeletal neoplasms. J Orthop Res 16: 8–14, 1998

169. Bentley H, Hamdy FC, Hart KA, Seid JM, Williams JL, Johnstone D, Russell RG: Expression of bone morphogenetic proteins in human prostatic adenocarcinoma and benign prostatic hyperplasia. Br J Cancer 66: 1159–1163, 1992

170. Barnes J, Anthony CT, Wall N, Steiner MS: Bone morphogenetic protein-6 expression in normal and malignant prostate. World J Urol 13: 337–343, 1995

171. Hamdy FC, Autzen P, Robinson MC, Horne CH, Neal DE, Robson CN: Immunolocalization and messenger RNA expression of bone morphogenetic protein-6 in human benign and malignant prostatic tissue. Cancer Res 57: 4427–4431, 1997

172. Kim IY, Lee DH, Ahn HJ, Tokunaga H, Song W, Devereaux LM, Jin D, Sampath TK, Morton RA: Expression of bone morphogenetic protein receptors type-IA, -IB and -II correlates with tumor grade in human prostate cancer tissues. Cancer Res 60: 2840–2844, 2000

173. Ide H, Katoh M, Sasaki H, Yoshida T, Aoki K, Nawa Y, Osada Y, Sugimura T, Terada M: Cloning of human bone morphogenetic protein type IB receptor (BMPR-IB) and its expression in prostate cancer in comparison with other BMPRs (published erratum appears in Oncogene 1997 Aug 28;15(9):1121). Oncogene 14: 1377–1382, 1997

174. Ide H, Yoshida T, Matsumoto N, Aoki K, Osada Y, Sugimura T, Terada M: Growth regulation of human prostate cancer cells by bone morphogenetic protein-2. Cancer Res 57: 5022–5027, 1997

175. Mundy GR, Yoneda T, Hiraga T: Preclinical studies with zoledronic acid and other bisphosphonates: Impact on the bone microenvironment. Semin Oncol 28: 35–44, 2001

176. Theriault RL, Hortobagyi GN: The evolving role of bisphosphonates. Semin Oncol 28: 284–290, 2001

177. Pelger RC, Hamdy NA, Zwinderman AH, Lycklama a Nijeholt AA, Papapoulos SE: Effects of the bisphosphonate olpadronate in patients with carcinoma of the prostate metastatic to the skeleton. Bone 22: 403–408, 1998

178. Garnero P, Buchs N, Zekri J, Rizzoli R, Coleman RE, Delmas PD: Markers of bone turnover for the management of patients with bone metastases from prostate cancer. Br J Cancer 82: 858–864, 2000

179. Heidenreich A, Hofmann R, Engelmann UH: The use of bisphosphonate for the palliative treatment of painful bone metastasis due to hormone refractory prostate cancer (In Process Citation). J Urol 165: 136–140, 2001

180. Stearns ME, Wang M: Effects of alendronate and taxol on PC-3 ML cell bone metastases in SCID mice. Inv Met 16: 116–131, 1996

181. Sun YC, Geldof AA, Newling DW, Rao BR: Progression delay of prostate tumor skeletal metastasis effects by bisphosphonates. J Urol 148: 1270–1273, 1992

182. Wang M, Stearns ME: Isolation and characterization of PC-3 human prostatic tumor sublines which preferentially metastasize to select organs in S.C.I.D. mice. Differentiation 48: 115–125, 1991

183. Boissier S, Ferreras M, Peyruchaud O, Magnetto S, Ebetino FH, Colombel M, Delmas P, Delaisse JM, Clezardin P: Bisphosphonates inhibit breast and prostate carcinoma cell invasion, an early event in the formation of bone metastases. Cancer Res 60: 2949–2954, 2000

184. Boissier S, Magnetto S, Frappart L, Cuzin B, Ebetino FH, Delmas PD, Clezardin P: Bisphosphonates inhibit prostate and breast carcinoma cell adhesion to unmineralized and mineralized bone extracellular matrices. Cancer Res 57: 3890–3894, 1997

185. Lee MV, Fong EM, Singer FR, Guenette RS: Bisphosphonate treatment inhibits the growth of prostate cancer cells. Cancer Res 61: 2602–2608, 2001

186. Diel IJ: Antitumour effects of bisphosphonates: first evidence and possible mechanisms. Drugs 59: 391–399, 2000

187. Hiraga T, Williams PJ, Mundy GR, Yoneda T: The bisphosphonate ibandronate promotes apoptosis in MDA-MB-231 human breast cancer cells in bone metastases. Cancer Res 61: 4418–4424, 2001

188. Smith PC, Hobish A, Lin D, Culig Z, Keller ET: Interleukin-6 and prostate cancer progression. Cytokine Growth Factor Rev 12: 33–40, 2001

189. Lum L, Wong BR, Josien R, Becherer JD, Erdjument-Bromage H, Schlondorff J, Tempst P, Choi Y, Blobel CP: Evidence for a role of a tumor necrosis factor-alpha (TNF-alpha)- converting enzyme-like protease in shedding of TRANCE, a TNF family member involved in osteoclastogenesis and dendritic cell survival. J Biol Chem 274: 13613–13618, 1999

190. Lacey DL, Timms E, Tan HL, Kelley MJ, Dunstan CR, Burgess T, Elliott R, Colombero A, Elliott G, Scully S, Hsu H, Sullivan J, Hawkins N, Davy E, Capparelli C, Eli A, Qian YX, Kaufman S, Sarosi I, Shalhoub V, Senaldi G, Guo J, Delaney J, Boyle WJ: Osteoprotegerin ligand is a cytokine that regulates osteoclast differentiation and activation. Cell 93: 165–176, 1998

191. Kong YY, Yoshida H, Sarosi I, Tan HL, Timms E, Capparelli C, Morony S, Oliveira-dos-Santos AJ, Van G, Itie A, Khoo W, Wakeham A, Dunstan CR, Lacey DL, Mak TW, Boyle WJ, Penninger JM: OPGL is a key regulator of osteoclastogenesis, lymphocyte development and lymph-node organogenesis. Nature 397: 315–323, 1999

192. Yasuda H, Shima N, Nakagawa N, Yamaguchi K, Kinosaki M, Mochizuki S, Tomoyasu A, Yano K, Goto M, Murakami A, Tsuda E, Morinaga T, Higashio K, Udagawa N, Takahashi N, Suda T: Osteoclast differentiation factor is a ligand for osteoprotegerin/osteoclastogenesis-inhibitory factor and is identical to TRANCE/RANKL. Proc Natl Acad Sci USA 95: 3597–3602, 1998

193. Fuller K, Wong B, Fox S, Choi Y, Chambers TJ: TRANCE is necessary and sufficient for osteoblast-mediated activation of bone resorption in osteoclasts. J Exp Med 188: 997–1001, 1998

212

194. Tsuda E, Goto M, Mochizuki S, Yano K, Kobayashi F, Morinaga T, Higashio K: Isolation of a novel cytokine from human fibroblasts that specifically inhibits osteoclastogenesis. Biochem Biophys Res Commun 234: 137–142, 1997

195. Tan KB, Harrop J, Reddy M, Young P, Terrett J, Emery J, Moore G, Truneh A: Characterization of a novel TNF-like ligand and recently described TNF ligand and TNF receptor superfamily genes and their constitutive and inducible expression in hematopoietic and non-hematopoietic cells. Gene 204: 35–46, 1997

196. Yasuda H, Shima N, Nakagawa N, Mochizuki SI, Yano K, Fujise N, Sato Y, Goto M, Yamaguchi K, Kuriyama M, Kanno T, Murakami A, Tsuda E, Morinaga T, Higashio K: Identity of osteoclastogenesis inhibitory factor (OCIF) and osteoprotegerin (OPG): a mechanism by which OPG/OCIF inhibits osteoclastogenesis in vitro. Endocrinology 139: 1329–1337, 1998

197. Kwon BS, Wang S, Udagawa N, Haridas V, Lee ZH, Kim KK, Oh KO, Greene J, Li Y, Su J, Gentz R, Aggarwal BB, Ni J: TR1, a new member of the tumor necrosis factor receptor superfamily, induces fibroblast proliferation and inhibits osteoclastogenesis and bone resorption. FASEB J 12: 845–854, 1998

198. Yun TJ, Chaudhary PM, Shu GL, Frazer JK, Ewings MK, Schwartz SM, Pascual V, Hood LE, Clark EA: OPG/FDCR-1, a TNF receptor family member, is expressed in lymphoid cells and is up-regulated by ligating CD40. J Immunol 161: 6113–6121, 1998

199. Hofbauer LC, Dunstan CR, Spelsberg TC, Riggs BL, Khosla S: Osteoprotegerin production by human osteoblast lineage cells is stimulated by vitamin D, bone morphogenetic protein-2, and cytokines. Biochem Biophys Res Commun 250: 776–781, 1998

200. Hofbauer LC, Heufelder AE: Osteoprotegerin and its cognate ligand: a new paradigm of osteoclastogenesis. Eur J Endocrinol 139: 152–154, 1998

201. Vidal NO, Brandstrom H, Jonsson KB, Ohlsson C: Osteoprotegerin mRNA is expressed in primary human osteoblast-like cells: down-regulation by glucocorticoids. J Endocrinol 159: 191–195, 1998

202. Kartsogiannis V, Zhou H, Horwood NJ, Thomas RJ, Hards DK, Quinn JM, Niforas P, Ng KW, Martin TJ, Gillespie MT: Localization of RANKL (receptor activator of NF kappa B ligand) mRNA and protein in skeletal and extraskeletal tissues. Bone 25: 525–534, 1999

203. Nagai M, Sato N: Reciprocal gene expression of osteoclastogenesis inhibitory factor and osteoclast differentiation factor regulates osteoclast formation. Biochem Biophys Res Commun 257: 719–723, 1999

204. Thomas GP, Baker SU, Eisman JA, Gardiner EM: Changing RANKL/OPG mRNA expression in differentiating murine primary osteoblasts. J Endocrinol 170: 451–460, 2001

205. Hofbauer LC, Heufelder AE, Erben RG: Osteoprotegerin, RANK, and RANK ligand: the good, the bad, and the ugly in rheumatoid arthritis. J Rheumatol 28: 685–687, 2001

206. Fazzalari NL, Kuliwaba JS, Atkins GJ, Forwood MR, Findlay DM: The ratio of messenger RNA levels of receptor activator of nuclear factor kappaB ligand to osteoprotegerin correlates with bone remodeling indices in normal human cancellous bone but not in osteoarthritis. J Bone Miner Res 16: 1015–1027, 2001

207. Yoneda T, Sasaki A, Mundy GR: Osteolytic bone metastasis in breast cancer. Breast Cancer Res Treat 32: 73–84, 1994

208. Akatsu T, Ono K, Katayama Y, Tamura T, Nishikawa M, Kugai N, Yamamoto M, Nagata N: The mouse mammary tumor cell line, MMT060562, produces prostaglandin E2 and leukemia inhibitory factor and supports osteoclast formation in vitro via a stromal cell-dependent pathway. J Bone Miner Res 13: 400–408, 1998

209. Mundy GR: Pathophysiology of cancer-associated hypercalcemia. Semin Oncol 17: 10–15, 1990

210. Roodman GD: Mechanisms of bone lesions in multiple myeloma and lymphoma. Cancer 80: 1557–1563, 1997

211. Thomas T, Lafage-Proust MH: Contribution of genetically modified mouse models to the elucidation of bone physiology. Rev Rhum Engl Ed 66: 728–735, 1999

212. Atkins GJ, Bouralexis S, Haynes DR, Graves SE, Geary SM, Evdokiou A, Zannettino AC, Hay S, Findlay DM: Osteoprotegerin inhibits osteoclast formation and bone resorbing activity in giant cell tumors of bone. Bone 28: 370–377, 2001

213. Han JH, Choi SJ, Kurihara N, Koide M, Oba Y, Roodman GD: Macrophage inflammatory protein-1alpha is an osteoclastogenic factor in myeloma that is independent of receptor activator of nuclear factor kappaB ligand. Blood 97: 3349–3353, 2001

214. Guise TA, Yin JJ, Taylor SD, Kumagai Y, Dallas M, Boyce BF, Yoneda T, Mundy GR: Evidence for a causal role of parathyroid hormone-related protein in the pathogenesis of human breast cancer-mediated osteolysis. J Clin Invest 98: 1544–1549, 1996

215. Sasaki A, Boyce BF, Story B, Wright KR, Chapman M, Boyce R, Mundy GR, Yoneda T: Bisphosphonate risedronate reduces metastatic human breast cancer burden in bone in nude mice. Cancer Res 55: 3551–3557, 1995

216. Michigami T, Ihara-Watanabe M, Yamazaki M, Ozono K: Receptor activator of nuclear factor kappaB ligand (RANKL) is a key molecule of osteoclast formation for bone metastasis in a newly developed model of human neuroblastoma. Cancer Res 61: 1637–1644, 2001

217. Oyajobi BO, Anderson DM, Traianedes K, Williams PJ, Yoneda T, Mundy GR: Therapeutic efficacy of a soluble receptor activator of nuclear factor kappaB-IgG Fc fusion protein in suppressing bone resorption and hypercalcemia in a model of humoral hypercalcemia of malignancy. Cancer Res 61: 2572–2578, 2001

218. John A, Tuszynski G: The role of matrix metalloproteinases in tumor angiogenesis and tumor metastasis. Pathol Oncol Res 7: 14–23, 2001

219. Boag AH, Young ID: Immunohistochemical analysis of type IV collagenase expression in prostatic hyperplasia and adenocarcinoma. Mod Pathol 6: 65–68, 1993

220. Bodey B, Bodey B, Jr., Siegel SE, Kaiser HE: Immunocytochemical detection of matrix metalloproteinase expression in prostate cancer. In vivo 15: 65–70, 2001

221. Festuccia C, Bologna M, Vicentini C, Tacconelli A, Miano R, Violini S, Mackay AR: Increased matrix metalloproteinase-9 secretion in short-term tissue cultures of prostatic tumor cells. Int J Cancer 69: 386–393, 1996

222. Hamdy FC, Fadlon EJ, Cottam D, Lawry J, Thurrell W, Silcocks PB, Anderson JB, Williams JL, Rees RC: Matrix metalloproteinase 9 expression in primary human prostatic adenocarcinoma and benign prostatic hyperplasia. Br J Cancer 69: 177–182, 1994

223. Hashimoto K, Kihira Y, Matuo Y, Usui T: Expression of matrix metalloproteinase-7 and tissue inhibitor of metalloproteinase-1 in human prostate. J Urol 160: 1872–1876, 1998

224. Montironi R, Fabris G, Lucarini G, Biagini G: Location of 72-kd metalloproteinase (type IV collagenase) in untreated prostatic adenocarcinoma. Pathol Res Pract 191: 1140–1146, 1995

225. Montironi R, Lucarini G, Castaldini C, Galluzzi CM, Biagini G, Fabris G: Immunohistochemical evaluation of type IV collagenase (72-kd metalloproteinase) in prostatic intraepithelial neoplasia. Anticancer Res 16: 2057–2062, 1996

226. Pajouh MS, Nagle RB, Breathnach R, Finch JS, Brawer MK, Bowden GT: Expression of metalloproteinase genes in human prostate cancer. J Cancer Res Clin Oncol 117: 144–150, 1991

227. Duivenvoorden WC, Hirte HW, Singh G: Use of tetracycline as an inhibitor of matrix metalloproteinase activity secreted by human bone-metastasizing cancer cells. Invasion Metastasis 17: 312–322, 1997

228. Sanchez-Sweatman OH, Orr FW, Singh G: Human metastatic prostate PC3 cell lines degrade bone using matrix metalloproteinases. Invasion Metastasis 18: 297–305, 1998

229. Lee J, Weber M, Mejia S, Bone E, Watson P, Orr W: A matrix metalloproteinase inhibitor, batimastat, retards the development of osteolytic bone metastases by MDA-MB-231 human breast cancer cells in Balb C nu/nu mice. Eur J Cancer 37: 106–113, 2001

230. Nemeth JA, Yousif R, Herzog M, Che M, Upadhyay J, Shekarriz B, Bhagat S, Mullins C, Fridman R, Cher ML: Matrix metalloproteinases activity, bone matrix turnover and tumor cell proliferation in prostate cancer bone metastasis. J Natl Cancer Inst 94: 17–25, 2002

231. Pirtskhalaishvili G, Nelson JB: Endothelium – derived factors as paracrine mediators of prostate cancer progression. Prostate 44: 77–87, 2000

232. Perkel VS, Mohan S, Baylink DJ, Linkhart TA: An inhibitory insulin-like growth factor binding protein (In-IGFBP) from human prostatic cell conditioned medium reveals N-terminal sequence identity with bone derived In-IGFBP. J Clin Endocrinol Metab 71: 533–535, 1990

233. Taguchi Y, Yamamoto M, Yamate T, Lin SC, Mocharla H, DeTogni P, Nakayama N, Boyce BF, Abe E, Manolagas SC: Interleukin-6-type cytokines stimulate mesenchymal progenitor differentiation toward the osteoblastic lineage. Proc Assoc Am Physicians 110: 559–574, 1998

234. Le Brun G, Aubin P, Soliman H, Ropiquet F, Villette JM, Berthon P, Creminon C, Cussenot O, Fiet J: Upregulation of endothelin 1 and its precursor by IL-1beta, TNF-alpha, and TGF-beta in the PC3 human prostate cancer cell line. Cytokine 11: 157–162, 1999

235. Goltzman D, Karaplis AC, Kremer R, Rabbani SA: Molecular basis of the spectrum of skeletal complications of neoplasia. Cancer 88: 2903–2908, 2000

Address for offprints: Evan T. Keller, Room 5304 CCGCB, 1500 East Medical Center Drive, Ann Arbor, MI 48109-0940 USA; *e-mail:* etkeller@umich.edu

Signal transduction targets in androgen-independent prostate cancer

Jian Zhou, Jessica Scholes and Jer-Tsong Hsieh
Department of Urology, University of Texas Southwestern Medical Center at Dallas, Dallas, TX, USA

Key words: prostate cancer, androgen-independent prostate cancer, signal transduction, growth factor, tumor suppressor

Abstract

Prostate cancer (PCa) first manifests as an androgen-dependent disease. Thus, androgen-deprivation therapy is a standard regimen for patients with metastatic PCa. Despite the initial success of androgen-deprivation therapy, PCa inevitably progresses from being androgen dependent (AD) to androgen independent (AI), and this marks the poor prognosis of this disease. Relapse of AIPCa becomes life threatening and accounts for the majority of mortality of PCa patients. Currently, no effective therapy is available for controlling AIPCa. Therefore, the challenge in providing a new intervention is to understand the fundamental changes that occur in AIPCa. Increasing evidence indicates that, under androgen-deprived milieu, several signal networks elicited by peptide growth factors dictate the AI phenotype of PCa. This review covers the latest studies investigating the potential involvement of autocrine growth factors in cell proliferation, survival, metastasis, and the reciprocal interaction with the androgen receptor pathway. In addition, loss of the negative feedback mechanism of the signal cascade further amplifies the effect of growth factors, and thus contributes significantly to the onset of AIPCa. The understanding of the signal target(s) in AIPCa should provide the new markers for prognosis and a new strategy for prevention and therapy.

Progression of androgen-independent prostate cancer

Clinical observations [1–3] indicate that eunuchs and prepubertal castrates do not develop prostate cancer (PCa). This suggests that all the steps of PCa carcinogenesis are prevented by prostatic atrophy associated with early castration or androgen deprivation. Animal models, first developed by Noble [4] and Pollard and Luckert [5] in which chronic administration of androgen and/or estrogen to certain strains of intact male rats caused PCa, further support these observations. Current effective therapeutic modalities, first developed by Huggins and Hodges in 1941 [6], interrupt the positive effect of growth stimulation by androgen. Androgen thus appears to be a 'pure' mitogen for the growth of PCa cells. Conversely, the morphogenic effect of androgen on normal prostatic epithelium must be impaired during the malignant process.

Despite the initial responsiveness of PCa toward androgen ablation, tumor cells invariably relapse to an androgen-refractory state that ultimately leads to mortality. Studies from the Shionogi mouse model [7] support the observation that androgen deprivation leads to a 90% regression of tumor mass (mainly androgen-dependent cells). But, recurrent tumors have a 500-fold increase in the number of androgen-independent (AI) cells over the fraction measured in the parent tumor. Using proliferation-associated antigens (Ki-67, PCNA, MIB 1) as markers, Bonkhoff and Remberger [8] estimated that approximately 70% of the proliferative activity is confined to basal cells in both normal and hyperplastic prostatic epithelia.

AIPCa cells thus appear resistant to a majority of chemotherapeutic agents that target rapidly cycling cells. These data indicate that the androgen eliciting differentiating pathway is often impaired in AIPCa, which may derive from the malignant transformation of 'stem cells' in the normal gland. Based on these findings, we believe that an effective therapy for AIPCa should focus on restoring the differentiation pathway that is operative in normal prostatic epithelia, but is often impaired in AIPCa cells.

M.L. Cher, K.V. Honn and A. Raz (eds.), Prostate Cancer: New Horizons in Research and Treatment, 215–226.
© 2002 *Kluwer Academic Publishers.*

Although the stem cells in the prostate are not well characterized, it is believed that certain basal cells may possess stem cell properties. Shortly after androgen deprivation, luminal epithelial cells in the prostate undergo apoptosis; the remaining epithelial cells are the AI basal cell population. Androgen administration can restore the normal acini/ductal structure and function in an involuted prostate by promoting the growth and differentiation of the remaining basal cell population [8,9]. Even after repeated administration of androgen to castrated animals, the prostate always re-grows to a previously programed organ size. This suggests that a limited number of stem cells from the basal cell population determine the ultimate growth potential of the gland [8–11].

The molecular signal(s) involved in this process are likely important in maintaining the homeostasis of the prostate gland. Imbalance in the homeostatic control of the signaling cascade in the stem cell may underlie the malignant phenotype of AIPCa cells. To better understand the biologic properties of AIPCa cells, we will elucidate: (a) the role of several key peptide growth factors that can stimulate cell growth, survival, and metastasis, (b) the intracellular pathways responsible for these processes, and (c) the cross-talk between these pathways and the steroid hormone-elicited pathway. In addition, we will discuss the potential impact of the loss of the negative feedback mechanism associated with these pathways on recurrent AIPCa.

Mitogenic signal pathways in AIPCa

Altered production of growth factors and/or aberrant expression of their receptors are usually associated with PCa cells. Increasing the production of autocrine growth factors is an important step for the appearance of AIPCa after androgen deprivation. For example, epidermal growth factor (EGF) is a mitogen required for normal prostate epithelial cells in both human and rat [12,13], and it is present, in a large amount, in human prostatic fluid [14]. Blocking EGF receptor (EGFR)-elicited signaling can inhibit the proliferation of both DU145 and LNCaP cells, which indicates the important involvement of the EGFR signal axis in the growth of PCa [15].

In the normal gland, the transforming growth factor-α (TGF-α), a ligand for EGFR, predominantly expresses in stromal cells [16]. However, the EGFR expresses in human prostatic epithelial cells with a higher expression in basal cells than luminal epithelia [17]. This suggests that TGF-α and EGFR have a paracrine interaction. In contrast, the autocrine interaction of EGF/TGF-α and its receptor has been shown to play an important role in the progression of PCa [18–20]. Particularly, increased autocrine production of EGF and/or TGF-α was found in several AIPCa cell lines including DU145. This caused the activation of EGFR as demonstrated by high levels of autophosphorylation of EGFR [19,21]. Furthermore, the addition of anti-EGFR antibody to DU145 cells can reduce EGFR autophosphorylation and subsequently inhibit cell proliferation [22].

In other cases, changing the receptor affinity in PCa allows cancer cells to utilize their own autocrine growth factor. In the Dunning tumor model, AT3 tumor cells expressed a different subclass of fibroblast growth factor receptor (FGFR) protein by switching exon IIIb (high affinity to keratinocyte growth factor [KGF]) to exon IIIc (high affinity to acidic FGF [aFGF] and basic FGF [bFGF]) as they acquire a more aggressive phenotype [23]. Similar exon switching has also been found in DU145 and its xenograft [24]. It is also found in PCa specimens, although incidence is low [25].

Autocrine production of FGF has been associated with the proliferation of AIPCa [23,26,27]. Moreover, AI tumors from Shionogi mice produce a bFGF-like protein [28]. In the Dunning tumor model, in concert with the switching of the receptor subtype in AT3 tumors, the increased steady-state levels of FGF-2, FGF-3, and FGF-5 mRNA were also found in these tumor cells [23].

Nerve growth factor (NGF) also appears to be a mitogen for AIPCa. For example, human prostate cell lines (TSU-Pr1, DU145, PC3, and LNCaP) are sensitive to NGF for proliferation [29,30]. Nevertheless, LNCaP does not produce NGF [31]. Since normal prostate stromal cells produce several active forms of NGF [32,33], this suggests that paracrine NGF could be a potent factor necessary for the growth of primary PCa. However, other AIPCa cell lines such as DU145, PC3, and TSU-Pr1 produce NGF in an autocrine manner [31], which indicates that paracrine and/or autocrine production of NGF contributes to the growth of AIPCa.

Immediately after autocrine growth factors bind to their specific receptor (protein receptor tyrosine kinase, PRTK), dimerization and autophosphorylation of the receptor promote interactions with cytoplasmic proteins. These interactions initiate a cascade of phosphorylation events through a variety of adapter proteins and kinases, which transduce the mitogenic signal by increasing gene expression in the nucleus (Figure 1).

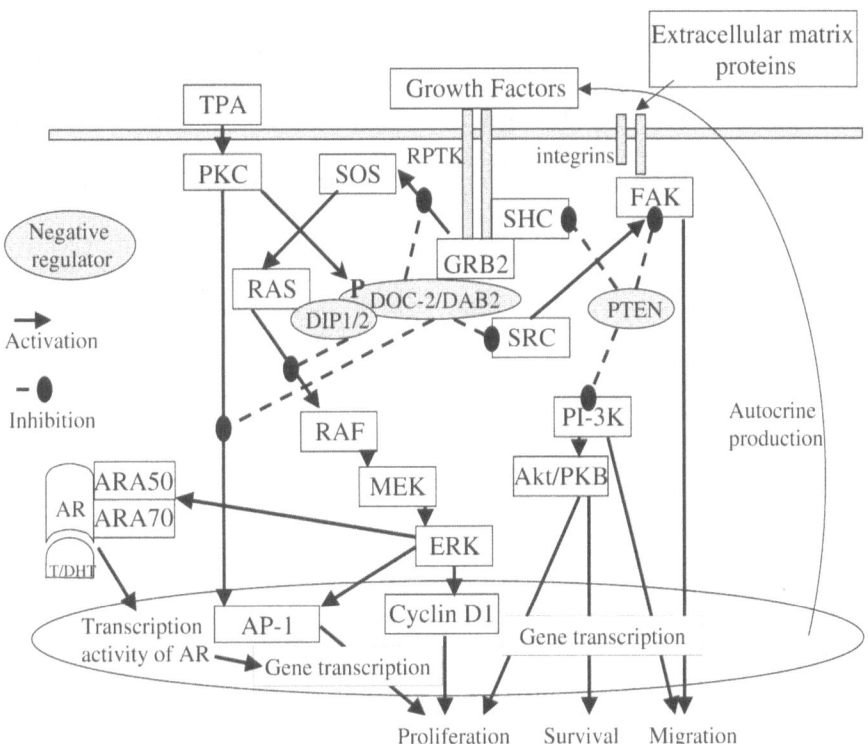

Figure 1. The homeostatic control of signal pathways in prostatic epithelium. The exogenous stimuli (such as hormones, growth factors, and extracellular matrix proteins) can elicit different specific signal cascades that activate gene transcription in the nucleus resulting in cell proliferation, survival, and migration. These signal networks are mainly modulated by protein–protein interaction and protein phosphorylation. Very often, the cross interaction between these pathways becomes more apparent in PCa cells, which underlies the autonomous growth of these cells. The presence of negative regulators prevents the constitutive activation of positive signals, which can maintain a delicate balance in normal cell. Conversely, loss of negative feedback regulators (such as DOC-2/DAB2 and PTEN) in PCa cells intensifies their malignant phenotype. T: testosterone, DHT: dihydrotestosterone.

The interaction between adapter proteins and their activated receptor can further initiate the translocation of a group of proteins, called guanine nucleotide exchange factors (GEFs such as SOS), which modulate the GTPase activity of G-protein such as RAS. Eventually, the GTP-binding RAS can activate a series of mitogen activated protein kinase (MAPK) reactions by Ser/Thr kinases (such as RAF [MAP kinase kinase kinase], ERK [MAP kinase]) and dual kinase (such as MEK [MAP kinase kinase]). MAP kinases can phosphorylate many transcriptional factors (e.g. EF-2) and cyclin (e.g. cyclin D1) is known to be involved in cell cycle regulation [34–36].

The *Ras* superfamily comprises nearly 50 currently known *Ras*-related genes, which encode GTP-binding proteins (i.e. G-protein), and RAS proteins are membrane-bound GTPase [34–36]. Furthermore, RAS proteins help control cell growth and differentiation,

but any one of many single amino acid mutations can produce highly oncogenic proteins. In animals, tumors induced by chemicals (e.g. nitrosomethylurea, dimethylbenzanthracene, or N-methyl-N-nitro-N-nitrosoguanidine) or physical manipulation (e.g. X-ray treatment) show about a 70% frequency of *Ras* mutation. This mutation is commonly associated with a point mutation at codon 12 or 61 [37–39]. Activating mutations in *Ras* oncogene occur in a variety of human tumors, such as in pancreatic (90%), colon (50%), thyroid (50%), and lung (30%) cancers [40].

In PCa, enhanced expression of RAS protein correlates with increased tumor grade [41]. Expression of RAS protein has also been assessed in primary and metastatic tumors. Reports [39–44] indicate that most metastatic tumors expressed RAS protein, while only a fifth of primary tumor do. Noticeably, in an androgen-deprived environment, the expression of oncogenic

Ras (V12ras) enhances ERK activation, cyclin D1 induction, and proliferation in LNCaP cells [45,46]. Moreover, suppressing RAS function by inhibiting its protein farnesylation using a peptidomimetic inhibitor (L-744,832) leads to a significant delay in the development of PCa in a xenograft model [47]. These data indicate that RAS protein plays a critical role in the progression of PCa. Nevertheless, *Ras* gene mutation is rare in PCa [42–44,48–50]. This implies that some other factor(s) may be involved in increasing RAS protein levels in PCa.

It also appears that RAF plays a functional role in PCa cells. Suppression of *Raf* gene expression by an anti-sense oligonucleotide induces apoptosis in PC3 and reduces tumor formation in nude mice [51,52]. Surprisingly, prolonged activation of RAF and MAPK are also able to induce cell cycle arrest in LNCaP cells through induction of p21$^{WAF1/CIP1}$ [53] or apoptosis [54]. These data suggest that perturbing a delicate balance of each component of the mitogenic signal cascade could adversely effect cell growth.

Overwhelming data demonstrate the critical role of the MAPK pathway in cell growth and malignant transformation [55–60]. In several PCa cell lines such as LNCaP and DU145 cells, inactivation of MAPK (e.g. ERK) by interrupting EGF binding to EGFR using a flavonoid antioxidant (Silibinin), decreases DNA synthesis and cell growth [61]. Using anti-phosphorylated ERK antibody, heightened activation of MAPK is often detected in high-grade PCa and AIPCa [59]. In AIPCa cell line such as DU145 cells, the constitutive phosphorylation of ERK2, a hallmark of MAPK activation is also observed [15]. However, this ERK2 activation can be blocked by several EGFR inhibitors such as Tyrphostin AG1748 and MAb-EGFR-528, indicating that the EGFR-elicited signal axis is critical for activating the MAPK pathway in AIPCa [15]. Therefore, it is likely that the increased activation of MAPK in high grade PCa and AIPCa is due to the stimulation of autocrine growth factors, which provides a growth advantage for the progression of these cancer cells.

Activation of cyclin D1, a key downstream effector protein in both MAPK and the protein kinase C (PKC)-elicited signal pathway, prompts cells entering S phase during cell cycle. For example, in LNCaP cells, both EGF and TPA (a PKC activator) can induce cyclin D1 in LNCaP cells [62]. Overexpression of cyclin D1 in LNCaP cells results in accelerated cell growth and increased *in vivo* tumorigenicity [63]. However, unlike breast cancer, cyclin D1 gene amplification is relatively rare in PCa cell lines [64]. Using quantitative

RT-PCR and Western analyses, Gumbiner et al. [65] demonstrate that no apparent increased cyclin D1 transcript and protein levels were observed in four prostate tumor cell lines and their xenografts tumors. However, an increased cyclin D1 transcript level was found in a small subset (4 out of 96) of clinical specimens derived from either stage C and D [65]. In another study using immunohistochemistry, cyclin D1 positive tumor (defined as identification of positive immunoreactivity in the nuclei of >20% of tumor cells) is 11% (10 of 86) of the primary cases compared with 68% for AI bone metastatic lesion prostate [66]. These data indicate that cyclin D1 may be involved in the onset of AIPCa.

Cell survival signals in AIPCa

Most mitogenic signals have a dual function involved not only in cell proliferation but also cell survival. For example, inhibition of MAPK activity by either Tyrphostin AG1748 (EGFR inhibitor) or PD98059 (MAPK inhibitor) enhances the G2/M cell cycle arrest and radiation-induced cell killing [67]. In addition, PTEN and the phosphatidylinositol triphosphate kinase (PI3-K) pathway have been implicated in the regulation of G1 growth arrest [68] and the regulation of cell survival. PTEN, a dual phosphatase for both phosphatidylinositol 3,4,5-triphosphate (PIP3) and tyrosine phosphoprotein, is frequently lost or mutated in AIPCa [69–72]. Loss of PTEN expression, mostly due to down-regulation of the gene by DNA hypermethylation, is found in PCa [72]. In the absence of PTEN, PIP3 phosphorylated by PI3-K accumulates in cells and it is an activator for Akt/PKB kinase, which promotes cell survival [73–75].

Recent data indicate that dephosphorylation of phosphoinositol-triphophate (PI3P) and focal adhesion kinase (FAK) by PTEN promotes apoptosis through inactivating the PI3-K/Akt cell survival pathway [74,75]. Also, activation of Akt can prevent TRAIL-induced apoptosis in LNCaP cells [76]. On the other hand, in LNCaP cells, the constitutive activation of PI3-K pathway due to PTEN mutation contributes to cell survival since inhibition of this pathway can cause cell apoptosis [77]. However, some data indicate that the PI3-K inhibitor-induced apoptosis in LNCaP cells can be reversed by activating EGFR and/or the androgen receptor (AR) [78], which suggests that the some pathway(s) parallel with the Akt/PKB pathway in PCa also contributes to cell survival.

Signal pathways involved in the metastasis of PCa

PCa cells have a high propensity to metastasize to bone, at which point AIPCa can arise and becomes a life-threatening disease. Metastasis requires not only cell mobility, but also the interaction between tumor cells and their surrounding environment. Several studies demonstrate that a growth factor and its receptor may be involved in this process. For example, overexpression of EGFR can increase the *in vivo* metastasis potential of DU145 cells [79]. Overexpression of Her-2/neu, a member of EGFR family, can facilitate the metastasis of a nontumorigenic rat prostate NbE cells to skeletal muscle in the rib [80]. Conversely, using EGFR-specific kinase inhibitor (PD153035) can reduce invasiveness of PCa using a transgenic adenocarcinoma mouse prostate (TRAMP) model [81]. These data indicate that the involvement of EGFR signaling in the metastasis of PCa.

The possible underlying mechanism for growth factor(s)-elicited PCa metastasis is due to the induction of cell migration. Rajan et al. [82] report that an EGF-like protein identified from several bone and leukemia cell lines acts as a potent chemoattractant, which increases cell migration of a PCa cell line (TSU-Pr1). This study suggests that the EGF-like molecule attracts PCa to invade or metastasize the peripheral lymph nodes and medullary bone. Concurrently, activation of the MAPK pathway is often associated with metastatic PCa [83,84]. It has been shown that the MAPK inhibitor can suppress the expression of the $\alpha 6$ integrin gene, a critical receptor for the interaction with matrix protein by the metastatic PCa, in both PC3 and LNCaP cells [85].

In LNCaP cells, increasing survival can also increase metastatic potential [86]. Conversely, PTEN can inhibit the PI-3K/Akt pathway by dephosphorylating PIP3, which leads to reduced cell motility [87,88]. Furthermore, PTEN can also inhibit cell migration by directly dephosphorylating FAK [89,90] and SRC homolog and collagen protein (SHC) [91] (Figure 1). The steady-state levels of FAK in three PCa cells (LNCaP, PC3, DU145) correlate with the cell migration capability [92]. Moreover, presence of the dominant negative FAK and inhibitor of SRC (oncogenic protein of Rous Sarcoma virus) protein can significantly inhibit migration of PCa [92], indicating that the involvement of integrin/matrix via SRC/FAK signaling is a key determinant for PCa metastasis. Similarly, overexpression of dominant negative SHC can inhibit

cell migration in a PTEN-negative giloblastoma cell-U-87MG [93].

Cross-talk between steroid hormone and growth factor-elicited signal pathways

Androgen is known as a key mitogen for primary PCa. In an androgen deprived milieu, it is possible that the AR in AIPCa can function through a ligand-independent fashion. Some data indicate that the ligand independent activation of AR could be achieved by mutation occurring in the ligand binding domain of AR and/or by associating with the growth factor-mediated signaling pathway. In AIPCa, AR mutation and amplification have been found in 20–40% of cases [94–96]. Also, increasing evidence indicate that there is interaction between AR and the peptide growth factor receptor signaling pathway. Activation of MAPK and protein kinase A (PKA) pathways can lead to the phosphorylation of AR, which increases its interaction with cofactors such as ARA50 or ARA70 and consequently enhance the transcription activity of AR [97,98]. This is consistent with data showing that the transcription activity of AR in LNCaP cells can be activated by several growth factors (insulin-like growth factor-1 [IGF-1], KGF, and EGF) [99] capable of initiating the MAPK pathway. Also, overexpression of Her-2/neu can induce AR activation through activation of the MAPK phosphorylation cascade [100,101]. Moreover, Sehgal et al. [102] indicate that androgen can induce amphiregulin, a ligand for EGFR, which could activate EGFR-mediated signal transduction. These data clearly indicate that reciprocal interaction between the AR and MAPK-mediated pathways may underlie the AI growth of PCa.

Loss of homeostatic control of the signal pathway in AIPCa

Despite the prevalence of positive signal(s) involved in the relapse of AIPCa, loss of negative feedback control in the signal network also significantly impact the onset of AIPCa. Loss of the tumor suppressor PTEN (Figure 1) has been implicated in proliferation, cell survival, and metastasis of PCa cells. The dual phosphatase activity of PTEN can dephosphorylate PIP3 which is required for activating the PI3-Kinsae/Akt pathway implicated in promoting proliferation and cell survival in PCa [77,78]. PTEN can also suppress cell

220

proliferation, survival, and migration of prostate cells by dephosphorylating tyrosine phosphoprotein such as FAK and SHC [89–91].

Based on animal models and clinical observation, we believe AIPCa possesses similar stem cell properties as the normal prostate gland. To unveil the fundamental changes that occur in AIPCa, we hypothesized that altered homeostatic control machinery, operative in normal prostatic basal cells, underlie the malignant phenotype of AIPCa. Our laboratory has screened cDNAs from the enriched basal cell population of the degenerated prostate gland. A candidate gene has recently been identified as DOC-2/DAB2 (differential-expressed in ovarian cancer-2/disabled 2), which was cloned from differential display as a potential tumor suppressor in ovarian cancer [103]. It encodes an 82 kDa phosphoprotein with a highly conserved sequence between human and rodent, which implies its important biological function. The N-terminal of DOC-2/DAB2 contains a homology domain (i.e. DAB domain) with the *disabled* (SRC-binding protein) gene involved in the differentiation of the neuron [104]. The C-terminal of DOC-2/DAB2 contains three proline-rich domains that can bind to SH3-containing protein [105]. Therefore, DOC-2/DAB2 appears to be a typical molecule involved in the signal network.

In the normal prostate, DOC-2/DAB2 is predominantly associated with basal epithelia cells when the prostate undergoes androgen-deprived degeneration [103]. Decreased expression of DOC-2/DAB2 has been found in several tumors including ovarian, choriocarcinoma, breast, and prostate. We also observed the absence of DOC-2/DAB2 in several PCa cell lines derived from AIPCa patients [103]. Increased expression of DOC-2/DAB2 can suppress cell growth and increase G1/Go growth arrest in a tumorigenic LNCaP subline (C4-20 cell). Similar results were observed in other cancer types [106–108]. In ovarian cancer, reintroducing DOC-2/DAB2 into cancer cells can reduce cell growth, tumorigenicity and suppress the serum induced *c-fos* gene expression [106–109]. These data indicate that DOC-2/DAB2 is a potent tumor suppressor.

The mechanism responsible for the loss of DOC-2/DAB2 in PCa is not fully understood. However, some evidence indicate that the expression of DOC-2/DAB2 is suppressed by the RAS-mediated pathway because DOC-2/DAB2 is down regulated at least 100-fold in RAS-transformed cells and such suppression can be reverted in the presence of MAPK inhibitor PD98059 [110]. Also, the gene transcription

of DOC-2/DAB2 can be modulated by either GATA-6 or retinoic acid during embryonic differentiation [111,112]. Noticeably, retinoic acid treatment can cause apoptosis in PCa cells [113,114]. However, the relationship of DOC-2/DAB2 and retinoic acid-induced apoptosis in PCa remains undetermined. Moreover, our data also demonstrate that DOC-2/DAB2 is induced during TPA-induced megakarocyte differentiation of K562 cells [115]. Based on these findings, we believe that the regulation DOC-2/DAB2 gene is associated with cell differentiation in several cell types including prostatic epithelia.

To examine the role of DOC-2/DAB2 in modulating signal transduction which may impact the phenotype of AIPCa cells, we first demonstrated that the presence of DOC-2/DAB2 is able to inhibit TPA-induced gene expression [116]. Moreover, DOC-2/DAB2 (Figure 1) can be rapidly phosphorylated by treatment of growth factor and TPA [116]. Therefore, we examined the impact of DOC-2/DAB2 phosphorylation on the effect of TPA in PCa cell lines such as LNCaP cells. It appears that the serine 24 in the N-terminal of DOC-2/DAB2 is the key phosphoamino acid residue in modulating PKC-elicited signal pathway, since the alteration of this residue abolishes the activity of AP-1 induced by TPA [115].

Recently, we identified a novel RAS-GTPase-activating protein (RAS-GAP) as a DOC-2/DAB2 interactive protein (DIP1/2) [117]. The human DIP1/2 gene locates at 9q33.1–33.3 [118] proximal to a potential tumor suppressor gene, TSC1 (Tuberous Sclerosis) [119]. It has also been reported [120] that a novel RAS-GAP gene fused to a myeloid/lymphoid leukemia gene in acute myeloid leukemia with chromosomal translocation [t(9;11)(q34; q23)]; DIP1/2 may be that candidate gene.

Using detailed biochemical analyses, we demonstrated that DIP1/2 is a typical RAS-GAP that hydrolyzes RAS-GTP (active RAS) to become RAS-GDP (inactive RAS). We further demonstrated that the interaction between DOC-2/DAB2 and DIP1/2 enhance the GAP activity in PCa cells (Figure 1), and, decreased expression of DIP1/2 is associated with several PCa cell lines derived from AIPCa patients. Apparently, one of the mechanisms of action of DOC-2/DAB2/DIP1/2 is to modulate RAS activity in AIPCa. In addition, the DAB domain of DOC-2/DAB2 directly associates with Smad and mad-related protein 2 and 3 (Smad2 and Smad3), which restores the transforming growth factor-β (TGF-β) signaling pathway in TGF-β mutant cells [121]. Thus, DOC-2/DAB2 appears to have multiple mechanisms of action that modulate the growth/differentiation of mammalian cells.

As shown previously, DOC-2/DAB2 interacts with GRB2 in mouse macrophage treated with colony stimulating factor-1 [105]. We further analyzed the functional role of the C-terminal of DOC-2/DAB2, particularly the proline rich domain, in growth factor-elicited signal transduction. In PCa, the expression of DOC-2/DAB2 prevents the SOS from binding GRB2 (Figure 1), which leads to the suppression of MAPK activation initiated by EGF [122]. Similar action of DOC-2/DAB2 is also observed in PC12 cells stimulated with neurotropin NT3 [122], suggesting that DOC-2/DAB2 is involved in the growth/differentiation of neuronal cells. Moreover, our preliminary data indicated that some other SH3-containing proteins such as SRC and NCK can interact with the DOC-2/DAB2 (Figure 1). The biologic implication of this interaction warrants further investigation. Nevertheless, the DOC-2/DAB2 complex represents a unique negative feedback machinery for balancing the signaling cascade elicited by exogenous stimuli. Altered expression of this complex underlies the onset of AIPCa.

Concluding remarks

Relapse of AIPCa signifies that PCa has become autonomous after androgen deprivation; the presence of peptide growth factors or cytokines becomes a prevalent mitogen for AIPCa. However, it is clear that these exogenous stimuli elicit various signal networks critical for cell proliferation, survival, and metastasis. Among these pathways, increased MAPK activation appears to predominate in the AIPCa cells. This is evidenced by several molecular markers such as RAS, ERK, and cyclin D1. Overwhelming *in vitro* and *in vivo* data demonstrate this relationship. Moreover, recent data also indicate the MAPK and AR pathways have a reciprocal interaction, which underlies the mechanism for the AI progression. Nevertheless, unlike other cancer types, the mutation rate of these key effectors (such as *Ras* and *cyclin D1*) is relatively low in PCa. Therefore, it is likely that other regulatory pathways such as the negative feedback mechanism are impaired in the PCa cells.

Several molecules were identified as a part of a negative regulatory network. PTEN is an excellent example of such a molecule because, (a) decreased or frequent loss of PTEN expression is found in PCa, and (b) loss of PTEN is known to increase the cell survival of PCa through the PI-3K/Akt pathway or through cell migration/metastasis through the SRC or FAK pathway. In addition, our laboratory identified a unique complex (DOC-2/DAB2/DIP1/2) that modulates the RAS and TGF-β mediated pathway. Since this complex can associate with many other effectors, it is possible to predict the potential impact of this complex on the progression of AIPCa.

The ultimate goal in studying the signal network in AIPCa is to identify marker(s) for early prognosis of AI disease and to develop specific agent(s) for disease intervention. Recent clinical approval of the c-ABL tyrosine kinase inhibitor (STI-571, Gleevec) marks the beginning of target-specific cancer therapy. In addition to the completion of the human genome project, in the foreseeable future, cancer therapy could be customized based upon an individual patient's genetic profile. Therefore, profiling signal transduction targets in AIPCa has tremendous clinical application.

Key unanswered questions

1. It appears that AIPCa contains a heterogeneous cell population. What are the critical signal networks operative in AIPCa cells?
2. AIPCa has a high propensity to grow in bone. What are the critical signal networks responsible for the interaction between these cells?
3. There is a significant overlapping in the signal cascade-elicited by many biologic responses. Are there key merging points in AIPCa?
4. What is the impact of different nerve growth factors on the progression of AIPCa?
5. It appears that a close interaction exists between AR and MAPK pathways. Can DOC-2/DAB2 complex modulate the AR-mediated signal transduction?
6. The presence of negative regulator is to prevent the constitutive activation of positive signal cascade elicited by stimuli. Therefore, what is the mechanism resulting in the association between these proteins immediately after the initial activation?
7. Loss of DOC-2/DAB2 expression is often found in AIPCa. What is the underlying mechanism(s) leading to the loss of DOC-2/DAB2 expression?
8. The underlying mechanism of negative feedback pathways is somewhat similar. Can these negative feedback pathways complement each other in AIPCa?

222

Acknowledgements

This work is supported by a grant from the National Institute of Health (DK 4765707). We also thank Andrew Webb for editing the manuscript.

References

1. Lipsett B: Interaction of drugs, hormones and nutrition in the causes of cancer. Cancer 43: 1967–1981, 1979
2. Wagenseil F: Chinesische eunuchen. Zeitschrift für Morphologie und Anthropologie 32: 416–468, 1933
3. Hamilton JB, Mestler GE: Mortality and survival: Comparison of eunuchs with intact men and women in a mentally retarded population. J Gerontol 24: 395–411, 1969
4. Noble RL: The development of prostatic adenocarcinoma in NB rats following prolonged sex hormone administration. Cancer Res 37: 1929–1933, 1977
5. Pollard M, Luckert PH: Production of autochtoneous prostate cancer in Lobound-Wistar rats by treatment with N-nitroso-N-methylurea and testosterone. JNCI 77: 583–587, 1986
6. Huggins C, Hodges CV: Studies on prostatic cancer I. The effect of castration of estrogen and of androgen injection on serum phosphatase in metastatic carcinoma of the prostate. Cancer Res 1: 293–297, 1941
7. Bruchovsky N, Rennie PS, Coldman AJ, Goldenberg SL, To M, Lawson D: The effects of androgen withdrawal on the stem cell composition of Shionogi carcinoma. Cancer Res 50: 2275–2282, 1990
8. Bonkohoff H, Remberger K: Differentiation pathways and histogenetic aspects of normal and abnormal prostatic growth: A stem cell model. Prostate 28: 98–106, 1996
9. Issacs JT, Coffey DS: Etiology and disease process of benign prostatic hyperplasia. Prostate, 2(Suppl): 33–50, 1989
10. Coffey DS, Walsh PC: Clinical and experimental studies of benign prostatic hyperplasia. Urol Clin North Am 17: 461–475, 1990
11. English HF, Santen RJ, Isaacs JT: Response of glandular versus basal rat ventral prostate. Prostate 11: 229–242, 1987
12. Mckeehan WL, Adams PS, Rosser MP: Direct mitogenic effects of insulin, epidermal growth factor and possibly prolactin, but not androgen, on normal rat prostate epithelial cells in serum-free primary cell culture. Cancer Res 44: 1998–2010, 1984
13. Peehl DM, Wong S, Bazinet M, Stamey TA: *In vitro* studies of human prostate epithelial cells. Growth Factors 1: 237–250, 1989
14. Gregory J, Willshire IR, Kavanagh JP, Blacklock NJ, Chowdury S, Richards RC: Urogastrone-epidermal growth factor concentration in prostatic fluid of normal individuals and patients with benign prostatic hypertrophy. Clin Sci 70: 359–363, 1986
15. Putz T, Cuilig Z, Eder IE, Nassler-Menardi C, Bartsch G, Grunicke H, Uberall F, Klocker H: Epidermal growth factor (EGF) receptor blockade inhibits the action of EGF, insulin-like growth factor I, and a protein kinase A activator on the mitogen-activated protein kinase pathway in prostate cancer cell lines. Cancer Res 59: 227–233, 1999
16. Cohen DW, Simak R, Fair WR, Melded J, Scher HI, Cordon-Cardo C: Expression of transforming growth factor-α and the epidermal growth factor receptor in human prostate tissue. J Urol 152: 2120–2124, 1994
17. Maygarden SJ, Novotny DB, Moul JW, Bae VL, Ware JL: Evaluation of cathepsin D and epidermal growth factor receptor in prostate carcinoma. Mod Pathol 7: 930–936, 1994
18. Scher HI, Sarkis A, Reuter V, Cohen D, Netto G, Petrylak D, Lianes P, Fuks Z, Mendelsohn J, Cordon-Cardo C: Changing pattern of expression of the epidermal growth factor receptor and transforming growth factor-α in the progression of prostatic neoplasms. Clin Cancer Res 1: 545–550, 1995
19. Connolly JM, Rose DP: Production of epidermal growth factor and transforming growth factor-α by the androgen-responsive LNCaP human prostate cancer cell line. Prostate 16: 209–218, 1990
20. Fong CJ, Sherwood ER, Mendelsohn J, Lee C, Kozlowski JM: Epidermal growth factor receptor monoclonal antibody inhibits constitutive receptor phosphorylation, reduces autonomous growth, and sensitizes androgen-independent prostatic carcinoma cells to tumor necrosis factor α. Cancer Res 52: 5887–5892, 1992
21. Connolly JM, Rose DP: Secretion of epidermal growth factor and related polypeptides by the Du145 human prostate cell line. Prostate 15: 177–186, 1989
22. MacDonald A, Habib FK: Divergent responses to epidermal growth factor in hormone sensitive and insensitive human prostate cancer cell lines. Br J Cancer 65: 177–182, 1992
23. Yan G, Fukabori Y, Mcbride G, Nikolaropolous S, McKeehan WL: Exon switching and activation of stromal and embryonic fibroblast growth factor (FGF)-FGF receptor genes in prostate epithelial cells accompany stromal independence and malignancy. Mol Cell Biol 13: 4513–4522, 1993
24. Carstens RP, Eaton JV, Krigman HR, Walther PJ, Garcia-Blanco MA: Alternative splicing of fibroblast growth factor receptor 2 (FGF-R2) in human prostate cancer. Oncogene 15: 3059–3065, 1997
25. Kwabi-Addo B, Ropiquet F, Giri D, Ittmann M: Alternative splicing of fibroblast growth factor receptors in human prostate cancer. Prostate 46: 163–172, 2001
26. Gleave M, Hsieh JT, Gao CA, von Eschenbach AC, Chung LW: Acceleration of human prostate cancer growth *in vivo* by factors produced by prostate and bone fibroblasts. Cancer Res 51: 3753–3761, 1991
27. Nakamoto T, Chang CS, Li AK, Chodak GW: Basic fibroblast growth factor in human prostate cancer cells. Cancer Res 52:571–577, 1992
28. Sato N, Watabe Y, Suzuki H, Shimazaki J: Progression of androgen-sensitive mouse tumor

(Shionogi cancinoma 115) to androgen-insensitive tumor after long-term removal of testosterone. Jpn J Cancer Res 84: 1300–1308, 1993

29. Pflug B, Djakiew D: Expression of p75NTR in a human prostate epithelial tumor cell line reduces nerve growth factor-induced cell growth by activation of programmed cell death. Mol Carcinog 23: 106–114, 1998

30. Angelsen A, Sandvik AK, Syversen U, Stridsberg M, Waldum HL: NGF-β, NE-cells and prostatic cancer cell lines. A study of neuroendocrine expression in the human prostatic cancer cell lines DU-145, PC-3, LNCaP, and TSU-pr1 following stimulation of the nerve growth factor-β. Scand J Urol Nephrol 32: 7–13, 1998

31. Dalal R, Djakiew D: Molecular characterization of neurotrophin expression and the corresponding tropomyosin receptor kinases (trks) in epithelial and stromal cells of the human prostate. Mol Cell Endocrinol 134: 15–22, 1997

32. Delsite R, Djakiew D: Characterization of nerve growth factor precursor protein expression by human prostate stromal cells: A role in selective neurotrophin stimulation of prostate epithelial cell growth. Prostate 41: 39–48, 1999

33. Djakiew D, Delsite R, Pflug B, Wrathall J, Lynch JH, Onoda M: Regulation of growth by a nerve growth factor-like protein which modulates paracrine interactions between a neoplastic epithelial cell line and stromal cells of the human prostate. Cancer Res 51: 3304–3310, 1991

34. Schlessinger J: SH2/SH3 signaling proteins. Curr Opin Genet Dev 4: 25–30, 1994

35. Seger R, Kreb EG: The MAPK siganling cascade. FASEB J 9: 726–735, 1995

36. Post GR, Brown JH: G protein-coupled receptors and signaling pathways regulating growth responses. FASEB J 10: 741–749, 1996

37. Bredel M, Pollack IF: The p21-Ras signal trnasduction pathway and growth regulation in human high-grade glioma. Brain Res Brain Res Rev 29: 232–249, 1999

38. Barbacid M: Ras genes. Annu Rev Biochem 56: 779–827, 1987

39. Nakazawa H, Aguelon AM, Yamasaki H: Identification and quantification of a carcinogen-induced molecular initiation event in cell transformation. Oncogene 7: 2295–2301, 1992

40. Bos JL: Ras oncogenes in human cancer: Review. Cancer Res 49: 4682–4689, 1989

41. Viola MV, Fromowitz F, Oravez S, Deb S, Finkel G, Lundy J, Hand P, Thor A, Schlom J: Expression of ras oncogene p21 in prostate cancer. N Engl J Med 314: 133–137, 1986

42. Sumiya H, Masai M, Akimoto S, Yatani R, Shimazaki J: Histochemical examination of expression of ras p21 protein and R 1881-binding protein in human prostatic cancers. Eur J Cancer 26: 786–789, 1990

43. Carter BS, Epstein JI, Isaacs WB: Ras gene mutation in human prostate cancer. Cancer Res 50: 6830–6832, 1990

44. Pergolizzi RG, Kreis W, Rottach C, Susin M, Broome JD: Mutational status of codons 12 and 13 of the N- and K-ras genes in tissue and cell lines derived from primary and metastatic prostate carcinomas. Cancer Invest 11: 25–32, 1993

45. Voeller HJ, Wilding G, Gelmann EP: v-rasH expression confers hormone-independent *in vitro* growth to LNCaP prostate carcinoma cells. Mol Endocrinol 5: 209–216, 1991

46. Fribourg AF, Knudsen KE, Strobeck MW, Lindhorst CM, Knudsen ES: Differential requirements for ras and the retinoblastoma tumor suppressor protein in the androgen dependence of prostatic adenocarcinoma cells. Cell Growth Differ 11: 361–372, 2000

47. Sirotnak FM, Sepp-Lorenzino L, Kohl NE, Rosen N, Scher HI: A peptidomimetic inhibitor of ras functionality markedly suppresses growth of human prostate tumor xenografts in mice. Prospects for long-term clinical utility. Cancer Chemother Pharmacol 46: 79–83, 2000

48. Gumerlock PH, Poonamallee UR, Meyers FJ, deVere White RW: Activated ras alleles in human carcinoma of the prostate are rare. Cancer Res 51: 1632–1637, 1991

49. Moul JW, Friedrichs PA, Lance RS, Theune SM, Chang EH: Infrequent RAS oncogene mutations in human prostate cancer. Prostate 20: 327–338, 1992

50. Ozen M, Pathak S: Genetic alterations in human prostate cancer: A review of current literature. Anticancer Res 20: 1905–1912, 2000

51. Lau QC, Brusselbach S, Muller R: Abrogation of c-Raf expression induces apoptosis in tumor cells. Oncogene 16: 1899–1902, 1998

52. Geiger T, Muller M, Monia BP, Fabbro D: Antitumor activity of a C-raf antisense oligonucleotide in combination with standard chemotherapeutic agents against various human tumors transplanted subcutaneously into nude mice. Clin Cancer Res 3: 1179–1185, 1997

53. Ravi RK, McMahon M, Yangang Z, Williams JR, Dillehay LE, Nelkin BD, Mabry M: Raf-1-induced cell cycle arrest in LNCaP human prostate cancer cells. J Cell Biochem 72: 458–469, 1999

54. Gschwend JE, Fair WR, Powell CT: Bryostatin 1 induces prolonged activation of extracellular regulated protein kinases in and apoptosis of LNCaP human prostate cancer cells overexpressing protein kinase c-α. Mol Pharmacol 57: 1224–1234, 2000

55. Cowley S, Paterson H, Kemp P, Marshall CJ: Activation of MAP kinase kinase is necessary and sufficient for PC12 differentiation and for transformation of NIH 3T3 cells. Cell 77: 841–852, 1994

56. Mansour SJ, Matten WT, Hermann AS, Candia JM, Rong S, Fukasawa K, Vande Woude GF, Ahn NG: Transformation of mammalian cells by constitutively active MAP kinase kinase. Science 265: 966–970, 1994

57. Magi-Galluzzi C, Mishra R, Fiorentino M, Montironi R, Yao H, Capodieci P, Wishnow K, Kaplan I, Stork PJ, Loda M: Mitogen-activated protein kinase phosphatase 1 is overexpressed in prostate cancers and is inversely related to apoptosis. Lab Invest 76: 37–51, 1997

58. Oka H, Chatani, Hoshino R, Ogawa O, Kakehi Y, Terachi T, Okada Y, Kawaichi M, Kohno M, Yoshida O: Constitutive activation of mitogen-activated protein (MAP) kinases in human renal cell carcinoma. Cancer Res 55: 4182–4187, 1995

59. Gioeli D, Mandell JW, Petroni GR, Frierson HF Jr, Weber MJ: Activation of mitogen-activated protein kinase

224

associated with prostate cancer progression. Cancer Res 59: 279–284, 1999

60. Sebolt-Leopold JS: Development of anticancer drugs targeting the MAP kinase pathway. Oncogene 19: 6594–6599, 2000

61. Sharma Y, Agarwal C, Singh AK, Agarwal R: Inhibitory effect of silibinin on ligand binding to erbB1 and associated mitogenic signaling, growth, and DNA synthesis in advanced human prostate carcinoma cells. Mol Carcinog 30: 224–236, 2001

62. Perry JE, Grossmann ME, Tindall DJ: Epidermal growth factor induces cyclin D1 in a human prostate cancer cell line. Prostate 35: 117–124, 1998

63. Chen Y, Martinez LA, LaCava M, Coghlan L, Conti CJ: Increased cell growth and tumorigenicity in human prostate LNCaP cells by overexpression to cyclin D1. Oncogene 16: 1913–1920, 1998

64. Han EK, Lim JT, Arber N, Rubin MA, Xing WQ, Weinstein IB: Cyclin D1 expression in human prostate carcinoma cell lines and primary tumors. Prostate 35: 95–101, 1998

65. Gumbiner LM, Gumerlock PH, Mack PC, Chi SG, deVere White RW, Mohler JL, Pretlow TG, Tricoli JV: Overexpression of cyclin D1 is rare in human prostate carcinoma. Prostate 38: 40–45, 1999

66. Drobnjak M, Osman I, Scher HI, Fazzari M, Cordon-Cardo C: Overexpression of cyclin D1 is associated with metastatic prostate cancer to bone. Clin Cancer Res 6: 1891–1895, 2000

67. Hagan M, Wang L, Hanley JR, Park JS, Dent P: Ionizing radiation-induced mitogen-activated protein (MAP) kinase activation in DU145 prostate carcinoma cells: MAP kinase inhibition enhances radiation-induced cell killing and G2/M-phase arrest. Radiat Res 153: 371–383, 2000

68. Ramaswamy S, Nakamura N, Vazquez F, Batt DB, Perera S, Roberts TM, Sellers WR: Regulation of G1 progression by the PTEN tumor suppressor protein is linked to inhibition of the phosphatidylinositol 3-kinase/Akt pathway. Proc Natl Acad Sci USA 96: 2110–2115, 1999

69. Li J, Yen C, Liaw D, Podsypanina K, Bose S, Wang SI, Puc J, Miliaresis C, Rodgers L, McCombie R, Bigner SH, Giovanella BC, Ittmann M, Tycko B, Hibshoosh H, Wigler MH, Parsons R: PTEN, a putative protein tyrosine phosphatase gene mutated in human brain, breast, and prostate cancer. Science 275: 1943–1947, 1997

70. Steck PA, Lin H, Langford LA, Jasser SA, Koul D, Yung WK, Pershouse MA: Functional and molecular analyses of 10q deletions in human gliomas. Genes Chromosomes Cancer 24: 135–143, 1999

71. Vlietstra RJ, van Alewijk DC, Hermans KG, van Steenbrugge GJ, Trapman J: Frequent inactivation of PTEN in prostate cancer cell lines and xenografts. Cancer Res 58: 2720–2723, 1998

72. Whang YE, Wu X, Suzuki H, Reiter RE, Tran C, Vessella RL, Said JW, Isaacs WB, Sawyers CL: Inactivation of the tumor suppressor PTEN/MMAC1 in advanced human prostate cancer through loss of expression. Proc Natl Acad Sci USA 95: 5246–5250, 1998

73. Stambolic V, Suzuki A, de la Pompa JL, Brothers GM, Mirtsos C, Sasaki T, Ruland J, Penninger JM, Siderovski DP, Mak TW: Negative regulation of PKB/Akt-dependent cell survival by the tumor suppressor PTEN. Cell 95: 29–39, 1998

74. Wu X, Senechal K, Neshat MS, Whang YE, Sawyers CL: The PTEN/MMAC1 tumor suppressor phosphatase functions as a negative regulator of the phosphoinositide 3-kinase/Akt pathway. Proc Natl Acad Sci USA 95: 15587–15591, 1998

75. Tamura M, Gu J, Danen EH, Takino T, Miyamoto S, Yamada KM: PTEN interactions with focal adhesion kinase and suppression of the extracellular matrix-dependent phosphatidylinositol 3-kinase/Akt cell survival pathway. J Biol Chem 274: 20693–20703, 1999

76. Nesterov A, Lu X, Johnson M, Miller GJ, Ivashchenko Y, Kraft AS: Elevated AKT activity protects the prostate cancer cell line LNCaP from TRAIL-induced apoptosis. J Biol Chem 276: 10767–10774, 2001

77. Lin J, Adam RM, Santiestevan E, Freeman MR: The phosphatidylinositol 3′-kinase pathway is a dominant growth factor-activated cell survival pathway in LNCaP human prostate carcinoma cells. Cancer Res 59: 2891–2897, 1999

78. Carson JP, Kulik G, Weber MJ: Antiapoptotic signaling in LNCaP prostate cancer cells: A survival signaling pathway independent of phosphatidylinositol 3′-kinase and Akt/protein kinase B. Cancer Res 59: 1449–1453, 1999

79. Turner T, Chen P, Goodly LJ, Wells A: EGF receptor signaling enhances in vivo invasiveness of DU-145 human prostate carcinoma cells. Clin Exp Metastasis 14: 409–418, 1996

80. Marengo SR, Sikes RA, Anezinis P, Chang SM, Chung LW: Metastasis induced by overexpression of p185neu-T after orthotopic injection into a prostatic epithelial cell line (NbE). Mol Carcinog 19: 165–175, 1997

81. Kassis J, Moellinger J, Lo H, Greenberg NM, Kim HG, Wells A: A role for phospholipase C-γ-mediated signaling in tumor cell invasion. Clin Cancer Res 5: 2251–2260, 1999

82. Rajan R, Vanderslice R, Kapur S, Lynch J, Thompson R, Djakiew D: Epidermal growth factor (EGF) promotes chemomigration of a human prostate tumor cell line, and EGF immunoreactive proteins are present at sites of metastasis in the stroma of lymph nodes and medullary bone. Prostate 28: 1–9, 1996

83. Krueger JS, Keshamouni VG, Atanaskova N, Reddy KB: Temporal and quantitative regulation of mitogen-activated protein kinase (MAPK) modulates cell motility and invasion. Oncogene 20: 4209–4218, 2001

84. Turner CE: Paxillin interactions. J Cell Sci 23: 4139–4140, 2000

85. Onishi T, Yamakawa K, Franco OE, Kawamura J, Watanabe M, Shiraishi T, Kitazawa S: Mitogen-activated protein kinase pathway is involved in α6 integrin gene expression in androgen-independent prostate cancer cells: role of proximal Sp1 consensus sequence. Biochim Biophy Acta 1538: 218–227, 2001

86. McConkey DJ, Greene G, Pettaway CA: Apoptosis resistance increases with metastatic potential in cells of the

human LNCaP prostate carcinoma line. Cancer Res 56: 5594–5599, 1996

87. Maehama T, Dixon JE: The tumor suppressor, PTEN/MMAC1, dephosphorylates the lipid second messenger, phosphatidylinositol 3,4,5-trisphosphate. J Biol Chem 273: 13375–13378, 1998

88. Morimoto AM, Tomlinson MG, Nakatani K, Bolen JB, Roth RA, Herbst R: The MMAC1 tumor suppressor phosphatase inhibits phospholipase C and integrin-linked kinase activity. Oncogene 19: 200–209, 2000

89. Tamura M, Gu J, Matsumoto K, Aota S, Parsons R, Yamada KM: Inhibition of cell migration, spreading, and focal adhesions by tumor suppressor PTEN. Science 280: 1614–1617, 1998

90. Tamura M, Gu J, Takino T, Yamada KM: Tumor suppressor PTEN inhibition of cell invasion, migration, and growth: Differential involvement of focal adhesion kinase and p130Cas. Cancer Res 59: 442–449, 1999

91. Gu J, Tamura M, Pankov R, Danen EH, Takino T, Matsumoto K, Yamada KM: Shc and FAK differentially regulate cell motility and directionality modulated by PTEN. J Cell Biol 146: 389–403, 1999

92. Slack JK, Adams RB, Rovin JD, Bissonette EA, Stoker CE, Parsons JT: Alterations in the focal adhesion kinase/Src signal transduction pathway correlate with increased migratory capacity of prostate carcinoma cells. Oncogene 20: 1152–1163, 2001

93. Gu J, Tamura M, Yamada KM: Tumor suppressor PTEN inhibits integrin- and growth factor-mediated mitogen-activated protein (MAP) kinase signaling pathways. J Cell Biol 143: 1375–1383, 1998

94. Gaddipati JP, McLeod DG, Heidenberg HB, Sesterhenn IA, Finger MJ, Moul JW, Srivastava S: Frequent detection of codon 877 mutation in the androgen receptor gene in advanced prostate cancers. Cancer Res 54: 2861–2864, 1994

95. Taplin ME, Bubley GJ, Shuster TD, Frantz ME, Spooner AE, Ogata GK, Keer HN, Balk SP: Mutation of the androgen-receptor gene in metastatic androgen-independent prostate cancer. N Engl J Med 332: 1393–1398, 1995

96. Visakorpi T, Hyytinen E, Koivisto P, Tanner M, Keinanen R, Palmberg C, Palotie A, Tammela T, Isola J, Kallioniemi OP: In vivo amplification of the androgen receptor gene and progression of human prostate cancer. Nat Genet 9: 401–406, 1995

97. Abreu-Martin MT, Chari A, Palladino AA, Craft NA, Sawyers CL: Mitogen-activated protein kinase kinase kinase 1 activates androgen receptor-dependent transcription and apoptosis in prostate cancer. Mol Cell Biol 19: 5143–5154, 1999

98. Chen T, Cho RW, Stork PJ, Weber MJ: Elevation of cyclic adenosine 3′,5′-monophosphate potentiates activation of mitogen-activated protein kinase by growth factors in LNCaP prostate cancer cells. Cancer Res 59: 213–218, 1999

99. Culig Z, Hobisch A, Cronauer MV, Radmayr C, Trapman J, Hittmair A, Bartsch G, Klocker H: Androgen receptor activation in prostatic tumor cell lines by insulin-like growth factor-I, keratinocyte growth factor, and epidermal growth factor. Cancer Res 54: 5474–5478, 1994

100. Craft N, Shostak Y, Carey M, Sawyers CL: A mechanism for hormone-independent prostate cancer through modulation of androgen receptor signaling by the HER-2/neu tyrosine kinase. Nat Med 5: 280–285, 1999

101. Yeh S, Lin HK, Kang HY, Thin TH, Lin MF, Chang C: From HER2/Neu signal cascade to androgen receptor and its coactivators: A novel pathway by induction of androgen target genes through MAP kinase in prostate cancer cells. Proc Natl Acad Sci USA 96: 5458–5463, 1999

102. Sehgal I, Bailey J, Hitzemann K, Pittelkow MR, Maihle NJ: Epidermal growth factor receptor-dependent stimulation of amphiregulin expression in androgen-stimulated human prostate cancer cells. Mol Biol Cell 5: 339–347, 1994

103. Tseng CP, Ely BD, Li Y, Pong RC, Hsieh JT: Regulation of rat DOC-2 gene during castration-induced rat ventral prostate degeneration and its growth inhibitory function in human prostatic carcinoma cells. Endocrinology 139: 3542–3553, 1998

104. Howell BW, Gertler FB, Cooper JA: Mouse disabled (mDab1): A Src binding protein implicated in neuronal development. EMBO J 16: 121–132, 1997

105. Xu XX, Yi T, Tang B, Lambeth JD: Disabled-2 (Dab2) is an SH3 domain-binding partner of Grb2. Oncogene 16: 1561–1569, 1998

106. Mok SC, Chan WY, Wong KK, Cheung KK, Lau CC, Ng SW, Baldini A, Colitti CV, Rock CO, Berkowitz RS: DOC-2, a candidate tumor suppressor gene in human epithelial ovarian cancer. Oncogene 16: 2381–2387, 1998

107. Fulop V, Colitti CV, Genest D, Berkowitz RS, Yiu GK, Ng SW, Szepesi J, Mok SC: DOC-2/hDab2, a candidate tumor suppressor gene involved in the development of gestational trophoblastic diseases. Oncogene 17: 419–424, 1998

108. Fazili Z, Sun W, Mittelstaedt S, Cohen C, Xu XX: Disabled-2 inactivation is an early step in ovarian tumorigenicity. Oncogene 18: 3104–3113, 1999

109. He J, Smith ER, Xu XX: Disabled-2 exerts its tumor suppressor activity by uncoupling c-Fos expression and MAP kinase activation. J Biol Chem 276: 26814–26818, 2001

110. Zuber J, Tchernitsa OI, Hinzmann B, Schmitz AC, Grips M, Hellriegel M, Sers C, Rosenthal A, Schafer R: A genome-wide survey of RAS transformation targets. Nat Genet 24: 144–1452, 2000

111. Morrisey EE, Musco S, Chen MY, Lu MM, Leiden JM, Parmacek MS: The gene encoding the mitogen-responsive phosphoprotein Dab2 is differentially regulated by GATA-6 and GATA-4 in the visceral endoderm. J Biol Chem 275: 19949–19954, 2000

112. Cho SY, Cho SY, Lee SH, Park SS: Differential expression of mouse Disabled 2 gene in retinoic acid-treated F9 embryonal carcinoma cells and early mouse embryos. Mol Cells 9: 179–184, 1999

113. Lu XP, Fanjul A, Picard N, Shroot B, Pfahl M: A selective retinoid with high activity against an androgen-resistant prostate cancer cell type. Int J Cancer 80: 272–278, 1999

114. Liang JY, Fontana JA, Rao JN, Ordonez JV, Dawson MI, Shroot B, Wilber JF, Feng P: Synthetic retinoid CD437

226

induces S-phase arrest and apoptosis in human prostate cancer cells LNCaP and PC-3. Prostate 38: 228–236, 1999

115. Tseng CP, Huang CH, Tseng CC, Lin MH, Hsieh JT, Tseng CH: Induction of disabled-2 gene during megakaryocyte differentiation of k562 cells. Biochem Biophys Res Commun 285: 129–135, 2001

116. Tseng CP, Ely BD, Pong RC, Wang Z, Zhou J, Hsieh JT: The role of DOC-2/DAB2 protein phosphorylation in the inhibition of AP-1 activity. An underlying mechanism of its tumor-suppressive function in prostate cancer. J Biol Chem 274: 31981–31986, 1999

117. Wang Z, Tseng CP, Pong RC, McConnell JD, Hsieh JT: A Novel RasGTPase activating protein that interacts with DOC-2/DAB2: A downstream effector leading to the suppression of prostate cancer. J Biol Chem (submitted), 2001

118. Chen H, Pong RC, Wang Z, Hsieh JT: Differential regulation of the human DIP1/2 gene in normal and malignant prostatic epithelia: Cloning and characterization of the DIP1/2 gene. Genomics (submittted), 2001

119. van Slegtenhorst M, de Hoogt R, Hermans C, Nellist M, Janssen B, Verhoef S, Lindhout D, van den Ouweland A, Halley D, Young J, Burley M, Jeremiah S, Woodward K, Nahmias J, Fox M, Ekong R, Osborne J, Wolfe J, Povey S, Snell RG, Cheadle JP, Jones AC, Tachataki M, Ravine D, Kwiatkowski DJ: Identification of the tuberous sclerosis gene TSC1 on chromosome 9q34. Science 277: 805–808, 1997

120. Genbank accession # AY032952.

121. Hocevar BA, Smine A, Xu XX, Howe PH: The adaptor molecule Disabled-2 links the transforming growth factor β receptors to the Smad pathway. EMBO J 20: 2789–2801, 2001

122. Zhou J, Hsieh JT: The inhibitory role of DOC-2/DAB2 in growth factor receptor-mediated signal cascade. DOC-2/DAB2-mediated inhibition of ERK phosphorylation via binding to Grb2. J Biol Chem 276: 27793–27798, 2001

Address for offprints: JT Hsieh, Department of Urology, University of Texas Southwestern Medical Center, 5323 Harry Hines Boulevard, Dallas, TX 75390-9110, USA; *Tel:* 214-648-3988; *Fax:* 214-648-8786; *e-mail:* jt.hsieh@utsouthwestern.edu

The diet, prostate inflammation, and the development of prostate cancer

William G. Nelson, Theodore L. DeWeese and Angelo M. DeMarzo
The Sidney Kimmel Cancer Center at Johns Hopkins, Baltimore, MD, USA

Key words: prostate cancer, glutathione *S*-transferases, proliferative inflammatory atrophy, oxidative stress

Summary

Evidence that somatic inactivation of *GSTP1*, encoding the human π-class glutathione *S*-transferase, may initiate prostatic carcinogenesis is reviewed along with epidemiological evidence implicating several environment and lifestyle factors, including the diet and sexually transmitted diseases, as prostate cancer risk factors. An integrated model is presented featuring *GSTP1* function as a 'caretaker' gene during the pathogenesis of prostate cancer, in which the early loss of GSTP1 activity renders prostate cells vulnerable to genome damage associated with chronic prostatic inflammation and repeated exposure to carcinogens. The model predicts that the critical prostate carcinogens will be those that are substrates for GSTP1 detoxification and are associated with high prostate cancer risk diet and lifestyle habits.

Both genetic and environmental factors likely contribute to the pathogenesis of human prostate cancer. In support of a role for inheritance in the development of prostate cancer, familial clusters of the disease have been reported, and segregation analyses have suggested that prostate cancer in some of these families is likely attributable to inheritance of prostate cancer susceptibility genes [1–3]. Over the past few years, a number of genetic loci have been identified that have been postulated to be responsible for inherited susceptibility to prostate cancer [4–17]. How do such genes lead to prostate cancer development? Until the suspected genes have been identified and characterized, the manner by which the genes increase prostate cancer risk will remain to be established. Nevertheless, in a recent study of cancer risks among 44,788 pairs of twins in Sweden, Denmark, and Finland [18], a statistically significant effect of genotype was observed only for some 42% of prostate cancer cases (with a 95% confidence interval of 29–50%), indicating that environment and lifestyle likely play a more dominant role than inheritance in the development of most prostate cancers.

A dominant role for environment and lifestyle in the development of life-threatening prostate cancer is further supported by ecological epidemiology data [19]. Prostate cancer incidence and mortality are well-known to vary greatly in different geographic regions of the world, with low risks of prostate cancer mortality characteristic of Asia and high risks of prostate cancer mortality characteristic of the US and Western Europe [19,20]. In addition, Asian immigrants to the US tend to adopt higher prostate cancer risks, strong evidence that the environment and lifestyle may be the major cause of life-threatening prostate cancer in the US [21,22]. How do the environment and lifestyle promote prostatic carcinogenesis? Insights into the earliest steps in the molecular pathogenesis of human prostate cancer have begun to provide a clue: prostate cancer development appears to be initiated by somatic inactivation of *GSTP1*, encoding the human π-class glutathione *S*-transferase [23–26]. Cancer cell DNA typically contains many somatic alterations, including mutations, deletions, amplifications, translocations, and hypermethylated CpG islands, that affect the function of critical genes and contribute to the malignant phenotype [27,28]. Critical genes targeted include oncogenes, which promote transformation when activated, and tumor suppressor genes, which fail to prevent transformation when inactivated. During the development of prostate cancer, *GSTP1* does not appear to function either as an oncogene, or as a tumor suppressor gene [25]. Instead, *GSTP1* likely acts as a 'caretaker' gene in prostate cells, which when inactivated, fails to prevent further somatic genome alterations upon chronic exposure to genome-damaging stresses [25,29]. In

M.L. Cher, K.V. Honn and A. Raz (eds.), Prostate Cancer: New Horizons in Research and Treatment, 227–240.
© 2002 *Kluwer Academic Publishers.*

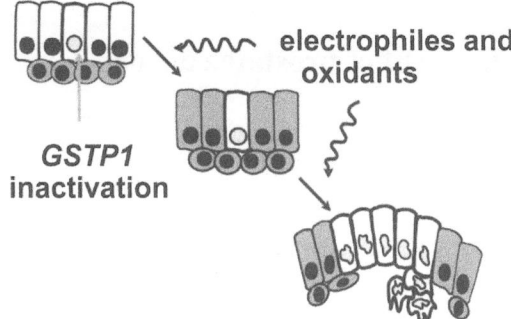

Figure 1. A new model for prostatic carcinogenesis. GSTP1 (gray) is constantly expressed in prostate basal epithelial cells, but can be induced in luminal epithelial cells upon exposure to reactive chemical species, including electrophiles and oxidants, that threaten genome damage. Loss of GSTP1 expression accompanying *GSTP1* CpG island hypermethylation increases vulnerability of luminal cells to neoplastic transformation and malignant progression.

this model of prostatic carcinogenesis, loss of *GSTP1* function increases the vulnerability of prostate cells to carcinogenic insults, contributed by environment and lifestyle, that promote prostate cancer development and progression (Figure 1).

Recognition that somatic inactivation of *GSTP1* may initiate prostatic carcinogenesis permits a reevaluation of the influence of environment and lifestyle on the development of life-threatening prostate cancer. Epidemiology studies have identified several environmental factors, including the diet, sexually transmitted diseases, and others, as candidate prostate cancer risk factors [30–32]. However, no specific prostate carcinogens have been identified. Glutathione *S*-transferases (GSTs), like GSTP1, are capable of detoxifying oxidant and electrophilic chemicals to prevent cell and genome damage [33]. If loss of *GSTP1* function plays a critical role in the pathogenesis of prostate cancer, we can expect that the relevant prostate carcinogens will be oxidants and electrophiles that (i) are substrates for GSTP1 detoxification, (ii) are associated with high prostate cancer risk diet and lifestyle habits, and (iii) are able to reach prostate cells with defective GSTP1 'caretaker' activity to inflict cell and genome injury. In this review, we consider the influence of environment and lifestyle on the development of life-threatening prostate cancer, focusing on the acquired vulnerability of prostate cells to carcinogens and other genome-damaging stresses associated with loss of *GSTP1* function.

The molecular pathogenesis of prostate cancer: Somatic inactivation of *GSTP1*

The pathogenesis of prostate cancer likely proceeds over at least 30 or more years. Small prostate cancers have been found in >30% of men aged 30–40 years, while diagnoses of clinically significant prostate cancers are typically made in men aged 60–70 years [34]. Prostate cancer cells typically contain a myriad of somatic genome alterations, including gene mutations, gene amplifications, gene deletions, chromosomal rearrangements, and changes in DNA methylation (see Figure 2) [35]. In addition, cancer cells from different prostate cancer cases, from different prostate cancer lesions in individual cases, or from different areas within the same prostate cancer lesions, often display marked differences in somatic genome changes [35,36]. This heterogeneity of somatic genome defects in prostate cancer cells, accumulating over decades, suggests that prostate cancers may arise as a consequence of either chronic or prolonged exposure to genome-damaging stresses, defective maintenance of genome integrity, or a combination of both processes. Furthermore, ongoing genomic instability in prostate cancer cells may be what leads to metastasis, progression to androgen independence after attempts at hormonal therapy, and other malignant behaviors [37–42].

Over the past several years, evidence has accumulated in support of the concept that somatic inactivation of *GSTP1*, most commonly by CpG island hypermethylation, may be the initiating somatic genome lesion for prostatic carcinogenesis, increasing the rate at which additional somatic genome alterations appear in response to exposure to genome-damaging stresses [23–26]. GSTs stereotypically provide an inducible defense against macromolecular damage by reactive chemical species [33]. In the normal prostate, GSTP1 polypeptides are selectively present in basal epithelial cells, with little, if any, enzyme detectable in non-stressed columnar epithelial cells (Figure 1). Nonetheless, *GSTP1* expression appears strikingly induced in columnar epithelial cells subjected to genome damaging stresses, such as those accompanying inflammation, commonly present in the human prostate. Proliferative inflammatory atrophy (PIA) lesions have been proposed to arise as a consequence of inflammatory injury to the prostate epithelium followed by exuberant epithelial cell proliferation/regeneration, and to give rise directly to prostatic intraepithelial neoplasia (PIN) lesions, known

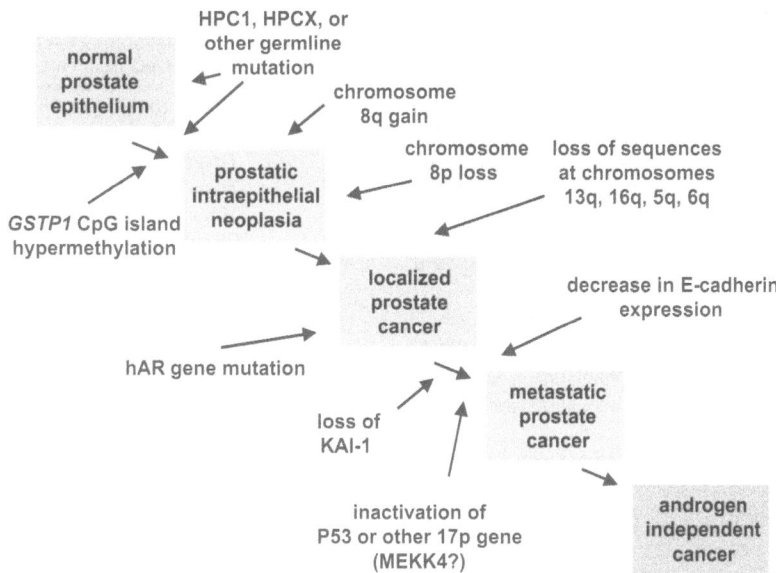

Figure 2. The molecular pathogenesis of prostate cancer. Somatic genome lesions accumulate during prostate cancer development. *GSTP1* CpG island hypermethylation appears to serve as the initiating somatic genome lesion.

precursors to prostate cancer [43,44]. In PIA lesions, atrophic luminal cells characteristically contain high levels of GSTP1 and other GSTs [43,45]. However, in PIN lesions, in contrast to PIA lesions, absent GSTP1 expression is a consistent finding [46]. Prostate cancer cells are also characteristically devoid of GSTP1. In almost all prostate cancer cases, the absence of GSTP1 expression can be attributed to somatic *GSTP1* CpG island hypermethylation, not present in DNA from normal tissues, but evident in DNA from some 70% of PIN lesions and >90% or prostate cancers [25,46]. As the most common somatic genome alteration yet reported for human prostate cancer, *GSTP1* CpG island hypermethylation, readily discriminated using various sensitive techniques, is an attractive candidate molecular biomarker for prostate cancer cells, under development for use in prostate cancer detection, diagnosis, and staging (Table 1) [23–25,46–54].

GSTP1 CpG island hypermethylation appears to prevent GSTP1 expression in prostate cancer cells via 'silencing' of *GSTP1* transcription. In support of this mechanism, LNCaP prostate cancer cells contain only hypermethylated *GSTP1* CpG island alleles, fail to express either *GSTP1* mRNA or GSTP1 polypeptides, and exhibit reduced *GSTP1* transcription, whereas treatment of LNCaP cells *in vitro* or *in vivo* with DNA methyltransferase inhibitors both reverses *GSTP1* CpG island hypermethylation and restores GSTP1

expression [24,25,55]. In addition, while unmethylated *GSTP1* transcriptional regulatory sequences readily promote abundant CAT reporter expression after transfection into LNCaP prostate cancer cells, *Sss*I CpG-methylase treatment of the *GSTP1* promoter before transfection leads to a marked reduction in CAT reporter expression [25,56]. Finally, detailed molecular pathology analyses have revealed, for almost all prostate cancer cases, that each of the cancer cells contains only hypermethylated *GSTP1* CpG island alleles, and each fails to express GSTP1 [25]. In contrast, for the two prostate cancer cases thus far described in which prostate cancer cells have been found to contain unmethylated *GSTP1* CpG island alleles, each of the prostate cancer cells displayed abundant GSTP1 expression [25,54]. CpG island hypermethylation has been proposed to repress gene transcription directly, via interference with transcriptional trans-activator binding, or indirectly, via the actions of $^{5-m}$C-binding proteins that affect chromatin structure, leading to a transcriptionally inactive chromatin conformation [57–63]. For the *GSTP1* CpG island, data collected thus far suggest that CpG island hypermethylation acts to repress *GSTP1* transcription indirectly [56]. Regardless of the mechanism by which CpG island hypermethylation prevents *GSTP1* transcription, because CpG methylation patterns are maintained through mitosis by the action of DNA methyltransferases,

Table 1. GSTP1 CpG island hypermethylation as a molecular biomarker for prostate cancer

Reference	Assay technique	GSTP1 CpG island hypermethylation*
Lee et al. (1994)	Southern blot	Tissue: 100% PCA; 0% BPH
Lee et al. (1997)	Restriction enzyme-PCR	Tissue: 91% PCA
Brooks et al. (1998)	Restriction enzyme-PCR	Tissue: 70% PIN
Santourlidis et al. (1999)	Restriction enzyme-PCR	Tissue: 75% PCA; 0% TCC
Millar et al. (1999)	Bisulfite genomic sequencing	Tissue: 83% PCA
Suh et al. (2000)	Restriction enzyme-PCR	Ejaculate: 44% PCA
Goessl et al. (2000)	Methylation-specific PCR	Tissue: 94% PCA; 0% BPH Urine: 36% PCA Ejaculate: 50% PCA Plasma: 50% PCA
Goessl et al. (2001)	Methylation-specific PCR	Urine: 73% PCA; 29% PIN; 2% BPH
Cairns et al. (2001)	Methylation-specific PCR	Tissue: 79% PCA Urine: 27% PCA
Lin et al. (2001)	Southern blot, restriction enzyme-PCR, bisulfite genomic sequencing	Tissue: 100% PCA
Goessl et al. (2001)	Methylation-specific PCR	Tissue: 90% PCA; 0% BPH Urine: 76% PCA Ejaculate: 50% PCA Plasma: 72% PCA
Jeronimo et al. (2001)	Quantitatitive methylation-specific PCR	Tissue: 91% PCA; 54% PIN; 29% BPH

*PCA-prostate cancer, BPH-benign prostatic hyperplasia, PIN-prostatic intraepithelial neoplasia, TCC-transitional cell carcinoma.

GSTP1 transcriptional 'silencing' associated with CpG island hypermethylation may be subject to selection during prostatic carcinogenesis. For this reason, the observation that most prostate cancers contain only prostate cancer cells with hypermethylated GSTP1 CpG island alleles may be evidence that loss of GSTP1 function likely provides some sort of selective growth or survival advantage at some point during the pathogenesis of prostate cancer.

Prostate cancer epidemiology: The diet, prostate inflammation, and prostate cancer risk

The etiology of prostate cancer has not been established. However, as mentioned previously, both prostate cancer incidence and mortality vary greatly in different geographic regions, with generally low risks of prostate cancer development characteristic of Asia, and generally high risks of prostate cancer development characteristic of the US and Western Europe [21,64–67]. Of note, prostate cancer risk among ethnic Asian immigrants to North America increases with duration of exposure to a Western lifestyle: Asian immigrants to North America have a higher risk of prostate cancer after living in North America for more than 25 years than after living in North America for less than 10 years [22]. Asian men born in the US have a risk for life-threatening prostate cancer development similar to Caucasian men. Of course, these epidemiological observations underscore the critical role for environment and lifestyle in fostering the epidemic of prostate cancer afflicting men in the US. The major environment and lifestyle factor modulating prostate cancer risk appears to be the diet. Clearly, stereotypical Asian diets are quite different from stereotypical Western diets. Unfortunately, whether the stereotypical Western diet makes an error of *commission* (e.g. over-consumption of dietary components increasing prostate cancer risks), an error of *omission* (e.g. under-consumption of dietary components decreasing prostate cancer risks), or *both* has been difficult to establish. Nonetheless, if specific dietary components could be demonstrated to change prostate cancer risks, the component could be *avoided* if it promoted prostate cancer and *provided* if it protected against prostate cancer as a rational prostate cancer prevention strategy.

Ecological, case-control, and cohort epidemiology studies all have long implicated fats and meats as candidate risks factors for prostate cancer (for a review, see [30]). The challenge for epidemiologists has been to ascertain whether increased prostate cancer risks might be attributable to total fat intake, to increased energy intake associated with high-fat diets, to intake of specific fats, or to intake of fats from specific sources, such as red meats. For example, in the Health Professionals

231

Follow-up Study, a prospective cohort of 51,529 men, total fat intake, adjusted for energy intake, appeared to confer increased risks (a relative risk of 1.79 for high *versus* low quintile of intake, with 95% confidence interval of 1.04–3.07) of prostate cancer development [68]. However, saturated fat intake *per se* did not appear to be responsible for the increased prostate cancer risks. Rather, animal fat intake (a relative risk of 1.63 with a 95% confidence interval of 0.95–2.78), particularly red meat intake (a relative risk of 2.64 with a 95% confidence interval of 1.21–5.77), may have been responsible for the observed prostate cancer risks associated with the high total fat diets. A deleterious effect of red meat consumption on prostate cancer risk has also been seen in the Physicians Health Study [69], a prospective cohort of 14,916 men (a relative risk of 2.5 for red meat consumption 5 times/week *versus* less than once/week with a 95% confidence interval of 0.9–6.7), and in a large cohort study in Hawaii [70], involving 20,316 men of varying ethnicities (a relative risk of 1.6 for highest *versus* lowest tertile of beef consumption with a 95% confidence interval of 1.1–2.4). Intriguingly, cooking of meats at high temperatures or on charcoal grills, is known to lead to the formation of heterocyclic amine carcinogens and/or polycyclic aromatic hydrocarbon carcinogens [71,72]. However, the level of intake of these carcinogenic substances has been difficult to estimate for epidemiologic studies of prostate cancer risk.

While chronic consumption of animal fats and red meats may promote prostate cancer, intake of vegetables may protect against prostate cancer development (for a review, see [31]). Among potentially protective vegetables, attention has been most intensively focused on tomatoes [73–76], which contain an α-carotenoid anti-oxidant, lycopene, and on cruciferous vegetables [76–78], which contain an anti-carcinogenic isothiocyanate, sulforaphane [79]. Lycopene, which appears in prostate tissues after tomato ingestion, can scavenge oxidant species, including nitric oxide, to prevent oxidative cell and genome damage [80–83]. In a study of 578 prostate cancer cases and 1294 controls from the Physician's Health Study cohort, high plasma lycopene levels were associated with a decrease in the risk of aggressive prostate cancer (a relative risk of 0.56 for high *versus* low quintile of lycopene plasma level with a 95% confidence interval of 0.34–0.91). Of interest, other anti-oxidants, selenium and vitamin E, have been found to attenuate prostate cancer development in randomized clinical trials [84–86]. Sulforaphane has been proposed to protect against

cancer development by increasing the expression of carcinogen-detoxification enzymes, including GSTs and quinone oxidoreductases, that help prevent genome damage mediated by carcinogens [79,87–89]. In a study of 628 prostate cancer cases and 602 controls from King County, Washington, cruciferous vegetable consumption, adjusted for total vegetable intake, was associated with diminished prostate cancer risks (a relative risk of 0.59 for 3 or more servings/week *versus* less than one serving/week with a 95% confidence interval of 0.39–0.90) [77].

In addition to the diet, environment and lifestyle factors affecting prostate cancer risk include sexually transmitted diseases, risk factors that might be modified to prevent prostate cancer [32]. However, unlike cancer of the uterine cervix, nasopharyngeal carcinoma, and Kaposi's sarcoma, it has been difficult to identify a specific pathogen responsible for the direct transformation of prostatic cells. Instead, prostatic inflammation associated with sexually transmitted infections may play a more important role in prostatic carcinogenesis. In a recent population-based study involving 981 prostate cancer cases (479 black men, 502 white men) and 1315 controls (594 black men, 721 white men), prostate cancer risks were increased among men (i) who reported a history of gonorrhoea or syphilis (a relative risk of 1.6 with a 95% confidence internal of 1.2–2.1), (ii) who reported three or more episodes of gonorrhea (a relative risk of 3.3 with a 95% confidence interval of 1.4–7.8), and (iii) who displayed serological evidence of syphilis (a relative risk of 1.8 with a 95% confidence interval of 1.0–3.5) [90]. Inflammation, known to inflict oxidative damage, has been thought to contribute to the pathogenesis of many human cancers [91]. Prostatitis, whether the result of an identified infection or idiopathic, very commonly afflicts men as they grow older in the US [92]. Whether chronic or recurrent prostatic inflammation contributes to prostate cancer development, or might explain differences in prostate cancer risks between different geographic regions, has not been ascertained.

A 'caretaker' role for *GSTP1* during prostatic carcinogenesis: The integration of prostate cancer molecular biology and epidemiology into a unified model

Rather than function as a tumor suppressor during prostatic carcinogenesis, *GSTP1* appears most likely to act as a 'caretaker' [29], defending prostate cells

232

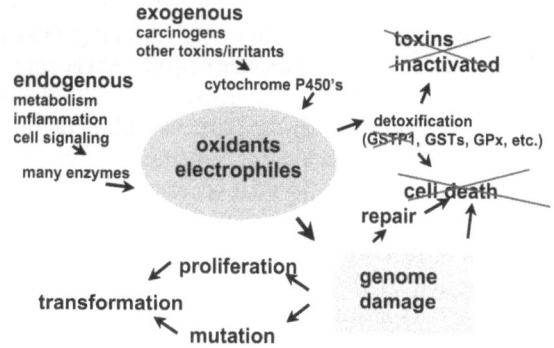

Figure 3. Loss of GSTP1 activity leads to a failure of cellular protection against oxidant and electrophilic carcinogens.

against genome damage mediated by carcinogens (Figure 3). GSTs have long been thought to protect against cancer development by catalyzing conjugation reactions between glutathione and a variety of reactive chemicals species, preventing carcinogen-induced cell and genome damage [33]. The enzymes are dimers composed of subunit polypeptides encoded by a complex collection of genes, organized into gene families α, μ, π, and θ. *GSTP1* encodes the single π-class GST subunit polypeptide; GSTP1-1 is a homodimer. The various different GSTs are normally expressed in different cells and tissues; however, GST activity can also be stereotypically induced in other cells and tissues in response to chemical stresses, via increases in *GST* subunit gene transcription [93,94]. The transcription factor Nrf2, binding to specific *cis*-regulatory sequences in *GST* subunit gene promoters, appears to play a critical role in activating *GST* subunit gene transcription in response to chemical stresses [95]. The inducible protection against reactive chemicals afforded by GSTs comprises a substantial barrier to chemical carcinogenesis. For example, mice carrying disrupted *Gstp1/2* genes, encoding the murine π-class GSTs, display increased skin tumorigenesis upon topical exposure to 7,12-dimethylbenz anthracene (DMBA) [96]. In addition, mice carrying disrupted *Nrf2* genes manifest increased gastric carcinogenesis upon exposure to benzo[a]pyrene [95]. By providing a barrier to cell and genome damage mediated by reactive chemicals, *GST* genes act as 'caretaker' genes for cancers arising as a consequence of carcinogen exposure.

As described above, prostate cancer epidemiology data have implicated heterocyclic amines (well-done meats), polycyclic aromatic hydrocarbons ('charbroiled' meats), and oxidants (inflammation) as candidate reactive chemicals that might threaten cell and

genome damage leading to prostate cancer development. If *GSTP1* 'caretaker' function provides a defense against such carcinogens, then the reactive chemical species ought to be substrates for GSTP1 detoxification. Recent data have suggested that heterocyclic amine carcinogens present in well-done meats may be detoxified by GSTP1 [97]. The heterocyclic aromatic amine carcinogen 2-amino-1-methyl-6-phenylimidazo[4,5-*b*]pyridine (PhIP) is known to cause mutations by adduction to DNA bases after metabolic activation by various cellular enzymes [71,98–101]. Rats fed PhIP have been reported to display mutations in prostate DNA and develop prostate cancer [102–104]. However, when LNCaP human prostate cancer cells devoid of GSTP1 were exposed to metabolically activated PhIP, high levels of PhIP-DNA adducts were detected, while LNCaP prostate cancer cells genetically modified to express GSTP1 exhibited substantial resistance to the formation of pro-mutagenic PhIP-DNA adducts [97]. Like the heterocyclic amine carcinogens, metabolically activated polycyclic aromatic hydrocarbon carcinogens are also GSTP1 substrates [105]. Of interest, polymorphic GSTP1 variants that are homodimers with subunit polypeptides containing isoleucine at amino acid 105, or containing valine at amino acid 105, appear to exhibit different catalytic properties when confronted with polycyclic aromatic hydrocarbons [106]. Furthermore, genetic epidemiology studies have suggested that homozygosity for *GSTP1val-105* alleles may increase breast cancer risks (a relative risk of 1.97 for *GSTP1val-105/val-105* with a 95% confidence interval of 0.77–5.02) [107]. The prostate cancer risks associated with homozygosity for *GSTP1val-105* alleles have not been established. Finally, new preliminary data have suggested that oxidants may also be substrates for GSTP1: upon prolonged exposure to an oxidative stress, LNCaP prostate cancer cells genetically modified to express GSTP1 suffered less oxidative genome damage than LNCaP prostate cancer cells devoid of GSTP1 activity (DeWeese et al. unpublished data).

Remarkably, loss of *GSTP1* 'caretaker' function may provide a selective growth or survival advantage upon exposure to certain carcinogens. Usually, increased sensitivity to the genome damaging actions of chemical carcinogens, such as that seen upon metabolically activated PhIP treatment of LNCaP prostate cancer cells devoid of GSTP1 *versus* LNCaP cells expressing GSTP1, is accompanied by increased sensitivity to the cytotoxic effects of the same carcinogens [97]. However, new preliminary data have revealed that when LNCaP prostate cancer cells, devoid of GSTP1 activity, are challenged by prolonged exposures to oxidant stresses, the cells appear to suffer much less cell death than LNCaP prostate cancer cells genetically modified to express GSTP1 (DeWeese et al. unpublished data). As a result, for LNCaP prostate cancer cells, loss of GSTP1 'caretaker' activity appeared to result in increased genome damage and decreased cell death upon oxidant exposure. Perhaps, this phenotype of oxidation damage 'tolerance' may provide PIN cells or prostate cancer cells a selective growth or survival advantage in the face of an oxidative stress like chronic prostate inflammation [26,43]. A similar phenotype of cell and genome damage 'tolerance' associated with loss of π-class GST activity has been reported for studies of mice exposed to acetaminophen overdoses, in which $Gstp1/2^{+/+}$ mice appeared to suffer markedly more hepatotoxicity than $Gstp1/2^{-/-}$ mice after administration of high doses of acetaminophen [108]. The mechanism(s) by which π-class GST activity might be coupled to cell death upon exposure to oxidants or to acetaminophen could potentially include glutathione 'bankruptcy' associated with π-class GST metabolism of reactive chemical species [108], toxification of the chemical species by π-class GST conjugation of the chemical species with glutathione [109], and/or potential modulation of stress-associated signal transduction pathways by π-class GSTs [110–113].

Thus, with loss of *GSTP1* 'caretaker' function as the initiating somatic genome lesion in the pathogenesis of prostate cancer, several features of the molecular pathogenesis of prostate cancer and several features of prostate cancer epidemiology can be integrated into a coherent model (Figure 4) [26]. In this model, the earliest steps in prostatic carcinogenesis occur as a result of prostatic inflammation, associated with prostatic infections or with idiopathic prostatitis, that leads to prostate cell oxidant injury and regeneration, resulting in the appearance of PIA lesions. The PIA cells, expressing high levels of GSTP1 and other oxidant protection enzymes, give rise to PIN cells, devoid of GSTP1, and ultimately to prostate cancer cells. With loss of *GSTP1* 'caretaker' function in the PIN cells and prostate cancer cells, decades of chronic oxidant stress, and of exposure to dietary heterocyclic amine and polycyclic aromatic hydrocarbons, lead to an accumulation of somatic genome alterations that drive malignant progression. Of interest, prostatic carcinogenesis may proceed via a similar pathway in rats, where both prostatic inflammation and heterocyclic

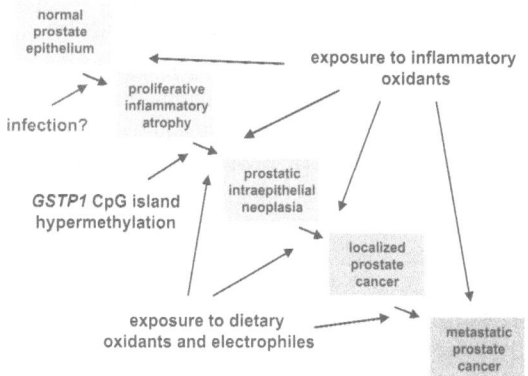

Figure 4. An integrated model for prostate cancer development featuring *GSTP1* inactivation in prostate cells in the face of exposure to inflammatory oxidants and dietary oxidants and electrophiles.

aromatic amine exposures have been reported to lead to prostatic neoplasia [102,103,114,115].

Rational strategies for prostate cancer prevention

To interrupt prostate cancer pathogenesis and prevent life-threatening prostate cancer, several rational approaches might be considered, including: (i) *attenuation* or *abrogation* of genome damaging stresses via avoidance of exogenous carcinogens (such as heterocyclic amines and polycyclic aromatic hydrocarbons) and/or reduction of endogenous carcinogenic stresses (such as inflammatory oxidants), (ii) *restoration* of *GSTP1* expression via treatment with inhibitors of CpG methylation, and (iii) *compensation* for inadequate GSTP1 activity via treatment with inducers of general GST activity. Some strategies for *attenuation* or *abrogation* of genome damaging stresses are already under evaluation for prostate cancer prevention. Antioxidant micronutrients, including vitamin E, selenium, and carotenoids, such as lycopene, might be expected to reduce oxidant damage to prostate cell DNA if used for prostate cancer prevention [73,74,116,117]. Each of these agents has reached human clinical studies. Selenium and vitamin E are to be tested in a large ($n = 32,400$) randomized trial (The Selenium and Vitamin E Chemoprevention Trial; SELECT) that is ongoing in the US to ascertain whether antioxidants selenium and vitamin E, alone or in combination, can reduce the incidence of prostate cancer in healthy men age 55 and older (age 50 and older for African–American men).

234

Early proof-of-principal clinical studies of lycopene, and/or tomato products, for prostate cancer have begun to be reported [118,119]. Anti-inflammatory agents might be expected to reduce inflammation-associated oxidant production in the prostate and reduce prostate cancer risks [120–122]. Several non-steroidal anti-inflammatory drugs are being examined as candidate drugs for prostate cancer prevention and/or treatment; 'proof-of-principle' clinical trials for prostate cancer are underway at Johns Hopkins featuring celecoxib (Celebrex®; Pharmacia) and sulindac.

Restoration of *GSTP1* function may be feasible as a prostate cancer prevention strategy (Figure 5). Silencing of *GSTP1* transcription in PIN and prostate cancer cells is likely maintained via the action of DNA methyltransferases, enzymes that could be targeted for therapeutic inhibition. We have collected data indicating that DNA methyltransferase inhibitors such as 5-aza-deoxycytidine and procainamide can restore GSTP1 expression in LNCaP prostate cancer cells *in vivo* [55]. These agents may be considered candidate prostate cancer prevention drugs. In addition, data have been reported revealing interactions both between [5-m]C-binding proteins and histone deacetylases (HDACs), and between DNA methyltransferases and HDACs, in effecting transcriptional repression [60–62,123]. Perhaps, combinations of drugs active at inhibiting DNA methyltransferases and at inhibiting chromatin-remodeling enzymes might prove useful in restoring high level GSTP1 expression in PIN or prostate cancer cells to slow life-threatening prostate cancer progression [61]. The key issue for development of this approach, especially if it is to be used for prostate cancer prevention as well as for prostate cancer treatment, will be whether restoration of *GSTP1*

expression (as well as the expression of other genes) can be accomplished with reasonable gene selectivity and with acceptable side effects. To this end, early phase I studies of combinations of the DNA methyltransferase inhibitor 5-aza-cytidine and the HDAC inhibitor phenylbutyrate have been initiated at Johns Hopkins.

Therapeutic *compensation* for inadequate 'caretaker' gene function may also hold promise for cancer prevention (Figure 6). Although *GSTP1* may be silenced early during the pathogenesis of prostate cancer, genes encoding other GST subunit polypeptides appear intact. As the genes encoding the other GST subunit polypeptides can be induced, via an Nrf2-dependent mechanism, this pathway can be exploited to better defend GSTP1-deficient prostate cells against injurious chemical stresses [93,94]. Augmentation of carcinogen-detoxification capacity, using a variety of such chemoprotective compounds, including isothiocyanates, 1,2-dithiole-3-thiones, terpenoids, etc., has been reported to prevent a variety of different cancers in different animal models by triggering the expression of carcinogen-detoxification enzymes [124]. Most or all of these compounds likely act to prevent cancer by activating carcinogen-detoxification enzyme gene expression via the Nrf2-dependent transcription induction pathway, as oltipraz, an anti-schistosomal 1,2-dithiole-3-thione compound known to protect against benzo[a]pyrene gastric carcinogenesis in murine models, had no effect on gastric tumor formation in mice carrying disrupted *Nrf2* alleles [95]. Induction of GST 'caretaker' activity in liver tissues, using oltipraz, a therapeutic inducer of GST activity, has been shown to reduce aflatoxin B_1

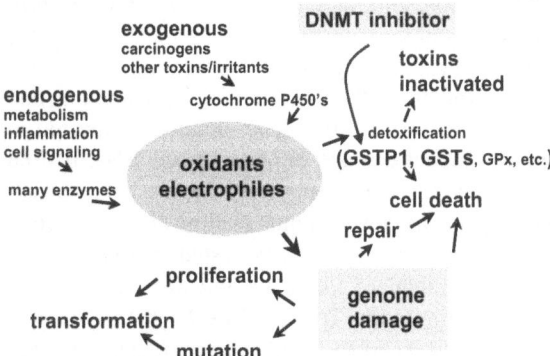

Figure 5. Therapeutic restoration of *GSTP1* function using DNA methyltransferase inhibitors.

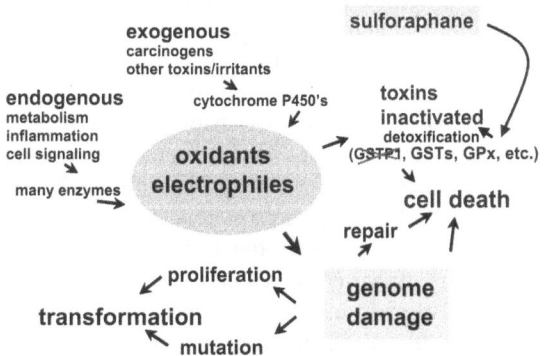

Figure 6. Therapeutic compensation for lack of GSTP1 activity using inducers of carcinogen detoxification enzymes, such as the isothiocyanate, sulforaphane, present in cruciferous vegetables.

damage when administered to a human clinical study cohort at high risk for aflatoxin exposure and liver cancer development in China [125–127]. Of greatest interest, many carcinogen-detoxification enzyme inducers have been detected in dietary components. For example, sulforaphane, an isothiocyanate that can trigger carcinogen-detoxification enzyme induction, is present in high amounts in cruciferous vegetables [79,87]. As described above, diets rich in carcinogen-inducers like sulforaphane have been associated with decreased cancer risks [77]. Early 'proof-of-principle' clinical trials of dietary carcinogen inducers as prevention for many different human cancers are currently underway [89,128].

Conclusions

Although both genes and the environment can contribute to the development of human prostate cancer, lifestyle factors, particularly the diet and possibly sexually transmitted diseases, likely play the dominant role in prostatic carcinogenesis. Loss of *GSTP1* 'caretaker' function, the earliest somatic genome alteration yet described for prostate cancer, appears to render prostate cells vulnerable to carcinogenic stresses. Heterocyclic amines, polycyclic aromatic hydrocarbons, and inflammatory oxidants, all carcinogens likely to be associated with high-risk prostate cancer diets and behaviors, are substrates for GSTP1 detoxification. In the absence of GSTP1 'caretaker' activity, chronic exposure to such carcinogens promotes an accumulation of somatic genome abnormalities, targeting oncogenes and tumor suppressor genes, that leads to life-threatening prostate cancer progression. Therapeutic strategies to *abrogate* genome damaging stresses, to *restore GSTP1* 'caretaker' function, or to *compensate* for inadequate *GSTP1* 'caretaker' gene function via induction of carcinogen-detoxification enzymes, might be expected to attenuate prostatic carcinogenesis.

Acknowledgement

William G. Nelson has a patent (US Patent 5,552,277) entitled 'Genetic Diagnosis of Prostate Cancer.'

References

1. Steinberg GD, Carter BS, Beaty TH, Childs B, Walsh PC: Family history and the risk of prostate cancer. Prostate 17: 337, 1990

2. Carter BS, Steinberg GD, Beaty TH, Childs B, Walsh PC: Familial risk factors for prostate cancer. Cancer Surv 11: 5, 1991

3. Carter BS, Beaty TH, Steinberg GD, Childs B, Walsh PC: Mendelian inheritance of familial prostate cancer. Proc Natl Acad Sci USA 89: 3367, 1992

4. Xu J, Zheng SL, Hawkins GA, Faith DA, Kelly B, Isaacs SD, Wiley KE, Chang B, Ewing CM, Bujnovszky P, Carpten JD, Bleecker ER, Walsh PC, Trent JM, Meyers DA, Isaacs WB: Linkage and association studies of prostate cancer susceptibility: evidence for linkage at 8p22-23. Am J Hum Genet 69: 341, 2001

5. Zheng SL, Xu J, Isaacs SD, Wiley K, Chang B, Bleecker ER, Walsh PC, Trent JM, Meyers DA, Isaacs WB: Evidence for a prostate cancer linkage to chromosome 20 in 159 hereditary prostate cancer families. Hum Genet 108: 430, 2001

6. Xu J, Zheng SL, Chang B, Smith JR, Carpten JD, Stine OC, Isaacs SD, Wiley KE, Henning L, Ewing C, Bujnovszky P, Bleeker ER, Walsh PC, Trent JM, Meyers DA, Isaacs WB: Linkage of prostate cancer susceptibility loci to chromosome 1. Hum Genet 108: 335, 2001

7. Xu J, Zheng SL, Carpten JD, Nupponen NN, Robbins CM, Mestre J, Moses TY, Faith DA, Kelly BD, Isaacs SD, Wiley KE, Ewing CM, Bujnovszky P, Chang B, Bailey-Wilson J, Bleecker ER, Walsh PC, Trent JM, Meyers DA, Isaacs WB: Evaluation of linkage and association of HPC2/ELAC2 in patients with familial or sporadic prostate cancer. Am J Hum Genet 68: 901, 2001

8. Gronberg H, Xu J, Smith JR, Carpten JD, Isaacs SD, Freije D, Bova GS, Danber JE, Bergh A, Walsh PC, Collins FS, Trent JM, Meyers DA, Isaacs WB: Early age at diagnosis in families providing evidence of linkage to the hereditary prostate cancer locus (HPC1) on chromosome 1. Cancer Res 57: 4707, 1997

9. Gronberg H, Isaacs SD, Smith JR, Carpten JD, Bova GS, Freije D, Xu J, Meyers DA, Collins FS, Trent JM, Walsh PC, Isaacs WB: Characteristics of prostate cancer in families potentially linked to the hereditary prostate cancer 1 (HPC1) locus. JAMA 278: 1251, 1997

10. Smith JR, Freije D, Carpten JD, Gronberg H, Xu J, Isaacs SD, Brownstein MJ, Bova GS, Guo H, Bujnovszky P, Nusskern DR, Damber JE, Bergh A, Emanuelsson M, Kallioniemi OP, Walker-Daniels J, Bailey-Wilson JE, Beaty TH, Meyers DA, Walsh PC, Collins FS, Trent JM, Isaacs WB: Major susceptibility locus for prostate cancer on chromosome 1 suggested by a genome-wide search. Science 274: 1371, 1996

11. Goode EL, Stanford JL, Peters MA, Janer M, Gibbs M, Kolb S, Badzioch MD, Hood L, Ostrander EA, Jarvik GP: Clinical characteristics of prostate cancer in an analysis of linkage to four putative susceptibility loci. Clin Cancer Res 7: 2739, 2001

12. Peters MA, Jarvik GP, Janer M, Chakrabarti L, Kolb S, Goode EL, Gibbs M, DuBois CC, Schuster EF, Hood L, Ostrander EA, Stanford JL: Genetic linkage analysis of prostate cancer families to Xq27-28. Hum Hered 51: 107, 2001

236

13. Gibbs M, Stanford JL, Jarvik GP, Janer M, Badzioch M, Peters MA, Goode EL, Kolb S, Chakrabarti L, Shook M, Basom R, Ostrander EA, Hood L: A genomic scan of families with prostate cancer identifies multiple regions of interest. Am J Hum Genet 67: 100, 2000

14. Gibbs M, Stanford JL, McIndoe RA, Jarvik GP, Kolb S, Goode EL, Chakrabarti L, Schuster EF, Buckley VA, Miller EL, Brandzel S, Li S, Hood L, Ostrander EA: Evidence for a rare prostate cancer-susceptibility locus at chromosome 1p36. Am J Hum Genet 64: 776, 1999

15. Xu J, Meyers D, Freije D, Isaacs S, Wiley K, Nusskern D, Ewing C, Wilkens E, Bujnovszky P, Bova GS, Walsh P, Isaacs W, Schleutker J, Matikainen M, Tammela T, Visakorpi T, Kallioniemi OP, Berry R, Schaid D, French A, McDonnell S, Schroeder J, Blute M, Thibodeau S, Trent J: Evidence for a prostate cancer susceptibility locus on the X chromosome. Nat Genet 20: 175, 1998

16. Berry R, Schroeder JJ, French AJ, McDonnell SK, Peterson BJ, Cunningham JM, Thibodeau SN, Schaid DJ: Evidence for a prostate cancer-susceptibility locus on chromosome 20. Am J Hum Genet 67: 82, 2000

17. Berthon P, Valeri A, Cohen-Akenine A, Drelon E, Paiss T, Wohr G, Latil A, Millasseau P, Mellah I, Cohen N, Blanche H, Bellane-Chantelot C, Demenais F, Teillac P, Le Duc A, de Petriconi R, Hautmann R, Chumakov I, Bachner L, Maitland NJ, Lidereau R, Vogel W, Fournier G, Mangin P, Cussenot O: Predisposing gene for early-onset prostate cancer, localized on chromosome 1q42.2-43. Am J Hum Genet 62: 1416, 1998

18. Lichtenstein P, Holm NV, Verkasalo PK, Iliadou A, Kaprio J, Koskenvuo M, Pukkala E, Skytthe A, Hemminki K: Environmental and heritable factors in the causation of cancer – analyses of cohorts of twins from Sweden, Denmark, and Finland. N Engl J Med 343: 78, 2000

19. Hsing AW, Devesa SS: Trends and patterns of prostate cancer: What do they suggest? Epidemiol Rev 23: 3, 2001

20. Hsing AW, Tsao L, Devesa SS: International trends and patterns of prostate cancer incidence and mortality. Int J Cancer 85: 60, 2000

21. Shimizu H, Ross RK, Bernstein L, Yatani R, Henderson BE, Mack TM: Cancers of the prostate and breast among Japanese and white immigrants in Los Angeles County. Br J Cancer 63: 963, 1991

22. Whittemore AS, Kolonel LN, Wu AH, John EM, Gallagher RP, Howe GR, Burch JD, Hankin J, Dreon DM, West DW: Prostate cancer in relation to diet, physical activity, and body size in blacks, whites, and Asians in the United States and Canada. J Natl Cancer Inst 87: 652, 1995

23. Lee WH, Isaacs WB, Bova GS, Nelson WG: CG island methylation changes near the GSTP1 gene in prostatic carcinoma cells detected using the polymerase chain reaction: a new prostate cancer biomarker. Cancer Epidemiol Biomarkers Prev 6: 443, 1997

24. Lee WH, Morton RA, Epstein JI, Brooks JD, Campbell PA, Bova GS, Hsieh WS, Isaacs WB, Nelson WG: Cytidine methylation of regulatory sequences near the pi-class glutathione S-transferase gene accompanies human prostatic carcinogenesis. Proc Natl Acad Sci USA 91: 11733, 1994

25. Lin X, Tascilar M, Lee WH, Vles WJ, Lee BH, Veeraswamy R, Asgari K, Freije D, van Rees B, Gage WR, Bova GS, Isaacs WB, Brooks JD, DeWeese TL, De Marzo AM, Nelson WG: GSTP1 CpG island hypermethylation is responsible for the absence of GSTP1 expression in human prostate cancer cells. Am J Pathol 159: 1815, 2001

26. Nelson WG, De Marzo AM, DeWeese TL: The molecular pathogenesis of prostate cancer: Implications for prostate cancer prevention. Urology 57: 39, 2001

27. Fearon ER, Vogelstein B: A genetic model for colorectal tumorigenesis. Cell 61: 759, 1990

28. Baylin SB, Herman JG: DNA hypermethylation in tumorigenesis: Epigenetics joins genetics. Trends Genet 16: 168, 2000

29. Kinzler KW, Vogelstein B: Cancer-susceptibility genes. Gatekeepers and caretakers (news; comment) (see comments). Nature 386: 761, 1997

30. Kolonel LN: Fat, meat, and prostate cancer. Epidemiol Rev 23: 72, 2001

31. Chan JM, Giovannucci EL: Vegetables, fruits, associated micronutrients, and risk of prostate cancer. Epidemiol Rev 23: 82, 2001

32. Strickler HD, Goedert JJ: Sexual behavior and evidence for an infectious cause of prostate cancer. Epidemiol Rev 23: 144, 2001

33. Hayes JD, Pulford DJ: The glutathione S-transferase supergene family: Regulation of GST and the contribution of the isoenzymes to cancer chemoprotection and drug resistance. Crit Rev Biochem Mol Biol 30: 445, 1995

34. Sakr WA, Grignon DJ, Crissman JD, Heilbrun LK, Cassin BJ, Pontes JJ, Haas GP: High grade prostatic intraepithelial neoplasia (HGPIN) and prostatic adenocarcinoma between the ages of 20–69: an autopsy study of 249 cases. In vivo 8: 439, 1994

35. Isaacs WB, Bova GS, Morton RA, Bussemakers MJ, Brooks JD, Ewing CM: Genetic alterations in prostate cancer. Cold Spring Harb Symp Quant Biol 59: 653, 1994

36. Ruijter ET, Miller GJ, van de Kaa CA, van Bokhoven A, Bussemakers MJ, Debruyne FM, Ruiter DJ, Schalken JA: Molecular analysis of multifocal prostate cancer lesions. J Pathol 188: 271, 1999

37. Suzuki H, Freije D, Nusskern DR, Okami K, Cairns P, Sidransky D, Isaacs WB, Bova GS: Interfocal heterogeneity of PTEN/MMAC1 gene alterations in multiple metastatic prostate cancer tissues. Cancer Res 58: 204, 1998

38. Cairns P, Okami K, Halachmi S, Halachmi N, Esteller M, Herman JG, Jen J, Isaacs WB, Bova GS, Sidransky D: Frequent inactivation of PTEN/MMAC1 in primary prostate cancer. Cancer Res 57: 4997, 1997

39. Jarrard DF, Bova GS, Ewing CM, Pin SS, Nguyen SH, Baylin SB, Cairns P, Sidransky D, Herman JG, Isaacs WB: Deletional, mutational, and methylation analyses of CDKN2 (p16/MTS1) in primary and metastatic prostate cancer. Genes Chromosomes Cancer 19: 90, 1997

40. Dong JT, Suzuki H, Pin SS, Bova GS, Schalken JA, Isaacs WB, Barrett JC, Isaacs JT: Down-regulation of the KAI1 metastasis suppressor gene during the progression of

human prostatic cancer infrequently involves gene mutation or allelic loss. Cancer Res 56: 4387, 1996

41. Cher ML, Bova GS, Moore DH, Small EJ, Carroll PR, Pin SS, Epstein JI, Isaacs WB, Jensen RH: Genetic alterations in untreated metastases and androgen-independent prostate cancer detected by comparative genomic hybridization and allelotyping. Cancer Res 56: 3091, 1996

42. Visakorpi T, Kallioniemi AH, Syvanen AC, Hyytinen ER, Karhu R, Tammela T, Isola JJ, Kallioniemi OP: Genetic changes in primary and recurrent prostate cancer by comparative genomic hybridization. Cancer Res 55: 342, 1995

43. De Marzo AM, Marchi VL, Epstein JI, Nelson WG: Proliferative inflammatory atrophy of the prostate: implications for prostatic carcinogenesis. Am J Pathol 155: 1985, 1999

44. Putzi MJ, De Marzo AM: Morphologic transitions between proliferative inflammatory atrophy and high-grade prostatic intraepithelial neoplasia (In process citation). Urology 56: 828, 2000

45. Parsons JK, Nelson CP, Gage WR, Nelson WG, Kensler TW, De Marzo AM: GSTA1 expression in normal, preneoplastic, and neoplastic human prostate tissue. Prostate 49: 30, 2001

46. Brooks JD, Weinstein M, Lin X, Sun Y, Pin SS, Bova GS, Epstein JI, Isaacs WB, Nelson WG: CG island methylation changes near the GSTP1 gene in prostatic intraepithelial neoplasia. Cancer Epidemiol Biomarkers Prev 7: 531, 1998

47. Cairns P, Esteller M, Herman JG, Schoenberg M, Jeronimo C, Sanchez-Cespedes M, Chow NH, Grasso M, Wu L, Westra WB, Sidransky D: Molecular detection of prostate cancer in urine by GSTP1 hypermethylation. Clin Cancer Res 7: 2727, 2001

48. Goessl C, Krause H, Muller M, Heicappell R, Schrader M, Sachsinger J, Miller K: Fluorescent methylation-specific polymerase chain reaction for DNA-based detection of prostate cancer in bodily fluids. Cancer Res 60: 5941, 2000

49. Goessl C, Muller M, Heicappell R, Krause H, Straub B, Schrader M, Miller K: DNA-based detection of prostate cancer in urine after prostatic massage. Urology 58: 335, 2001

50. Goessl C, Muller M, Heicappell R, Krause H, Miller K: DNA-based detection of prostate cancer in blood, urine, and ejaculates. Ann N Y Acad Sci 945: 51, 2001

51. Jeronimo C, Usadel H, Henrique R, Oliveira J, Lopes C, Nelson WG, Sidransky D: Quantitation of GSTP1 methylation in non-neoplastic prostatic tissue and organ-confined prostate adenocarcinoma. J Natl Cancer Inst 93: 1747, 2001

52. Suh CI, Shanafelt T, May DJ, Shroyer KR, Bobak JB, Crawford ED, Miller GJ, Markham N, Glode LM: Comparison of telomerase activity and GSTP1 promoter methylation in ejaculate as potential screening tests for prostate cancer. Mol Cell Probes 14: 211, 2000

53. Santourlidis S, Florl A, Ackermann R, Wirtz HC, Schulz WA: High frequency of alterations in DNA methylation in adenocarcinoma of the prostate. Prostate 39: 166, 1999

54. Millar DS, Ow KK, Paul CL, Russell PJ, Molloy PL, Clark SJ: Detailed methylation analysis of the glutathione S-transferase pi (GSTP1) gene in prostate cancer. Oncogene 18: 1313, 1999

55. Lin X, Asgari K, Putzi MJ, Gage WR, Yu X, Cornblatt BS, Kumar A, Piantadosi S, DeWeese TL, De Marzo AM, Nelson WG: Reversal of GSTP1 CpG island hypermethylation and reactivation of pi-class glutathione S-transferase (GSTP1) expression in human prostate cancer cells by treatment with procainamide. Cancer Res 61: 8611, 2001

56. Singal R, van Wert J, Bashambu M: Cytosine methylation represses glutathione S-transferase P1 (GSTP1) gene expression in human prostate cancer cells. Cancer Res 61: 4820, 2001

57. Ng HH, Jeppesen P, Bird A: Active repression of methylated genes by the chromosomal protein MBD1. Mol Cell Biol 20: 1394, 2000

58. Zhang Y, Ng HH, Erdjument-Bromage H, Tempst P, Bird A, Reinberg D: Analysis of the NuRD subunits reveals a histone deacetylase core complex and a connection with DNA methylation. Genes Dev 13: 1924, 1999

59. Mielnicki LM, Ying AM, Head KL, Asch HL, Asch BB: Epigenetic regulation of gelsolin expression in human breast cancer cells. Exp Cell Res 249: 161, 1999

60. Jones PL, Veenstra GJ, Wade PA, Vermaak D, Kass SU, Landsberger N, Strouboulis J, Wolffe AP: Methylated DNA and MeCP2 recruit histone deacetylase to repress transcription. Nat Genet 19: 187, 1998

61. Cameron EE, Bachman KE, Myohanen S, Herman JG, Baylin SB: Synergy of demethylation and histone deacetylase inhibition in the re-expression of genes silenced in cancer. Nat Genet 21: 103, 1999

62. Nan X, Ng HH, Johnson CA, Laherty CD, Turner BM, Eisenman RN, Bird A: Transcriptional repression by the methyl-CpG-binding protein MeCP2 involves a histone deacetylase complex. Nature 393: 386, 1998

63. Pikaart MJ, Recillas-Targa F, Felsenfeld G: Loss of transcriptional activity of a transgene is accompanied by DNA methylation and histone deacetylation and is prevented by insulators. Genes Dev 12: 2852, 1998

64. Brawley OW, Knopf K, Thompson I: The epidemiology of prostate cancer part II: the risk factors. Semin Urol Oncol 16: 193, 1998

65. Carter BS, Carter HB, Isaacs JT: Epidemiologic evidence regarding predisposing factors to prostate cancer. Prostate 16: 187, 1990

66. Haenszel W, Kurihara M: Studies of Japanese migrants. I. Mortality from cancer and other diseases among Japanese in the United States. J Natl Cancer Inst 40: 43, 1968

67. Danley KL, Richardson JL, Bernstein L, Langholz B, Ross RK: Prostate cancer: Trends in mortality and stage-specific incidence rates by racial/ethnic group in Los Angeles County, California (United States). Cancer Causes Control 6: 492, 1995

68. Giovannucci E, Rimm EB, Colditz GA, Stampfer MJ, Ascherio A, Chute CC, Willett WC: A prospective study of dietary fat and risk of prostate cancer. J Natl Cancer Inst 85: 1571, 1993

69. Gann PH, Hennekens CH, Sacks FM, Grodstein F, Giovannucci EL, Stampfer MJ: Prospective study of plasma fatty acids and risk of prostate cancer. J Natl Cancer Inst 86: 281, 1994

70. Le Marchand L, Kolonel LN, Wilkens LR, Myers BC, Hirohata T: Animal fat consumption and prostate cancer: A prospective study in Hawaii. Epidemiology 5: 276, 1994

71. Gross GA, Turesky RJ, Fay LB, Stillwell WG, Skipper PL, Tannenbaum SR: Heterocyclic aromatic amine formation in grilled bacon, beef and fish and in grill scrapings. Carcinogenesis 14: 2313, 1993

72. Lijinsky W, Shubik P: Benzo(a)pyrene and other polynuclear hydrocarbons in charcoal-broiled meat. Science 145: 53, 1964

73. Gann PH, Ma J, Giovannucci E, Willett W, Sacks FM, Hennekens CH, Stampfer MJ: Lower prostate cancer risk in men with elevated plasma lycopene levels: Results of a prospective analysis. Cancer Res 59: 1225, 1999

74. Giovannucci E, Ascherio A, Rimm EB, Stampfer MJ, Colditz GA, Willett WC: Intake of carotenoids and retinol in relation to risk of prostate cancer. J Natl Cancer Inst 87: 1767, 1995

75. Giovannucci E: Tomatoes, tomato-based products, lycopene, and cancer: Review of the epidemiologic literature. J Natl Cancer Inst 91: 317, 1999

76. Jain MG, Hislop GT, Howe GR, Ghadirian P: Plant foods, antioxidants, and prostate cancer risk: Findings from case-control studies in Canada. Nutr Cancer 34: 173, 1999

77. Cohen JH, Kristal AR, Stanford JL: Fruit and vegetable intakes and prostate cancer risk. J Natl Cancer Inst 92: 61, 2000

78. Kolonel LN, Hankin JH, Whittemore AS, Wu AH, Gallagher RP, Wilkens LR, John EM, Howe GR, Dreon DM, West DW, Paffenbarger RS Jr: Vegetables, fruits, legumes and prostate cancer: A multiethnic case-control study. Cancer Epidemiol Biomarkers Prev 9: 795, 2000

79. Zhang Y, Talalay P, Cho CG, Posner GH: A major inducer of anticarcinogenic protective enzymes from broccoli: Isolation and elucidation of structure. Proc Natl Acad Sci USA 89: 2399, 1992

80. Clinton SK: The dietary antioxidant network and prostate carcinoma. Cancer 86: 1629, 1999

81. Christen S, Woodall AA, Shigenaga MK, Southwell-Keely PT, Duncan MW, Ames BN: Gamma-tocopherol traps mutagenic electrophiles such as NO(X) and complements alpha-tocopherol: Physiological implications. Proc Natl Acad Sci USA 94: 3217, 1997

82. Freeman VL, Meydani M, Yong S, Pyle J, Wan Y, Arvizu-Durazo R, Liao Y: Prostatic levels of tocopherols, carotenoids, and retinol in relation to plasma levels and self-reported usual dietary intake. Am J Epidemiol 151: 109, 2000

83. Clinton SK, Emenhiser C, Schwartz SJ, Bostwick DG, Williams AW, Moore BJ, Erdman JW Jr: Cis-trans lycopene isomers, carotenoids, and retinol in the human prostate. Cancer Epidemiol Biomarkers Prev 5: 823, 1996

84. Clark LC, Combs GF Jr, Turnbull BW, Slate EH, Chalker DK, Chow J, Davis LS, Glover RA, Graham GF, Gross EG, Krongrad A, Lesher JL Jr, Park HK, Sanders BB Jr, Smith CL, Taylor JR: Effects of selenium supplementation for cancer prevention in patients with carcinoma of the skin. A randomized controlled trial. Nutritional Prevention of Cancer Study Group (see comments) (published erratum appears in JAMA 1997 May 21; 277(19): 1520). JAMA 276: 1957, 1996

85. Clark LC, Dalkin B, Krongrad A, Combs GF Jr, Turnbull BW, Slate EH, Witherington R, Herlong JH, Janosko E, Carpenter D, Borosso C, Falk S, Rounder J: Decreased incidence of prostate cancer with selenium supplementation: Results of a double-blind cancer prevention trial. Br J Urol 81: 730, 1998

86. Heinonen OP, Albanes D, Virtamo J, Taylor PR, Huttunen JK, Hartman AM, Haapakoski J, Malila N, Rautalahti M, Ripatti S, Maenpaa H, Teerenhovi L, Koss L, Virolainen M, Edwards BK: Prostate cancer and supplementation with alpha-tocopherol and beta-carotene: Incidence and mortality in a controlled trial (see comments). J Natl Cancer Inst 90: 440, 1998

87. Zhang Y, Kensler TW, Cho CG, Posner GH, Talalay P: Anticarcinogenic activities of sulforaphane and structurally related synthetic norbornyl isothiocyanates. Proc Natl Acad Sci USA 91: 3147, 1994

88. Fahey JW, Zhang Y, Talalay P: Broccoli sprouts: An exceptionally rich source of inducers of enzymes that protect against chemical carcinogens. Proc Natl Acad Sci USA 94: 10,367, 1997

89. Shapiro TA, Fahey JW, Wade KL, Stephenson KK, Talalay P: Chemoprotective glucosinolates and isothiocyanates of broccoli sprouts: Metabolism and excretion in humans. Cancer Epidemiol Biomarkers Prev 10: 501, 2001

90. Hayes RB, Pottern LM, Strickler H, Rabkin C, Pope V, Swanson GM, Greenberg RS, Schoenberg JB, Liff J, Schwartz AG, Hoover RN, Fraumeni JF Jr: Sexual behaviour, STDs and risks for prostate cancer. Br J Cancer 82: 718, 2000

91. Ames BN, Gold LS, Willett WC: The causes and prevention of cancer. Proc Natl Acad Sci USA 92: 5258, 1995

92. Roberts RO, Lieber MM, Rhodes T, Girman CJ, Bostwick DG, Jacobsen SJ: Prevalence of a physician-assigned diagnosis of prostatitis: The olmsted county study of urinary symptoms and health status among men. Urology 51: 578, 1998

93. Rushmore TH, King RG, Paulson KE, Pickett CB: Regulation of glutathione S-transferase Ya subunit gene expression: Identification of a unique xenobiotic-responsive element controlling inducible expression by planar aromatic compounds. Proc Natl Acad Sci USA 87: 3826, 1990

94. Rushmore TH, Pickett CB: Transcriptional regulation of the rat glutathione S-transferase Ya subunit gene. Characterization of a xenobiotic-responsive element controlling inducible expression by phenolic antioxidants. J Biol Chem 265: 14648, 1990

95. Ramos-Gomez M, Kwak MK, Dolan PM, Itoh K, Yamamoto M, Talalay P, Kensler TW: From the Cover: Sensitivity to carcinogenesis is increased and chemoprotective efficacy of enzyme inducers is lost in nrf2 transcription factor-deficient mice. Proc Natl Acad Sci USA 98: 3410, 2001

96. Henderson CJ, Smith AG, Ure J, Brown K, Bacon EJ, Wolf CR: Increased skin tumorigenesis in mice lacking pi

class glutathione S-transferases. Proc Natl Acad Sci USA 95: 5275, 1998

97. Nelson CP, Kidd LC, Sauvageot J, Isaacs WB, De Marzo AM, Groopman JD, Nelson WG, Kensler TW: Protection against 2-hydroxyamino-1-methyl-6-phenylimidazo[4,5-b]pyridine cytotoxicity and DNA adduct formation in human prostate by glutathione S-transferase P1. Cancer Res 61: 103, 2001

98. Morgenthaler PM, Holzhauser D: Analysis of mutations induced by 2-amino-1-methyl-6-phenylimidazo[4,5-b]pyridine (PhIP) in human lymphoblastoid cells. Carcinogenesis 16: 713, 1995

99. Nagaoka H, Wakabayashi K, Kim SB, Kim IS, Tanaka Y, Ochiai M, Tada A, Nukaya H, Sugimura T, Nagao M: Adduct formation at C-8 of guanine on in vitro reaction of the ultimate form of 2-amino-1-methyl-6-phenylimidazo[4,5-b]pyridine with 2′-deoxyguanosine and its phosphate esters. Jpn J Cancer Res 83: 1025, 1992

100. Knize MG, Sinha R, Rothman N, Brown ED, Salmon CP, Levander OA, Cunningham PL, Felton JS: Heterocyclic amine content in fast-food meat products. Food Chem Toxicol 33: 545, 1995

101. Davis CD, Schut HA, Snyderwine EG: Adduction of the heterocyclic amine food mutagens IQ and PhIP to mitochondrial and nuclear DNA in the liver of Fischer-344 rats. Carcinogenesis 15: 641, 1994

102. Shirai T, Sano M, Tamano S, Takahashi S, Hirose M, Futakuchi M, Hasegawa R, Imaida K, Matsumoto K, Wakabayashi K, Sugimura T, Ito N: The prostate: A target for carcinogenicity of 2-amino-1-methyl-6-phenylimidazo[4,5-b]pyridine (PhIP) derived from cooked foods. Cancer Res 57: 195, 1997

103. Shirai T, Cui L, Takahashi S, Futakuchi M, Asamoto M, Kato K, Ito N: Carcinogenicity of 2-amino-1-methyl-6-phenylimidazo [4,5-b]pyridine (PhIP) in the rat prostate and induction of invasive carcinomas by subsequent treatment with testosterone propionate. Cancer Lett 143: 217, 1999

104. Stuart GR, Holcroft J, de Boer JG, Glickman BW: Prostate mutations in rats induced by the suspected human carcinogen 2-amino-1-methyl-6-phenylimidazo[4,5-b]pyridine. Cancer Res 60: 266, 2000

105. Fields WR, Morrow CS, Doss AJ, Sundberg K, Jernstrom B, Townsend AJ: Overexpression of stably transfected human glutathione S-transferase P1-1 protects against DNA damage by benzo[a]pyrene diol-epoxide in human T47D cells. Mol Pharmacol 54: 298, 1998

106. Sundberg K, Johansson AS, Stenberg G, Widersten M, Seidel A, Mannervik B, Jernstrom B: Differences in the catalytic efficiencies of allelic variants of glutathione transferase P1-1 towards carcinogenic diol epoxides of polycyclic aromatic hydrocarbons. Carcinogenesis 19: 433, 1998

107. Helzlsouer KJ, Selmin O, Huang HY, Strickland PT, Hoffman S, Alberg AJ, Watson M, Comstock GW, Bell D: Association between glutathione S-transferase M1, P1, and T1 genetic polymorphisms and development of breast cancer. J Natl Cancer Inst 90: 512, 1998

108. Henderson CJ, Wolf CR, Kitteringham N, Powell H, Otto D, Park BK: Increased resistance to acetaminophen hepatotoxicity in mice lacking glutathione S-transferase Pi. Proc Natl Acad Sci USA 97: 12,741, 2000

109. Diah SK, Smitherman PK, Townsend AJ, Morrow CS: Detoxification of 1-chloro-2,4-dinitrobenzene in MCF7 breast cancer cells expressing glutathione S-transferase P1-1 and/or multidrug resistance protein 1. Toxicol Appl Pharmacol 157: 85, 1999

110. Adler V, Yin Z, Fuchs SY, Benezra M, Rosario L, Tew KD, Pincus MR, Sardana M, Henderson CJ, Wolf CR, Davis RJ, Ronai Z: Regulation of JNK signaling by GSTp. Embo J 18: 1321, 1999

111. Wang T, Arifoglu P, Ronai Z, Tew KD: Glutathione S-transferase P1-1 (GSTP1-1) Inhibits c-Jun N-terminal Kinase (JNK1) signaling through interaction with the C terminus. J Biol Chem 276: 20999, 2001

112. Yin Z, Ivanov VN, Habelhah H, Tew K, Ronai Z: Glutathione S-transferase p elicits protection against H2O2-induced cell death via coordinated regulation of stress kinases. Cancer Res 60: 4053, 2000

113. Ruscoe JE, Rosario LA, Wang T, Gate L, Arifoglu P, Wolf CR, Henderson CJ, Ronai Z, Tew KD: Pharmacologic or genetic manipulation of glutathione S-transferase P1-1 (GSTpi) influences cell proliferation pathways. J Pharmacol Exp Ther 298: 339, 2001

114. Reznik G, Hamlin MH II, Ward JM, Stinson SF: Prostatic hyperplasia and neoplasia in aging F344 rats. Prostate 2: 261, 1981

115. Gilardoni MB, Rabinovich GA, Oviedo M, Depiante-Depaoli M: Prostate cancer induction in autoimmune rats and modulation of T cell apoptosis. J Exp Clin Cancer Res 18: 493, 1999

116. Yoshizawa K, Willett WC, Morris SJ, Stampfer MJ, Spiegelman D, Rimm EB, Giovannucci E: Study of prediagnostic selenium level in toenails and the risk of advanced prostate cancer (see comments). J Natl Cancer Inst 90: 1219, 1998

117. Helzlsouer KJ, Huang HY, Alberg AJ, Hoffman S, Burke A, Norkus EP, Morris JS, Comstock GW: Association between alpha-tocopherol, gamma-tocopherol, selenium, and subsequent prostate cancer. J Natl Cancer Inst 92: 2018, 2000

118. Kucuk O, Sarkar FH, Sakr W, Djuric Z, Pollak MN, Khachik F, Li YW, Banerjee M, Grignon D, Bertram JS, Crissman JD, Pontes EJ, Wood DP Jr: Phase II randomized clinical trial of lycopene supplementation before radical prostatectomy. Cancer Epidemiol Biomarkers Prev 10: 861, 2001

119. Chen L, Stacewicz-Sapuntzakis M, Duncan C, Sharifi R, Ghosh L, Breemen Rv R, Ashton D, Bowen PE: Oxidative DNA damage in prostate cancer patients consuming tomato sauce-based entrees as a whole-food intervention. J Natl Cancer Inst 93: 1872, 2001

120. Wechter WJ, Leipold DD, Murray ED Jr, Quiggle D, McCracken JD, Barrios RS, Greenberg NM: E-7869 (R-flurbiprofen) inhibits progression of prostate cancer in the TRAMP mouse. Cancer Res 60: 2203, 2000

240

121. Nelson JE, Harris RE: Inverse association of prostate cancer and non-steroidal anti-inflammatory drugs (NSAIDs): Results of a case-control study. Oncol Rep 7: 169, 2000

122. Nelson WG, Wilding G: Prostate cancer prevention agent development: Criteria and pipeline for candidate chemoprevention agents. Urology 57: 56, 2001

123. Rountree MR, Bachman KE, Baylin SB: DNMT1 binds HDAC2 and a new co-repressor, DMAP1, to form a complex at replication foci. Nat Genet 25: 269, 2000

124. Kensler TW: Chemoprevention by inducers of carcinogen detoxication enzymes. Environ Health Perspect 105 Suppl(4): 965, 1997

125. Wang JS, Shen X, He X, Zhu YR, Zhang BC, Wang JB, Qian GS, Kuang SY, Zarba A, Egner PA, Jacobson LP, Munoz A, Helzlsouer KJ, Groopman JD, Kensler TW: Protective alterations in phase 1 and 2 metabolism of aflatoxin B1 by oltipraz in residents of Qidong, People's Republic of China. J Natl Cancer Inst 91: 347, 1999

126. Jacobson LP, Zhang BC, Zhu YR, Wang JB, Wu Y, Zhang QN, Yu LY, Qian GS, Kuang SY, Li YF, Fang X, Zarba A, Chen B, Enger C, Davidson NE, Gorman MB, Gordon GB, Prochaska HJ, Egner PA, Groopman JD, Munoz A, Helzlsouer KJ, Kensler TW: Oltipraz chemoprevention trial in Qidong, People's Republic of China: Study design and clinical outcomes. Cancer Epidemiol Biomarkers Prev 6: 257, 1997

127. Kensler TW, He X, Otieno M, Egner PA, Jacobson LP, Chen B, Wang JS, Zhu YR, Zhang BC, Wang JB, Wu Y, Zhang QN, Qian GS, Kuang SY, Fang X, Li YF, Yu LY, Prochaska HJ, Davidson NE, Gordon GB, Gorman MB, Zarba A, Enger C, Munoz A, Helzlsouer KJ: Oltipraz chemoprevention trial in Qidong, People's Republic of China: Modulation of serum aflatoxin albumin adduct biomarkers. Cancer Epidemiol Biomarkers Prev 7: 127, 1998

128. Shapiro TA, Fahey JW, Wade KL, Stephenson KK, Talalay P: Human metabolism and excretion of cancer chemoprotective glucosinolates and isothiocyanates of cruciferous vegetables. Cancer Epidemiol Biomarkers Prev 7: 1091, 1998

Prostate cancer diagnosis, staging and survival

Vivek Narain, Michael L. Cher and David P. Wood Jr.
*Department of Urology, Wayne State University School of Medicine and The Prostate Program of
The Barbara Ann Karmanos Cancer Institute, Detroit, MI, USA*

Key words: prostate cancer, survival, diagnosis

Summary

Prostate cancer is the most common malignancy in men and the second most common cancer related death. Through research, we have found that African–American men and men with a family history of prostate cancer have a significantly higher risk of prostate cancer. In the 90's the mortality rate from prostate cancer decreased, presumably due to PSA testing. Patients with organ-confined tumors, particularly if they have a moderate Gleason score have an excellent chance of long-term survival with radical prostatectomy or external beam radiation therapy. Advances in detecting micrometastatic disease are needed to further impact on this disease.

Introduction

Prostate cancer is the most common non-dermatologic malignancy diagnosed among men in the United States with an estimated 198,100 new cases during 2001 [1]. One in 6 American males is expected to be diagnosed with this disease during his lifetime. Prostate cancer accounts for 31% of all newly diagnosed cancer in US in 2001, and 11% of all cancer deaths in US, making it the second leading cause of cancer deaths in men [1]. A substantial proportion of patients will develop metastatic disease at some point in their course and approximately 31,500 of all prostate cancer patients will die of their disease in 2001 [1]. Prostate cancer accounts for almost as many deaths among men as breast cancer causes among women. The clinical course of metastatic disease is characteristically progressive and fatal with a median overall survival between 24 and 36 months. Studies in Scandinavia have shown that a 70-year-old man with clinically-localized prostate cancer treated with non-curative intent has a 50% chance of dying of (not with) prostate cancer. The probability of dying from prostate cancer is close to 100% in younger age (50–55 years) groups [2]. Because prostate cancer is more common in older men, prostate cancer ranks 21st among cancers in years of potential life lost [3]. The age-adjusted death rate from prostate cancer increased

by over 20% between 1973 and 1991 [4]. The lifetime risk of dying from prostate cancer is 3.4% for American men [3].

Due to the introduction of serum prostate-specific antigen (PSA) testing, the incidence of prostate cancer increased substantially during the period 1988–1992. This test resulted in a tremendous increase of diagnoses in asymptomatic men. Since 1992–1993, prostate cancer incidence rates have declined and have leveled off. Although the prostate cancer incidence curves appear to have peaked in 1992 and 1993, the current incidence rate remains substantially increased compared with the pre-PSA era [5].

Despite the widespread use of PSA testing, there is continued debate regarding its overall benefit. Currently, there is minimal evidence that PSA-screening decreases prostate-cancer mortality or improves survival. Whether early detection does more good than harm is a matter of some controversy. As a result, conflicting recommendations have been issued by various professional organizations. The US Preventive Services Task Force, the American College of Surgeons, the American Society of Internal Medicine, the National Cancer Institute, the American Association of Family Practioners, and the American College of Preventive Medicine all indicate that routine screening for prostate cancer is not recommended [6]. Conversely, a

M.L. Cher, K.V. Honn and A. Raz (eds.), Prostate Cancer: New Horizons in Research and Treatment, 241–251.

recent report of a large randomized study of screening indicated that a screening strategy that included serum-PSA testing and digital rectal examination (DRE) resulted in significantly fewer deaths from prostate cancer. Labrie et al. [7] showed that men in the prostate cancer screening arm had a significantly less likelihood of dying from prostate cancer than men randomized to standard care. Catalona et al. [8] showed that screening leads to a more favorable impact on prognosis by reducing the incidence of advanced disease. If PSA screening does identify clinically-significant prostate cancer as opposed to latent or clinically-insignificant tumors, and if current treatment is effective, then mortality and survival would be expected to improve. Indeed, two separate studies have confirmed that mortality rates are decreasing since the introduction of PSA testing [9,10,11]. Thus, evidence is beginning to accumulate in support of early detection. Several ongoing trials of early detection and treatment should eventually confirm these findings.

The American Cancer Society recommends that beginning at age 50, the PSA test and the DRE should be offered annually to men who have a life-expectancy of at least 10 years. Men at high risk (African American men and men who have a first degree relative who was diagnosed with prostate cancer at a young age) should begin testing at age 45 [1]. The American Urological Association and the American College of Radiology similarly endorse the American Cancer Society's recommendations [10,11]. An immediate checkup should be performed on any man who suddenly develops persistent urinary symptoms. A yearly examination can help avoid the potentially serious consequences of advanced prostate cancer.

Risk factors

Risk factors for prostate cancer include age, family history of prostate cancer, African American race, and possibly dietary fat intake [12]. Age and race remain the strongest risk factors yet identified for prostate cancer from epidemiologic studies.

More than 70% of all prostate cancers are diagnosed in men over age 65 [1]. The prevalence of incidental prostate cancer detected at autopsy is 30% for men over age 50 years. Incidence rates for non-organ-confined prostate cancer increase dramatically with age, from 82/100,000 for men from 50 to 54 years of age to 1326/100,000 for men from 70 to 74 years of age [13].

The reported prevalence of histologic prostate cancer in men without previously known prostate cancer during their lifetimes is 10–42% at age 50–59, 17–38% at age 60–69, 25–66% at age 70–79, and 18–100% at age 80 and older [14–17]. Sakr et al. [18] found that even men aged 30–49 years had foci of histologic prostate cancer present on careful evaluation at autopsy.

In the United States, African American men (AAM) have a substantially higher incidence of prostate cancer compared to age matched Caucasian men [19]. Of all racial and ethnic groups studied, AAM have the highest rate of cancers of the prostate (180.6 per 100,000). In comparison, the incidence of prostate cancer is 134.7 and 24.2 per 100,000 in Caucasian American men (CAM) and American Korean men, respectively. Moreover, the prostate cancer mortality rate for AAM (53.7 per 100,000) is twice as high as the rate for CAM (24.1 per 100,000) [19].

Many studies have reported that a positive family history of prostate cancer is considered a significant risk factor for the development of the disease. Age-adjusted relative risks for prostate cancer were 2.4 and 2.1 for men with a first or a second degree relative affected with prostate cancer, respectively [20]. Up to 13% of patients diagnosed with prostate cancer have a positive family history compared with 5.7% of age-matched population controls [20]. There is also a trend of increasing risk in incidence with increasing number of affected family members with prostate cancer.

Linkage studies done in Swedish and American families have demonstrated a major susceptibility locus for prostate cancer on chromosome 1 in the q24–25 region, also known as Hereditary Prostate Cancer 1 (HPC1) locus [21]. It is estimated that within Sweden as many as 50% of early-onset families have evidence of linkage to the HPC1 region [22]. Evidence for linkage to HPC1, however, is provided primarily by large (five or more members affected) families with an early average age (<65) of diagnosis. Inherited alterations at this locus have also been linked to higher grade tumors and more advanced stage disease [23]. Recently, other potential hereditary prostate cancer loci have been found at chromosome 1p36, chromosome 1q42.2–43, and the chromosome Xq27–28. It is estimated that the cancer susceptibility locus on X chromosome accounts for approximately 16% of hereditary prostate cancer cases and suggests an X-linked mode of inheritance [24].

The role of diet as a risk factor remains undetermined. While definite evidence is lacking, men may be able to lower their risk of developing and dying from prostate cancer by eating diets low in saturated fats (especially red meat) and calcium and high in tomatoes and tomato sauce (lycopenes), soy (isoflavones), vitamin E, and selenium [25]. Agent Orange, a defoliant utilized in the Vietnam War, has been associated with increased risk of prostate cancer. Other putative risk factors such as occupation, sexual behavior, infectious agents, vasectomy, cigarette smoking, and benign prostate conditions have not been demonstrated to alter the risk of prostate cancer [12].

Diagnostic modalities

The triad of DRE, serum PSA, and trans-rectal ultrasound (TRUS)-directed prostatic biopsy is used in the detection of prostate cancer [26]. Many authors have shown that DRE and serum PSA are the most useful and cost-effective first-line tests for assessing the risk of prostate cancer in an individual [27]. Others believe that serum PSA alone can be used efficiently as a screening test for prostate cancer, thus keeping the more costly and less well-tolerated DRE and TRUS as second step procedures [27]. With a combination of yearly PSA levels and DRE, close to 90% of prostate cancers can be diagnosed at a clinically-localized stage.

Digital rectal examination

DRE is the oldest detection test for prostate cancer. Physicians have traditionally used digital rectal examination in early detection efforts, despite a lack of evidence from controlled studies showing that the procedure reduces disease-specific mortality or net morbidity rates for prostate or rectal cancer [28]. In relatively unselected populations, 7–15% of men older than 50 years of age may have a suspicious DRE if the criteria for abnormal results are broadened to include induration and marked asymmetry in addition to frank nodularity [29].

The sensitivity of DRE is limited, however, because the examining finger can palpate only the posterior and lateral aspects of the gland. Studies suggest that 25–35% of tumors occur in portions of the prostate not accessible to the examining finger [30]. In addition, Stage T1 tumors, by definition, are non-palpable. DRE has a sensitivity of 55–68% in detecting prostate cancer in asymptomatic men [31,32] but values as low as 18–22% have also been reported in studies using

different screening protocols [6,7]. The DRE also has limited specificity, producing a large proportion of false-positive results. The reported positive predictive value in asymptomatic men is 6–33% [29,32] but appears to be somewhat higher when performed by urologists rather than by general practitioners [33] and varies relatively little with age.

Abnormal results on DRE increase the odds of finding a clinically significant intracapsular prostate tumor (>0.5 ml) 1.5- to 2-fold and increase the odds of extracapsular disease 3- to 9-fold [34]. In general, DRE misses a substantial proportion of cancers and detects most cancers at a more advanced pathologic stage when treatment is less likely effective.

Prostate-specific antigen

PSA has revolutionized the management of prostate cancer since its introduction into clinical practice in the 1980s. It is used not only in detection but also in staging of this common disease. Serum PSA has also been shown to be helpful in monitoring therapeutic response following different modalities.

PSA is a glycoprotein, serine protease, specific for prostatic epithelium and periurethral glands [35]. In screening studies, a serum PSA value greater than 4 ng/ml has a reported sensitivity of over 80% in detecting prostate cancer in asymptomatic men [32]. Approximately 2–3% of men screened for prostate cancer using serum PSA blood test will have prostate cancer [31]. In most screening studies involving asymptomatic men, the reported positive predictive value of an elevated serum PSA in detecting prostate cancer is 28–35% [8,32]. The positive predictive value of an elevated serum PSA when DRE is negative appears to be about 20% [36]. Ninety percent of cancers detected due to an elevated serum PSA level will be clinically localized and two-thirds will be found to be pathologically organ-confined if the prostate is removed [37].

Despite the impressive results of initial studies, PSA alone is not a perfect screening tool. Although a serum PSA level of 4.0 ng/ml or higher traditionally has been considered abnormal, the use of this cutoff point will miss approximately 21% of patients with prostate cancer. Also, many patients with benign prostatic conditions have elevations in serum PSA level; about 25% of men with benign prostatic hypertrophy (BPH) and no malignancy have an elevated serum PSA level [38]. Even though serum PSA testing has clearly

244

revolutionized early detection, a relatively large number of men continue to undergo TRUS-guided biopsy and are never found to have cancer.

Approximately 25% of the men with a serum PSA level between 4.0 and 10.0 ng/mL and normal DRE will harbor prostate cancer. Several techniques have been proposed to enhance the specificity of the PSA test in order to avoid unnecessary prostate biopsies in this subset of patients. PSA exists in multiple forms in the serum, and although most is complexed to protease inhibitors, a small fraction remains unbound. The percentage of free-PSA (free/total PSA ratio) is lower in men with prostate cancer. A recent prospective, multi-center clinical trial of the Hybritech (San Diego, Calif.) percent free-PSA assay demonstrated that a cutoff value of less than 25% free-PSA yielded a 95% cancer detection rate in men with total serum PSA levels between 4.0 and 10.0 ng/ml [39].

The serum concentration of PSA appears to be influenced by total prostate volume; thus some investigators have suggested that PSA density (the PSA concentration divided by the gland volume as measured by TRUS) may help differentiate benign from malignant disease [40]. In theory, this calculation corrects for the proportion of serum PSA elevation due to benign prostatic enlargement. According to these studies, a PSA density greater than 0.15 ng/ml may be more predictive of cancer. Other studies suggest that the rate of change (PSA velocity), rather than the actual PSA level, is a better predictor of the presence of prostate cancer. An increase of 0.75 ng/ml or higher per year has a reported specificity of 90% and 100% in distinguishing prostate cancer from BPH and normal glands, respectively [41]. Serum PSA values tend to increase with age, and investigators have therefore proposed age-specific PSA reference ranges (ASRRs) [42] (Table 1). ASRRs increase the specificity of PSA to detect prostate cancer. Investigators at Walter Reed Medical Center have shown that AAM with newly diagnosed prostate cancer have higher serum PSA values than do Caucasians, even after correcting for

stage, grade and tumor volume, and have subsequently developed different ASRRs for the AAM [43]. These data have not been universally accepted and different cutoffs have been advocated by other authors [44,45].

The use of PSA testing in conjunction with DRE in early detection programs for prostate cancer has been linked to a marked increase in the detection of localized disease and a simultaneous decline in both regional and metastatic prostate cancer. Improved understanding of the circulating molecular forms of the PSA molecule have further enhanced our ability to detect, stage, and monitor prostate cancer. Population-based data from the metropolitan Detroit Surveillance, Epidemiology, and End Results (SEER) Program supported the trend of early detection of prostate cancer due to rise in the routine use of serum PSA as a screening test for prostate cancer [46]. Local-stage cancer demonstrated the largest increase in incidence. The incidence of local-stage disease rose from a rate of 56.5 per 100,000 men in 1982 to a high of 167.9 per 100,000 in 1992 and then declined to a rate of 129.6 per 100,000 in 1996. With regard to grade, the incidence rate for moderately differentiated prostate cancers was the highest in 1993 at a rate of 122.9 per 100,000, rising from the 1982 rate of 22.8 per 100,000, and had been close to 100 per 100,000 for the years 1994 to 1996. The rates of the well- and poorly-differentiated cancers also increased at the same time as the moderately-differentiated cancers, although not nearly to the same extent, and have since dropped to the pre-1989 levels. The proportion of moderately-differentiated prostate cancer rose from 24.5% in 1982 to 61.7% in 1996. Stage-specific analysis showed that the proportion of moderately-differentiated cancers increased most dramatically in local-stage and regional-stage; however, distant-stage showed minimal change with grade over time. These data have provided important evidence that prostate cancer identified with serum PSA testing is more likely to be moderately- or well-differentiated and confined to the prostate.

Table 1. 'Normal' serum PSA values using traditional and age-specific reference ranges (ASRR)

Age (Years)	Traditional PSA normal for all men (ng/ml)	Traditional ASRRs [42] (ng/ml)	Walter Reed ASRRs [43] (ng/ml)	
			Caucasian	African–American
40–49	0–4.0	0–2.5	0–2.5	0–2.5
50–59	0–4.0	0–3.5	0–3.5	0–4.0
60–69	0–4.0	0–4.5	0–3.5	0–4.5
70–79	0–4.0	0–6.5	0–3.5	0–5.5

Transrectal ultrasound and needle biopsy

Sextant biopsy of the prostate under TRUS guidance, introduced a little more than 10 years ago, has revolutionized our ability to detect carcinoma of the prostate. Prostate biopsy methods have improved significantly. First, a smaller 18-guage biopsy needle has replaced a more traumatic 14-guage needle. Second, transrectal ultrasound-guided biopsy has replaced digital-guided transperineal biopsy. The smaller needle has resulted in less post-biopsy complications and allowed for more biopsies in one session, but it also provides less than half the tissue per needle as core compared with the 14-guage biopsy. However, based on a correlation study of prostate needle biopsies and matched prostatectomies, the accuracy of the 18-guage needle biopsy was similar to that reported with 14-guage biopsies.

Years of experience have shown that TRUS-directed spring-loaded biopsy, although very useful, has several limitations [47]. Prospective TRUS imaging data have demonstrated that biopsies directed toward irregularities on the image may be only slightly superior to random biopsies with regard to cancer detection [48]. Thus, the original lesion-directed biopsy has led to the development of the six-core, or sextant biopsy technique. Today, the trend is to increase the number of biopsies in order to compensate for the limitations of the imaging. At least, eight to ten biopsies are recommended to sample the prostate gland more adequately in an effort to increase diagnostic yield. Sextant biopsies plus additional biopsies directed more laterally is currently the preferred approach by many investigators. This technique has improved detection rates significantly [49].

Staging modalities

For surgeons, the goal of preoperative staging is to exclude those patients who are unlikely to be rendered disease-free following radical prostatectomy. The majority of urologists obtain routine CT, MRI, and radionuclide bone scans on all candidates for radical prostatectomy. It is generally assumed that the presence of gross capsular penetration, seminal vesicle invasion, lymph node metastases and systemic metastases diminish the probability of a surgical cure. Gross seminal vesicle invasion and extracapsular penetration (clinical stage T3 disease) are likely to be detected at the time of DRE, CT, TRUS, or MRI. However, extraprostatic disease is often detected only

histologically; current clinical staging techniques lack the sensitivity for detecting microscopic capsular penetration or seminal vesicle invasion.

In terms of staging, cross-sectional imaging studies have also provided little useful information for the majority of patients. CT scan is routinely used to detect pelvic lymph node metastasis. The detection of nodal metastases with CT scan is based on size criteria, with a nodal size of 1.0 cm often used as the upper limit of normal. However, reactive- and tumor-bearing lymph nodes frequently have a similar appearance; metastatic disease is generally not detected in non-enlarged lymph nodes, and nodal enlargement may not be due to metastases but due to reactive hyperplasia. In fact, up to 45% of metastatic lymph nodes are less than 0.4 cm in diameter [50]. Only 1% of the positive-staging pelvic lymph-adenectomies are found to have sufficient volume of nodal disease to be detected by CT. Tiguert et al. [51] found that lymph node size could not be used as a surrogate marker for the presence of lymph node metastasis. In that series, even though no patients had enlarged lymph nodes by CT criteria (greater than 1.5 cm), 8% of patients with lymph node metastasis and 12% of patients without lymph node metastasis had nodes with an axial dimension greater than 1.5 cm on final pathologic specimen. Therefore, CT is not a reasonable staging modality for identifying pelvic lymph node metastasis in patients with clinically-localized carcinoma of the prostate. Similarly, pelvic MRI has not been able to detect micrometastatic lymph node metastasis.

The ^{111}In-capromab pendetide scan, also known as the ProstaScint scan (Cytogen Corporation, Princeton, NJ) utilizes a radiolabeled monoclonal antibody directed toward an intracellular epitope (N-terminus) of the prostate-specific membrane antigen (PSMA) molecule. It is used to identify residual prostate cancer in the prostate bed or metastasis to lymphatic tissue, soft tissue, or bone [52]. It also has the potential to detect metastatic disease or local recurrence of prostate cancer. However, there are little published data regarding the use of this agent and, histologic confirmation of the results of the scan is lacking. Large-scale clinical trials with histologic confirmation of imaging findings are necessary before routine use of this agent in clinical practice can be recommended. Nonetheless, antibody-based imaging is an exciting and potentially useful approach, and results may improve as better antibodies are developed.

In men likely to have metastatic disease, a radionuclide bone scan is warranted and remains the most effective study to evaluate the patient for bone metastasis. The primary limitation of a radionuclide bone scan for identifying skeletal metastasis is its lack of specificity. Chybowski et al. [53] reported that radionuclide bone scans were always negative in subjects with serum PSA levels lower than 15 ng/ml. Therefore, routine use of bone scan on patients with PSA levels lower than 15 ng/ml is unnecessary provided the tumor is not poorly-differentiated and there are no musculoskeletal symptoms.

The ability to detect malignant spread at its earliest stage has been made possible by the advent of reverse transcriptase polymerase chain reaction (RT-PCR) assay. The underlying premise of the RT-PCR technique is that detection of prostate-specific mRNA in either the peripheral circulation or the bone marrow implies the existence of circulating prostate cells. Wood et al. [54] found PSA RT-PCR status to be a significant predictor for disease-free survival based on a multivariate analysis including serum PSA, and biopsy Gleason score. Similarly, Gao et al. [55] noted a positive correlation between the presence of circulating prostate cells in the bone marrow and PSA recurrence after radical prostatectomy. Although RT-PCR can detect the presence of a PSA-expressing cell, the assay does not provide information on tumor-specific molecular alterations that may have predictive power in identifying patients destined to develop overt metastasis. Phenotypic analysis of individual micrometastatic cells is a promising approach to give a more complete picture of this disease process including staging and prognostic information [56,57].

Endorectal surface coil magnetic resonance imaging is presently being touted as an accurate means of detecting periprostatic extension of prostate cancer. In a prospective study by Ogura et al., [58] the dynamic substraction technique was found to have an accuracy rate of 72% for tumor localization in the prostate gland, 84% for extracapsular extension, and 97% for seminal vesicle invasion. The accuracy of MRI in differentiating stage T2 from stage T3 was 82%. These results are very encouraging and deserve more attention.

Several investigators have examined the correlations between the preoperative serum PSA value, Gleason Score, clinical stage, and final pathologic stage [59,60]. All of the preoperative clinical factors are independently predictive of pathologic stage. Multivariate analyses have demonstrated that the predictive value of pathologic stage is increased when all 3 factors are considered simultaneously. Currently, the composite nomogram published by Partin et al. [61] provides

the best reference in evaluating pathologic stage when selecting a candidate for radical prostatectomy.

Survival

In the past two decades, success in early detection has been paralleled by technical improvements in radiation and surgery as therapy for localized cancer of the prostate. Improvements in surgical techniques, as well as in radiation methodologies and novel therapeutic approaches have also decreased the morbidity associated with the disease. Unfortunately, the most common cause of death from prostate cancer continues to be hormone-refractory metastatic disease.

We recently examined the influence of clinical and pathological parameters on survival after radical prostatectomy as monotherapy in the PSA era. The series included 1053 consecutive patients who underwent radical retropubic prostatectomy with bilateral lymph node dissection for clinically-localized prostate cancer at Wayne State University from 1990 to 1999 by full-time academic staff. Biochemical recurrence of disease was defined as a post-operative serum PSA > 0.4 ng/ml, with a rising trend.

Overall, the 10-year disease-free survival (DFS) was 82% with a mean follow-up of 48 months for the entire cohort. The 10-year DFS estimates for organ-confined disease, positive surgical margins, seminal vesicle invasion, and lymph node metastasis, were 96%, 82%, 43%, and 24%, respectively, $p = 0.0001$ (Figure 1).

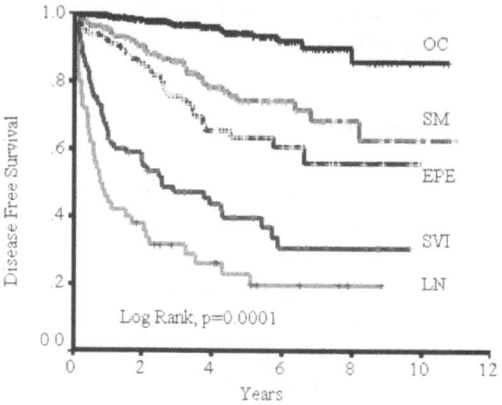

Figure 1. Kaplan–Meier curve for disease-free survival according to pathologic stage in patients undergoing radical retropubic prostatectomy at Wayne State University between 1900 and 1999. (OC = Organ confined, SM = Positive Surgical Margins, EPE = Extra-Prostatic Extension, SVI = Seminal Vesicle Invasion, LN = Positive Lymph Nodes).

In our study, both the biopsy and prostatectomy Gleason score correlated with overall disease-free survival, however, the correlation was stronger with the surgical specimens. The 8-year disease-free survival rates for biopsy Gleason score <7, 7, and >7 were 75%, 59%, and 50%, respectively ($p = 0.001$). The 8-year disease-free survival rates were 90%, 62%, and 28%, respectively, for prostatectomy Gleason score <7, 7, and >7 ($p = 0.001$) (Figures 2 and 3). When the overall disease-free survival was compared between biopsy and prostatectomy Gleason <7, the prostatectomy

Gleason had significant predictive advantage over the biopsy Gleason score ($p = 0.001$). While the overall disease-free survival was similar between biopsy and prostatectomy Gleason 7 ($p = 0.12$), a significantly worse disease-free survival was noted for prostatectomy Gleason >7 when compared to biopsy Gleason >7 ($p = 0.02$). These data demonstrate an inherent sampling problem when investigators attempt to use biopsy tissue to develop prognostic markers. The issue is that the small volume of tissue sampled by needle biopsy may sometimes fail to be representative of the true status of disease.

The vast majority of our patients were clinically staged preoperatively as T2a (45%) followed by T1c (30%), T2b (22%), and T1a-b (3%) (Table 2). Over the last 10 years, the percentage of patients with pathological organ-confined disease undergoing surgery has doubled with a concurrent increase in clinical T1c disease by almost 24-fold. While only 30% of patients operated in 1990–1991 had organ-confined disease in the final pathologic specimen, aggressive early detection strategies have allowed organ-confined disease rates of 60% over the last 2 years (Figure 4).

Interestingly, early detection and aggressive treatment can lessen some of the ethnic disparities noted

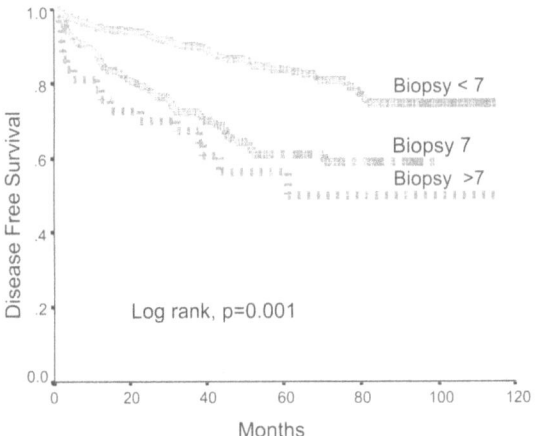

Figure 2. Kaplan–Meier curve for disease-free survival comparing biopsy Gleason score < 7, 7, >7, in patients undergoing radical retropubic prostatectomy at Wayne State University between 1900 and 1999.

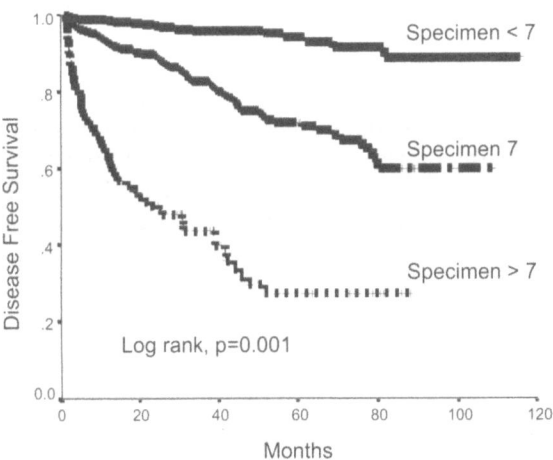

Figure 3. Kaplan–Meier curve for disease-free survival comparing specimen Gleason score <7, 7, >7, in patients undergoing radical retropubic prostatectomy for prostate cancer at Wayne State University between 1900 and 1999.

Table 2. Preoperative clinical staging in patients who underwent radical prostatectomy at Wayne State University between 1990 and 1999

Clinical stage	No (%)	PSA	No (%)
T1a-b	28 (3)	0–4	166 (16)
T1c	309 (30)	4–9	582 (56)
T2a	472 (45)	10–19	192 (18)
T2b	234 (22)	≥20	103 (10)

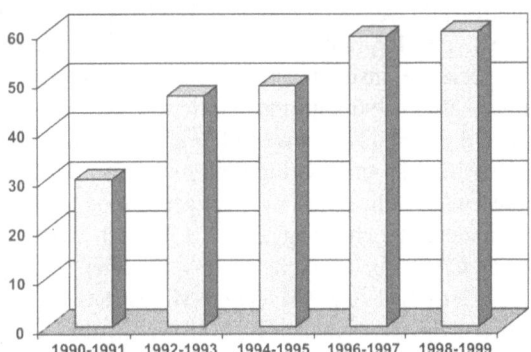

Figure 4. Organ-confined rate in patients undergoing radical retropubic prostatectomy at Wayne State University between 1900 and 1999.

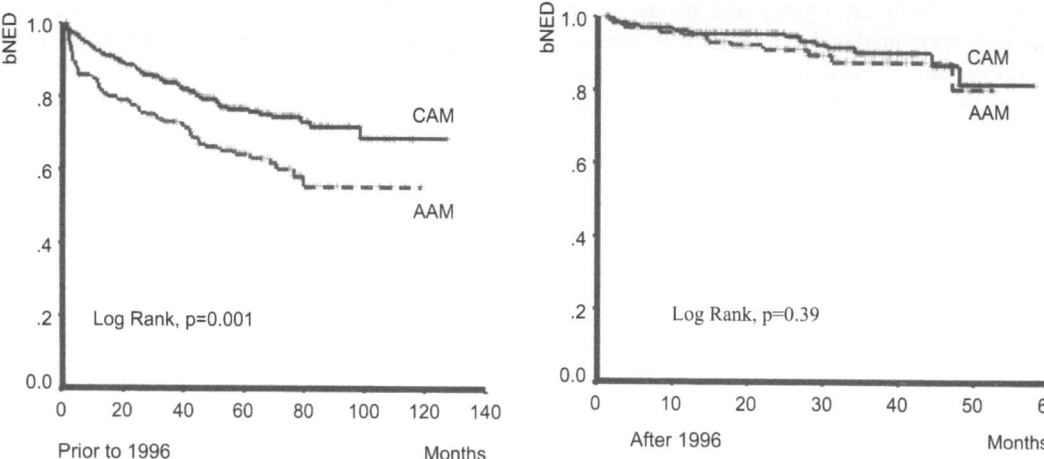

Figure 5. Kaplan–Meier curve for disease free survival between African American Males and Caucasian American Males before (left) and after (right) 1996 in patients undergoing radical retropubic prostatectomy at Wayne State University between 1900 and 1999.

among prostate cancer patients. In our study, a shift in stage was observed in both AAM and CAM groups, however, it was more pronounced in AAM. Non-palpable disease was present in only 16% of AAM undergoing surgery prior to 1996, compared to 44% of AAM undergoing surgery after 1996. Pathologically organ-confined disease was present in 37% of AAM treated prior to 1996 and 58% afterward ($p = 0.001$). The same phenomenon occurred in CAM where organ-confined disease rates for patients undergoing surgery before and after 1996 were 48% and 62%, respectively ($p = 0.004$).

The disease-free survival differences between CAM and AAM, were significant for patients undergoing surgery prior to 1996 but not afterwards (Figure 5). The calculated cancer-recurrence-free median probabilities at 42 months for patients undergoing surgery prior to 1996 were 81% and 68% for CAM and AAM, respectively (log-rank $p = 0.001$). These differences have become insignificant for patients undergoing surgery after 1996 with median disease-free survival probabilities at 42 months of 90% and 88% for CAM and AAM, respectively (log-rank $p = 0.39$). Furthermore, AAM who underwent surgery prior to 1996 experienced biochemical relapses almost twice as fast as CAM, for example: by 2 years after surgery, 22% *versus* 12% of AAM and CAM, respectively had recorded elevations in their PSA. However, after 1996, the overall recurrence rate by 2 years was 6%, and the disproportionate difference between AAM and CAM had narrowed to 1.9%.

The multivariate Cox proportional hazards model for patients undergoing surgery prior to 1996 indicated that pathological stage, specimen Gleason score, PSA and race all provided unique predictive information about cancer recurrence. However, race was not a significant predictor in the multivariate analysis of after 1996, while the other variables sustained their independence.

In conclusion, the life-expectancy of the patient, the natural history and curability of the prostate cancer, and the morbidity of treatment should all be considered prior to deciding appropriate management for an individual patient. Present literature provides strong evidence that clinical diagnosis of prostate cancer has a clinically significant impact on survival and that radical prostatectomy cures prostate cancer. Because of inherent uncertainties in life expectancy and biologic activity of different cancers, a randomized study will never provide a definitive recommendation for an individual patient. Thus, the patient and his priorities will always play a pivotal role in decisions related to the management of clinically-localized prostate disease.

References

1. Cancer Facts & Figures 2001, American Cancer Society http://www.cancer.org/downloads/STT/F&F2001.pdf accessed Dec 16, 2001
2. Aus G. Hugosson J, Norlen L: Long-term survival among men with conservatively treated localized prostate cancer. J Urol 154: 460–465, 1995

3. Ries LAG, Hankey BF, Miller BA: Cancer Statistics Review 1973–1988. Bethesda: National Cancer Institute (NIH Publication No. 91-2789), 1991

4. Ries LAG, Miller BA, Hankey BF, Kosary CL, Harras A, Edwards BK (eds) SEER Cancer Statistics Review, 1973–1991: Tables and Graphs. Bethesda: National Cancer Institute, 371 (NIH Publication No. 94-2789.), 1994

5. Schwartz KL, Severson RK, Gurney JG, Montie JE: Trends in the stage specific incidence of prostate carcinoma in the Detroit metropolitan area, 1973–1994. Cancer 15: 1260–1266, 1996

6. Wilt TJ, Partin MR, Liang BA: Outcome-based practice: Early detection and treatment of prostate cancer. Hosp Phys 37(2): 54–67, 2001

7. Labrie F, Dupont A, Candas B: Decrease of prostate cancer death by screening: First data from the Quebec prospective and randomized study. Proc Am Soc Clin Oncol, 1998, Los Angeles, California.

8. Catalona WJ, Smith DS, Ratliff TL, Basler JW: Detection of organ-confined prostate cancer is increased through prostate-specific antigen-based screening. JAMA 270: 948–954, 1993

9. Bartsch G, Horninger W, Klocker H, Oberaigner W, Severi G, Robertson C, Boyle P: Decrease in prostate cancer mortality following introduction of prostate specific antigen (PSA) screening in the federal state of Tyrol, Austria. (Abstract) J Urol 163 (Suppl 4): 88, Abstract 387, 2000

10. American Foundation for Urologic Disease. Prostate cancer resource guide. 1999–2000 edition. http://www.afud.org/pca/pcaindex.html accessed Dec 16, 2001

11. Mettlin C, Jones G, Averett H, Gusberg SB, Murphy GP: Defining and updating the American Cancer Society guidelines for the cancer-related checkup: Prostate and endometrial cancers. CA Cancer J Clin 43: 42–46, 1993

12. Pienta KJ, Esper RS: Risk factors for prostate cancer: Ann Intern Med 118: 793–803, 1993

13. Ries LA, Kosary CL, Hankey BF: SEER cancer statistics review, 1973–1994; tables and graphs. Bethesda (MD); US National Cancer Institute; NIH Publication No. 97-2789, 1997

14. Breslow N, Chan CW, Dhom G, Drury RA, Franks LM, Gellei B, Lee YS, Lundberg S, Sparke B, Sternby NH, Tulinius H: Latent carcinoma of prostate at autopsy in seven areas. Int J Cancer 20: 680–688, 1977

15. Edwards CN, Steinthorsson E, Nicholson D: An autopsy study of latent prostatic cancer. Cancer 6: 531–554, 1953

16. Halpert B, Schmalhorst WR: Carcinoma of the prostate in patients 70 to 79 years old. Cancer 19: 695–698, 1966

17. Scott R Jr, Mutchnik DL, Laskowski TZ, Schmalhorst WR: Carcinoma of the prostate in elderly men: Incidence, growth characteristics and clinical significance. J Urol 101(4): 602–607, 1969

18. Sakr WA, Haas GP, Cassin BF, Pontes JE, Crissman JD: The frequency of carcinoma and intraepithelial neoplasia of the prostate in young male patients. J Urol 150: 379–385, 1993

19. Parker SL, Davis KJ, Wingo PA, Ries LA, Heath CW Jr.: Cancer Statistics by Race and Ethnicity. CA Cancer J Clin 48(1): 31–48, 1998

20. Spitz MR, Currier RD, Fueger JJ, Babaian RJ, Newell GR: Familial patterns of prostate cancer: A case-control analysis. J Urol 146(5): 1305–1307, 1991

21. Smith JR, Freije D, Carpten JD, Gronberg H, Xu J, Isaacs SD, Brownstein MJ, Bova GS, Guo H, Bujnovszky P, Nusskern DR, Damber JE, Bergh A, Emanuelsson M, Kallioniemi OP, Walker-Daniels J, Bailey-Wilson JE, Beaty TH, Meyers DA, Walsh PC, Collins FS, Trent JM, Isaacs WB: Major susceptibility locus for prostate cancer on chromosome 1 suggested by a genome-wide search. Science 274(5291): 1371–1374, 1996

22. Gronberg H, Smith J, Emanuelsson M, Jonsson BA, Bergh A, Carpten J, Isaacs W, Xu J, Meyers D, Trent J, Damber JE: In Swedish families with hereditary prostate cancer, linkage to the HPC1 locus on chromosome 1q2-25 is restricted to families with early-onset prostate cancer. Am J Hum Genet 65(1): 134–140, 1999

23. Gronberg H, Isaacs SD, Smith JR, Carpten JD, Bova GS, Freije D, Xu J, Meyers DA, Collins FS, Trent JM, Walsh PC, Isaacs WB: Characteristics of prostate cancer in families potentially linked to the hereditary prostate cancer 1 (HPC1) locus. JAMA 278(15): 1251–1255, 1997

24. Xu J, Meyers D, Freije D, Isaacs S, Wiley K, Nusskern D, Ewing C, Wilkens E, Bujnovszky P, Bova GS, Walsh P, Isaacs W, Schleutker J, Matikainen M, Tammela T, Visakorpi T, Kallioniemi OP, Berry R, Schaid D, French A, McDonnell S, Schroeder J, Blute M, Thibodeau S, Trent J: Evidence for a prostate cancer susceptibility locus on the X chromosome. Nat Genet. 20(2): 175–179, 1998

25. Gann, PH: Diet and prostate cancer risk: The embarrassment of riches. Cancer Causes Control 9: 541–543, 1998

26. Littrup PJ, Kane RA, Mettlin CJ, Murphy GP, Lee F, Toi A, Badalament R, Babaian R: Cost effective prostate cancer detection. Cancer 74(12): 3146–3158, 1994

27. Candas B, Cusan L, Gomez J-L, Diamond P, Suburu RE, Levesque J, Brousseau G, Belanger A, Labrie F: Evaluation of prostate specific antigen and digital rectal examination as screening tests for prostate cancer. Prostate 45(1): 19–35, 2000

28. Gerber GS, Thompson IM, Thisted R, Chodak GW: Disease-specific survival following routine prostate cancer screening by digital rectal examination. JAMA 269(1): 61–64, 1993

29. Richie JP, Catalona WJ, Ahmann FR, Hudson MA, Scardino PT, Flanigan RC, deKernion JB, Ratliff TL, Kavoussi LR, Dalkin BL: Effect of patient age on early detection of prostate cancer with serum prostate-specific antigen and digital rectal examination. Urology 42(4): 365–374, 1993

30. McNeal JE, Bostwick DG, Kindrachuk RA, Redwine EA, Freiha FS, Stamey TA: Patterns of progression in prostate cancer. Lancet 1(8472): 60–63, 1986

31. Catalona WJ, Smith DS, Ratliff TL, Dodds KM, Coplen DE, Yuan JJ, Petros JA, Andriole GL: Measurement of prostate-specific antigen in serum as a screening test for prostate cancer. N Engl J Med 324(17): 1156–1161, 1991

32. Catalona WJ, Richie JP, Ahmann FR, Hudson MA, Scardino PT, Flanigan RC, deKernion JB, Ratliff TL,

Kavoussi LR, Dalkin BL: Comparison of digital rectal examination and serum prostate specific antigen in the early detection of prostate cancer: Results of a multicenter clinical trial of 6,630 men. J Urol 151(5): 1283–1290,1994

33. Pedersen KV, Carlsson P, Varenhorst E, Lofman O, Berglund K: Screening for carcinoma of the prostate by digital rectal examination in a randomly selected population. BMJ 300(6731): 1041–1044, 1990

34. Coley CM, Barry MJ, Fleming C, Mulley AG. Early detection of prostate cancer. Part I: Prior probability and effectiveness of tests. American College of Physicians. Ann Intern Med 126(5): 394–406, 1997

35. Elgamal AA, Van de Voorde W, Van Poppel H, Lauweryns J, Baert L: Immunihistochemical localization of prostate-specific markers within the accessory male sex glands of Cowper, Littre, and Morgagni. Urol 44(1): 84–90, 1994

36. Andriole GL, Catalona WJ: Using PSA to screen for prostate cancer: The Washington University experience. Urol Clin North Am 20(4): 647–651, 1993

37. Brawer MK, Chetner MP, Beatie J, Buchner DM, Vessella RL, Lange PH: Screening for prostatic carcinoma with prostate specific antigen. J Urol 147(3 Pt 2): 841–845, 1992

38. Oesterling JE: Prostate-specific antigen: A critical assessment of the most useful tumor marker for adenocarcinoma of the prostate. J Urol 145: 907–923, 1991

39. Catalona WJ, Partin AW, Slawin KM, Brawer MK, Flanigan RC, Patel A, Richie JP, deKernion JB, Walsh PC, Scardino PT, Lange PH, Subong EN, Parson RE, Gasior GH, Loveland KG, Southwick PC: Use of the percentage free prostate-specific antigen to enhance differentiation of prostate cancer from benign prostatic disease: A prospective multicenter clinical trial. JAMA 279(19): 1542–1547, 1998

40. Semjonow A, Hamm M, Rathert P, Hertle L: Prostate-specific antigen corrected for prostate volume improves differentiation of benign prostatic hyperplasia and organ-confined prostatic cancer. Br J Urol 73(5): 538–543, 1994

41. Carter HB, Pearson JD, Metter EJ, Brant LJ, Chan DW, Andres R, Fozard JL, Walsh PC: Longitudinal evaluation of prostate-specific antigen levels in men with and without prostate disease. JAMA 267(16): 2215–2220, 1992

42. Oesterling JE, Jacobsen SJ, Chute CG, Guess HA, Girman CJ, Panser LA, Lieber MM: Serum prostate-specific antigen in a community-based population of healthy men: Established of age-specific reference ranges. JAMA 270(7): 860–864, 1993

43. Moul JW: Use, Interpretation, and Prognostic Value of Total and Free PSA tests. Mediguide Urol 12(2): 1–8, 1999

44. Powell IJ, Banerjee M, Novallo M, Sakr W, Grignon D, Wood DP, Pontes JE: Should the age specific prostate specific antigen cutoff for prostate cancer biopsy be higher for black than for white men older than 50 years? J Urol 163(1): 146–149, 2000

45. Smith DS, Catalona, WJ, Bullock AD: Lower total PSA cutoffs for cancer screening in African American men. Urol 157(suppl): 160 Abstract No. 618, 1997

46. Schwartz KL, Grignon DJ, Sakr WA, Wood DP Jr: Prostate cancer histologic trends in the metropolitan Detroit area, 1982 to 1996, Urology 53(4): 769–774,1999

47. Aarnink RG, Beerlage, HP, De La Rosette JJ, Debruyne FM, Wijkstra H: Transrectal ultrasound of the prostate: innovations and future applications. J Urol 159: 1568–1579, 1998

48. Halpern EJ, Strup SE: Using gray-scale and color and power Dopler sonography to detect prostatic cancer. AJR Am J Roentgenol 174(3): 623–627, 2000

49. Chang JJ, Shinohara K, Bhargava V, Presti JC Jr: Prospective evaluation of lateral biopsies of the peripheral zone for prostate cancer detection. J Urol 160 (6 Pt 1): 2111–2114, 1998

50. Davis GL: Sensitivity of frozen section examination of pelvic lymph nodes for metastatic prostate carcinoma. Cancer 76: 661–668, 1995

51. Tiguert R, Gheiler EL, Tefilli MV, Oskanian P, Banerjee M, Grignon DJ, Sakr W, Pontes JE, Wood DP Jr: Lymph node size does not correlate with the presence of prostate cancer matastasis. Urology 53(2): 367–371, 1999

52. Sodee DB, Conant R, Chalfant M, Miron S, Klein E, Bahnson R, Spirnak JP, Carlin B, Bellon EM, Rogers B: Preliminary imaging results using IN-III labeled CYT-356 (Prostascint) in the detection of recurrent prostate cancer. Clin Nucl Med 21(10): 759–769, 1996

53. Chybowski FM, Keller JJ, Bergstralh EJ, Oesterling JE: Predicting radionuclide bone scan findings in patients with newly diagnosed untreated prostate cancer: Prostate specific antigen is superior to all other clinical parameters. J Urol 145(2): 313–318, 1991

54. Wood DP, Banerjee M: Presence of circulating prostate cells in the bone marrow of patients undergoing radical prostatectomy is predictive of disease free survival. J Clin Oncol 15(12): 3451–3457, 1997

55. Gao CL, Dean RC, Pinto A, Mooneyhan R, Connelly RR, McLeod DG, Srivastava S, Moul JW: Detection of circulating prostate specific antigen expressing prostatic cells in the bone marrow of radical prostatectomy patients by sensitive reverse transcriptase polymerase chain reaction. J Urol 161(4): 1070–1076, 1999

56. Cher ML, de Oliveira JG, Beaman AA, Nemeth JA, Hussain M, Wood DP Jr: Cellular proliferation and prevalence of micrometastatic cells in the bone marrow of patients with clinically localized prostate cancer. Clin Cancer Res 5(9): 2421–2425, 1999

57. Bianco FJ Jr, Wood DP Jr, Gomes de Oliveira J, Nemeth JA, Beaman AA, Cher ML: Proliferation of prostate cancer cells in the bone marrow predicts recurrence in patients with localized prostate cancer. Prostate 49(4): 235–242, 2001

58. Ogura K, Maekawa S, Okubo K, Aoki Y, Okada T, Oda K, Watanabe Y, Tsukayam C, Arai Y: Dynamic endorectal magnetic resonance imaging for local staging and detection of neurovascular bundle involvement of prostate cancer: Correlation with histopathologic results. Urology 57: 721–726, 2001

59. Partin AW, Yoo J, Carter HB, Pearson JD, Chan DW, Epstein JI, Walsh PC: The use of prostate-specific antigen, clinical stage, and Gleason score to predict pathological stage in men with localized prostate cancer. J Urol 150(1): 110–114, 1993

60. Badalament RA, Miller MC, Peller PA, Young DC, Bahn DK, Kochie P, O'Dowd GJ, Veltri RW: An algorithm for predicting non-organ confined prostate cancer using the results obtained from sextant core biopsies with prostate-specific antigen level. J Urol 156(4): 1375–1380, 1996

61. Partin AW, Kattan MW, Subong EN, Walsh PC, Wojno KJ, Oesterling JE, Scardino PT, Pearson JD: Combination of prostate specific antigen, clinical stage, and Gleason score to predict pathological stage of logical prostate cancer. JAMA 277(18): 1445–1451, 1997.

Address for offprints: David P. Wood Jr., Department of Urology, Wayne State University, 4160 John R., Suite 1017, Detroit, MI 48201, USA; *Tel:* (313) 745-7381; *Fax:* (313) 745-0464; *E-mail:* dwood@med.wayne.edu

Surgery for prostate cancer: Rationale, technique and outcomes

Tracy M. Downs, Christopher J. Kane, Gary D. Grossfeld, Maxwell V. Meng and Peter R. Carroll
Department of Urology and UCSF/Mt. Zion Comprehensive Cancer Center, UCSF Prostate Cancer SPORE, University of California, San Francisco, CA, USA

Key words: prostate cancer, prostatectomy, technique and outcomes

Summary

Prostate cancer is the most common non-cutaneous malignancy in men and poses a substantial risk to the life and health of patients. Treatment options for patients with prostate cancer are plentiful. Radical prostatectomy is one option that can be performed using several different surgical approaches. It can be performed with limited risk of complications and is likely to be curative in patients with organ-confined disease and those with limited extracapsular extension.

I. Rationale

Introduction

The case for early prostate cancer detection is supported by the following: the disease is burdensome; prostate specific antigen (PSA) improves detection of clinically important tumors without significantly increasing the detection of unimportant tumors; most PSA-detected tumors are curable using current techniques; and there is no cure for metastatic disease [1]. Treatment options for patients with prostate cancer are plentiful [2]. Radical prostatectomy is one option. The rationale supporting radical prostatectomy includes the following: (1) it is likely to be curative for organ-confined cancers and many cancers with limited disease beyond the prostate capsule (extracapsular extension), (2) a large number of cancers currently detected are curable using this technique, (3) morbidity associated with radical prostatectomy is limited when performed by experienced surgeons and (4) adjuvant therapy can be delivered safely and efficiently in selected, high-risk patients.

Radical prostatectomy can be performed through a lower abdominal incision (radical retropubic prostatectomy (RRP)), a perineal incision (radical perineal prostatectomy) or laparoscopically. Although, there are proponents for each technique, the endpoints for all are similar and include cancer cure and maintenance of acceptable urinary function and, if possible, potency in those potent before the procedure.

Prostate cancer staging and grading systems

A patient's prostate-specific antigen level, clinical tumor stage and Gleason grade provide valuable information to clinicians. The Tumor-Node-Metastases (TNM) system is used for the staging of prostate cancer (Table 1). The Gleason grade or score is a histologic grading system, which is used to characterize the aggressiveness of the malignancy. Cancers are graded on a scale ranging from 1 to 5, with 1, the most well-differentiated tumors and 5, representing poorly-differentiated tumors. The two most frequent architectural patterns of prostate cancer growth are assessed and the grades added (Gleason summary score) together to give an overall score from 2 to 10. Gleason summary 7 tumors have a significantly-worse prognosis than Gleason summary scores ≤6 but are not as aggressive as Gleason summary 8–10 cancers.

Patient selection

Radical prostatectomy should be considered in those patients with either organ-confined disease or those with limited extracapsular extension in which a clear or negative surgical margin is possible [2]. Such patients would include those with low- and intermediate-risk cancers defined by T1/T2 disease associated with serum PSA concentrations <10 ng/ml and no primary high-grade components (i.e. Gleason grade 4 or 5). Patients whose cancers have features of more-advanced, but non-metastatic disease may

M.L. Cher, K.V. Honn and A. Raz (eds.), Prostate Cancer: New Horizons in Research and Treatment, 253–268.
© 2002 *Kluwer Academic Publishers.*

Table 1. 1997 American Joint Committee on Cancer/International Union Against Cancer: Tumor-Node-Metastasis (TNM) Prostate Cancer Staging System [85]

Stage	Definition
Primary tumor, Clinical (T)	
TX	–Primary tumor cannot be assessed
T0	–No evidence of primary tumor
T1	–Clinically inapparent tumor not palpable nor visible by imaging
	–T1a: Tumor incidental histologic finding in 5% or less of tissue resected
	–T1b: Tumor incidental histologic finding in more than 5% of tissue resected
	–T1c: Tumor identified by needle biopsy (e.g. because of elevated prostate specific antigen levels)
T2	–Tumor confined within the prostate
	–T2a: Tumor involves one lobe
	–T2b: Tumor involves both lobes
T3	–Tumor extends through the prostate capsule
	–T3a: Extracapsular extension (unilateral or bilateral)
	–T3b: Tumor invades seminal vesicle(s)
T4	–Tumor is fixed or invades adjacent structures other than seminal vesicles, bladder neck or external sphincter, rectum, levator muscles, and/or pelvic wall.
Primary tumor, Pathologic (pT)	
pT2	–Organ confined
	–pT2a: Unilateral
	–pT2b: Bilateral
pT3	–Extraprostatic extension
	–pT3a: Extraprostatic extension
	–pT3b: Seminal vesicle invasion
pT4	–Invasion of bladder, rectum
Regional lymph nodes (N)	
NX	–Regional lymph nodes cannot be assessed
N0	–No regional lymph node metastasis
N1	–Metastasis in regional lymph node or nodes
Distant metastases (M)	
MX	–Distant metastasis cannot be assessed
M0	–No distant metastasis
M1	–Distant metastasis
	–M1a: Nonregional lymph nodes(s)
	–M1b: Bone(s)
	–M1c: Other site(s)

be candidates for the procedure. This would include patients whose cancers are of high grade, but low T stage (T1–T3a) and are associated with low serum PSA concentrations (<15 ng/ml). Although high-risk patients (T3b, Gleason sum 8, 9 or 10, or serum PSA >20 ng/ml) can undergo the procedure with acceptable morbidity and excellent rates of local control, long-term cure is less likely and such patients should be advised that adjuvant therapy might be necessary [3]. Such patients are at high risk of distant failure and should be considered for alternative techniques or adjuvant therapy following surgery.

Patients with low-risk cancers should be advised that excellent outcomes might be achieved with a variety of techniques, including surgery, radiation therapy and watchful waiting in selected patients. Although progression may occur slowly in the low-risk patient population, eventual treatment is likely in those who are young or have elevated or rising serum PSA levels [4]. Intermediate-risk patients are challenging as their disease has a high risk of progression if left untreated and somewhere between 30% and 60% may fail on the basis of serial PSA testing, despite standard therapy. More precise markers of progression would be beneficial to better select patients for treatment in this patient population.

Transrectal ultrasound guided prostate needle biopsy is the standard diagnostic tool used to make the diagnosis of prostate cancer. D'Amico and colleagues tested the hypothesis that the percent of positive prostate biopsies obtained, at the time of transrectal ultrasound guided biopsy, provides clinically-relevant information about early biochemical PSA failure following radical prostatectomy [5]. Controlling for the known prognostic factors of pretreatment, PSA and cancer grade and stage, they showed that the percent of positive biopsies (<34%, 34–50% and >50%) was an independent predictor of time to PSA-failure following surgery. Specifically, the majority of patients (80%) in the intermediate-risk group could be classified as either a low- (86–93%) or high-risk (8–11%) biochemical relapse-free survival cohort. Patients who are to undergo the procedure should be in good physical health and have a long life expectancy.

Indications for pelvic lymphadenectomy

Contemporary series of patients with localized prostate cancers suggest that few patients harbor lymphatic disease (4–9%) and the risk of lymph node metastases can be quantitated using preoperative parameters. Although lymphadenectomy is generally not considered a therapeutic intervention, in most patients, information gained may alter initial treatment decisions and certainly identifies patients who may be candidates for immediate adjuvant therapy. Whereas patients at intermediate- to high-risk of lymph-node metastases benefit from lymphadenectomy, those at low-risk may forgo lymphadenectomy and be treated with radical prostatectomy alone [6–8]. Meng and Carroll [9] suggested that lymph-node dissection is unnecessary in the subset of patients in which the risk of lymph-node involvement is less than 18%. The anticipated risk of lymph-node metastases can be calculated from the several nomograms or equations currently available.

II. Surgical management of prostate cancer

Technique of radical retropubic prostatectomy

Most often, radical prostatectomy is performed using general anesthesia. Some advocate the use of either epidural or spinal anesthesia in addition to a general anesthetic to decrease intraoperative blood loss and improve postoperative pain management. The use of Ketorolac, a non-steroidal anti-inflammatory medication, in the postoperative period may be beneficial [10–12]. Donation of autologous blood is offered to patients, but given the limited blood loss noted by most experienced surgeons, it may not be necessary [13–15].

The contemporary technique of RRP has been developed and refined by Walsh et al. [16,17]. Appreciating the anatomic relationships and pelvic regional anatomy is essential (Figure 1). Patients may be positioned supine or in the very low lithotomy position. A 6–8-cm lower midline abdominal incision is less-morbid for the patient compared to longer incisions and provides adequate exposure. A fixed retractor facilitates exposure of the prostate and regional anatomy. Lymphadenectomy may be performed selectively as described [9]. Exposure to the prostate is undertaken by first incising the endopelvic fascia from just lateral to the puboprostatic ligaments along the lateral edge of the prostate (Figure 2). Fibers of the levator ani are separated from the apex of the prostate. The pubprostatic ligaments, which provide anterior support of the urethra, are left intact over the urethra, but any attachments to the prostate are incised (Figure 3). Preservation of the

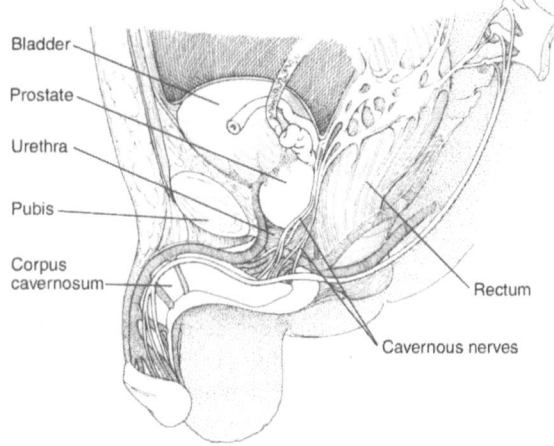

Figure 1. Sagittal section through the male pelvis.

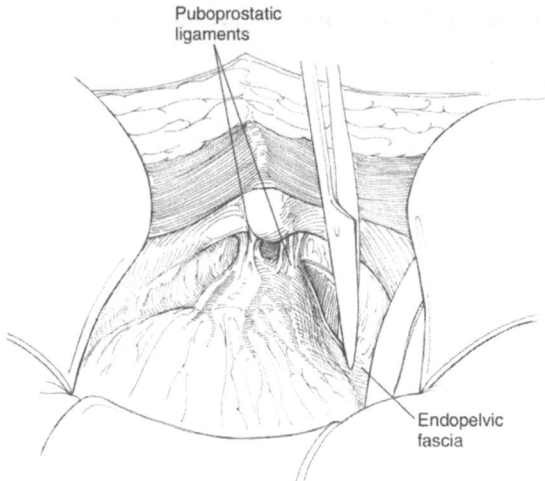

Figure 2. Incision in the endopelvic fascia is made just lateral to the puboprostatic ligaments. The incision is continued alongside the lateral edge of the prostate and extends to the base of the prostate proximally.

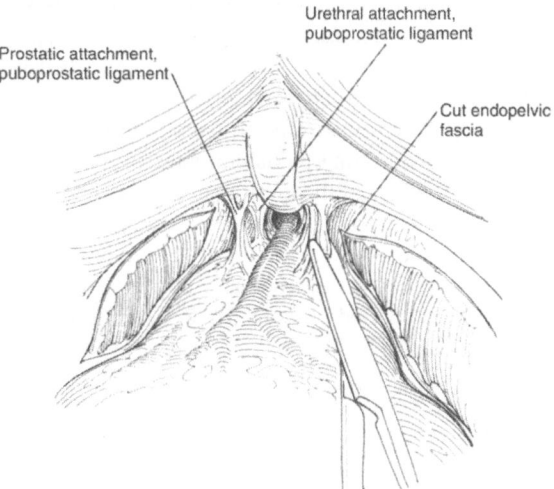

Figure 3. The pubo-prostatic ligaments are cut at their insertion into the anterior surface of the prostate. They are left intact over the urethra.

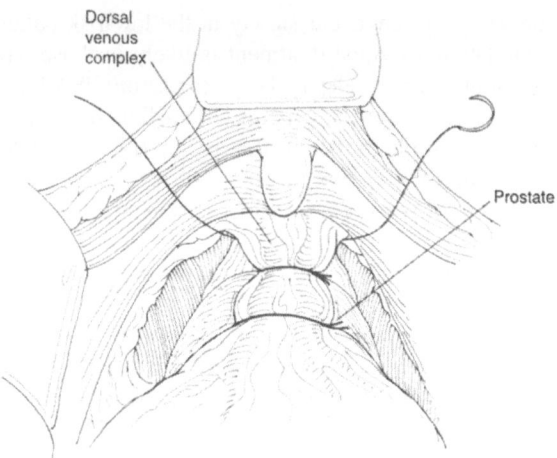

Figure 4. The dorsal vein complex is gathered proximally and distally with absorbable suture material.

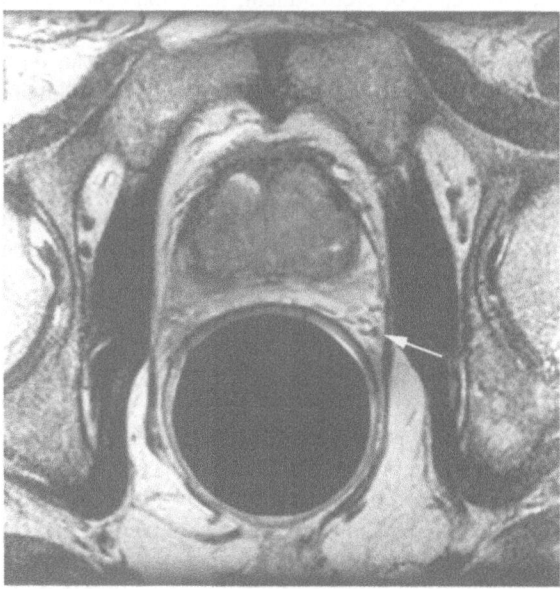

Figure 5. Endorectal MRI at the mid-portion of the prostate. The posterolateral course of the neurovascular bundles is noted (arrow).

pubprostatic (pubourethral) ligaments may facilitate earlier and more complete return of urinary continence compared to the use of previous techniques, which incised them over the urethra [18]. Next, the fascia, and overlying dorsal vein complex is gathered and suture ligated to facilitate exposure of the prostate, prevent bleeding from the complex, and to allow clear access to the urethra (Figure 4) [19].

The nerves and arterial blood supply (neurovascular bundles) crucial to potency run posterolaterally along either side of the prostate (Figure 5). In selected patients, the neurovascular bundle can be spared in an effort to preserve potency without sacrificing cancer control [17,20]. Conversely, extracapsular extension, when it does occur, may occur in the region(s) of the neurovascular bundles. These bundles should be preserved cautiously in those at high risk of extracapsular extension. The risk of extracapsular extension can be quantified using pretreatment nomograms or equations described previously. Such patients include those with multiple positive biopsies on a single side of the prostate, high-volume disease within a biopsy core, induration in the area of the neurovascular bundle or high-grade disease.

During nerve-sparing radical prostatectomy, the lateral prostatic fascia should be incised anterior to the bundles and the neurovascular bundles should be separated from the prostatic capsule before the urethra is incised. The incision in the lateral prostatic fascia is best made not at the apex of the prostate, but more proximally near the mid-portion of the prostate (Figure 6) [21]. Early experience with the use of a nerve-stimulation device during surgery, for the identification of the neurovascular bundles has yielded varied results and its usefulness during radical prostatectomy has yet to be determined [22,23].

Recent studies have suggested that intraoperative frozen section (IFS) analysis may be used to better determine the status of the surgical margin in patients undergoing nerve-sparing radical prostatecotmy [24]. We recently examined the use of IFS analysis in 101 patients undergoing nerve-sparing radical prostatectomy at the University of California, San Francisco (UCSF). IFS analysis was performed on the surgical margin thought to be at risk for tumor involvement based on the results of systematic prostate biopsy, transrectal ultrasound or intraoperative inspection. If the frozen section was positive, additional tissue (including the neurovascular bundle when appropriate)

was subsequently removed. IFS results were identical to those obtained on the final, permanent section in 92 of the 101(91%) cases. Of the 15 patients with a positive frozen section, 11 had identical findings on the permanent pathologic sections. In this group with positive-IFS, twelve (80%) had no evidence of tumor in additionally resected tissue. The positive and negative predictive values for the IFS technique were 73% and 94%, respectively. The risk of recurrence in patients with either positive or negative IFS findings was similar. These data suggest that IFS may be applied during radical prostatectomy to spare the neurovascular bundles in select patients.

Once the neurovascular bundles have been separated unilaterally or bilaterally from the prostatic capsule (in cases of nerve-sparing surgery), the urethral incision can be performed. Next, an anterior incision is made and the Foley catheter is grasped and pulled into the wound before being cut distally (Figure 7). The posterior portion of the urethra can be incised sharply under direct vision. Once the posterior portion of the urethra and sphincter have been cut, the rectourethralis muscle and Denonvilliers' fascia are identified [25].

The lateral pedicles, containing branches of the prostatic and rectal arteries are ligated alongside the prostate. Dissection proceeds superiorly or cranially exposing Denonvilliers' fascia over the seminal vesicles and ampullae of the vas deferens (Figure 8). After the fascia has been incised, the ampullae are clipped or tied before being cut and each seminal vesicle is excised in its entirety. The prostate is then separated from the bladder neck circumferentially. Bladder neck preservation may allow for earlier and more complete return of urinary continence compared to techniques

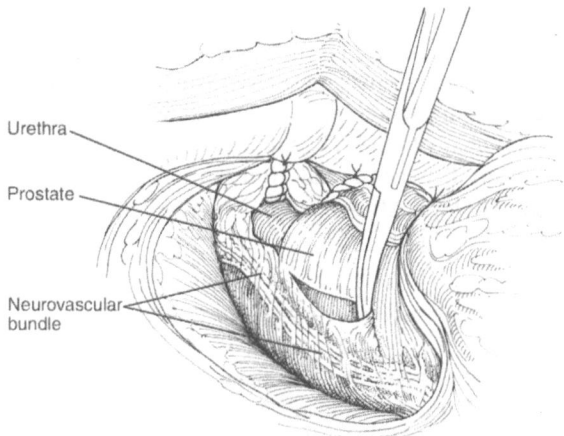

Figure 6. The lateral prostatic fascia is incised and the neurovascular bundle(s) is gently dropped posteriorly away from the prostatic capsule.

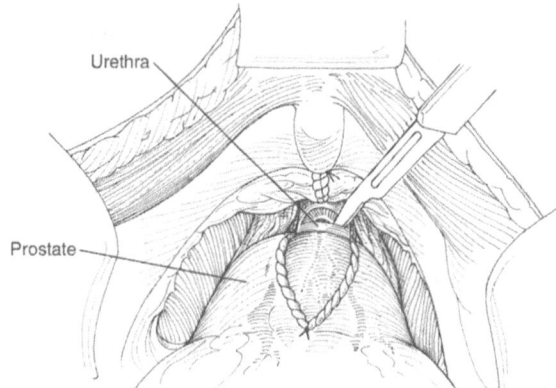

Figure 7. The anterior surface of the urethra in incised exposing the urethral catheter, which is grasped and cut.

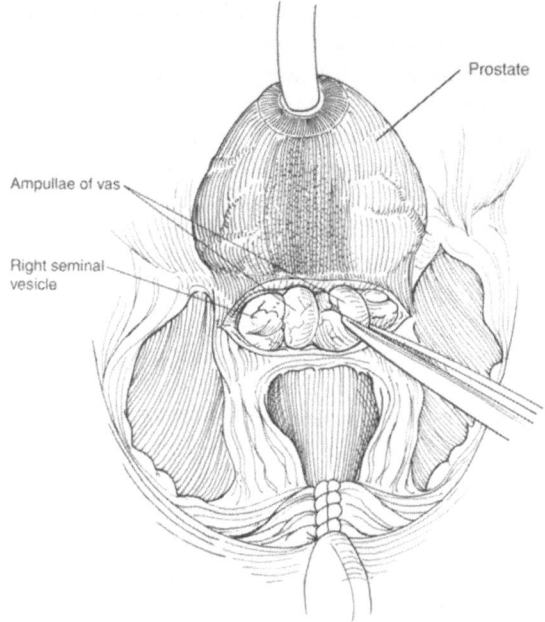

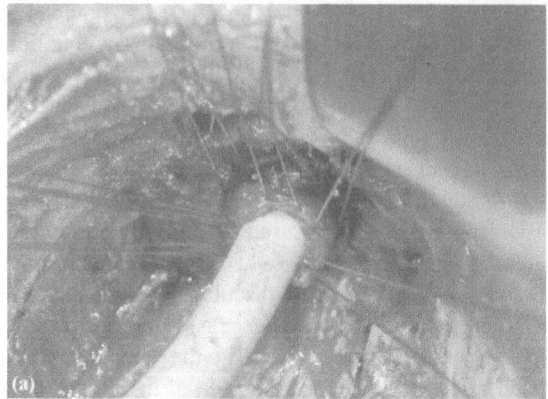

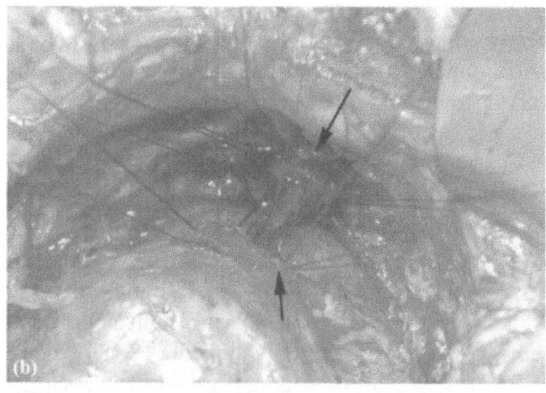

Figure 8. Denovillier's fascia is incised over the seminal vesicles and ampullae of the vas deferens.

whereby the bladder neck is excised more extensively [26]. The bladder neck can be narrowed in a 'racket handle' fashion, if necessary, using a continuous 4–0 or 3–0 absorbable suture.

The bladder neck is sutured to the urethra using interrupted 3–0 or 4–0 suture material over a 16 or 18 Fr. urethral catheter. The sutures should include only the cut end of the urethra and not the levator musculature or nerve fibers (Figure 9). A closed drainage system is placed and the wound is closed; the drain is usually removed on the second postoperative day. As patients are usually hospitalized for only 2 days, it may be best to close the skin using fine running subcuticular sutures rather than staples to avoid an early return visit for staple removal.

Patients thought to be at an increased risk of postoperative urinary incontinence (i.e. advanced age, previous radiation, and cancer at the apex requiring wide excision) may be candidates for autologous fascial sling placement at the time of radical prostatectomy. A strip of rectus fascia measuring approximately 1/8 cm is harvested and the ends of the fascia are plicated with 2–0 absorbable or non-absorbable suture. After the vesico-urethral anastamosis is completed, the sling is carefully placed underneath the anastamosis using a right-angled clamp, at the level of the anastamosis and external sphincter and not more

Figure 9. (a) The distal sphincteric continence mechanism is well preserved and eight absorbable sutures are placed for the anastamosis (intra-operative photograph). (b) The new bladder to urethral anastamosis is brought down into the pelvis and the sutures tied between the bladder and urethra (arrows, intra-operative photograph).

proximally. The free suture ends are placed through the ipsilateral rectus fascia. The rectus fascia is closed inferiorly using interrupted absorbable suture material and the sling sutures are tied loosely, without tension, on the rectus fascia. The urethral catheter is removed generally between 5 and 10 days following the procedure [27]. Contrast studies are not necessary before catheter removal.

Technique of radical perineal prostatectomy

Young performed the first radical perineal prostatectomy (RPP) in 1904 and many modifications have been made since then [28–30]. While the majority of patients with newly diagnosed prostate cancer, are good candidates for either a perineal or retropubic radical prostatectomy, there are certain instances when one approach may be favored. Instances where the perineal approach might be favored would include patients with a history of renal transplantation, prior extensive bladder surgery or the morbidly-obese patients. Instances where the retropubic approach might be a better option would include patients with large prostate size (> 100–120 g), history of perineal or rectal surgery or rectocutaneous fistulae and patients who cannot be placed in an exaggerated dorsal lithotomy position. Previously it was thought RPP had distinct advantages over RRP such as lower blood loss (by avoiding Santorini's plexus), less patient-discomfort, quicker return of bowel function and shorter hospitalization [31–33]. One disadvantage with the perineal approach was the requirement of two surgical incisions, one for the lymph-node dissection and the other for the radical prostatectomy. Laparoscopic pelvic lymph-node dissection has eliminated the need for this second incision and with current nomograms and lymph-node predictive models, pelvic lymph-node dissection can be eliminated in selected patients [9,34].

Several contemporary studies have compared the relative merits of radical perineal and RRP [32,33,35]. Each study reported lower blood loss and fewer blood transfusions with the perineal approach. The average blood loss in these studies was 1138–2000 ml in the RRP groups compared to 415–802 ml in the RPP groups [32,33,35]. The investigators concluded that in similar patient populations, RPP offers equivalent clinical outcomes, while causing significantly less blood loss. Sullivan et al. in an non-randomized study reported improved clinical outcomes for RPP compared to RRP in terms of a shorter hospital stay (4.5 days vs. 6.7 days), quicker return to a regular diet (2.3 days vs. 5.1 days) and fewer days of parenteral analgesics (1.7 days vs. 3.8 days) [32]. However, RRP series show that when the operation is performed by experienced surgeons that equivalent or improved outcomes compared to the perineal approach can be achieved in terms of low blood loss, less patient discomfort and shorter hospitalization.

The incontinence rate following RPP ranges from 4% to 8% [33,36–39]. During the perineal dissection the puboprostatic ligaments are left intact around the membranous urethra and this may contribute to maintenance of urinary continence. In patients with 'good' preoperative potency who underwent nerve-sparing procedures, 70% remained potent in one series [37].

Positive surgical margins have been detected in 9–44% of radical perineal prostatectomy series [32–35,37,40]. Weldon et al. [37] reported the pattern of positive surgical margins in 200 consecutive radical perineal prostatectomies for clinical stage T1/T2 adenocarcinoma of the prostate. The overall positive surgical margin rate was 44% in this series. With the perineal approach, there appears to be fewer positive apical margins (7% RPP vs. 10–48% RRP) and posterolateral margins (16% RPP vs. 26–44% RRP) but more positive anterior margins (25% RPP vs. 2–10% RRP) [41–43]. New onset of fecal incontinence (18%) and rectal injuries (0–11%) may be more common with the perineal approach [44]. Anastomotic strictures may be more common with the retropubic approach (4% RRP vs. 2% RPP). In summary, RPP and RRP have very similar outcomes and surgeon experience may be the most important reason for selecting one approach over the other.

Technique of laparoscopic radical prostatectomy

The first report of laparoscopic radical prostatectomy (LAPRP) by Schussler et al. [45] in 1997 demonstrated the feasability of the procedure. Guillonneau et al. [46] reported the results of 40 patients who had LAPRP performed at the Institut Mutualiste Montsouris, Paris, France. Their operative time averaged 4.5 h, catheter time was 7.6 days and the transfusion rate was 17.5%. They reported a 17.5% positive margin rate with 89.7% undetectable serum PSA at one month of follow-up.

After induction of general anesthesia, an oral-gastric tube is placed, which is removed immediately following the operation, and the patient is placed in the supine or low lithotomy position with the legs spread to allow rectal or perineal access.

We use a five-port technique with the first being a 12-mm port placed infraumbilically. The ports are placed in a fan distribution with two, 12-mm ports lateral to the rectus abdominus muscles, in a line 2–5 cm inferior to the infraumbilical port and two, 5-mm ports 3 cm medial to the anterior superior iliac spines (Figure 10). The primary surgeon works from the patient's left side through the left iliac and left pararectus ports. The patient is placed in Trendelenberg position and a transverse peritoneal incision is made in the pouch of Douglas. The vas deferens is clipped and transected on each side and the seminal vesicles are dissected circumferentially. A transverse incision is made in Denonvillier's fascia at the seminal-vesicle–prostate junction allowing access between the fascia and the anterior perirectal fat. After filling the bladder with 200 ml of sterile water a peritoneal incision is made in the anterior abdominal peritoneum

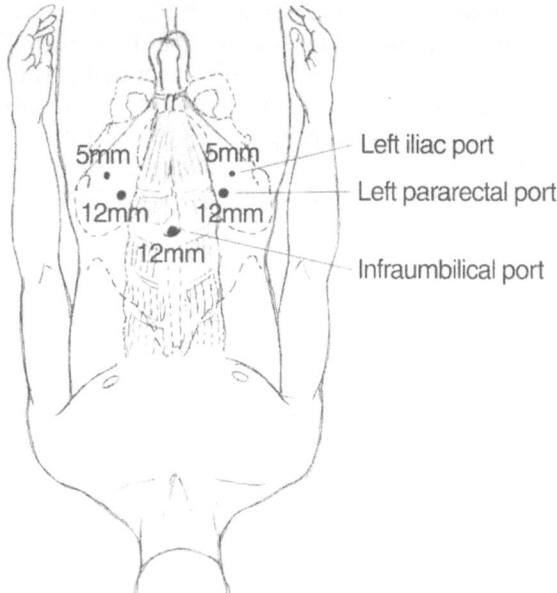

Figure 10. Positioning of ports for laparoscopic radical prostatectomy.

starting lateral to one obliterated umbilical artery, across the urachus and extending lateral to the other obliterated umbilical artery. The endopelvic fascia is incised preserving the puboprostatic ligaments. Next, an endoscopic babcock clamp is used to bunch the dorsal venous complex and an articulating endoscopic gastrointestinal anastomotic stapler (Endo-GIA, US Surgical, Norwalk, CT) is placed as distal as possible on the dorsal vein; care is taken not to include the urethra in the stapler. The anterior bladder neck is incised and the Foley catheter balloon is deflated and the tip grasped. Next, the posterior bladder neck is transected. For a nerve-sparing procedure, the lateral prostatic fascia can be visualized and incised antegrade so that the neurovascular bundle can be visualized. As the prostate is retracted posteriorly, the apical dissection is performed until the anterior surface of the urethra is identified. The anterior urethra is sharply divided, the catheter is withdrawn and gently lifted by the assistant allowing the posterior portion of the urethra to be visualized and transected. With cranial retraction on the prostate, the rectourethralis attachments are divided and the remaining attachments between the prostate and prostatic pedicles or Denonvillier's fascia are divided. The free specimen is placed in the left lower abdomen for retrieval at the end of the case.

The vesico-urethral anastomosis is then performed using either a running or an interrupted anastomosis.

The specimen is retrieved and delivered through the infraumbilical port, enlarging it if necessary. A closed suction drain is placed, utilizing one of the 5-mm ports. Subcuticular skin closure is performed and small dressings are placed.

Numerous centers worldwide are now performing laparoscopic radical prostatectomy, however the true benefits, if any, of LAPRP over standard radical prostatectomy are not clear. The potential benefit of more precise dissection due to the magnification and illumination of the laparoscope exists, but significant improvements in most clinical outcomes have not been seen yet. Factors which LAPRP may achieve similar results to standard open radical prostatectomy are cancer control, urinary continence and potency preservation. Areas in which LAPRP may improve upon results from standard open prostatectomy include less postoperative pain, earlier return to full activities, and less blood loss. Currently, LAPRP appears to be associated with longer operative times, operating room charges, and total cost of hospitalization.

III. Outcomes

Cancer control

Contemporary methods of radical prostatectomy for patients with clinically localized disease are generally associated with excellent outcomes (Tables 2–4). Survival may be reported in several ways: overall survival, cause-specific survival and biochemical relapse-free survival. Paulson et al. [47] reported a 90% cancer specific survival at 13.5 years after radical perineal prostatectomy for patients with organ confined and specimen confined disease. In an independent analysis of men treated with RRP at the Mayo Clinic, Zincke et al. [48,49] reported crude and cause specific survival rates of 75% and 90%, respectively. The crude survival rates at ten and fifteen years after surgery were similar to those of age-matched men from the general population without prostate cancer.

However, between 22% and 50% of patients thought to have organ-confined prostate cancer at the time of surgery are later found to have disease beyond the prostate based on a careful review of the surgical specimen [50–53]. Given the protracted nature of prostate cancer and the fact that residual and/or recurrent disease may respond to salvage or secondary therapy such as radiation or androgen deprivation, postoperative follow-up with serum PSA testing has become an

Table 2. Biochemical relapse-free survival following radical prostatectomy

Institution	N	5-yr (%)	10-yr (%)	Outcome (ng/ml)	Follow-up (yr)
Washington Univ. et al. [56]	925	78	61	PSA < 0.6	2.3 (mean)
Duke et al. [59]	1319	65–70	—	PSA < 0.5	4 (median)
Baylor et al. [58]	500	77	74	PSA < 0.4	2.7 (median)
UCLA et al. [60]	601	69	47	PSA < 0.4	2.8 (median)
		86	78	clinically free of disease	
Mayo Clinic et al. [48]	3170	70	52	PSA < 0.2	5.0 (mean)
		85	72	clinically free of disease	
Cleveland Clinic et al. [50]	423	59	—	PSA < 0.2	4.3 (median)
		84	—	clinically free of disease	
John Hopkins et al. [62]	2404	84	74	PSA < 0.2	6.3 (mean)
UCSF	666	78	—	PSA < 0.2	3.1 (mean)

Table 3. Summary of RPP series

Series	N	PSA* (ng/ml)	Clinical stage	Gleason grade	EBL (ml)	Hospitalization (days)	Continence (%)	Potency (%)	Positive margins (%)	Biochemical relapse-free survival (%)	Mean follow-up (months)
Frazier et al. [33]	122	NA	B (85%)	NA	565	12	96	77	29	NA	NA
Lance et al. [35]	190	6.93	97% (≤T2b)	NA	802#	NA	65	8	43	82	42.9
Sullivan et al. [32]	138	6.48	98% (≤T2b)	5.27	416	4.5	72	NA	9	70	30
Weldo et al. [34]	200	12.2	T1 (16%) T2 (84%)	≤6 (79%)	NA	NA	NA	NA	44	79	35
Weldo et al. [37]	220	11.4	T1 (16%) T2 (82%)	≤6 (73%)	645	NA	95	70	NA	NA	NA
Parra et al. [40]	500	NA	NA	NA	270	1.5	94	47	16	NA	NA

*Mean value; #Median.

Table 4. Summary of LAPRP series

Series	N	Time (h)	EBL (ml)	Transfusion rate (%)	Conversion (%)	Positive margin (%)	Continence (%)	Potency with Bilat. nerve-sparing (%)	Hospitalization (days)
Schussler et al. [45]	9	9.4	640	0	0	11	67	50	7.3
Raboy et al. [86]	2	4.8	500	50	0	50	NA	NA	2.5
Guillonneau and Vallencien [87]	120	4.0	402	10	5.8	15	72	45	6.6
Abbou et al. [88]	43	4.3	NA	4.7	0	27.9	84	14	7.2
Van Velthoven et al. [89]	22	6.7	490	31	23	23	NA	NA	NA
Rassweiler et al. [90]	180	4.5	1230	31	4.4	16	97 (12 mo)	NA	10
Tuerk et al. [91]	152	4.4	185	1.3	0	23.4	92	NA	NA
Zippe et al. [92]	50	5.4	225	2	2	20	76	31	1.6

important endpoint in follow-up. Virtually all recurrent clinical and metastatic disease is preceded by a rising PSA, and only a few sporadic cases of recurrence have been reported in the absence of a detectable serum PSA level. Biochemical failure is defined as either the persistence of a detectable PSA after surgery or the development of a detectable PSA in those with a previously undetectable postoperative level. What constitutes a detectable serum PSA varies among investigators and the use of ultra- or hypersensitive PSA assays improves the lead-time for early detection of recurrence [54,55].

Radical retropubic prostatectomy is associated with overall five- and ten-year actuarial biochemical progression-free survival rates ranging from 59–83% and 47–74%, respectively [48,50,56,57–61]. Biochemical relapse-free survival following RPP ranges from 70% to 82.4% with mean follow-up of 30 months to 42.9 months [32,34,35]. Biochemical relapse typically occurs prior to any evidence of clinical disease recurrence. This is reflected by higher clinical disease-free rates at 84–86% (5 year) and 72–78% (10 year). The variability in outcomes across different series and techniques most likely reflects differences in patient selection and definition of biochemical failure and, to a lesser extent, variations in surgical technique.

In two contemporary RRP series from the Cleveland Clinic and John Hopkins Hospital, totaling more than two thousand patients, no patients showed signs of clinical disease in the absence of PSA failure [50,57]. Following biochemical (PSA) failure, up to 68% of men progressed to detectable clinical disease at a median follow-up of 19 months. With adjuvant therapy such as radiation or androgen deprivation at the time of PSA failure, the rate of progression to clinical disease was reportedly lower at 21% [50]. Metastatic disease following PSA failure occured in 34% of patients without adjuvant or salvage therapy, and investigators reported a median actuarial time to metastases of eight years from the time of PSA failure [57]. For those who develop metastatic disease, the median actuarial time to death in one series was five years from the date of metastasis.

Johns Hopkins recently reported their long-term biochemical disease-free and cancer-specific survival in 2404 patients managed with radical prostatectomy [62]. Mean follow-up was 6.3 ± 4.2 years (range, 1–17 yr) and 26% of patients ($n = 621$) were followed for at least 10 years. The overall actuarial PSA progression-free, metastasis-free and cancer-specific survival at 5-, 10-, and 15-years was 84%, 74%, 66%; 96%, 90%, 82%, and 99%, 96%, 90%, respectively.

Patients with clinical stage $\leq$T2 had a 5-, 10-, and 15-year recurrence-free actuarial survival rate of 86%, 76%, and 71% compared to 60%, 49% in patients with T3a disease (15-yr data not available for T3a patients). For patients stratified into pre-treatment PSA values of $\leq$4 ng/ml, 4.1–10 ng/ml, 10.1–20 ng/ml, and >20 ng/ml risk groups, 5-, 10-, and 15-year recurrence-free actuarial survival rates were 94%, 91%, 67%; 89%, 79%, 75%; 73%, 57%, 54%, and 60%, 48%, 48%, respectively. Patients stratified based upon post-operative Gleason-score of $\leq$6, 7(3 + 4), 7(4 + 3), and 8–10 had 5-, 10-, and 15-year recurrence-free actuarial survival rates of 98%, 94%, 86%; 81%, 60%, 59%; 53%, 33%, 33%, and 44%, 29%, 15%, respectively. The Gleason 7(4 + 3) group had progression-free survival rates similar to the Gleason 8–10 group. Patients with pathologically organ confined disease (i.e. $\leq$pT2) had a 5-, 10-, and 15-year recurrence-free actuarial survival rate of 97%, 93%, and 84%, respectively.

The kinetics of biochemical recurrence correlates with the pattern of relapse. Patel et al. [63] found that patients with PSA doubling times of six months or greater had an 80% clinically disease-free rate at a mean follow-up of 58 months as compared to 64% in those with PSA doubling-times of less than six months. Furthermore, patients who progressed to aggressive distant metastatic disease had a shorter median PSA doubling time than those with only biochemical failure or local disease recurrence (4.3 vs. 11.7 months, respectively) [64].

General complications

Contemporary methods of radical prostatectomy are associated with limited morbidity. Perioperative mortality is exceedingly rare, at approximately 0.2% [20,48]. Intra-operative rectal injury and the need for a colostomy has decreased from 1% and 0.2%, respectively, prior to 1988 to 0.6% and 0.06%, currently. Similarly, complications such as myocardial infarction (0.1–0.4%), deep venous thrombosis (1.1%), pulmonary embolism (0.75%), blood transfusions (<5%), anastamotic stricture (4%), inguinal hernia (1%), and incisional hernia (0.6%) are becoming more uncommon. Complication rates are likely to decrease with further experience and refinements in technique [65].

Urinary function

After radical prostatectomy, immediate postoperative incontinence may occur in up to 80% of patients. More contemporary series report a much lower rate of immediate incontinence [20,66]. The wide variability in postradical prostatectomy incontinence rates reported in the literature is due to contemporary improvements in surgical technique and differing definitions over what constitutes urinary continence. Approximately 90% of men who undergo radical prostatectomy will be continent at one year when continence is defined as no regular use of pads and/or no leakage with moderate exercise. Severe and persistent incontinence defined as leakage with normal activity or the need for three or more pads per day occurs in 1–6% of patients. Such patients may be candidates for use of an artificial sphincter or periurethral collagen injection [67].

At UCSF, a contemporary cohort of patients ($n = 217$) underwent radical retropubic prostatectomy and were surveyed anonymously using a detailed validated questionnaire. Overall continence, one year after radical prostatectomy was 98% as defined above. Average time to continence was two to four weeks. Immediate continence was achieved in 23% of men. Over half (55%) of men were continent by one month.

Sexual function

Return of potency after radical prostatectomy is not only a function of technique (i.e. nerve-sparing procedure) but is also dependent on others factors. Rabbani et al. [68] studied 314 consecutive men managed with radical prostatectomy to determine predictors of the recovery of sexual function following surgery. Patient age, preoperative potency status and extent of neurovascular bundle preservation were predictive of potency recovery. At 3 years following the operation, 76%, 56% and 47% of those ages <60, 60–65 and >65 years of age were potent. Not surprisingly men with only partial erections preoperatively and those who underwent unilateral nerve-sparing surgery were less likely to recover potency, 47% and 25%, respectively. All studies suggest that the patients most likely to benefit from nerve-sparing surgery are those who are young, potent, sexually active and have focal disease. It also appears that return of spontaneous erections following nerve-sparing surgery may be improved with early use of either sildenafil or intracavernous injection therapy [69–71]. Sural nerve grafting at the time of radical prostatectomy in those patients where resection of the neurovascular bundle is necessary to achieve adequate surgical margins has been described [72]. However, given the considerable shift from higher-stage disease (T2) to lower-stage disease (T1), most

patients currently undergoing radical prostatectomy are candidates for preservation of their neurovascular bundles, which is likely to result in better preservation of sexual function than the use of sural nerve grafts.

Potency following radical prostatectomy can be restored in a variety of ways. Men who have undergone nerve-sparing surgery who have not regained erections adequate for vaginal penetration may be excellent candidates for the use of sildenafil. Approximately, 43–75% of such patients may respond to this drug favorably [69–71]. For those who do not respond to sildenafil or are not candidates for it, use of either intraurethral or intracorporeal therapy will likely result in adequate return of potency. Uses of vacuum erection devices and, less commonly, insertion of a penile prosthesis are other alternatives.

IV. Neoadjuvant and adjuvant therapy

A significant number of men who undergo standard local treatment for prostate cancer will experience biochemical recurrence. The risk of biochemical and clinical recurrence is related to cancer stage, volume and grade, preoperative serum PSA, and surgical margin status.

The effects of neoadjuvant androgen deprivation therapy may be evaluated by its ability to reduce prostate volume (i.e. down sizing), lower clinical and pathologic tumor stage (i.e. down staging),) as well as to reduce the incidence of positive surgical margins.

For locally-advanced (clinical stage T3) prostate cancer, neoadjuvant hormonal therapy has been effective in reducing serum PSA and prostate volume but less successful in accomplishing pathologic downstaging.

Several studies have also examined the incidence of positive surgical margins in those with cT2 and cT3 disease. Two studies failed to demonstrate an advantage to neoadjuvant therapy for cT3 disease in terms of surgical margin status as well as disease progression as measured by biochemical relapse-free survival, disease-free survival, or cause-specific survival [73,74].

For localized (T1/T2) prostate cancer, preoperative androgen ablation reduces the rates of positive margins but has not translated into improved long-term PSA-free survival (Tables 5 and 6). Soloway and colleagues reported the 5-year results of a multi-institutional study in which patients with cT2bNxM$_0$ received neoadjuvant androgen ablation prior to radical prostatectomy [75]. In this prospective randomized trial, 138 patients

Table 5. Impact of 3 months of neoadjuvant androgen deprivation therapy on the rate of positive surgical margins in patients with cT1/cT2 prostate cancer

Series	Patients (N)	Control group (%)	Neoadjuvant group (%)
Goldenberg et al. [93]	213	65	28
Schulman et al. [94]	402	37	13
Soloway et al. [95]	282	48	18
Labrie et al. [96]	161	34	8
Lee et al. [97]	258	49	15
Fair et al. [98]	114	36	17
Fair et al. [99]	141	34	8
Meyer et al. [100]	680	47	25
Pedersen et al. [101]	111	46	24

Table 6. Impact of 3 months of neoadjuvant androgen deprivation therapy on PSA recurrence rates in patients with cT1/cT2 prostate cancer

Series	Patients (N)	Control group (%)	Neoadjuvant group (%)	Follow-up (months)
Aus et al. [102]	122	41	35	38
Meyer et al. [100]	680	30	35	38
Klotz et al. [103]	213	30	40	36
Fair et al. [99]	194	16	11	29
Schulman et al. [94]	398	32.5	26.4	48
Soloway et al. [104]	255	32	35	60

received 3 months of leuprolide plus flutamide before radical prostatectomy and 144 patients underwent radical prostatectomy only (controls). Patients were followed every 6 months with PSA testing for 5 years and biochemical recurrence was defined as a PSA > 0.4 ng/ml. The neoadjuvant hormonal therapy group had a statistically significant lower-incidence of positive surgical margins (18%) compared to 48% in the surgery only cohort ($p < 0.001$). The biochemical recurrence-free rate at 5-years was no different in the neoadjuvant hormonal therapy group (64.8%) than in the surgery only group (67.6%). The impact of positive surgical margins on biochemical disease-free survival was not significantly different in patients with (SM+, 46.2% failure) or without positive surgical margins (SM−, 33% failure) in the neoadjuvant hormonal therapy group ($p = 0.310$). In the surgery only cohort, patients with positive surgical margins had

a higher rate of PSA recurrence (51.7%) compared with patients with negative surgical margins (17.4%) ($p < 0.001$). While most trials to date have used 3 months of androgen deprivation before surgery, some suggest that extending the length of time of neoadjuvant androgen deprivation before surgery may translate into improved outcomes [76,77]. A Canadian Urologic Oncology Group trial evaluated 3 *versus* 8 months of neoadjuvant androgen deprivation therapy before radical prostatectomy. The positive margin rate in the 8-month neoadjuvant hormonal therapy group was significantly lower that the 3-month group (12% vs. 23%, respectively, $p = 0.0106$) [78]. Longer follow-up of this randomized trial is required to determine if more extensive (8 months) neoadjuvant hormonal therapy alters biochemical recurrence rates. While the role of neoadjuvant therapy remains unclear, it is clear that there is no substitute for careful preoperative risk assessment and meticulous surgical technique.

Standard second or adjuvant treatment options following radical prostatectomy include radiation therapy with or without androgen deprivation or androgen deprivation therapy alone. Adjuvant treatment, if given, can be tailored to the risk of relapse as well as to the pattern of biochemical relapse, local *versus* distant. Distant relapse may be more likely in those with high-grade disease, lymph-node metastasis, and very high pretreatment PSA, as well as those patients who fail to have their serum PSA fall to undetectable levels immediately after surgery. Patients at high risk of distant relapse are also ideal candidates for experimental adjuvant systemic therapy.

Radiation therapy may be given following surgery on the basis of a detectable, but low serum PSA (i.e. ≤1.5 ng/ml) with a prolonged PSA doubling time (i.e. >6–12 months) or based on adverse disease characteristics, such as positive surgical margins [79,80,81–84]. The actual likelihood of achieving an undetectable serum PSA with therapeutic radiation in those who have failed biochemically after surgery is approaching 43%. Adjuvant radiation therapy in those at high risk of biochemical recurrence (i.e. positive surgical margins) appears to decrease the risk of biochemical failure, but may not have a substantive effect on disease-specific survival.

Conclusion

In summary, radical prostatectomy is a safe operation and an effective procedure for properly selected patients. Major complications are rare and decrease with the surgeon's experience. With current refinements in the technique, significant urinary incontinence is rare and preservation of potency is possible in selected patients. Adjuvant therapy in selected patients may further improve long-term, cause-specific and biochemical relapse-free survival.

Acknowledgements

The authors wish to acknowledge that this study was supported by the National Institutes of Health/NCI, UCSF Prostate Cancer SPORE, grant number 1 P50 C89520, and a generous gift to the Prostate Cancer Center from the UCSF Prostate Cancer Center Advocates Group.

References

1. Walsh PC: Prostate cancer kills: Strategy to reduce deaths (see comments). Urology 44: 463–466, 1994

2. Thompson IM: Counseling patients with newly diagnosed prostate cancer. Oncology (Huntingt) 14: 119–126, 131; Discussion 135–136, 2000

3. Amling CL, Leibovich BC, Lerner SE, Bergstralh EJ, Blute ML, Myers RP, Zincke H: Primary surgical therapy for clinical stage T3 adenocarcinoma of the prostate. Semin Urol Oncol 15: 215–221, 1997

4. Koppie TM, Grossfeld GD, Miller D, Yu J, Stier D, Broering JM, Lubeck D, Henning JM, Flanders SC, Carroll PR: (in press) Patterns of treatment in patients with prostate cancer initially managed with surveillance: results from the CaPSURE database. J Urol

5. D'Amico AV, Whittington R, Malkowicz SB, Schultz D, Fondurulia J, Chen MH, Tomaszewski JE, Renshaw AA, Wein A, Richie JP: Clinical utility of the percentage of positive prostate biopsies in defining biochemical outcome after radical prostatectomy for patients with clinically localized prostate cancer (see comments). J Clin Oncol 18: 1164–1172, 2000

6. Bishoff JT, Reyes A, Thompson IM, Harris MJ, St Clair SR, Gomella L, Butzin CA: Pelvic lymphadenectomy can be omitted in selected patients with carcinoma of the prostate: Development of a system of patient selection. Urology 45: 270–274, 1995

7. Narayan P, Fournier G, Gajendran V, Leidich R, Lo R, Wolf JS Jr, Jacob G, Nicolaisen G, Palmer K, Freiha F: Utility of preoperative serum prostate-specific antigen concentration and biopsy Gleason score in predicting risk of pelvic lymph-node metastases in prostate cancer. Urology 44: 519–524, 1994

8. Partin A, Kattan M, Subong E, Walsh P, Wojno K, Oesterling J, Scardino P, Pearson J: Combination of prostate-specific antigen, clinincal stage, and Gleason Score to predict pathological stage of localized prostate cancer. A multi-institutional update. JAMA 277: 1445–1551, 1997

9. Meng MV, Carroll PR: When is pelvic lymph node dissection necessary before radical prostatectomy? A decision analysis. J Urol 164: 1235–1240, 2000

10. Frank E, Sood OP, Torjman M, Mulholland SG, Gomella LG: Postoperative epidural analgesia following radical retropubic prostatectomy: Outcome assessment. J Surg Oncol 67: 117–120, 1998

11. Gottschalk A, Smith DS, Jobes DR, Kennedy SK, Lally SE, Noble VE, Grugan KF, Seifert HA, Cheung A, Malkowicz SB, Gutsche BB, Wein AJ: Preemptive epidural analgesia and recovery from radical prostatectomy: A randomized controlled trial (see comments). Jama 279: 1076–1082, 1998

12. Reinhart DI: Minimising the adverse effects of ketorolac. Drug Saf 22: 487–497, 2000

13. Goad JR, Eastham JA, Fitzgerald KB, Kattan MW, Collini MP, Yawn DH, Scardino PT: Radical retropubic prostatectomy: Limited benefit of autologous blood donation. J Urol 154: 2103–2109, 1995

14. O'Hara JF Jr, Sprung J, Klein EA, Dilger JA, Domen RE, Piedmonte MR: Use of preoperative autologous blood donation in patients undergoing radical retropubic prostatectomy. Urology 54: 130–134, 1999

15. Noldus J, Gonnermann D, Huland H: Autologous blood transfusion in radical prostatectomy: Results in 263 patients. Eur Urol 27: 213–217, 1995

16. Walsh PC: Radical prostatectomy: A procedure in evolution. Semin Oncol 21: 662–671, 1994

17. Walsh PC, Partin AW, Epstein JI: Cancer control and quality of life following anatomical radical retropubic prostatectomy: Results at 10 years (see comments). J Urol 152: 1831–1836, 1994

18. Steiner MS: The puboprostatic ligament and the male urethral suspensory mechanism: An anatomic study. Urology 44: 530–534, 1994

19. Koch MO: Management of the dorsal vein complex during radical retropubic prostatectomy. Semin Urol Oncol 18: 33–37, 2000

20. Catalona WJ, Carvalhal GF, Mager DE, Smith DS: Potency, continence and complication rates in 1,870 consecutive radical retropubic prostatectomies. J Urol 162: 433–438, 1999

21. Ghavamian R, Zincke H: An updated simplified approach to nerve-sparing radical retropubic prostatectomy. BJU Int 84: 160–163, 1999

22. Klotz L: Neurostimulation during radical prostatectomy: Improving nerve-sparing techniques. Semin Urol Oncol 18: 46–50, 2000

23. Klotz L: Intraoperative cavernous nerve stimulation during nerve sparing radical prostatectomy: How and when? Curr Opin Urol 10: 239–243, 2000

24. Cangiano TG, Litwin MS, Naitoh J, Dorey F, deKernion JB: Intraoperative frozen section monitoring of nerve sparing radical retropubic prostatectomy. J Urol 162: 655–658, 1999

25. Steiner MS: Anatomic basis for the continence-preserving radical retropubic prostatectomy. Semin Urol Oncol 18: 9–18, 2000

26. Soloway MS, Neulander E: Bladder-neck preservation during radical retropubic prostatectomy. Semin Urol Oncol 18: 51–56, 2000

27. DeMarco RT, Bihrle R, Foster RS: Early catheter removal following radical retropubic prostatectomy. Semin Urol Oncol 18: 57–59, 2000

28. Weldon VE, Tavel FR: Potency-sparing radical perineal prostatectomy: Anatomy, surgical technique and initial results. J Urol 140: 559–562, 1988

29. Paulson DF: Radical perineal prostatectomy. Urol Clin N Am 7: 847, 1980

30. Belt E: Radical perineal prostatectomy in early carcinoma of the prostate. J Urol 48: 287, 1942

31. Scolieri MJ, Resnick MI: The technique of radical perineal prostatectomy. Urol Clin N Am 28: 521–533, 2001

32. Sullivan LD, Weir MJ, Kinahan JF, Taylor DL: A comparison of the relative merits of radical perineal and radical retropubic prostatectomy. BJU International 85: 95–100, 2000

33. Frazier HA, Robertson JE, Paulson DF: Radical prostatectomy: The pros and cons of the perineal versus retropubic approach. J Urol 147: 888–890, 1992

34. Weldon VE, Tavel FR, Neuwirth H, Cohen R: Patterns of positive specimen margins and detectable prostate specific antigen after radical perineal prostatectomy. J Urol 153: 1565–1569, 1995

35. Lance RS, Freidrichs PA, Kane CJ, Powell CR, Pulos E, Moul JW, Mcleod DG, Cornum RL, Thrasher JB: A comparison of radical retropubic with perineal prostatectomy for localized prostate cancer within the uniformed services urology research group. BJU International 87: 61–65, 2001

36. Zippe CD, Rackley RR: Non-nerve sparing radical prostatectomy in the elderly patient: Perineal vs. retropubic approach (abstract 359). J Urol 155: 400A, 1996

37. Weldon VE, Tavel FR, Neuwirth H: Continence, potency and morbidity after radical perineal prostatectomy. J Urol 153: 1565, 1997

38. Thomas R, Steele R, Smith R: One-Stage laparoscopic pelvic lymphadenectomy and radical perineal prostatectomy. J Urol 152: 1174, 1994

39. Gibbons RP, Correa RJJ, Brannen GE: Total prostatectomy for localized prostate cancer. J Urol 131: 73, 1984

40. Parra RO: Analysis of an experience with 500 radical perineal prostatectomies in localized prostate cancer (Abstract). J Urol 163: 284–285, 2000

41. Rosen MA, Goldstone L, Lapin S, Wheeler T, Scardino PT: Frequency and location of extracapsular extension and positive surgical margins in radical prostatectomy specimens. J Urol 148: 331, 1992

42. Stamey TA, Villers AA, McNeal JE, Link PC, Freiha FS: Positive surgical margins at radical prostatectomy: Importance of the apical dissection. J Urol 143: 1166, 1990

43. Epstein JI, Pizov G, Walsh PC: Correlation of pathologic findings with progression after radical retropubic prostatectomy. Cancer 71: 3582, 1993

44. Bishoff JT, Motley G, Optenberg SA, Stein CR, Moon KA, Browning SM, Sabanegh E, Foley JP, Thompson IM: Incidence of fecal and urinary incontinence following radical perineal and retropubic prostatectomy in a national population. J Urol 160: 454–458, 1998

45. Schuessler W, Schulman P, Clayman R, Kavoussin L: Laparoscopic radical prostatectomy: Initial short-term experience. Urology 50: 854–857, 1997

46. Guillonneau B, Cathelineau X, Barrett E, Rozet F, Vallencien G: Laparoscopic radical prostatectomy: Technical and early oncological assessment of 40 operations. Eur Urol 36: 14–20, 1999

47. Paulson DF: Impact of radical prostatectomy in the management of clinically localized disease. J Urol 152: 1826–1830, 1994

48. Zincke H, Oesterling JE, Blute ML, Bergstralh EJ, Myers RP, Barrett DM: Long-term (15 years) results after radical prostatectomy for clinically localized (stage T2c or lower) prostate cancer (see comments). J Urol 152: 1850–1857, 1994

49. Zincke H, Bergstralh EJ, Blute ML, Myers RP, Barrett DM, Lieber MM, Martin SK, Oesterling JE: Radical prostatectomy for clinically localized prostate cancer: Long-term results of 1,143 patients from a single institution (see comments). J Clin Oncol 12: 2254–2263, 1994

50. Kupelian PA, Katcher J, Levin HS, Klein EA: Stage T1-2 prostate cancer: A multivariate analysis of factors affecting biochemical and clinical failures after radical prostatectomy. Int J Radiat Oncol Biol Phys 37: 1043–1052, 1997

51. Partin AW, Kattan MW, Subong EN, Walsh PC, Wojno KJ, Oesterling JE, Scardino PT, Pearson JD: Combination of prostate-specific antigen, clinical stage, and Gleason score to predict pathological stage of localized prostate cancer. A multi-institutional update (see comments) (published erratum appears in JAMA 1997 July 9; 278(2): 118). Jama 277: 1445–1451, 1997

52. Badalament RA, Miller MC, Peller PA, Young DC, Bahn DK, Kochie P, O'Dowd GJ, Veltri RW: An algorithm for predicting nonorgan confined prostate cancer using the results obtained from sextant core biopsies with prostate specific antigen level. J Urol 156: 1375–1380, 1996

53. Grossfeld GD, Chang JJ, Broering JM, Miller DP, Yu J, Flanders SC, Carroll PR: Does the completeness of prostate sampling predict outcome for patients undergoing radical prostatectomy?: Data from the CAPSURE database. Urology 56: 430–435, 2000

54. Haese A, Huland E, Graefen M, Huland H: Supersensitive PSA-analysis after radical prostatectomy: A powerful tool to reduce the time gap between surgery and evidence of biochemical failure. Anticancer Res 19: 2641–2644, 1999

55. Yu H, Diamandis EP, Prestigiacomo AF, Stamey TA: Ultrasensitive assay of prostate-specific antigen used for early detection of prostate cancer relapse and estimation of tumor-doubling time after radical prostatectomy. Clin Chem 41: 430–434, 1995

56. Catalona WJ, Smith DS: 5-year tumor recurrence rates after anatomical radical retropubic prostatectomy for prostate cancer (see comments). J Urol 152: 1837–1842, 1994

57. Pound CR, Partin AW, Eisenberger MA, Chan DW, Pearson JD, Walsh PC: Natural history of progression after PSA elevation following radical prostatectomy (see comments). Jama 281: 1591–1597, 1999

58. Ohori M, Wheeler TM, Kattan MW, Goto Y, Scardino PT: Prognostic significance of positive surgical margins in radical prostatectomy specimens. J Urol 154: 1818–1824, 1995

59. Iselin CE, Box JW, Vollmer RT, Layfield LJ, Robertson JE, Paulson DF: Surgical control of clinically localized prostate carcinoma is equivalent in African–American and white males. Cancer 83: 2353–2360, 1998

60. Trapasso JG, deKernion JB, Smith RB, Dorey F: The incidence and significance of detectable levels of serum prostate specific antigen after radical prostatectomy (see comments). J Urol 152: 1821–1825, 1994

61. Partin AW, Pound CR, Clemens JQ, Epstein JI, Walsh PC: Serum PSA after anatomic radical prostatectomy. The Johns Hopkins experience after 10 years. Urol Clin North Am 20: 713–725, 1993

62. Han M, Partin A, Pound C, Epstein JI, Walsh PC: Long-term biochemical disease-free and cancer-specific survival following anatomic radical retropubic prostatectomy. The 15-year Johns Hopkins experience. Urol Clin N Am 28: 555–565, 2001

63. Patel A, Dorey F, Franklin J, deKernion JB: Recurrence patterns after radical retropubic prostatectomy: Clinical usefulness of prostate specific antigen doubling times and log slope prostate specific antigen (see comments). J Urol 158: 1441–1445, 1997

64. Partin AW, Pearson JD, Landis PK, Carter HB, Pound CR, Clemens JQ, Epstein JI, Walsh PC: Evaluation of serum prostate-specific antigen velocity after radical prostatectomy to distinguish local recurrence from distant metastases. Urology 43: 649–659, 1994

65. Thompson IM, Middleton RG, Optenberg SA, Austenfeld MS, Smalley SR, Cooner WH, Correa RJ Jr, Miller HC Jr, Oesterling JE, Resnick MI, Wasson JH, Roehrborn CG: Have complication rates decreased after treatment for localized prostate cancer? J Urol 162: 107–112, 1999

66. Goluboff ET, Saidi JA, Mazer S, Bagiella E, Heitjan DF, Benson MC, Olsson CA: Urinary continence after radical prostatectomy: The Columbia experience. J Urol 159: 1276–1280, 1998

67. Wahle GR: Urinary incontinence after radical prostatectomy. Semin Urol Oncol 18: 66–70, 2000

68. Rabbani F, Stapleton AM, Kattan MW, Wheeler TM, Scardino PT: Factors predicting recovery of erections after radical prostatectomy (in process citation). J Urol 164: 1929–1934, 2000

69. Zippe CD, Jhaveri FM, Klein EA, Kedia S, Pasqualotto FF, Kedia A, Agarwal A, Montague DK, Lakin MM: Role of Viagra after radical prostatectomy. Urology 55: 241–245, 2000

70. Zippe CD, Kedia S, Kedia AW, Pasqualotto F: Sildenafil citrate (Viagra) after radical retropubic prostatectomy: Pro (editorial). Urology 54: 583–586, 1999

71. Blander DS, Sanchez-Ortiz RF, Wein AJ, Broderick GA: Efficacy of sildenafil in erectile dysfunction after radical prostatectomy (in process citation). Int J Impot Res 12: 165–168, 2000

72. Kim ED, Scardino PT, Hampel O, Mills NL, Wheeler TM, Nath RK: Interposition of sural nerve restores function of cavernous nerves resected during radical prostatectomy. J Urol 161: 188–192, 1999

73. Witjes WP, Schulman CC, Debruyne FM: Preliminary results of a prospective randomized study comparing radical prostatectomy *versus* radical prostatectomy associated with neoadjuvant hormonal combination therapy in T2-3 N0 M0 prostatic carcinoma. The european study group on neoadjuvant treatment of prostate cancer. Urology 49: 65–69, 1997

74. Van Poppel H, De Ridder D, Elgamal AA, Van de Voorde W, Werbrouck P, Ackaert K, Oyen R, Pittomvils G, Baert L: Neoadjuvant hormonal therapy before radical prostatectomy decreases the number of positive surgical margins in stage T2 prostate cancer: Interim results of a prospective randomized trial. The Belgian Uro-Oncological Study Group. J Urol 154: 429–434, 1995

75. Soloway M, Pareek K, Rooholiah S, Wajsman Z, Mcleod D, Wood DJ, Puras-Baez A: Neoadjuvant androgen ablation before radical prostatectomy in cT2bNxMo prostate cancer: 5-year results. J Urol 167: 112–116, 2002

76. Gleave ME, Goldenberg SL, Jones EC, Bruchovsky N, Kinahan J, Sullivan LD: Optimal duration of neoadjuvant androgen withdrawal therapy before radical prostatectomy in clinically confined prostate cancer. Semin Urol Oncol 14: 39–45; Discussion 46–47, 1996

77. Gleave ME, La Bianca SE, Goldenberg SL, Jones EC, Bruchovsky N, Sullivan LD: Long-term neoadjuvant hormone therapy prior to radical prostatectomy: Evaluation of risk for biochemical recurrence at 5-year follow-up. Urology 56: 289–294, 2000

78. Gleave M, Goldenberg S, Chin J, Warner J, Saad F, Klotz L, Jewett M, Kassabian V, Chetner M, Dupont C, Van Rensselaer S: Randomized comparative study of 3 *versus* 8-month neoadjuvant hormonal therapy before radical prostatectomy: Biochemical and pathological effects. J Urol 166: 500–507, 2001

79. McCarthy JF, Catalona WJ, Hudson MA: Effect of radiation therapy on detectable serum prostate specific antigen levels following radical prostatectomy: Early *versus* delayed treatment. J Urol 151: 1575–1578, 1994

80. Petrovich Z, Lieskovsky G, Langholz B, Luxton G, Jozsef G, Skinner DG: Radiotherapy following radical prostatectomy in patients with adenocarcinoma of the prostate. Int J Radiat Oncol Biol Phys 21: 949–954, 1991

81. Zietman AL, Coen JJ, Shipley WU, Althausen AF: Adjuvant irradiation after radical prostatectomy for adenocarcinoma of prostate: Analysis of freedom from PSA failure. Urology 42: 292–298; Discussion 298–299, 1993

82. Coetzee LJ, Hars V, Paulson DF: Postoperative prostate-specific antigen as a prognostic indicator in patients with margin-positive prostate cancer, undergoing adjuvant radiotherapy after radical prostatectomy. Urology 47: 232–235, 1996

83. Gibbons RP, Cole BS, Richardson RG, Correa RJ Jr, Brannen GE, Mason JT, Taylor WJ, Hafermann MD: Adjuvant radiotherapy following radical prostatectomy: Results and complications. J Urol 135: 65–68, 1986

84. Syndikus I, Pickles T, Kostashuk E, Sullivan LD: Post-operative radiotherapy for stage pT3 carcinoma of the prostate: Improved local control (see comments). J Urol 155: 1983–1986, 1996

85. Fleming I, Cooper J, Henson D: Manual for Staging of Cancer Lippincott-Raven, Philadelphia, 1997

86. Raboy A, Albert P, Ferzli: Early experience with extraperitoneal endoscopic radical retropubic prostatectomy. Surg Endosc 12: 1264–1267, 1998

87. Guillonneau B, Vallencien G: Laparoscopic radical prostatectomy: The Montsouris experience. J Urol 163: 418–422, 2000

88. Abbou CC, Salomon L, Hoznek A, Antiphon P, Cicco A, Saint F, Alame W, Bellot J, Chopin DK: Laparoscopic radical prostatectomy: Preliminary results. Urology 55: 630–634, 2000

89. van Velthoven R, Peltier A, Hawaux E, Vendewalle J: Transperitoneal laparoscopic anatomic radical prostatectomy, preliminary results. J Urol 163: 141, Abstract 621, 2000

90. Rassweiler J, Sentker L, Seeman O, Hatzinger M, Rumpelt H: Laparoscopic radical prostatectomy with the heilbronn technique: An analysis of the first 180 cases. J Urol 166: 2101–2108, 2001

91. Turek I, Degar S, Winkelman B, Loening S: Laparoscopic radical prostatectomy- the Berlin experience. J Urol 165: 326, Abstract 1340, 2001

92. Zippe CD, Meraney A, Sung G, Gill I: Laparoscopic prostatectomy in the USA: Cleveland clinic series of 50 patients. J Urol, 165: 326, abstract 1341, 2001

93. Goldenberg SL, Klotz LH, Srigley J, Jewett MA, Mador D, Fradet Y, Barkin J, Chin J, Paquin JM, Bullock MJ, Laplante S: Randomized, prospective, controlled study comparing radical prostatectomy alone and neoadjuvant androgen withdrawal in the treatment of localized prostate cancer Canadian Urologic Oncology Group (see comments). J Urol 156: 873–877, 1996

94. Schulman C, Debruyne F, Forster G, Selvaggi F, Zlotta A, Witjes W: 4-year follow-upresults of a European prospective randomized study on neoadjuvant hormonal therapy prior to radical prostatectomy in T2-3N0M0 prostate cancer. Eur Urol 38: 706–713, 2000

95. Soloway M, Sharifi R, Wajsman Z, Mcleod DG, Wood DJ, Puras-Baez A: Randomized prospective study comparing radical prostatectomy alone versus radical prostatectomy preceded by androgen blockade in clinical stage B2

(T2bNxM0) prostate cancer. The Lupron Depot Neoadjuvant Prostate Cancer Study Group. J Urol 154: 424–428, 1995

96. Labrie F, Cusan L, Gomez J, Diamond P, Suburu R, Lemay M, Tetu B, Fradet Y, Candas B: Down-staging of early stage prostate cancer before radical prostatectomy: The first randomized trial of neoadjuvant combination therapy with flutamide and a luteinizing hormone-releasing hormone agonist. Urology 44A: 29–36, 1994

97. Lee F, Siders D, McHug T, Solomon M, LKlamerus M: Long term follow-up of stages T@-T3 prostate cancer pretreated with androgen ablation therapy prior to radical prostatectomy. Anticancer Res 17: 1507–1510, 1997

98. Fair WR, Scher HI: Neoadjuvant hormonal therapy plus surgery for prostate cancer. The MSKCC experience. Surg Oncol Clin N Am 6: 831–846, 1997

99. Fair WR, Cookson MS, Stroumbakis N, Cohen D, Aprikian AG, Wang Y, Russo P, Soloway SM, Sogani P, Sheinfeld J, Herr H, Dalgabni G, Begg CB, Heston WD, Reuter VE: The indications, rationale, and results of neoadjuvant androgen deprivation in the treatment of prostatic cancer: Memorial Sloan-Kettering Cancer Center results. Urology 49: 46–55, 1997

100. Meyer F, Moore L, Bairati I, Lacombe L, Tetu B, Fradet Y: Neoadjuvant hormonal therapy before radical prostatectomy and risk of prostate specific antigen failure. J Urol 162: 2024–2028, 1999

101. Pedersen K, Lundberg S, Hugosson J: Neoadjuvant hormonal treatment with triptorelin versus no treatment prior to radical prostatectomy: A prospective randomized multicenter study. J Urol 153: 391A, 1995

102. Aus G, Abrahamsson P-A, Ahlgren G: Hormonal treatment before radical prostatectomy: A 3-year followup. J Urol 159: 2013–2016, 1998

103. Klotz LH, Goldenberg SL, Jewett M, Barkin J, Chetner M, Fradet Y, Chin J, Laplante S: CUOG randomized trial of neoadjuvant androgen ablation before radical prostatectomy: 36-month post-treatment PSA results. Canadian Urologic Oncology Group. Urology 53: 757–763, 1999

104. Soloway M: Radical prostatectomy alone versus radical prostatectomy preceded by three months androgen blockade in cT2b prostate cancer: 60 mon results. The Lupron Depot Neoadjuvant Prostate Cancer Study Group. J Urol 167: 113–116, 2002

Address for offprints: Peter R. Carroll, Professor and Chair, Department of Urology, University of California, San Francisco, San Francisco, CA 94143-0738, USA; *Tel*: (415) 476-1611; *Fax*: (415) 476-8849; *E-mail*: pcarroll@urol.ucsf.edu

The future of cancer imaging

David A. Benaron
Stanford University School of Medicine, Palo Alto, CA, USA

Predictions are hard to make. . . especially about the future. Yogi Berra (1925–).

Key words: CT, MRI, optical imaging, contrast agents, MRSI, PET, monoclonal antibody, molecular imaging, functional imaging, review

Summary

Conventional (anatomical, structural) imaging is insensitive to the presence of cancer, often failing to yield the very information needed for accurate diagnosis and staging, for proper treatment selection and monitoring or for effective follow-up after treatment. This, fortunately, is changing. Newer techniques, already in clinical testing, are rapidly pushing clinical imaging in the same direction as the rest of medicine: away from simple detection of the gross structural end-effects of disease, and toward a patient-specific approach based on physiologic, histologic, antigenic, molecular, and (ultimately) genetic markers of disease. By 2010, unimodal, nonspecific, and insensitive radiological images may look as primitive to us as the first Roentgen radiographs. In some cases, these new scans will be so seamlessly integrated into therapeutic treatment that they may not even be thought of as imaging *per se*. This chapter looks forward to see how imaging for oncology may look in the coming decade, focusing upon near-term trends and techniques by selecting those already demonstrated *in vivo* in at least animals or which are now under human study, and thus which have moved far enough that they have already begun to impact patient care, or are likely to begin do so in the near future.

I. The present imperfect

For much of the 20th century, medical imaging aimed for faster and increasingly detailed anatomic snapshots of the human body. Such structural images now play a central role in how cancer is diagnosed, staged, and managed. Recently, this imaging paradigm culminated in the realization of the 'Visible Human Project' [1], a precise and highly detailed anatomic catalog of the CT and MRI appearance of an anatomically normal, though recently deceased, human subject [2].

Yet, when it comes to the clinical management of an individual, a living oncology patient, such 'traditional' imaging often fails to provide accurate, basic information necessary to manage the patient's disease optimally (such as true metastatic extent), let alone provide the molecular and genetic information that will be increasingly needed to guide therapeutic choices. In fact, if a deceased patient is sufficient to provide the images, then *de facto* issues such as cell function, gene expression, antigenic appearance, metabolism, and other aspects of physiology are clearly not significant contributors to the integrity of the final image.

Consider the following statistics:

- *Diagnosis: small primary tumors go undetected* For many cancers, an internal, aggressive, noncalcified tumor under containing fewer than 500,000 cells (i.e., under 2 mm wide) is likely to pass undetected through most body-region scans, including CT, MRI, ultrasound, radionuclide, and metabolic PET. At this size, a tumor has effectively undergone 19 cell doublings – about halfway through doubling toward a predicted lethal load of 10^{10}–10^{12} cells – and is likely to be sufficiently repleted with gene defects so that it will undergo continued and uninterrupted growth if not treated.

- *Staging: metastatic disease underdiagnosed* For the reasons stated above, patients with negative scans for metastases at initial presentation routinely go on to develop, and die from, metastatic cancer. For example, about 20% of women with breast cancer clinically confined to the breast and lymph nodes (low and intermediate risk), and the majority of men with local margin-positivity after prostatectomy, will go on to have a recurrence of their disease, despite initially negative bone and body imaging scans. Even though it did not appear in the image, undetected residual and/or metastatic cancer must have been present at the time of the initial scanning.

- *Margins: residual disease common after surgery* After surgical resection, 30% or more of patients with breast or prostate cancer have residual disease in the surgical field [3,4], undetected by even real-time surgical imaging, but yet which will be found on gross and histochemical pathology in the days or weeks after the surgery has been completed, and the patient has been closed and sent home. Cancer recurrence rates are $2.5 \times$ higher in multivariate analysis if the margins are positive [5,6] and these patients are significantly more likely to die of their disease.

- *Therapy: treatment response poorly measured* 'Measurable disease,' a common yardstick for monitoring response to treatment, is absent after surgical excision of many tumors. Because of this, the standard of care is to blindly treat with chemotherapy selected by convention using prior retrospective studies, and to consider this treatment a success or failure only in retrospect (i.e., success is when a patient survives 5 years, and failure is when a relapse occurs).

Even when residual tumor can be imaged, such scans may not be helpful in evaluating therapy. A bone scan, commonly used to guide therapy in breast, prostate, and other cancers metastatic to the bone, will often remain uninterpretable for months following the initiation of therapy. Bone scans show the same response for both bone healing as well as for tumor growth (bone lysis with its attendant increase in reactionary osteogenesis), and will therefore often fail to confirm a significant response to chemotherapy, even up to 6 months after an ultimately 'successful' chemotherapy regimen

has been initiated. Similarly, a hepatic parenchymal scar or peritoneal fibrosis after tumor treatment may be radiologically indistinguishable from recurrent or untreated disease, with assessment made only by invasive biopsy or surgical sampling or, more commonly, by following its progression over time.

How can conventional oncology imaging be so far off the mark?

One reason is that 'conventional' radiologic approaches, while now computer-assisted and technologically far advanced from the first X-rays, still typically produce their images based upon bulk features of the tissue. The resulting anatomic signal is therefore epiphenomenal, being merely an expression of the sum of nonspecific interactions of the imaging source with the tissues structure, physiology and/or pathology. Thus, the degree to which a tumor can be visualized on conventional CT, MRI, or ultrasound is merely a function of the ability of that tumor to differentially scatter, absorb, or emit radiation as compared to the surrounding tissue and inherent background noise. It is not surprising, then, that this signal has little specificity and sensitivity for the detection of tumor, for while conventional tumor imaging sources are, at least in part, a function of cell density, microcalcifications, and the like, these effects are no more a signature of cancer *per se* than the density of a liver on a plain film is a reliable predictor of its synthetic function.

Equally important, while the lethality of many solid tumors is due to the physical crowding or bulk effects of the tumor, the majority of diagnosis, treatment selection, treatment monitoring, and follow-up, involves decisions in which the physical, bulk characteristics of the tumor are, not the driving question. Rather, the questions that require answers are those of tumor presence vs. absence, of type and grade and distribution, and of gene expression, cell function, and receptor positivity.

As a result, oncology in particular has gone looking for methods that dovetail with the emphasis in medicine: gene-specific or receptor-specific therapies, minimally invasive treatments for early-diagnosed tumors, stage-specific treatment options.

II. Trends in imaging

Paralleling changes in much of medicine, tumor imaging has been moving away from nonspecific imaging, and toward specific imaging: patient-specific, disease-specific, and cell-specific. Driving this change are four trends:

- *Patient-specific medicine* The trend in oncology, as in medicine in general, is away from nonspecific diagnosis and treatment, and toward patient-specific therapy. As cell receptor status and gene expression become used with increasing frequency to manage the oncology patient, the diagnosis and treatment for cancer becomes dependent on identifying the molecular and genetic makeup of the tumor (for breast cancer, this is currently a palate of PR, ER, Her2-neu positivity, and perhaps a mitotic rate assay such as Ki-66, or others, depending upon institution), rather than upon the anatomic and pathologic grade of the tumor.
- *Specific markers* New markers are becoming available at a dizzying pace as a result of biochemical advances and the genome project [7,8]. Gene chips and other tools are allowing such markers to begin to be correlated with clinical stage, tumor aggressiveness, outcome, and response to treatment, while drug discovery seeks to use these identified markers as specific targets for new pharmaceutical agents. From an imaging point of view, such markers are important as the anatomic, or bulk effects, of tumors are absent at the early or minimal residual disease stages of cancer, while genetic disturbances and receptor abnormalities remain present in small tumor populations, and can be tumor-specific, stage-specific, and response-specific.
- *Novel sensors* New sensors have allowed for new types of scanners, such as portable optical imagers for visible and near-infrared photon detection. Examples of such new sensors include activatable contrast agents and genetic expression elements which can be used to produce or amplify local contrast in imaging studies. Advances in computing power, which has continued to double the power every 18 months without increases in cost, make increasingly complex calculation- and graphics-heavy imaging software routine, and possible in real-time or near-real-time.
- *Less-invasive medicine* Last, the trend in medicine for the past 20 years has been toward reduced invasiveness. More sensitive imaging allows diagnosis and therapy to be physically targeted to the tumor, as well as allows less invasive monitoring of therapeutic response. Local, regionally limited surgical procedures (such as lumpectomy, local ablation, endoscopic approaches) now permit confined islands of disease, if located, to be treated quickly and effectively.

III. New roles for imaging

The role of imaging is changing. Imaging will become less of a tool for initial gross staging. Instead, it will become more frequent and integrate more effectively and seamlessly with patient management at all stages of oncology diagnosis, treatment, and follow-up. Sensitive and specific imaging will allow for a more proactive role for imaging in the following areas.

Diagnosis

At diagnosis, imaging will yield more sensitive detection of cancer, including optimally imaging such features as receptor status, gene expression, and tumor grade now obtained only through biopsy and analysis by pathology microscopy, immunohistochemistry, and PCR. The lower limit for tumor detection is improving. For example, while the lower limit of tumor detection in human subjects is currently about 500,000 cells (2–3 mm diameter tumor), optical methods have moved the lower limit of tumor detection in animal models down to fewer than 1,000 cells, noninvasively and specifically imaged [9]. The ability to image receptor status *in vivo* has been demonstrated using antigenically targeted probes, such as those targeted to somatostatin [10]. More specific scans will also play a role in avoiding invasive evaluations. The majority of all biopsies are negative, therefore a reduction in invasive evaluations will be a benefit of more specific scans [11].

Despite such improvements, there will always be some degree of a lag between the identification of new markers via molecular biology and the ability to image those markers, and thus there will likely continue to be a need for tissue samples to allow for testing of the latest markers for optimal selection of therapy, as well as for banking of tissue, to allow for testing of future markers when these become available.

Staging

Staging will become more accurate, thus profoundly influencing patient segmentation and treatment

272

selection. Surgical staging procedures, such as nodal biopsy, may be able to be reduced using imaging (or perhaps replaced entirely if tissue for pathology has already been obtained), with imaging follow-up used to ensure accuracy of a negative scan.

One step toward this scenario – limiting the size of lymphatic staging by better imaging of the sentinel nodes – has been achieved using radioemitter-based colloid imaging for melanoma and breast, and this has led to a decrease in the physical extent of the surgical procedure, and to reduced morbidity and a minimal loss of diagnostic accuracy (though with an unknown effect of long-term outcome [12]).

The next step is replacing the nonspecific radioemitter with a specific and highly sensitive marker or reporter for tumor in the nodes. For breast cancer, if this can be achieved, then only tumor-positive nodes would be therapeutically removed (and sent to pathology), while the majority of women would be able to forego the therapeutic nodal biopsy altogether. Further, the detection of mediastinal (as opposed to axillary) nodes would be improved, perhaps leading to elective removal of those mediastinal nodes using a minimally invasive parasternal procedure.

Therapeutic monitoring and feedback

Early, course-correcting treatment feedback will become standard-of-care for many therapies, especially when good alternative therapies exist. Rather than perform a bone scan months down the road after treatment is initiated, tumor response will be evaluated with scans during the first treatment doses. For example, MR spectroscopic imaging (MRSI) and/or PET imaging before and after treatment to look for changes in cell metabolism consistent with a response has already been studied as a potential method to identify responders from non-responders months before current methods can do so [13–16]. Sequential scans may also be able to identify the emergence of resistance during ongoing treatment, such that the treatment may be changed before the patient presents with clinical signs of treatment failure. Optical imaging has detected emergence of resistance in animal models of disease within days to weeks [9], while MRI and PET have been used to image apoptosis in animals [17], and in some instances in humans [18].

Another aspect of therapeutic monitoring is the measurement of chemotherapy levels in the patient's tissues, or in the tumor itself, using noninvasive or minimally-invasive imaging techniques [19–23]. This would allow for patient-specific dosing, based upon the actual tumor or tissue levels in a given patient, rather than blindly based upon body surface area or weight.

Using such approaches, gene therapies can be immediately evaluated for efficacy of gene expression, and followed on an ongoing basis for continued expression and/or tumor effect. Similarly, cell trafficking may be followed, again as markers of anti-tumor activity or to help assess clinical response.

Such early and ongoing treatment response feedback likely to be cost effective. While the cost effectiveness of oncologic screening tests has been hotly debated, such as with routine mammography [24–26], a patient under treatment can immediately balance the imaging costs against the cost of the therapy. Newer chemotherapy agents are significantly more expensive than the older agents; therefore an early feedback scan to measure treatment effect would prevent further use of an expensive agent that would otherwise ultimately be without effect. Under this view, such treatment response imaging scans may become a required part of care. Further, the patient can then rapidly be switched to another, and hopefully more active chemotherapeutic agent, which is likely to have a positive impact on overall response rates, survival time, and cost of care.

Image guidance

Image guided therapies will expand as the sensitivity of images to small regions of disease increases. Our group has been development real-time tumor imaging systems sensitive to the antigenic presence of residual tumor in the surgical field. Preliminary data from our group [67,246] and others [9] suggest that such scans may lower the detectability limit of disease to 100 μm islands. Such a tool, deployed in the operating room, directly impacts the 30% of breast and prostate cancer patients with residual disease in the surgical field after treatment, and could potentially allow for reduction or even elimination of the presence of positive-margins, indicating residual tumor, after surgical resection.

We and others have also been developing real-time sensors embedded into the surgical tools themselves, to give feedback during the surgical process [174,248]. Both of these approaches could lead to more effective treatment, and as well as enabling more minimally invasive treatment procedures.

Follow-up

Many cancer patients are at high risk for relapse. While there are again economic issues that have been used to argue for the limitation of access to follow-up imaging techniques, such imaging is already standard for some cancers (such as lymphoma). Increases in the sensitivity of follow-up scans will likely increase the benefit and applicability of such scans. For example, six months after node-negative scans in the breast cancer patient who avoided a nodal dissection due to negative initial, a repeat scan may be indicated to catch those patients with early disease too small to be detected on the first pass.

Drug discovery

Imaging is playing an increasing role in the discovery and development of new agents, both in humans and animals. The same imaging agents that can be used for imaging targets in humans can be used during drug discovery and development for use in imaging animals. Thus, better animal imaging permits for better and more rapid drug discovery, as well as for better basic research [27].

Specific systems for imaging animals have been made available for micro (small animal) CT [28,29], PET [30,31], MRI, and optical luciferase [32] and green fluorescent protein (GFP) [33] imaging. Supported by the NCI, our group is developing for commercial release an imaging system for the real-time *in vivo* imaging of optical markers and reporters in animals and humans in room light [67].

In addition to these imaging systems, designer animals, with desired combinations of knockout target genes and add-in reporter genes, are playing an increasing role in the drug discovery process. Animals with reporter genes tied to specific imaging modalities are already being created. For example, animals could be bred with a cells of T-cell origin expressing a reporter gene, such that T-cell trafficking can be imaged without further animal design or development (discussed further under Cell Tracking).

IV. The new tumor signals

The goal of the imaging will become more focused on specificity through selection of an imaging signal directly related to the identification and characterization of a target tissue.

The sources of imaging signal from tumor may be inherent or non-native. Native signals include the oxygenation of hemoglobin (lower in most tumors than in surrounding tissues), biochemical metabolite and cellular energetics substrate concentrations (known to be altered in cancer), and nuclear size and density measures.

However, not every pathologic or physiologic change has an inherent, strong, and identifiable signal. In such cases, medical imaging has historically turned to contrast agents to supplement a weak or absent native contrast, in order to create a strong, specific, and detectable imaging signal.

Both exogenously delivered and internally expressed contrast agents have been used. Some of these molecules generate their own signal, such as radiopharmaceuticals which generate a high-energy photon during a nuclear decay, or optical luciferase emitters which spontaneously generate visible to infrared photons.

From the largest scale (microns) to the smallest (angstroms), these new markers can be grouped as follows.

High-resolution anatomic markers

While traditional, gross anatomic imaging may become less useful over time, structural imaging still holds out new promise with the development of high resolution anatomic markers. In fact, some, such as Donald Coffey, at Johns Hopkins, argue that, at the cellular level 'morphology recapitulates oncogenesis' [34,35] – namely that cell morphology defects are critical to tumor imaging, as these morphologic changes reflect the very cellular defects in sensing, inhibition, and structure that allow a cell to become malignant in the first place.

Imaging and sensing at the sub-10-μm level can allow for radiologic imaging with details similar to those provided by gross microscopy. Such study of the nuclear size, shape, and density was an early strength of microscopy, and has well-known correspondence to changes in nuclear content, ploidy, and packing. Certain nuclear changes are pathognomonic for cancer, while the appearance of abnormal glandular structures in luminal epithelial tissues can, by itself, be diagnostic for the presence of adenocarcinoma. While such diagnostic features do not characterize tissue receptor status, they can be used in real-time to direct biopsy for further diagnosis, or to guide the gross removal of tissue already diagnosed as cancerous.

An example of one such high-resolution anatomic imaging technique is optical coherence tomography (OCT, discussed under Selected Techniques). Developed in the early 1990s [36], this technique uses light to produce noninvasive cross-sectional images with a resolution in the Z (depth) axis of $2–10\,\mu m$. OCT can be performed through a needle or endoscope catheter, to produce images as shown in Figure 1.

Such high-resolution OCT images could be used to direct biopsy, where the accuracy of current needle biopsy is limited by sampling error. Due to the randomness of biopsy, there is risk that the biopsy will miss the intended lesion (and thus a biopsy will be falsely negative when in fact the patient has cancer). This is a non-trivial issue. In prostate biopsy, random, regionally targeted, and multiple [37] biopsy remains the preferred method of prostate cancer diagnosis, and still even multiple prostate biopsy will miss up to 30% of cancer present at the time of biopsy [38–40]. Tumors of the prostate do not show up well on ultrasound, MRI, or CT, making guidance using conventional systems difficult. As only 1 in 20 lesions seen on ultrasound are cancerous (5% Specificity, 80% Sensitivity), directing a biopsy needle at dark spots (hypoechoic regions) on the ultrasound misses cancer more often than does a random 'blind' stick. The effect is that aiming at what is seen on the ultrasound yields worse results than random sampling [41,42]. Prostate biopsies are thus, in effect, performed blindly. Similarly, breast biopsy is now performed using an open incision in 70% of cases due to the risk of missing a cancer using a needle biopsy. Last, such high resolution images could also be used to direct biopsy of Barrett's Esophagus, a patchy disease requiring multiple biopsy attempts to guide the biopsy to locations where abnormal cells are seen.

Another example of a high-resolution anatomic marker is nuclear density and sizing determined by light scattering spectroscopy (LSS), an optical technique, as shown in Figure 2. In LSS imaging (discussed under Selected Techniques), a mucosal surface is optically imaged, and an overlay of nuclear size or nuclear density is generated. Such a technique fulfills the needs of a biopsy guidance system, as the entire imaged surface is analyzed, not just the site of a needle biopsy. Importantly, this approach may be useful therapeutically, allowing for feedback during surgery to reduce the incidence of positive margins.

Both of these techniques, OCT structural imaging and LSS nuclear sizing, provide valuable high-resolution information about the cell morphology, and thus distinguish themselves from the more traditional structural techniques that image bulk structural effects on a scale of 10–1000 times larger than the cells themselves.

Functional markers

Functional markers are a first step away from conventional anatomic markers, and toward more specific imaging. Functional markers work on the basis of dynamic features, such as capillary leak, lymphatic transport, blood oxygenation, and blood flow. In a sense, these features are not much different than anatomic probes which provide their signal by bulk phenomenon, but functional markers improve upon conventional techniques by providing a signal that is (at least in part) dependent upon the biology of living tissue.

An example of a functional marker is the tissue or vascular transit time of injected indocyanine green (ICG), an FDA-approved injectable contrast agent [43,44], and which shows a signal, likely due to increased retention and capillary leak of neovasculature in cancer, or by co-transport with albumin in the lymph after extracellular injection. An optical image of ICG in spontaneous dog mammary tumors is shown in Figure 3.

Another type of functional marker is colloid, used in lymphatic mapping. Colloid follows the lymphatic draining the extracellular fluid, and thus identifies the lymph node or nodes which drain that tissue, termed the sentinel node, and can be radiolabeled or optically labeled. The identification of such sentinel node or nodes has been performed using functionally targeted radioactive tracers for breast cancer [45] and melanoma [46], and has since enabled the development of limited nodal resections, called sentinel lymph node biopsies [47,48], as a cancer staging and therapeutic procedure. We have used albumin and PEG macromolecules, each labeled with cyanine dyes to track lymphatic flow in mice, to label lymph nodes, and to label tumors, as shown in Figure 4, and anticipate testing this agent in humans in the near future [67].

Similarly, radiolabeled Tc-Sestamibi [49], a cationic, lipophilic agent which concentrates in some tumors [50], likely accumulating in the negatively charged, hypoxic mitochondria [51], can be used to

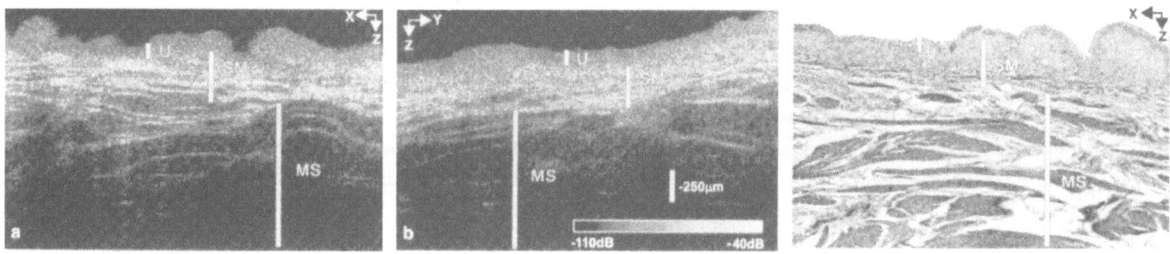

Figure 1. *Ex vivo* two-dimensional Optical Coherence Tomography (OCT) images of fresh porcine bladder. OCT images from the surface down, much like an ultrasound image, yielding a two-dimensional image of surface position and the tissue at depth. The structures seen in the OCT images (right) correspond to those seen in the H&E panel (left). Image size 4 mm × 4 mm. The urothelium (U), submucosa (SM) and muscularis (MS) layer of the urinary bladder wall are clearly seen, as indicated by white bars. Modified from Pan et al. [242].

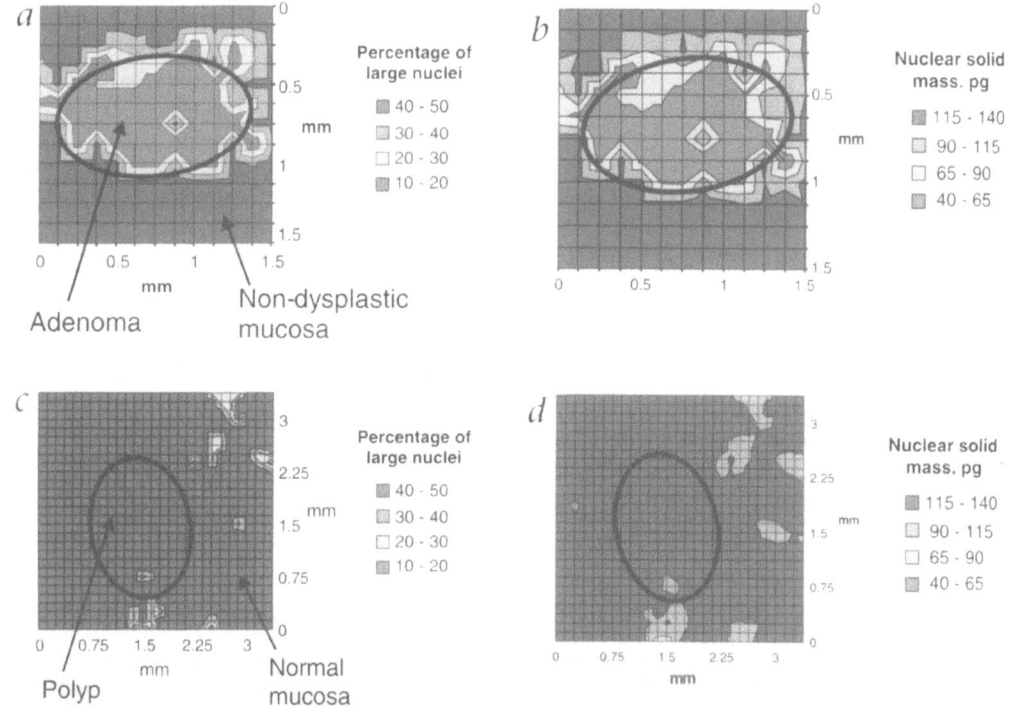

Figure 2. Optical Light Scattering Spectroscopy (LSS) images of nuclear size and density. In these images, (a and b) an adenoma shows as red, having a high percentage of large nuclei and high solid nuclear mass. In contrast, (c and d) a polyp is not visible by percent large nuclei, nor by high nuclear solid mass. These images required about 10 min to collect in a noninvasive, noncontact manner. From Gurjar et al. (2001) [243].

reject the need for biopsy in patients with dense or calcified breasts who otherwise would have gone on to have an invasive biopsy after a questionable or indeterminate mammogram [11]. Sestamibi could be similarly labeled using a fluorescent dye; other agents, such as an octapeptide analog of somatostatin, have been coupled to optical dyes and imaged *in vivo* using optical methods [52,53].

Antigenic probes

Antigenic probes typically recognize and bind to extracellular, and in some cases intracellular, domains. While most cancers do not externally express novel markers, many markers are overexpressed or upregulated in tumors. Targeted antibodies have been demonstrated effective *in vivo* for both diagnostic and

276

therapeutic purposes. Target binding sites for cancer include those antigens and receptors expressed or overexpressed in cancer as compared to normal tissue, such as PSMA [54,55] in the prostate; CEA; MUC1 and other mucins; mammaglobin, HER-2/neu, EGF-R, ER, PR, and others in breast. Some receptors internalize, allowing intracellular delivery of the agent. Although early attempts at such targeting produced high levels of nonspecific binding, high immunogenic-

ity, and short half-lives [56], significant improvements have allowed clinical utility to be reached for several targeted agents [57]. At least 24 therapeutic antibodies are in clinical trials, 10 have been approved by the US Food and Drug Administration for various chronic diseases, and 200 others are in preclinical development.

Examples of successful clinical application of monoclonal antibodies *in vivo* include, in breast, EGF-like sites (Her-2/neu) are used to target therapy, while targeted lymphoscintigraphy after intravenous or local injection helps to identify patients with axillary involvement [58,59]. In the lung, a ^{99}Tc-labeled agents targeted toward somatostatin receptor-bearing pulmonary masses was approved by the FDA in 1999 for the localization of lung cancer. Last, two monoclonal agents are approved for colorectal cancer. When used in addition to CT scanning, one of these (CEA-Scan) increased preoperative identification of resectable patients by 40% and identified twice as many non-resectable patients as CT alone [60]. Many agents have side-effects or have failed as therapeutic agents due to cross-reactivity (such as cardiotoxicity of Her-2-neu). However, such cross-reactivity does not prevent low doses of a targeted imaging agent being used. Thus, there is a rich pool of agents to choose from, including agents no longer being used as therapeutic agents.

The successful delivery of such agents to tissues for therapeutic purposes confirms the concept that such agents can be used in lower concentration for imaging. Results to date have been mixed, but the images appear

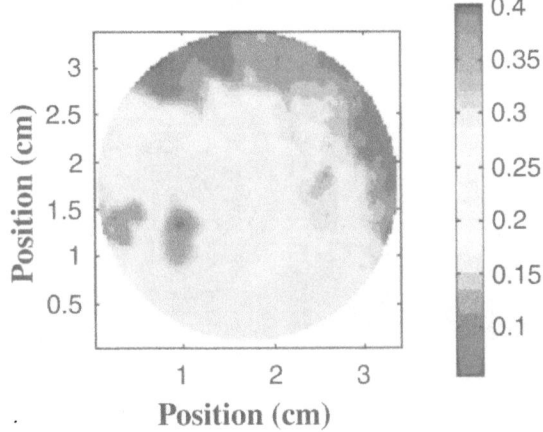

Figure 3. A optical canine breast image made after injection of a fluorescent optical contrast. The image was collected optically. A spontaneous canine mammary tumor shows up as red–dark red, due to retention of the contrast agent in the neovasculature and/or capillary leakage. Image provided by Sevick-Muraca et al. (1999).

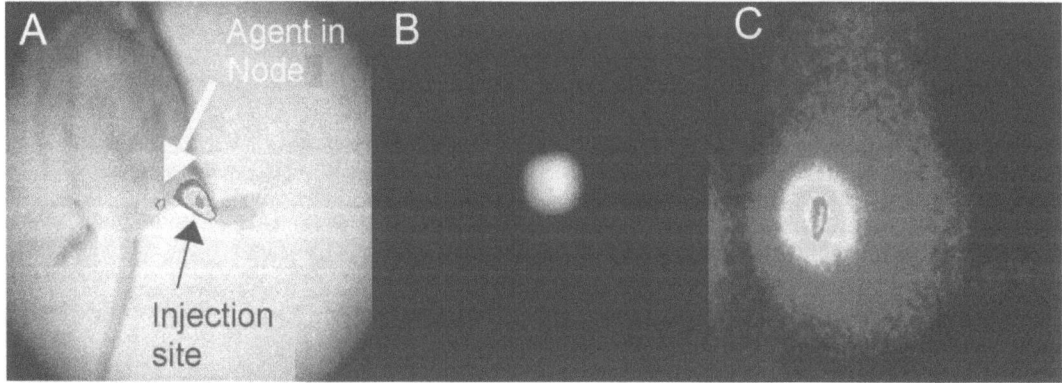

Figure 4. Optical contrast images collected in room light. (A) A subcutaneous injection of PEG conjugated to cyanine dyes for lymphatic tracking shows a lymph node in real time. (B) A 5 mm breast lymph node model at 2 cm depth is seen in real-time in this room light image. (C) One frame from a real-time optical fluorescence cine in which a 5 mm tumor model is imaged in real-time in a moving mouse. Importantly, these images were collected in room light, using a camera developed under National Cancer Institute support allowing trace fluorescence to be imaged in real-time during interventional surgical procedures. Images from Benaron et al. (2001) [65].

to be improving as better and more specific antigens and antibodies are identified. About 1,000–10,000 copies can be delivered to a target cell expressing a surface receptor (such receptors are typically expressed with between 10^5 and 10^7 copies per cell surface). However, distribution of large antigenic agents into these tissues is often patchy and uneven, particularly into tumors which frequently have heterogeneous blood flow, poorly perfused and hypoxic regions, and possibly necrotic centers. As a result of the limited numbers of copies that can be delivered per cell, and the patchy distribution, the resolution of antigenic approaches in humans using radionuclides has been typically no better than 3–4 mm. SPECT is 2-orders of magnitude less sensitive than PET, but the spatial resolution can be better than 2 mm.

While novel disease-specific markers for tumors are not common in non-hematopoetic malignancies [245], there are many tissue-class-specific antigens which are unique, and are not typically expressed on other tissues (or are expressed elsewhere in a limited fashion). Of importance, malignant cells often continue to express class-markers which are characteristic of or specific to the normal tissue from which the tumor originated [245]. Thus, the appearance of these tissue-class-specific markers at a body site where these markers are not normally found implies both the presence of tumor and a metastasis of that tumor. Class-based agents are also potentially useful for cellular tracking of hematopoetic subsets, in which a subclass of cells exhibits a unique and differentiating combination of surface markers, such as white cell subclasses.

A partial list of known tissue-class-specific or tissue-class-restricted (less specific) molecules are shown in Table 1.

One example of class-based imaging using the antigens normally expressed by the parent is use of the J591 antibody, developed by Bander and colleagues at Cornell, and targeted to an extracellular domain of the PSMA membrane protein. As the target is extracellular, this antibody binds to intact, viable LNCaP cells *in vitro* (unlike ProstaScint antibody, 7E11, which binds to an intracellular domain of PSMA and thus will not bind to intact cells). Studies have consistently shown that PSMA is highly restricted to prostate epithelial cells and a few other tissues. The background signal from other targets of the antibody has been inconsequential when compared to prostate expression of J591 labeling. While some other normal tissues that express substantially lower levels of PSMA include some renal tubules, duodenum, astrocytes and salivary

Table 1. Tissue-class-specific tumor markers

Breast Adenocarcinoma	Muc-1*
	Carcinoembryonic antigen (CEA, nonspecific)
	Cytokeratin-19
Follicular thyroid carcinomas	Thyroglobulin
	Thyroid Peroxidase
Gastrointestinal adenocarcinoma	CEA*
	Cytokeratin-20
Hepatocellular carcinoma	Alpha-fetoprotein (AFP)
	Albumin
Lung adenocarcinoma	CEA*
	Muc-1
	Cytokeratin-19
	Surfactant Protein
Melanoma	Tyrosinase
	MART-I
	GAGE*
Neuroblastoma	Tyrosine Hydroxylase
	PGP 9.5
	GAGE* (also found in melanoma)
Prostate adenocarcinoma	PSMA* (also found in neovasculature)
	PTI-1*
Uterine cervical adenocarcinoma	Squamous cell carcinoma antigen (SCC)

Modified from Ghossein et al. [245] and others. * = class-restricted (appearing in a limited number, but more than one, tissue class).

gland, assays have demonstrated that the level of PSMA expression in these other tissues is approximately 2–3 decades lower than in prostate cancer. Beyond the limited normal tissue expression and substantially lower levels of expression, these non-prostate sites are significantly less accessible to circulating mAb and do not represent confounding *in vivo* targets. Further, when used as an imaging agent for local cancer, binding to non-prostate tissues, far removed from the surgical field, may be less relevant. This is confirmed by nuclear medicine scan in humans that show high tumor binding, and low levels elsewhere.

Of note, J591 mAbs are also reactive with vascular endothelium within a wide variety of carcinomas, including lung, colon, breast, and others, but not with normal vascular endothelium. Thus, these mAbs antibodies may prove useful for *in vivo* targeting of prostate cancer, as well as to the vascular compartment of a wide variety of carcinomas, possibly making J591 cancer-specific for other types of tumors in which the tissue does not display PSMA antigen in its normal state. This would allow for J591 antibody to be used in the sensitive detection of other types of cancers still contained within the primary organ. A humanized version, named huJ591, is now under testing as a radionuclide agent bound to ^{111}In and ^{131}I labeled forms of J591.

Another example of a use of class-based antigenic targeting is the use of specific agents for improving lymph node scans. The success of interoperative lymphatic mapping depends upon accurate identification of the sentinel node [61]. Nonspecific targeting of lymphnodes includes such agents as Isosulfan blue dye [62], carbon particles [61], albumin [63], radio- and/or dye-labeled liposomes [64], and synthetic macromolecules [65]. Lymphotic imaging has typically been via nuclear medicine techniques, however MRI [66] and optical methods [67] have been reported. Image-targeted lymphotic surgery allows for a limited region of resection, without loss, or with minimal loss, of staging accuracy [68–71]. Even better would be a targeted agent, able to indicate whether a node contained tumor or not, which could in theory allow the 69% of women with negative nodes to bypass the procedure entirely. Markers targeted toward tumor cells include CEA for colorectal cancer [72] and others [73,74].

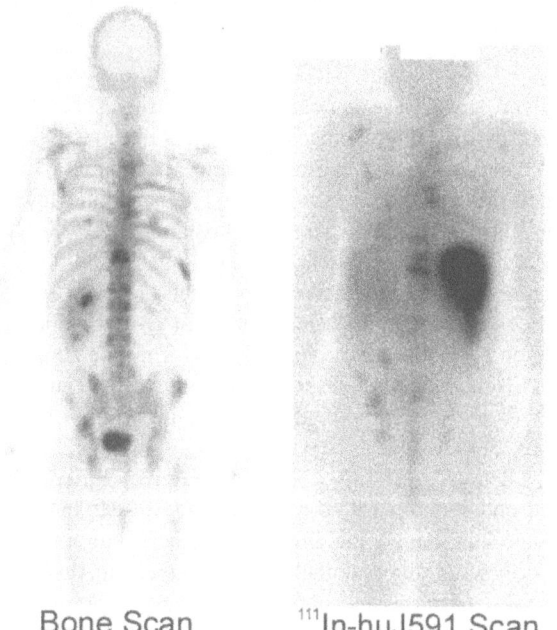

Bone Scan   ^{111}In-huJ591 Scan

Figure 5. Images using PSMA-targeted antibody hJ-591. A standard posterior-view radionuclide bone scan (left) shows comparable lesions to an image made using ^{111}In-labeled huJ591 antibody in the same human subject. (Source: S. Goldsmith, N. Bander, Cornell Univ.).

Antigenic probes are being explored as tools to permit selective use of lymphatic biopsy procedures, particularly in melanoma and breast cancer. The goal would be to avoid nodal dissection in the majority of patients who, in retrospect, did not require a nodal dissection. For example, PET has been investigated as a method for segmenting breast cancer patients into those that should have sentinel nodal biopsy, and those who can skip the procedure altogether, using ^{18}F-FDG [76]. In recent studies, a negative predictive value of 67% was seen (i.e., a negative result was correct only two-thirds of the time), and given that that a lymph node resection itself (e.g., the surgery itself, independent of other therapy) is believed to improve survival by 4–16% [12], it was concluded that PET is not yet ready for use as a selection tool.

It remains likely that, as long as micrometastases can influence recurrence and survival, that tools such as PET, CT, and MRI alone will not have sufficient sensitivity to allow for imaging-only determination of the presence, location, and size of metastases; however, optical methods now under investigation may have sufficiently high sensitivity that they may be able to fulfill this role, and multiple trials for such optical methods are in planning or are underway. For example, our group is developing targeted cyanine dyes, such as cytokeratin-targeted and MIBI targeted agents, for sentinel lymph node staging.

Limitations to a tissue-class-based approach do exist. First, tumors are heterogeneous, with significant genetic instability and variation, and thus many antigenic markers may be lost. Second, treatment, such as hormonal therapy, can deplete cell populations expressing certain native markers, or result in up- or down-regulation of groups of genes, including those responsible for the diagnostic imaging marker [75]. Next, tumor cells often demonstrate developmental regression toward a more pluripotent, but differently marked, stem cell line, and in this process markers may change. Last, as normal tissue(s), by definition, express these class-specific markers, metastatic tumor too close to, or located within, the normal tissue will most likely become undetectable, as the signal will be lost in noise.

Metabolic spectroscopy

Metabolic probes rely on imaging agents involving certain enzymatic pathways or transport functions of the cell. Traditionally, such probes have been metabolic homologs which accumulate at the site of a specific metabolic activity. Examples of such probes are ^{18}F-fluorodeoxyglucose ([18]FDG) in PET and ^{11}C-thymidine in radionuclide scans, both of which accumulate in tumor cells due a relatively higher metabolic rate. Equivalent fluorescence-based analogs are under study for optical imaging, such as with a fluorescent deoxyglucose.

Newer techniques are now introducing the localization of spectroscopy, but without the requirement for exogenous labeled probes. Two methods of performing spectroscopy are optical spectroscopic methods (including elastic and Raman spectroscopy) and MRSI [77–83], each allowing for the imaging of biochemical intermediates, cell components, and cellular energetics.

An example of proton magnetic resonance spectroscopic imaging is shown (^{1}H-MRSI is further described under Selected Techniques). In this example, a two-dimensional grid placed over each conventional MR image slices marks the boundaries of spectroscopic analysis of each grid voxel for agents such as choline (Cho), a structural component of cells which produces a stronger signal in tumor, creatine (Cr), a marker of cellular energetics which falls in tumor, and N-acetyl aspartate (NAA), a marker of neuronal integrity which falls in tumor. In brain tumor, the Choline : NAA ratio and creatine levels allow differentiation of normal tissue, tumor, and necrotic tissue, as shown in Figure 6.

Metabolic changes can be very sensitive and early indicators of treatment response. As such, metabolic approaches show promise for the monitoring, and perhaps ultimately selection, of treatment.

Molecular probes

Advances in gene mapping, and in methods to identify small molecules and targets involved in cell signaling and physiology, have led to the discovery of a large number of potential labeling targets for contrast imaging. In theory, any marker can be targeted as a contrast site provided that the agent can be delivered in sufficient concentration and for a sufficient time that imaging can occur.

Several recent reviews have focused on this emerging area of molecular imaging [84–87]. Broadly, molecular imaging is defined as the *in vivo* imaging, characterization, and measurement of biologic processes at the cellular and molecular imaging. This is usually (though not always) held to be in contradistinction to antigenic imaging, in which surface markers, but not the pathways themselves, are imaged using antigenic probes.

Molecular probes have several key advantages. First, molecules are small, and thus unlike antibody-targeted therapies, they achieve a distribution more quickly. In one study comparing antibody-targeted and small peptide-targeted optical agents, the octapeptide somatostatin analog achieved good imaging distributions in 15 min to several hours after injection, while the antibody-targeted agents required 1–2 days to reach a similar distribution [88]. Next, molecules are, in general, more easily labeled, stored, and reproducibly synthesized, all requirements for regulatory approval of imaging agents.

While optical methods can image femtomolar (sub-picomolar) concentrations [89] and detect rare single-cell events, this is not true for MRI and PET. Both MRI and PET require amplification of the signal in order for low concentrations to become detectable. Multiple amplification strategies have been developed, with some appropriate only for animal use, and others well suited to translation toward human imaging.

Amplification strategies for MRI, PET, and optical imaging include the following:

- *Trapping* Trapping implies a one-way localization into a tissue or cell compartment. An agent may be trapped by metabolic conversion or receptor-mediated internalization, such that a concentration of an intermediate accumulates over time.
- *Expression* An imaging agent can be inducibly expressed, such as by the genetic expression of a GFP gene, which results in hundreds of mRNA messages, and therefore in thousands of GFP copies per cell. Such probes can detect gene expression at a very low level. A clever modification of this is the expression of a gene which codes for an unusual metabolite, such as for expression of arginine kinase (AK), the prokaryotic correlate of creatine kinase (CK). The existence of AK in a eukaryote must come from a transfected expressible element, while AK can be detected using ^{31}P-MRSI [94].
- *Activation* An imaging agent may be in a dormant phase, and switched on (or even switched off) in response to interaction with a target molecule, enzyme, or receptor. Such agents are known for MRI [90] and optical methods [91,92]. An example of activation is the near-infrared activatable fluorescent probes devised by Weissleder and colleagues [92,93]. This agent here is initially self-quenching, but becomes brightly fluorescent after

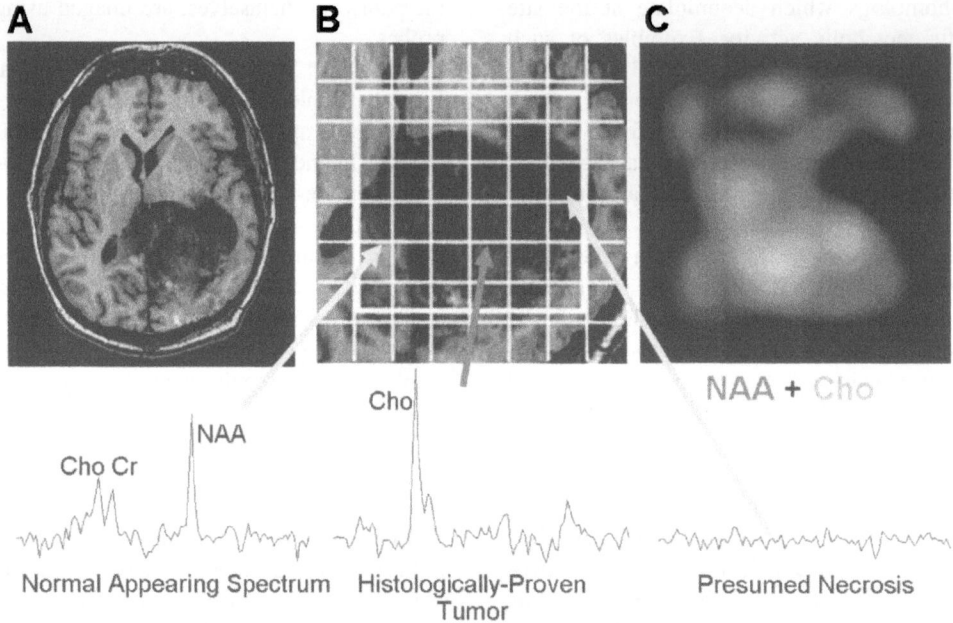

Figure 6. MRSI images from a brain tumor. (A) Conventional MRI image of a brain tumor before surgery. (B) A grid for spectroscopic analysis is overlayed on a region of the MRI scan in A, with MRSI spectra from three regions shown (arrows). (C) NAA is shown in red, choline in green. Regions of solid tumor appear green, normal brain tissue appears red-yellow, and necrotic tissue appears black. Modified from Vigneron et al. (2001) [82].

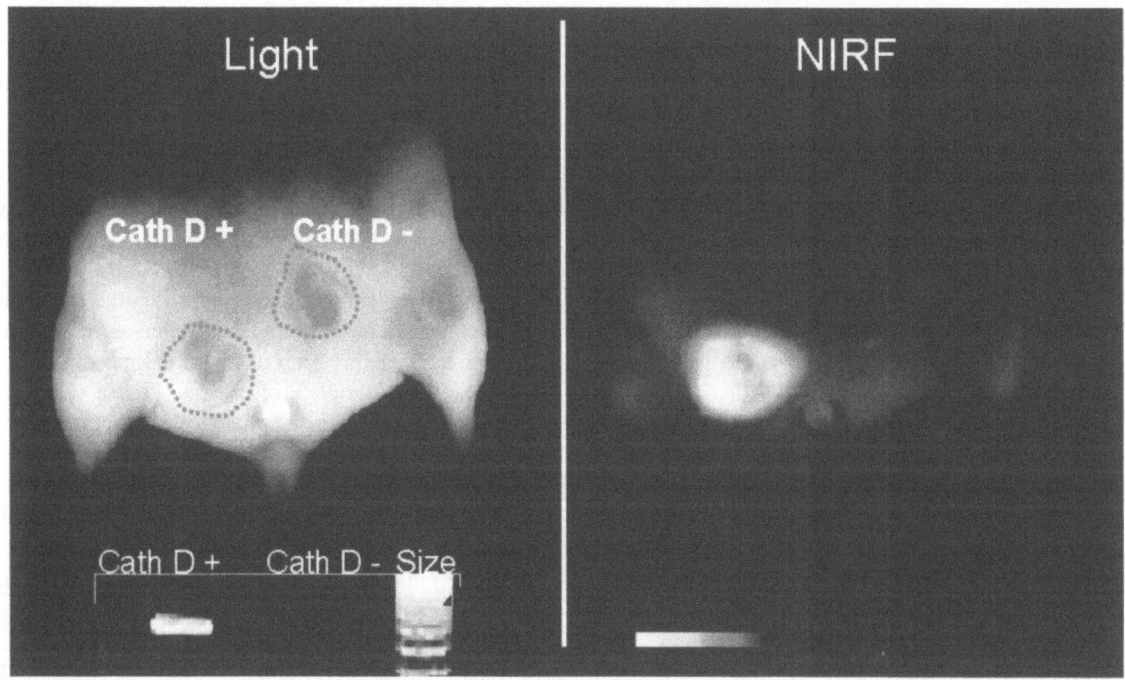

Figure 7. An activatable near-infrared fluorescent (NIRF) probe which is cleaved and activates in the presence of Cathepsin D. (Left) White light image showing the location of two tumors. (Right) Noninvasive NIRF image of dye activation *in vivo*. From Tung et al., Cancer Research (2001) [93].

action by Cathepsin-D (Cat D) on an integrated Cat D cleavage site in the reporter molecule, as shown in Figure 7.

• *Combinations of the above* More than one approach can be used. For example, a dormant gene membrane translocator can be turned-on in a target cell (such as a tumor), producing mRNA coding for the translocator. Gene expression produces thousands of membrane-bound translocator proteins, which allows for the internalization and trapping of an extracellular contrast agent, excluded from cells not bearing the translocator on their cell surface. An example of using an expressed reporter molecule to concentrate a contrast agent is the use of an expressible transferrin receptor (see Figure 8). As MRSI can detect metabolites, unusual but detectable metabolites can also be the end product for imaging. Although outside of the conventional H-based MRI, recombinant adenovirus encoding AK (the invertebrate homolog to the vertebrate CK) produces a detectable phosphoarginine in ^{31}P-MRI [94].

Cell tracking

Any of the above amplifications or labeling strategies can be used to label a specific class of cell. For example, white blood cell tracking [95] using cell-surface antigens may be used for imaging inflammation. Tracking of other blood-borne cells has also been reported [96–99]. Alternatively, a T-cell subset imaging mouse could be created by collecting that particular T-cell subset from a bone marrow sample in a mouse bred to express luciferase in every cell line, followed by transplantation of the harvested T-cell subset into the marrow of an identical, but luciferase negative, mouse, thus producing a mouse in which every CD4+ T-cell expresses luciferase, but no other cell line in the mouse expresses luciferase, or even has the genetic capacity to do so.

Tumor cell tracking has been performed using PET [100], MRI [101], and optical GFP [102] and luciferase [9] imaging. As one example of cell tracking, using genetically expressed elements such as GFP, developmental subsets (such as neuronal elements) or tumor cells can be imaged. An image showing tracking and imaging of individual glioma cells in a living mouse is shown in Figure 9 [103].

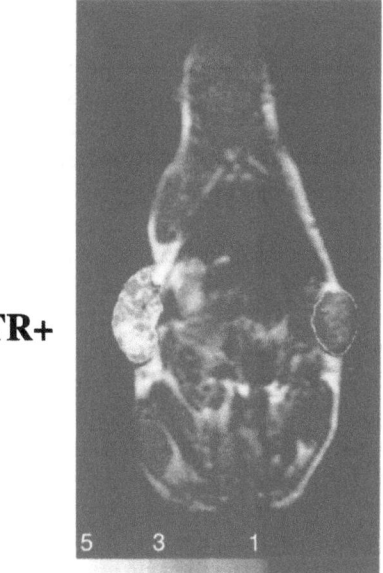

ETR+   ETR-

Figure 8. In vivo T1-weighted MR imaging of genetic expression. In this image, an engineered transferrin receptor (ETR) is transfected and expressed in a tumor cell line, which becomes detectable when a paramagnetic transferrin ligand probe is injected. (Left) With ETR expression, addition of the transferrin ligand produces a strong signal. (Right) In the absence of ETR expression, a control tumor does not enhance with ligand injection. From Weissleder et al. (2000) [244].

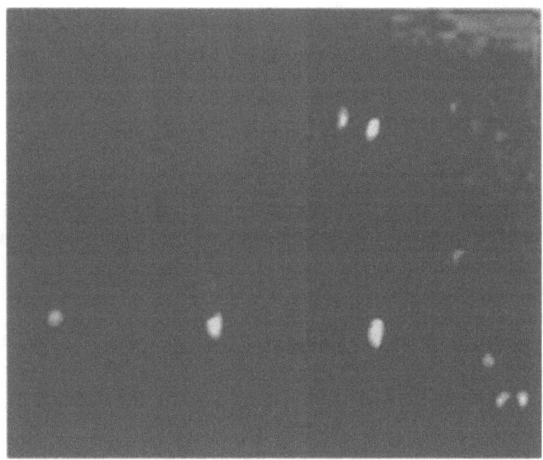

Figure 9. In vivo optical tracking and imaging of single glioma cells constitutively expressing GFP. The ability to externally image and identify single glioma cells labeled with GFP *in vivo* illustrates the power and sensitivity of optical techniques. From Yang et al. (2002) [103].

V. Selected near-term clinical techniques

The contrast sources, both intrinsic signals and extrinsic agents, as described above are being moved toward clinical use in several areas. In this article, selected techniques that extend the reach of current imaging, and are in or are moving toward clinical use, are discussed in more detail.

The methods described below are summarized in Table 2. By family, these areas are as follows:

Magnetic resonance

Conventional (anatomic) MRI has high spatial resolution, but cannot reliably distinguish tumor from other tissues, such as necrotic tissue or even normal tissue in some cases. In the brain, a T_2-weighted image may encompass a tumor, but also reflects nonspecific effects such as edema and inflammation. Such factors produce considerable uncertainties in margins, which limits the utility of the technique for defining treatment targets [82]. In the prostate, the staging accuracy of tumor in the peripheral zone has been reported to be only 70% [110]. However, MRI cannot reliably distinguish between stromal benign prostatic hyperplasia from prostate adenocarcinoma, as a result of the overlap in their signal intensities [104], and post-biopsy hemorrhage, scar, prostatitis, or interglandular dysplasia can be indistinguishable from prostate cancer in 50% of cases [105]. This remains true, even with high-resolution local prostate imaging coils [106,107].

Newer techniques are extending the sensitivity of MRI. Using MRSI, metabolic intermediates and cell energetic markers can be imaged. Using activatable or expressible MRI contrast amplification, localized functional enhancement can be achieved and even genetic expression can be imaged, as discussed below.

Table 2. Newer, more specific and sensitive methods of imaging fall into 3 families: MRI, PET/nuclear med, and optical imaging.

Family/ Method	Sensing method	Depth limit (mm)	Lower size limit* (mm)	Lower concentration limit*	Time/Scan (sec or min)
MRI					
MRSI	Spectroscopic MRI	None	2	100 μM	10–20 min
Genetic expression	T_1 MRI or Novel-metabolite MRSI	None	2	n/a	10 sec to 10 min
Activatable	Switchable water access to Gd-DTPA	None	2	n/a	10 sec to 10 min
PET/SPECT					
Radiolabeled mAb	Beta-decay (1 positron → 2 photons)	Minimal limitation	3	n/a	10–30 min
^{18}F-FDG	Alpha-decay (1 photon)	Minimal limitation	5	n/a	5–20 min
Optical					
Optical coherence tomography	Single-scattered photons	2–3	0.002	n/a	0.05 sec per frame
Luciferase	Bioluminescence	50–70	0.05	<1 pM	0.5–5 min
Optical contrast	Fluorescence	30–50	10% of depth	1 pM	0.01 sec to 5 min
Nuclear sizing	Optical scattering	2	0.1	n/a	10–20 min
Raman	Raman spectroscopy	5	5*	10 μM	1–10 min
Diffuse optical tomography	Optical absorbance and/or scattering	20–50	10% of depth	<1 μM	0.05 sec to 20 min

The source of the signal, the level of minimum detection, and advantages and disadvantages are summarized above. *Size and concentration limits for studies in human subjects. Animal imager limits are potentially lower due to smaller bore size and/or higher power due to absence of human safety exposure limits.

Magnetic resonance spectroscopy imaging

More detailed metabolic information is available from proton MRI than is conventionally displayed. The information typically shown to the radiologist is only a small subset of the data made available by the core technique, nuclear magnetic resonance (NMR). The displayed imaged typically seen represents various characteristics of the NMR signal of the protons in water (or sometimes fat) as the signal varies by relative concentration and environment (intra/extracellular ratios, diffusibility, etc.).

The MRI signal can be improved, without augmentation from an exogenous contrast agent, as contrast is provided by native metabolites and components of the tissue itself. MRSI takes advantage of the chemical signatures in the detected signal, most commonly in the ^{1}H or ^{31}P spectrum [108]. Local variations in the environment for each of these atoms produces variations in the resonant emissions, which are translated into images that can be related to the concentration of the various molecular species producing the signals. An abbreviated list of these agents now detectable is shown in Table 3.

Advantages of this approach are that cellular metabolism can be monitored, and that (at least for ^{1}H analysis) the detection requires only software package updates for many conventional MRI instruments. Major disadvantages include the high magnetic field

Table 3. Molecules detectable by MR ^{1}H and ^{31}P Spectroscopic Imaging (MRSI)

^{1}H Proton spectroscopy	^{31}P Phosphorous spectroscopy
Choline	ATP/ADP/AMP/adenosine
Creatine	Creatine/phosphocreatine
Citrate	Inorganic phosphorous
Lactate	Phosphoarginine[a]
Glutamate, glutamine	Phospholipids[b]
Asparate/asparagine	
Lipid	
Water	
Polyamines, ethanolamines	

The list is abbreviated, as high-resolution techniques ($> 3T$) are beginning to reliably detect a long list of metabolites. Significant differences have been found in these components between benign and malignant tumors, with tumor typically showing increased choline to creatine ratios and/or increased lactate in the ^{1}H spectrum, and/or showing decreased energy reserves in the ^{31}P spectrum. [a] = Phosphoarginine not native in eukaryotes, expressed using transfected Arginine Kinase (AK). [b] = specific phospholipids include sphingomyelin, phosphatidylcholine, phosphatidylserine, phosphatidic acid, phosphatidylglycerol, and alkylacylphosphatidylcholine.

required for the best resolution ($>2T$), the requirement for high micromolar to millimolar concentrations (thus making expressed custom agents more difficult to detect), and the long imaging times required for small voxel size.

Using proton spectroscopy alone, such techniques can identify tissues by type [109], as well as differentiate tumor from non-tumor in the prostate [110] and brain [111], with the possibility of prostate [112,113], brain [114,115], breast [116,117], tumor grading. Three-dimensional techniques have the ability to provide greater spatial localization, as well as better resolution of the component peaks [118].

Metabolite levels measured by MRSI are tumor and tissue specific. In prostate, citrate is a normal component of healthy prostate tissue, showing the highest level of citrate of any tissue in the human body [119,120], while during oncogenesis, the level of citrate in these cells falls to undetectable levels [120]. In contrast, brain tumors typically show decreased *N*-acetyl aspartate signal [121] (NAA), suggestive of a reduction in neuronal cell density (as anti-NAA radiolabeled antibodies have shown NAA to be confined in the brain to neurons [122]), and a higher choline signal, attributed to altered membrane phospholipids metabolism, mobility, and/or composition [111]. Significantly, even in the lowest grade brain tumors, NAA levels were reduced to low or undetectable levels, as compared to FDG-PET [123,124]. In some tumors, high lactate signals are also variably seen.

A set of MRSI spectra from prostate cancer [125] is shown in Figure 10 (such spectra can also be used to generate color overlay images, highlighting malignant tissues, as shown earlier in Figure 6).

This MRSI signal is now being studied as an endpoint in chemoprevention trials [13]. MRSI has also been used to target therapy in pre-treatment planning, such as to increase local radiation in prostate brachytherapy in regions with high choline:citrate ratios [126].

MRI molecular amplification strategies

MRI, if given an appropriate signal, can image with resolution down to the $10\,\mu m$ level in animal models [127]. However, because of low sensitivity, MRI is usually limited to the mM level, such as blood-oxygen level determination (BOLD) imaging of the paramagnetic deoxyhemoglobin. In comparison, an antibody binding to surface receptors in tumor usually achieves a level in the picomolar range, at best. Therefore, to

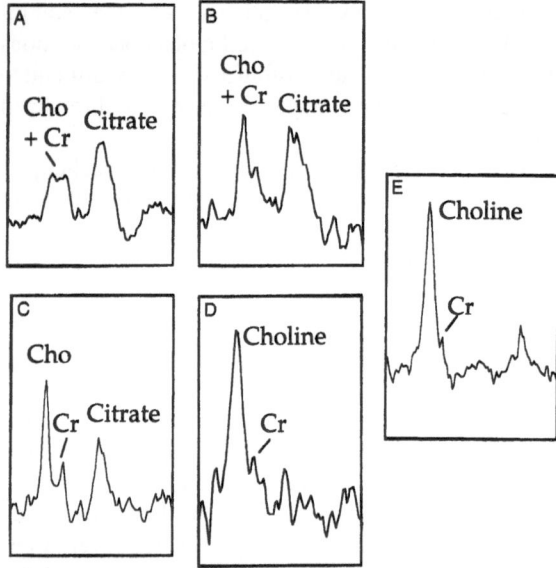

Figure 10. MRSI spectra obtained *in vivo* show changes with grade of prostate cancer. Prostate cancer Gleason grades (A) 5, (B) 6, (C) 7, (D) 8, and (E) prostate cancer metastatic to brain. Imaging volume is 0.24 cm³. From Kurhanewicz et al. (2000) [125].

detect molecular events using MRI, an amplification strategy is often employed [128].

One MRI amplification strategy is to use certain intrinsic enzymes to create a T_1-weighted signal. This has been exploited in melanomas using tyrosinase which binds iron to produce enhanced signal in some native melanomas [129–131], β-galactosidase which can cleave-design substrates shielding water from gadolinium, allowing the signal to turn on [132], and in polymers with detectable MRI signal [133]. For example, insertion of human tyrosinase cDNA into cells results in an 8-fold signal enhancement, attributed to the enhanced iron sequestration by melanin [134].

An alternative strategy is to produce a pump that concentrates an exogenous imaging agent, such as the human transferrin receptor [135,136], modified to prevent the iron-mediated feedback that would otherwise limit signal *in vivo* [244].

As with all genetically expressed reporter systems, the system has the potential of being inherited by progeny of a parent cell, and thus can stably label a growing population.

PET/SPECT

In radionuclide imaging, an imaging reporter generates a single high-energy photon during nuclear decay of an unstable intermediate, with targeting of the radionuclide to achieve specificity, usually achieved with antibodies (labeled with 99mTc or 111In) or by molecules that preferentially accumulate at target locations (such as at sites of increased bone turnover with 99mTc-methylenediphosphonate, somatostatin receptors with 111In-Octreotide, hypoxic tissues with 99mTc-sestamibi, lymphomas with 67Ga-chloride, or brain tumors and osteosarcomas with 201Tl). In contrast, PET emitters are also single-atom reporters, but these elements decay with by positron emission, which produces two high-energy photons. PET emitters include the basic organic compound building blocks O, C, N, and (as there is no hydrogen PET emitter) F. Such atoms are readily incorporated into biological molecules that are enzymatic or receptor substrate analogs, such as 18F-fluorodeoxyglucose (FDG) or 11C-thymidine. Accumulation of PET reporters can be controlled by the transport or enzymatic process targeted by the reporter, usually through intracellular trapping (such as by trapping of phosphorylated FDG in the cell or incorporation of thymidine into DNA). Positron emitters are also known for other atoms, including Cu, Zn, K, Br, Rb, I, P, Fe, and Ga.

An advantage to PET over chelated, targeted radionuclides is the small size of the PET reporter molecules, which allows rapid diffusion or transport into tissues, cells, and even into the cell nucleus. Nearly any molecule can be modified to be a reporter, including pharmaceuticals and metabolites.

A significant disadvantage to all nuclear agents is that each reporter molecule reports only once, and this reporting occurs over hours to days (radionuclides) or minutes to hours (PET) for each molecule. As a result, the fraction of PET emitters which produce a signal during any given imaging period is small, and therefore a large number of molecules must be localized at the imaging site in order to produce a detectable signal. Further, the molecule itself, even if metabolized for excretion, will contain the imaging atom and produce an imaging signal nonspecifically, and therefore this method is prone to a significant and nonspecific background signal.

Antigenic radionuclide targeting

The results for tumor staging using these agents have been uneven. In some tumors, PET images have demonstrated value and/or correlate well with stage and grade [137–139], while in others the correlation has not been reliable, or the data are inconclusive [140–143]. In lung cancer, few multi-center, controlled PET trials have been published and verified. Multiple small studies have shown that FDP-PET can distinguish malignant from benign solitary pulmonary nodules with a sensitivity of 80–100%, though the study samples have been sufficiently small and variable that the results are currently inconclusive. In the assessment of mediastinal involvement in non-small cell lung cancer, a meta-analysis has shown FDG-PET to have a sensitivity and specificity similar to mediastinoscopy [144] and to be able to detect distant metastases not seen with conventional imaging techniques in 10% of cases, changing tumor stage and influencing surgical and chemotherapeutic choices [145–147]. In melanoma, PET has detected occult regional nodal involvement [148,149]. In lymphoma, PET can detect nodal involvement up to 6 months earlier than for conventional imaging, and influence patient management in 22% of cases [150].

Nuclear medicine agents have been used to image apoptosis. In apoptosis, cells execute a programmed sequence of cell death. One of the earliest events in programmed cell death is the externalization of phosphatidylserine, a membrane phospholipid normally restricted to the inner leaflet of the lipid bilayer. Annexin V, an endogenous human protein with a high affinity for membrane bound phosphatidylserine, can be used *in vitro* to detect apoptosis before other well described morphologic or nuclear changes associated with programmed cell death. Nuclear medicine agents, either ^{99m}Tc-p-annexin-V (Apomate™) [151] or other agents [152] and MRI agents [17] have been used to image apoptosis, in some cases in patients [18]. Such events may be useful in determination of tumor response to chemotherapy.

Imaging gene expression

Many of the amplification strategies listed for MRI can be applied to PET imaging [153,154].

In PET reporter gene systems, the protein products of the reporter genes are transmembrane pumps or intracellular/nuclear enzymes which modify otherwise diffusible substrates, and produce a gene-expression-dependent or metabolism-dependent trapping of PET probes [155,156]. Examples in which a transmembrane pump concentrates an exogenous imaging agent include dopamine D_2R receptors. D_2R has been used in adenoviral delivery systems and imaged by PET following systemic injection of a positron-labeled ligand

FESP (3-(2'-^{18}F-fluoroethyl)-spiperone) and subsequent D_2R-dependent FESP sequestration. A mutant D_2R receptor gene, which does not modulate cyclic AMP levels, has been described, allowing the reporter function to operate independently of cell signaling and metabolism [157]. Other PET agents are under development for other gene systems, including somatostatin [158], Iodine [159] (some breast cancers are believed to demonstrate increased avidity to iodine), as well as synthetic receptors engineered for internally bound ligands [160,161].

Expressible trapping agents include herpes simplex virus type-1 thymidine kinase reporter gene expression, which relies upon ^{18}F-FHBG or other PET agents as reporter probes [162–164]. Early human studies suggest that this agent functions well in human subjects [165]. An HSV1-Tk/GFP (TKGFP) was also recently used to monitor transcriptional activation of p53-dependent genes, and DNA damage-induced up-regulation of p53 transcriptional activity was correlated with the expression of p53-dependent downstream genes (such as p21) in wild-type p53 cells, but not in p53 −/− cells [166].

Optical imaging

While most of us consider the interior of our bodies to be dark, the human body is not impermeable to light. In fact, if you walked outside on a sunny day, there would be sufficient light under your skull to comfortably read this page [167]. You can see this effect by shining a red laser pointer against your finger. The fingertip glows red, demonstrating that much of the light, while scattered and redirected, still passes through the finger [168].

The key appeal of optics is its inherent low-end sensitivity, which is unmatched by any other *in vivo* imaging technique. For example, while MRI and MRSI require micromolar concentrations of contrast agents, optical methods can detect concentrations which are sub-picomolar [89]. Also, while 500,000-cell tumors are at the limit of human *in vivo* MRI, PET, and CT detection, as few as 100 internal luciferase-labeled tumor cells *in vivo* can be visualized from the outside an animal. In fact, single cells labeled with GFP have been tracked *in vivo* [169]. Last, in terms of spatial resolution, OCT provides the highest resolution of any *in vivo* imaging method, optical or otherwise [198].

Other advantages of optical methods include the ability to monitor multiple independent optical reporters simultaneously *in vivo* based upon wavelength, the absence of radioactive intermediates, and the relative simplicity of the imaging hardware as compared to MRI and PET equipment.

The major disadvantage of optical approaches is a limited penetration. Red and infrared light lose about 90% of their intensity with each centimeter traveled through tissue, while blue-green light loses 90% of signal for each 0.1–1 mm traveled. As a result, even the most deeply penetrating infrared optical signals are lost at between 4 and 8 cm of tissue depth from the imaging sensor (at the shallower end of this range for systems requiring illumination, such as fluorescence, and at the deeper end of this range for systems requiring only detection, such as red luciferase bioluminescence). In part, it is this limitation that ultimately is most likely to limit use of optical techniques *in vivo*. Nevertheless, the high sensitivity of optical approaches has led to a rapid adoption in animal models, with human applications following shortly behind.

Why are optical approaches potentially so sensitive when used at relatively shallow depths? Consider a comparison of an optical dye and a radionuclide, both targeted toward the same extracellular surface receptor on a tumor. Once losses are considered, the minimum detectable number of cells for a nuclear scan is 200,000, while this minimum number is 1–10 cells for an optical scan, as summarized in Table 4.

Multiple methods of contrast are available for optical imaging. These mechanisms of contrast using optics have comparable parallels to more conventional types of imaging, as shown in Table 5.

Table 4. Sensitivity of optical methods is over 1000-fold higher than comparable nuclear medicine agents

	Radioemitter	Optical dye
For each cell		
Emission time	3.5 days	10 μsec
No. of contrast molecules	1000	1000
Time per photon	7 min	10 per sec
Scans	1	1000–10,000
Image time	35 min	1 sec
Counts/image/cell (no loss)	5	1,000,000+
For each image		
Imaging loss	10^5	10^7
Counts/cell/scan	5×10^{-6}	0.1
Minimum detectable cells	200,000	1–10

Here, the minimal detectable signal from an antibody-targeted Technetium-labeled radionuclide is 10,000-fold less than that for a similarly targeted fluorescent optical marker. A thallium-based marker decays at random, with a half-life of 3.5 days, therefore for 1000 molecules attaching per cell, a radioemitter produces one photon every 7 min, equivalent to 5 photons produced from a single cell in a 35 min scan. In contrast, a stimulated dye decays in nanoseconds to milliseconds, 1000 photons in 10 μsec, or an average of one photon every 10 per sec. The illumination may be pulsed 1000 times a second, producing 1 million photons per second from a single illuminated cell. In practice, for surface or near-surface conditions, optical imaging methods can be more than 1000 times as sensitive as CT, MRI, or PET imaging, and falls by about 10-fold for every centimeter of depth. Even if a shorter lifetime emitter is used, optics remains more sensitive than other methods due to the combination of a short cycle time of an optical marker (microseconds) and the ability to repeatedly cycle the optical reporter, limited only by bleaching. Modified from Benaron (2001) [246].

Optical spectroscopy

Optics, like MRI, is at heart a spectroscopic approach. The behavior of light in tissues is wavelength-specific, with respect to absorbance, fluorescence, scattering, and other optical effects. Use of multiple wavelengths of light can allow for quantitation of multiple cell elements, including blood, water, and fat content [170,171].

Clinical application of optical methods has allowed for quantitation of hemoglobin oxygenation noninvasively in the brain [172,173,248], muscle [173,175–177], tumors [172], and in the gastrointestinal tract (via endoscopy), as well as been shown to detect or image functional changes in brain hemoglobin concentration and saturation through the intact skull during cognition in adults [178,179] and sensation perception

in infants [179,180]. These measurements of cognition have been correlated with fMRI measures in the same subjects [179], and underscore the sensitivity of optical techniques.

Spectroscopic optical methods provide for absolute quantitation of the capillary or 'tissue' level saturation of hemoglobin with oxygen [181]. This value is sensitive to hypoxia, whether due to impaired flow, increased consumption, or low arterial oxygen content. In many tissues measured, the oxygenation of the normal tissue is surprisingly well regulated, with an average saturation of 71% and a tight control range (s.d. = +/−3%) in many tissues. The sensitivity of hemoglobin-imaging techniques has been demonstrated by the imaging of localized changes in cortical oxygenation in the brain, measured through the intact adult skull, during cognition and sensory tasks [179,180].

Table 5. Optical markers have parallels to other standard imaging methods

	Absorbing dye	Scattering agent	Fluorescent emitters	Bioluminescent reporter
Comparable method	CT w/contrast	Ultrasound w/bubbles	MRI w/Gd-DTPA	PET w/*FD-Glu
Optical agents	Hb, ICG	Nuclear sizing, terminal cell swelling	GFP, RFP, ICG and Cyanine derivatives	Bioluminescence (e.g., luciferases), chemiluminescence
Major advantages	Native contrast, spectroscopy	High morphological sensitivity	Probes easily transferred to human clinical use	High detection sensitivity
Major drawbacks	Bulk tissue only, signal for lost for trace disease	Bulk tissue only, signal for lost for trace disease	Good partitioning or activatable agent required for high sensitivity	Requires genetic engineering

After Benaron (2001) [247].

In contrast, to normal tissues, the oxygen supply in tumors is poorly regulated, producing local changes in oxygenation and blood content. This physical size of this perturbation radius exceeds the radius of the tumor itself. Thus, a 100 μm tumor can potentially influence oxygenation for 1 mm or more surrounding the tumor, providing signal strength to the optical signal, and providing a mechanism by which small tumors can be imaged. An oxygenation image from a breast tumor model is shown in Figure 11. Recently, we have introduced a clinical system for spectroscopically monitoring oxygenation *in vivo* using needle, catheter, endoscopic, or surface probes [182]. This device is under study for mapping oxygenation in tumors, and is expected to be submitted for U.S. FDA approval by the close of 2002.

There are other native contrast agents in the body besides hemoglobin. Many biological compounds, such as NADH, melanin, and others are fluorescent. Use of native fluorescence has been proposed as a possible tumor signal, and many groups have investigated using these signals *in vivo* for tumor diagnosis and imaging [183–188]. Combination approaches incorporating fluorescence as one of several optical measures have allowed for high sensitivity and specificity in surface cancers [189].

Fluorescence lifetime approaches are being explored [190,191], in which a native or exogenous contrast agent has the lifetime of its fluorescence altered based upon oxygen levels, pH, or other local environmental characteristics to provide imaging contrast.

Last, there are techniques to detect chemical compounds more specifically, such as Raman spectroscopy.

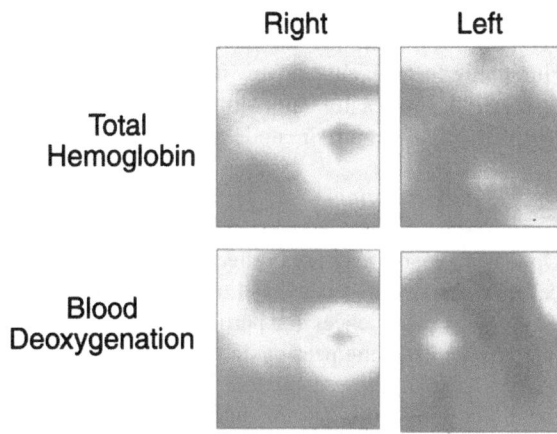

Figure 11. Breast model total hemoglobin and oxygenation imaged using a fast optical system developed by Chance et al. The right breast (with a suspicious lesion) shows a region of increased total hemoglobin and blood deoxygenation. The left breast (with no suspicious area) shows no comparable lesion. Image provided by Chance et al. (1999).

Raman spectroscopy detects the inelastic collisions of photons with molecules; that is, the light escaping has had its energy reduced (and thus its wavelength increased) by an amount related to the molecular bond it interacted with. This effect produces very specific and narrow spectroscopic bands which are unique to different chemical species. Raman techniques have been used to detect calcium deposits [192], to identify vascular plaques [193,194], and to identify cancer [195,196]. A drawback of this approach is that Raman events occur at a low frequency (about 1 in 10^6), although surface-enhanced and other approaches can intensity Raman signals.

288

Optical coherence tomography

Optical coherence tomography [36,197,198] is a technique that is the optical parallel to acoustic ultrasonography. The key advantage of this technique is that it allows for high-resolution scans across a mucosal surface, or from within a needle, with a resolution of 2–10 μm down to depths of 2 mm (e.g., see Figure 2). At this time, OCT is the single highest resolution imaging approach that is commercially available for imaging living tissues at depth (excluding surface confocal microscopy).

Images can be collected at video rates. Images appear very similar to ultrasound images, save that the full depth of the image usually covers less than 2 mm. OCT has demonstrated high resolution in several clinical applications, especially in the eye [199], bladder [242,200], gastrointestinal tract [201–203] and blood vessels [204]. Commercial instruments from Zeiss Humphrey Instruments are now in use in ophthalmology, while devices for onocologic, endoscopic, and radiologic applications are under development.

Optical nuclear sizing

Optical nuclear sizing uses reflected light to estimate cell nuclear size and density. Long and widely used in the physical sciences for particle size quantitation in the chemical engineering lab and manufacturing process control, these approaches have been adapted for direct application to cell, nuclear, and mitochondrial sizing *in vivo* by Backman and Feld [205,243], Bigio and Mourant [206,207], Sevick [208,209], and others [210,211]. Sizing relies on the influence of scattering particles in the tissue and the varying effect they have based upon the wavelength of the light. Although early work suggested that the mitochondria are a major source of light scattering [210], more recent work has suggested that the nuclear size and cell membranes influence scattering more strongly [205,211]. This is key, as it has been long recognized that changes in the nuclei or epithelial cells are among the most important structural correlates of dysplasia and carcinoma [212]. Nuclear changes arise from errors and variability in chromatin content and packing, which are nearly universal in tumors; cell size and morphology also vary in tumor cells.

In vivo, optical sizing has allowed for noninvasive extraction of nuclear size and nuclear fraction distributions from intact tissue *in vivo* as an image. The basic principle is shown in Figure 12 (images using this technique are shown previously in Figure 2).

Optical contrast agents

Optical contrast agents and reporters can add extraordinary sensitivity and specificity to an image. There are two basic types of optical agents: contrast agents and reporters.

Contrast agents interact with, and modify, light supplied externally to the tissues. Examples of this type include such as with GFP or ICG. Reporters, discussed in the next section spontaneously generate light, producing their light using the energy provided by metabolic substrates.

Optical contrast agents, as compared to optical reporters, have the advantages that many MRI and PET contrast agents can be adapted to produce corresponding optical equivalents, that no genetic engineering is required (thought this can be used, with good effect), and that these agents are the most easily adapted for human use. Multiple groups are developing optical contrast agents [43,44,52,213–218], including our group [67].

Non-targeted functional imaging optical agents can achieve localization in tumors due to physiological characteristics, such as delayed vascular transit or increased capillary leakage [43,44,52,219]. For example, a cyanine dye, injected intravenously, has been shown to localize in tumors after 2 h, with clearance of the dye from the remainder of sites in less than 24 h, leaving a deposition of dye which can be noninvasively imaged, as shown in Figure 13. Other examples of optical functional imaging agents include Isosulfan Blue, a dye used for the visual targeting of sentinel lymph node surgery [67,220].

Targeted optical contrast agents have been demonstrated using antigenic and molecular probes methods, with examples of such dyes shown in Figure 14. For example, Somatostatin-receptor targeting has allowed for imaging of somatostatin-receptor positive tumor-bearing rodents [52,88]. We have used prostate-specific membrane antigen (PSMA) for targeting metastatic prostate tumors [67]. Targeting can also be achieved through activation, such as with this optical agent that becomes fluorescent when a peptide linkage within the dye is cleaved by specific enzymatic interactions (an image of a cleavable dye *in vivo* is shown previously in Figure 7).

Active drugs themselves can be highly optically active, and thus can function both as both therapeutic agents as well as contrast agents. Paralleling the methods used to produce trapped contrast agents in MRI and PET, porphyrin precursors can be made to accumulate in many tumors. The concentration of such agents by

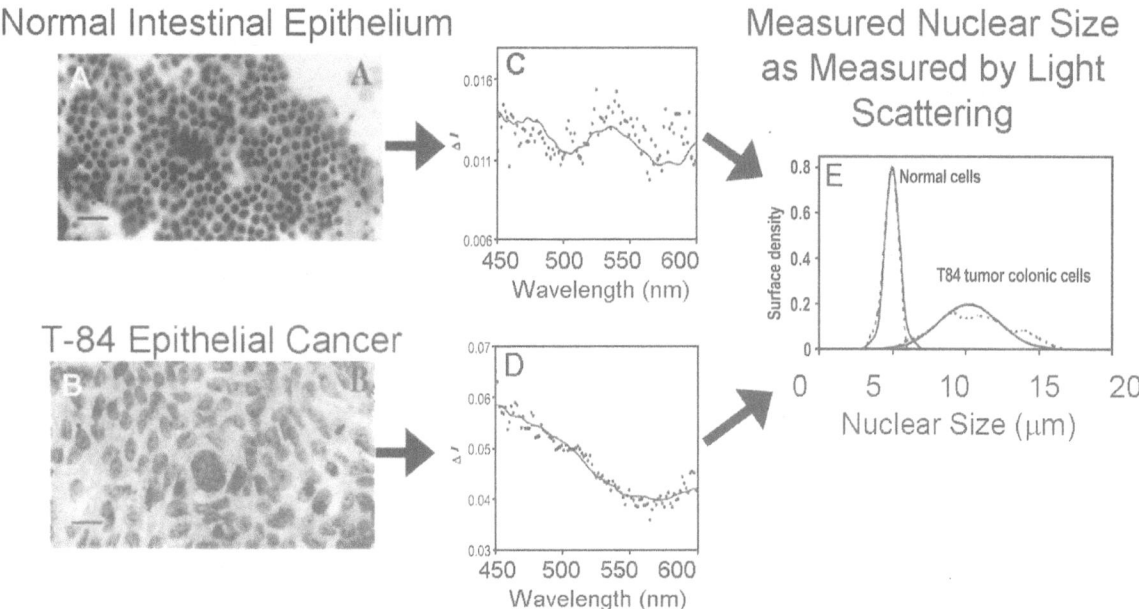

Figure 12. Particle sizing by Light Scattering Spectroscopy. In this method, normal intestinal epithelium shows (A) homogenous nuclei and narrow cell size ranges, producing (C) an optical spectrum that varies by wavelength while (E) after analysis yields a nuclear size range of about 5–8 mm. In contrast, T-84 epithelial cancer shows (B) enlarged and variably sized nuclei, producing (D) an optical spectrum that varies by wavelength which (E) after analysis yields an enlarged and variable nuclear size range of 6–14 μm. Modified from Backman et al. (1999) [205].

metabolically active tissues forms the basis of photodynamic therapies. The same characteristics allowing these agents to react with light for PDT treatment also allow these drugs to function as optical contrast agents [221–223], as shown in Figure 15.

Optical reporters

Reporters spontaneously generate light, producing their light using the energy provided by metabolic substrates. Examples of this type include luciferases [224,225], and chemiluminescent [226–228] agents.

In 1994, we first proposed that luciferase imaging, previously used to label tissues *in vivo* but analyzed after sacrificing test animals and collecting light from homogenated extracts, could be used *in vivo* to label infectious agents, to monitor gene expression, to follow tumor load, and to perform cell tracking *in vivo* [229]. This has since been confirmed by us and other groups, and *in vivo* bioluminescence has evolved into a standard technique in microbiology, oncology, and *in vivo* gene expression monitoring.

The key advantage of luminescent techniques is an inherent high sensitivity. In *ex vivo* techniques, optical methods are used to identify even single cells out of large populations, such as when using cell sorters to remove rare tumor cells from bone marrow aspirates. This level of detection has been shown to be transferable *in vivo*. For example, using genetically expressed GFP, individual glioma cells in a living mouse have been individually tracked *in vivo* (shown previously in Figure 9). Also, human cervical carcinoma cells (HeLa) labeled with luciferase and injected intraperitoneally allowed detection of as few as 100 tumor cells in peritoneum, a 10,000-fold improvement over conventional imaging detection [9]. Viral expression has also been tracked using this method, with HIV replication imaged in multi-well chambers [224].

Luciferase methods have allowed for treatment response to be imaged in microbiology [225] and oncology [9] in animal models of disease. Importantly, emergence of resistance can be seen as 'hot-spots' that develop in the center of regions with otherwise decreasing counts, as shown in Figure 16. This not only provides sensitive methods to study this response, but in addition the optical signal can be used for targeting.

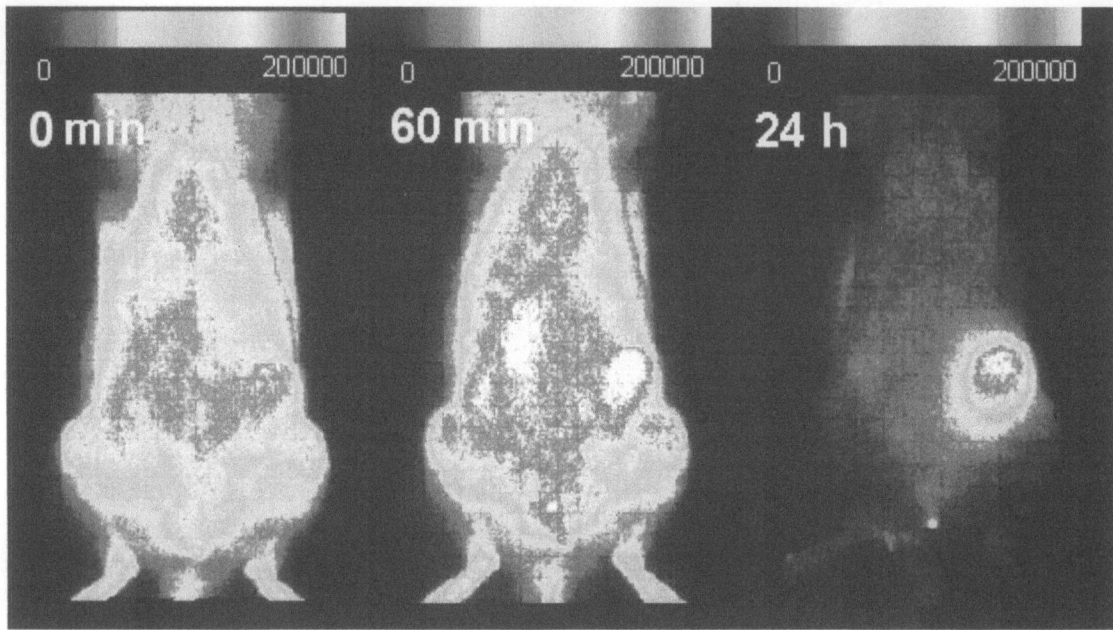

Figure 13. Optical image of a cyanine dye leaking from the vasculature in a mouse. Images obtained of MTLn-3 breast tumor in a rat, labeled by i.v. injection of optical contrast at 1 min, 60 min, and 24 h post-injection. Image provided by Licha et al. (2000).

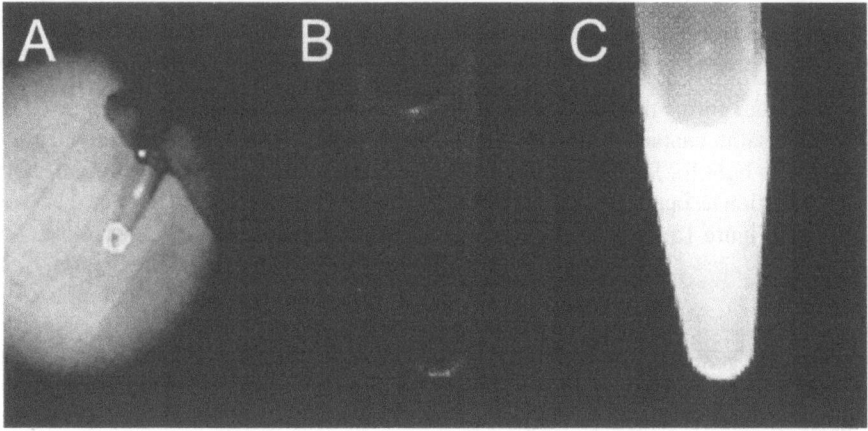

Figure 14. Two targeted optical dyes. (A) An antigenically targeted fluorescent dye, produced by our group for human use and targeted toward PSMA, as seen using a camera we developed for room light use. The concentration of dye in the tube is similar to that which can be achieved in tissue, or 1000 copies per cell. (B) A tube of enzymatically activatable optical dye, in which fluorescence is self-quenched prior to cleavage of a protein linkage by Caspase-3, after which the fluorescent substantially increases. (C) The dye is fluorescent in the presence of Caspase-3. In the presence of a Caspase-3 inhibitor, the activatable dye does not become fluorescent. (A) from Benaron et al. (2000) [67], (B) and (C) modified from Tung CH [93], in Weissleder et al. (2001) [85].

Simultaneous monitoring of multiple reporters

Because optical methods are potentially spectroscopic, multiple wavelengths can be used for independent reporter systems. For example, two different luciferase-based reporters, each responding to a different molecular signal, allow for multiple receptors to be simultaneously and independently monitored [230], while separation by wavelength allows for discrimination of even spatially overlapping signals [231], as

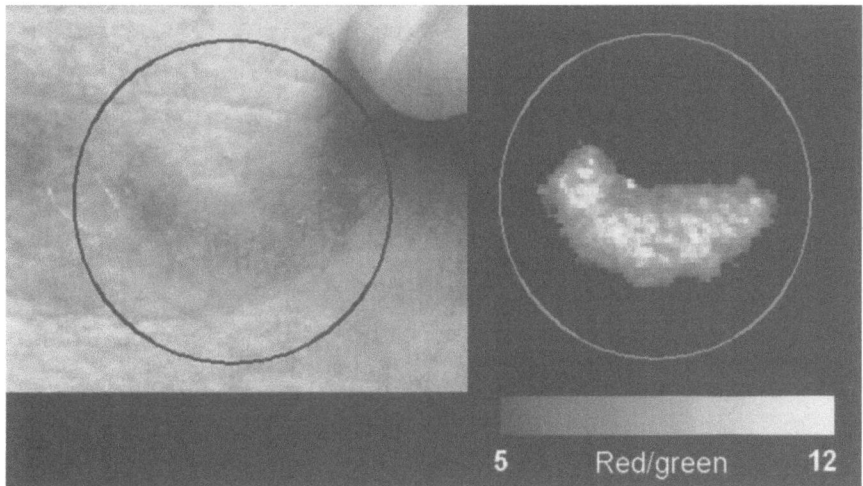

Figure 15. Photofrin® (porfimer sodium), a mixture of porphyrin derivatives used in photodynamic therapy, preferentially accumulates in metabolically active tissue, such as melanomas. (Left) A cutaneous human melanoma as seen by eye in room light after injection of Photofrin®, prior to photodynamic therapy treatment. (Right) A fluorescence red : green ratio image, demonstrating image contrast achieved based upon porphyrin trapping in the actively metabolic cutaneous melanoma. Using newer imaging techniques, this approach should be possible *in vivo* at depths of up to 4–6 cm. Image provided by Klinteberg and Svanberg, Lund (1999).

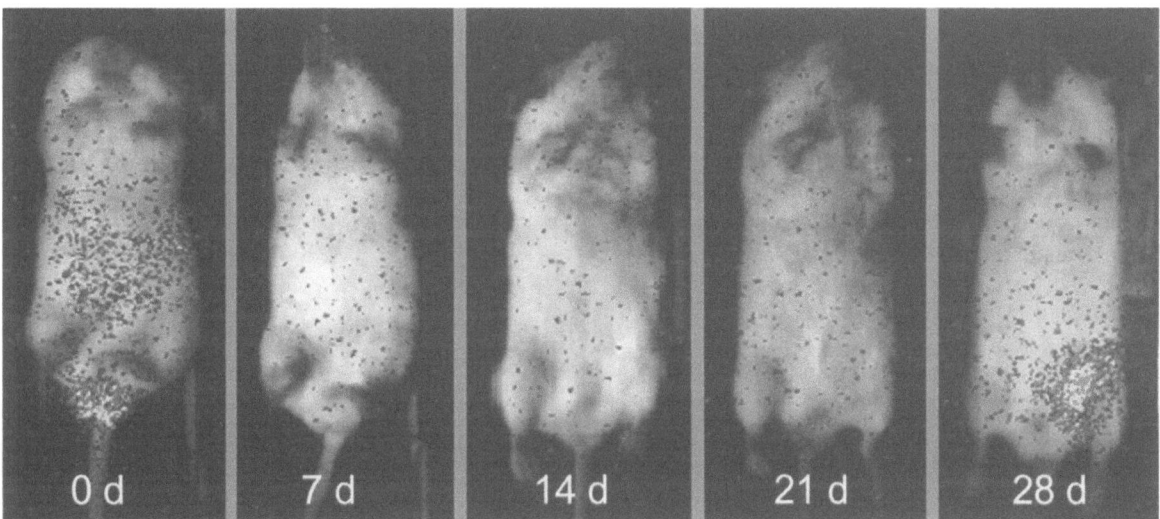

Figure 16. Quantitative imaging of tumor response using luciferase. An intraperitoneal tumor, labeled with luciferase, is injected by tail vein on day 0. During treatment with Cisplatin, the optical signal regresses, and then resurges on day 28, consistent with the development of resistance. Cell counts of under 1000 cells can be detected and imaged in 5 min. Image from Edinger et al. (2000) [9].

shown in Figure 17. Separation of multiple reporters can be achieved using reporters of different wavelengths. In a multi-wavelength approach, the number of independent channels monitored by optical methods is limited only by the full-width half-maximum of the wavelength spread of the optical reporter, taking into consideration the wavelength distortions caused by transmission through tissue (in which the longer wavelengths are relatively better transmitted and preserved). Some optical reporters can be quite narrow in their emission spectrum. For example, quantum dots can fluoresce with FWHM of 20 nm in theory (often

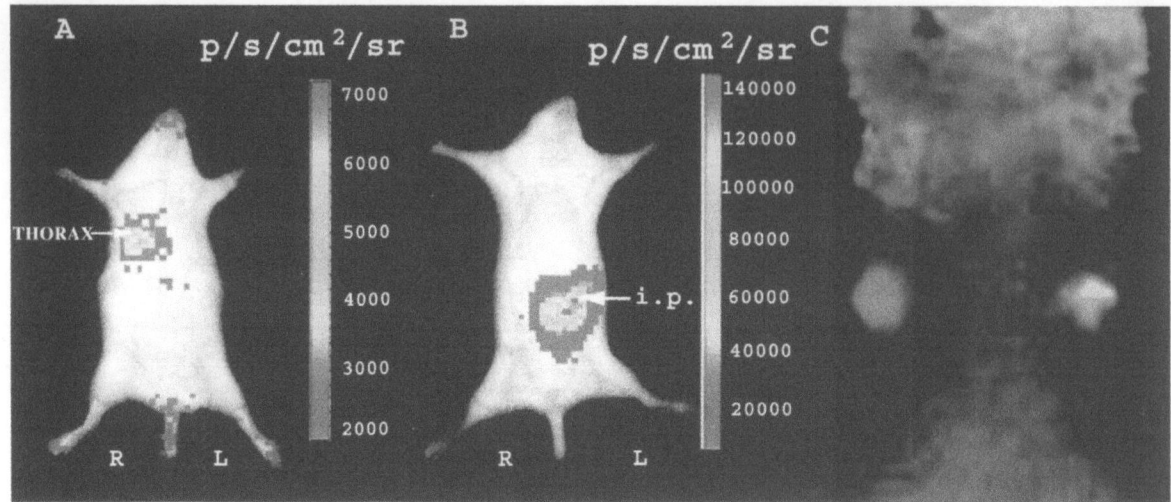

Figure 17. Dual optical reporter systems allow two molecular or genetic pathways to be simultaneously and independently monitoring using optical imaging. In this system, a dual reporter system in shown in which (A) a thoracic Renilla luciferase reporter and (B) an intraperitoneal firefly luciferase reporter can be independently switched on and off, with clear separation of the signals. From Bhaumik et al. (2002) [230]. (C) red and green fluorescent protein signals can be separated by wavelength, even when simultaneously produced. "From Anticancer [169]".

50–100 nm in practice), suggesting that 5 or more independent channels are attainable. In theory, MRSI could achieve a similar method by producing different substrates from each reporter, while separation of multiple nuclear medicine channels based upon the energy of the photon released is possible, but more difficult. Combinations, such as optical and PET imaging, have been demonstrated [166].

Optical gene expression and cell tracking

Many of the same approaches that are successful for allowing gene expression to be imaged using MRI and PET, also allow for the optical detection and imaging of gene expression. Optical agents can be linked to gene expression [232], or constitutively expressed to produce cell tracking signals [233]. Both optical contrast agents and optical reporters can be used in such techniques. An optical image of glioma cell tracking is shown previously in Figure 9.

Optical Instrumentation

Unlike CT, MRI, and PET, for which there are commercial systems and accepted imaging standards, a major hurdle for optical imaging is that, the vast majority of the human-directed or animal-directed optical imaging systems are in academic institutions, and differ widely

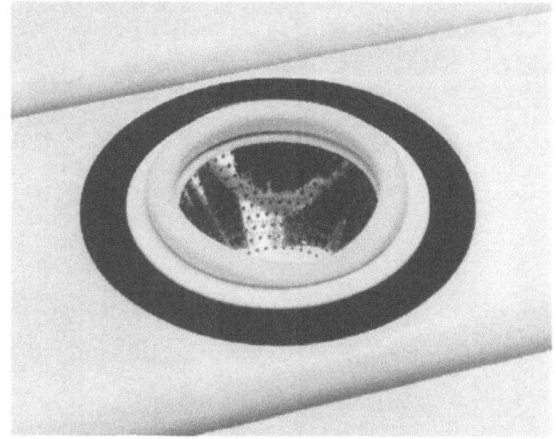

Figure 18. The breast imaging cup of a prototype commercial imaging device for the breast. The cup is filled with an index-matching solution, and the breast is suspended in the cup while the patient lies prone on the imaging table. Image provided by van der Mark, Philips Research (1997) [234].

from institution to institution. There are only a few commercial imaging platforms for animals or humans, such as the IVIS™ system for imaging luciferase activity in animal models from Xenogen, and an OCT system for ophthalmology from Humphrey. This lack of an approved imaging platform prevents new optical imaging agents from reaching regulatory submission, as an agent cannot be validated without an accompanying imaging platform, and platforms are not commercialized due to the absence of agents.

Major imaging companies such as Phillips [234] and Siemens [235] have considered commercializing optical imaging systems, and have created prototype designs for commercial imaging systems. A prototype optical imaging cup from an optical breast imaging device developed at Phillips is shown in Figure 18.

The NIH and NCI have recently offered support for the development of such optical systems, and multiple alternative systems are being developed. Since 1998, our group has been developing a commercial instrument, named Palomar™, for real-time imaging of fluorescent agents *in vivo* in human subjects, and clinical testing is expected to begin later this year. We suspect that a simple, non-tomographic, planar camera-based approach will allow for a relevant and manufacturable clinical whole-body imaging system to be constructed.

VI. New questions raised

As with any new technique, new information leads to new problems. As the sensitivity and specificity of imaging grows, and treatment becomes more patient-specific, the following questions become less clear, rather than more clear.

When is a diagnosis of cancer made?

On a gross slide, pathologists are in general (though not complete) agreement as to knowing cancer when they see it, stain it, or label it. However, *in vivo*, this line is likely to be far less clear. In one post-mortem study, 11% of patients in the pathology lab have at least one undiagnosed cancer at autopsy [236]. Separately, we also know that the majority of asymptomatic men above the age of 65 have either prostate cancer or high-grade PIN [237,238]. This problem is likely to compound when extended to many organ systems. The number of patients with precancerous lesions somewhere in their body could conceivably approach 100%. What if all of these nodules, dysplasias, precancers, or frank carcinomas can be seen on imaging, what then? The situation is likely to get even more complicated if precancerous changes can be imaged.

Such radiologic sensitivity will be a dual-edged sword. Overdiagnosis is risky, and carries both health, social, psychological, and economic costs. One example of such risks occurred when cardiac stress and thallium perfusion tests first became available. At that time, many healthy executives sought 'state of the art' examinations as part of their comprehensive health plans. When abnormalities were found on these scans of otherwise asymptomatic executives, a significant number underwent cardiac catheterization, a non-benign procedure, which led to serious complications in about one percent of these otherwise healthy adults. Now, the use of such tests in asymptomatic patients is discouraged. If high degrees of sensitivity to cancer are developed, care will need to be taken in deciding whom to image, and then as to how and when a diagnosis of cancer is made.

What constitutes metastatic disease?

Careful and early diagnosis, staging, and treatment selection will only serve to increase treatment success. However, we know that rare but detectable tumor cells in the bone marrow and the peripheral blood are not uncommon in many cancers, including breast, lung, and colorectal carcinomas [239,240]. These distant metastases are associated with clinical risk. In one study of PMA transcripts in pelvic lymph nodes at the time of prostatectomy by reverse-transcriptase PCR, only 30% of the PCR-negative patients demonstrated future local or distant recurrence, compared with 88% of the PCR-positive patients [241]. Thus, such 'molecularly positive' patients suffered recurrence significantly more often, despite negative images, while many patients that did recur were PCR negative as well.

Would an imaging technique based on antigenic markers detect such PCR-positive cells, or even identify pockets of positive cells in otherwise PCR-negative patients? If discrete islands of cells are seen, locally-ablative therapy could conceivably be targeted at distant image-positive sites – and would this alter the rate of clinical relapse? And how should distally marker-positive, but otherwise imaging-negative, patients be treated – as metastasis-free or distantly-diseased?

Such questions will challenge our current neat staging definitions of the patient with cancer. Thresholds will need to be considered, and new treatment decision trees will need to be implemented.

What is imaging?

Last, what is 'imaging'? The answer to this question may seem obvious now, but the borders between imaging and sensing, imaging and therapy, and imaging

294

and feedback control are blurring. As a comparison, in 1950 an equally obvious question would have been "what is a phone?" now, the speaker, mouthpiece, and even the cord that defined the phone are optional, and phone-like features are embedded features in devices as varied as pagers to web browsers to pacemakers. Imaging will likely follow a similar evolutionary trend, with both imagers, as well as the contrast agents we use, changing.

Imaging systems of the future may be so integrated within other devices that they may not be recognizable to us as imagers. How would one classify a molecular-probe-based imaging tool which operates as a surgical tool to remove tumor in an automated manner, with the image not even visible to a physician user, who merely inserts the device into a tumor. Or, how would one describe a circulating nanoagent that runs on glucose, and emits light in response to contact with gram negative bacteria, with this light captured outside of the body by a bedside camera, continuously on, to produce a real-time readout of the location, cell number, and type of impending infection, including antibiotic recommendations?

The power of multimodal methods will also likely grow. Already, combinations such as CT to image structure combined with PET to image function, all within the same device, are already under testing. Images from these systems will likely make the current unimodal images seem as antique as the first Roentgenograms from 100 years ago.

Such advances will challenge what we think of as imaging.

Biographical note

David Benaron, MD is on academic faculty at the School of Medicine at Stanford University, where he established the Biomedical Optics Laboratory in 1990. Dr. Benaron is a founder of Xenogen Corporation (www.xenogen.com), a biotechnology concern that develops and markets tools for drug discovery in the living organism, and of Spectros Corporation (www.spectros.com), a biotechnology concern that develops and marketing optical tools for clinical use imaging and therapeutic use. He holds equity in both, and receives financial compensation from spectros.

References

1. Proceedings of The Third Visible Human Project Conference, National Institutes of Health, RA Banvard, editor, 5–6 October 2000, National Library of Medicine. See also www.nlm.nih.gov/research/visible
2. For the MRI atlas, the subject was a convicted felon, imaged, with his consent, shortly after lethal injection.
3. Abbas F, Kaplan M, Soloway MS: Induction androgen deprivation therapy before radical prostatectomy for prostate cancer – initial results. Br J Urol 77(3): 423–428, 1996
4. Beck NE, Bradburn MJ, Vincenti AC, Rainsbury RM: Detection of residual disease following breast-conserving surgery. Br J Surg 85: 1273–1276, 1998
5. Eastham JA, Kattan MW, Rogers E, Goad JR, Ohori M, Boone TB, Scardino PT: Risk factors for urinary incontinence after radical prostatectomy. J Urol 156(5): 1707–1713, 1996
6. Fesseha T, Sakr W, Banerjee M, Wood DP, Pontes JE: Prognostic implications of a positive apical margin in radical prostatectomy specimens. J Urol 158: 2176–2179, 1997
7. Marshall E: Human genome: rival genome sequencers celebrate a milestone together. Science 288: 2294–2295, 2000
8. Pennnisi E: Human genome: finally, the book of life and instructions for navigating it. Science 288: 2304–2307, 2000
9. Edinger M, Sweeney TJ, Tucker AA, Olomu AB, Negrin RS, Contag CH: Noninvasive assessment of tumor cell proliferation in animal models. Neoplasia 1(4): 303–310, 1999
10. Termanini B, Gibril F, Reynolds JC, Doppman JL, Chen CC, Stewart CA, Sutliff VE, Jensen RT: Value of somatostatin receptor scintigraphy: a prospective study in gastrinoma of its effect on clinical management. Gastroenterology 112(2): 335–347, 1997
11. Allen MW, Hendi P, Schwimmer J, Bassett L, Gambhir SS: Decision analysis for the cost effectiveness of sestamibi scintimammography in minimizing unnecessary biopsies. Q J Null Med 44(2): 168–185, 2000
12. Krag D: Why perform randomized clinical trials for sentinel node surgery for breast cancer? Am J Surg 182(4): 411–413, 2001
13. Kurhanewicz J, Swanson MG, Wood PJ, Vigneron DB: Magnetic resonance imaging and spectroscopic imaging: Improved patient selection and potential for metabolic intermediate endpoints in prostate cancer chemoprevention trials. Urology 57(4 Suppl 1): 124–128, 2001
14. Kallen K, Burtscher IM, Holtas S, Ryding E, Rosen I: 201Thallium SPECT and 1H-MRS compared with MRI in chemotherapy monitoring of high-grade malignant astrocytomas. J Neuro-Oncol 46(2): 173–185, 2000
15. Kallen K, Geijer B, Malmstrom P, Andersson AM, Holtas S, Ryding E, Rosen I: Quantitative 201Tl SPET imaging in the follow-up of treatment for brain tumour: a sensitive tool for the early identification of response to chemotherapy? Nucl Med Commun 21(3): 259–267, 2000
16. Bokemeyer C, Kollmannsberger C, Oechsle K, Dohmen BM, Pfannenberg A, Claussen CD, Bares R, Kanz L: Early prediction of treatment response to high-dose salvage chemotherapy in patients with relapsed germ cell cancer using [(18)F]FDG PET. Br J Cancer 86(4): 506–511, 2002

17. Zhao M, Beauregard DA, Loizou L, Davletov B, Brindle KM: Non-invasive detection of apoptosis using magnetic resonance imaging and a targeted contrast agent. Nat Med 7(11): 1241–1244, 2001

18. Hofstra L, Dumont EA, Thimister PW, Heidendal GA, DeBruine AP, Elenbaas TW, Boersma HH, van Heerde WL, Reutelingsperger CP: in vivo detection of apoptosis in an intracardiac tumor. JAMA 285(14): 1841–1842, 2001

19. Griffiths JR, Glickson JD: Monitoring pharmacokinetics of anticancer drugs: non-invasive investigation using magnetic resonance spectroscopy. Adv Drug Deliv Rev 41(1): 75–89, 2000

20. Chen DM, Hawkins BL, Glickson JD: Proton nuclear magnetic resonances study of bleomycin in aqueous solution. Assignment of resonances. Biochemistry 16(12): 2731–2738, 1977

21. Bigio IJ, Mourant JR, Los G: Noninvasive, in-situ measurement of drug concentrations in tissue using optical spectroscopy. J Gravit Physiol 6(1): 173–175, 1999

22. Mourant JR, Johnson TM, Los G, Bigio IJ: Non-invasive measurement of chemotherapy drug concentrations in tissue: preliminary demonstrations of in vivo measurements. Phys Med Biol 44(5): 1397–1417, 1999

23. Front D, Israel O, Iosilevsky G, Even-Sapir E, Frenkel A, Kolodny GM, Feinsod M: SPECT quantitation of cobalt-57 bleomycin delivery to human brain tumors. J Nucl Med 29(2): 187–194, 1988

24. Feig SA: Current status of screening mammography. Obstet Gynecol Clin North Am 29(1): 123–136, 2002

25. Kerlikowske K, Salzmann P, Phillips KA, Cauley JA, Cummings SR: Continuing screening mammography in women aged 70–79 years: impact on life expectancy and cost-effectiveness. JAMA 282(22): 2156–2163, 1999

26. Rosenquist CJ, Lindfors KK: Screening mammography beginning at age 40 years: a reappraisal of cost-effectiveness. Cancer 82(11): 2235–2240, 1998

27. Budinger TF, Benaron DA, Koretsky AP: Imaging transgenic animals. Annu Rev Biomed Eng 1: 611–648, 1999

28. ImTek, Inc MicroCT, cited in: Paulus MJ, Gleason SS, Kennel SJ, Hunsicker PR, Johnson DK: High resolution X-ray computed tomography: an emerging tool for small animal cancer research. Neoplasia 2(1–2): 62–70, 2000 (Review)

29. ScanCo System, cited in: Muller R, Van Campenhout H, Van Damme B, Van Der Perre G, Dequeker J, Hildebrand T, Ruegsegger P: Morphometric analysis of human bone biopsies: a quantitative structural comparison of histological sections and micro-computed tomography. Bone 23(1): 59–66, 1998

30. Chatziioannou AF, Cherry SR, Shao Y, Silverman RW, Meadors K, Farquhar TH, Pedarsani M, Phelps ME: Performance evaluation of microPET: a high-resolution lutetium oxyorthosilicate PET scanner for animal imaging. J Nucl Med 40(7): 1164–1175, 1999

31. Tai C, Chatziioannou A, Siegel S, Young J, Newport D, Goble RN, Nutt RE, Cherry SR: Performance evaluation of the microPET P4: a PET system dedicated to animal imaging. Phys Med Biol 46(7): 1845–1862, 2001

32. IVIS™ System, Xenogen Corporation, Alameda, California

33. AntiCancer, San Diego, California

34. Coffey D: Special Lecture. Presented at the CaP CURE 7th Annual Scientific retreat, Lake Tahoe, NV, September 21–24, 2000

35. Getzenberg RH, Pienta KJ, Huang EYW, Coffey DS: Identification of Nuclear Matrix Proteins in the Cancer and Normal Rat Prostate. Cancer Res. 51: 6514–6520, 1991

36. Huang D, Swanson EA, Lin CP, Schuman JS, Stinson WG, Chang W, Hee MR, Flotte T, Gregory K, Pulafito CA, Fujimoto JG: Optical coherence tomography. Science 254: 1178–1181, 1991

37. Initially sextant biopsy, but now often decant, or dodecant, or higher sample numbers in order to improve the statistical reliability of a negative result; the reliability of an unequivocal positive result is generally not in question

38. Keech DW, Catalona WJ, Smith DS: Serial prostatic biopsies in men with persistently elevated serum prostate specific antigen values. J Urol 151: 1571–1574, 1994

39. Ellis WJ, Brawer MK: Repeat prostate needle biopsy. Who Needs it? J Urol 153: 1496–1498, 1995

40. Roehrborn CG, Pickens GJ, Snaders JS: Diagnostic yield of repeated transrectal ultrasound-guided biopsies stratified by specific histopathologic diagnoses and prostate-specific antigen levels. Urology 47: 347–352, 1996

41. Hammerer P, Huland H: Systematic sextant biopsies in 651 patients referred for prostate evaluation. J Urol 151(1): 99–102, 1994

42. Terris MK, Freiha FS, McNeal JE et al.: Efficacy of transrectal ultrasound for identification of clinically undetected prostate cancer. J Urol 146: 78–83, 1991

43. Reynolds JS, Troy TL, Mayer RH, Thompson AB, Waters DJ, Cornell KK, Snyder PW, Sevick-Muraca EM: Imaging of spontaneous canine mammary tumors using fluorescent contrast agents. Photochem Photobiol 70(1): 87–94, 1999

44. Gurfinkel M, Thompson AB, Ralston W, Troy TL, Moore AL, Moore TA, Gust JD, Tatman D, Reynolds JS, Muggenburg B, Nikula K, Pandey R, Mayer RH, Hawrysz DJ, Sevick-Muraca EM: Pharmacokinetics of ICG and HPPH-car for the detection of normal and tumor tissue using fluorescence, near-infrared reflectance imaging: a case study. Photochem Photobiol 72(1): 94–102, 2000

45. Alex JC, Krag DN: Gamma-probe guided localization of lymph nodes. Surg Oncol 2(3): 137–143, 1993

46. Alex JC, Weaver DL, Fairbank JT, Rankin BS, Krag DN: Gamma-probe-guided lymph node localization in malignant melanoma. Surg Oncol 2(5): 303–308, 1993

47. Krag DN, Weaver DL, Alex JC, Fairbank JT: Surgical resection and radiolocalization of the sentinel lymph node in breast cancer using a gamma probe. Surg Oncol 2(6): 335–339, 1993 (with discussion, p 340)

48. Glass LF, Messina JL, Cruse W, Wells K, Rapaport D, Miliotes G, Berman C, Reintgen D, Fenske NA: The use of intraoperative radiolymphoscintigraphy for sentinel node biopsy in patients with malignant melanoma. Dermatol Surg 22(8): 715–720, 1996

49. The compound ^{99m}Tc-methoxyisobutyl isonitrile, Cardiolite, Du Pont Pharmaceuticals, Wilmington, DE

50. Muller ST, Guth-Tougelides B, Crutzig H: imaging of malignant tumors with MIBI-99mTc Spect. J Nucl Med 28: 562P, 1987 (Abstract)

51. Chiu ML, Kronauge JF, Piwnica-Worms D: Effect of mitochondrial and plasma membrane potentials on accumulation of hexakis (2-methoxyisobutylisonitrile) technetium(I) in cultured mouse fibroblasts. J Nucl Med 31(10): 1646–1653, 1990

52. Becker A, Hessenius C, Licha K, Ebert B, Sukowski U, Semmler W, Wiedenmann B, Grotzinger C: Receptor-targeted optical imaging of tumors with near-infrared fluorescent ligands. Nat Biotechnol 19(4): 327–331, 2001

53. Becker A, Hessenius C, Bhargava S, Grotzinger C, Licha K, Schneider-Mergener J, Wiedenmann B, Semmler W: Cyanine dye labeled vasoactive intestinal peptide and somatostatin analog for optical detection of gastroenteropancreatic tumors. Ann NY Acad Sci 921: 275–278, 2000

54. Fair WR, Israeli RS, Heston DW: Prostate specfic membrane antigen. Prostate 32: 140–148, 1997

55. Petronis JD, Regan F, Lin K: Indium-111 Capromab pendetide imaging to detect recurrent and metastatic prostate cancer. Clin Nucl Med 23(10): 672–677, 1998

56. Jain RK: Physiological barriers to delivery of monocolonal antibodies and other macromolecules in tumors. Cancer Res 50(Suppl): 814s–819s, 1990

57. Delaloye AB, Delaloye B: Tumor imaging with monoclonal antibodies. Sem Nucl Med 2: 144–164, 1995

58. Paganelli G, De Cicco C, Cremonesi M et al.: Optimized sentinel node scintigraphy in breast cancer. Quart J Nucl Med 42: 49–53, 1998

59. Bombardieri E, Crippa F, Maffioli L: Nuclear medicine approaches for detection of axillary lymph node metastases. Quart J Nucl Med 42: 54–65, 1998

60. Moffat FL, Pinsky CM, Hammershaimb L, Petrelli NJ, Patt YZ, Whaley FS, Goldenberg DM: The Immunomedics Study Group. Clinical utility of external immunoscintigraphy with the IMMU-4 technetium-99m-Fab' antibody fragment in patients undergoing surgery for carcinoma of the colon and rectum. Results of a pivotal, Phase III trial. J Clin Oncol 14: 2295–2305, 1996

61. Lucci A, Turner RR, Morton DL: Carbon dye as an adjunct to isosulfan blue dye for sentinel lymph node dissection. Surgery 126(1): 48–53, 1999

62. Morton DL, Wen DR, Wong JH, Economon JS, Cagle LA, Sotrm FK: Technical details of interoperative lymphatic mapping for early stage melanoma. Arch Surg 127: 392–399, 1992

63. Edreira MM, Colobo LL, Perez JH, Sajaroff EO, Castiglia SG: in vivo evaluation of three different 99mTc-labelled radiopharmaceuticals for sentinel lymph node identification. Nuc Med Commun 22(5): 499–504, 2001

64. Phillips WT, Klipper R, Goins B: Use of 99mTc-labeled liposomes encapsulating blue dye for identification of the sentinel lymph node. J Nuc Med 42(3): 446–451, 2001

65. Benaron DA, Scardino PT, Bander NR, Talmi YT: Optical dyes for real-time trace cancer imaging. Presented at 7th Annual CaP CURE scientific retreat, 21–24, August 2000, Lake Tahoe, NV

66. Torchia MG, Nason R, Danzinger R, Lewis JM, Thliveris JA: Interstitial MR lymphangiography for the detection of sentinel lymph nodes. J Surg Oncol 78(3): 151–156, 2001

67. Benaron DA, Scardino PT, Talmi YT, Bander NR: Targeted optical dyes for real-time trace cancer imaging. Presented at 8th Annual CaP CURE scientific retreat, 6–9, August 2001, Lake Tahoe, NV

68. Giulano AE, Jones RC, Brennan M, Statman R: Sentinel lymphadenectomy in breast cancer. J Clin Oncol 15: 2345–2350, 1997

69. Krag D, Weaver D, Ashikaga T, Moffat F, Klimberg VS, Shriver C, Feldman S, Kusminsky R, Gadd M, Kuhn J, Harlow S, Beitsch P: The sentinel node in breast cancer – a multicenter validation study N Engl J Med 339(14): 941–946, 1998

70. Krag DN, Meijer DL, Weaver DL et al.: Minimal access surgery for staging of malignant melanoma. Arch Surg 130: 654–660, 1995

71. Miltenburg DM, Miller C, Karamlou TB, Brunicardi FC: Meta-analysis of sentinel lymph node biopsy in breast cancer. J Surg Res 84(2): 138–142, 1999

72. Lechner P, Lind P, Snyder M, Haushofer H: Probe-guided surgery for colorectal cancer. Recent Res Cancer Res 157: 273–280, 2000

73. Vera DR, Wallace AM, Hoh CK, Mattrey RF: A synthetic macromolecule for sentinel node detection: of 99mTc-DTPA-Mannosyl-Dextran. J Nucl Med 42(6): 951–959, 2001

74. We are investigating use of an optical reporter dye, solubilized in lymphatic fluids using PEG, as well as targeted using cytokeratin for breast, or muc-1 for melanoma

75. Young CYF, Montogomery BT, Andrews PE, Qui SD, Bilhartz DL, Tindall DJ: Hormonal regulation of prostate-specific antigen messenger RNA in human prostatic adenocarcinoma cell line LNCaP. Cancer Res 51: 3748–3752, 1991

76. Guller U, Nitzsche EU, Schirp U, Viehl CT, Torhorst J, Moch H, Langer I, Marti WR, Oertli D, Harder F, Zuber M: Selective axillary surgery in breast cancer patients based on positron emission tomography with 18F-fluoro-2-deoxy-D-glucose: not yet! Breast Cancer Res Treat 71(2): 171–173, 2002

77. Bruhn H, Frahm J, Gyngell ML, Merboldt KD, Hanicke W, Sauter R, Hamburger C: Noninvasive differentiation of tumors with use of localized H-1 MR spectroscopy in vivo: initial experience in patients with cerebral tumors. Radiology 172(2): 541–548, 1989

78. Glickson JD: Clinical NMR spectroscopy of tumors. Current status and future directions. Invest Radiol 24(12): 1011–1006, 1989

79. Langkowski JH, Wieland J, Bomsdorf H, Leibfritz D, Westphal M, Offermann W, Maas R: Pre-operative localized in vivo proton spectroscopy in cerebral tumors at 4.0 Tesla – first results. Magn Reson Imaging 7(5): 547–555, 1989

80. Demaerel P, Johannik K, Van Hecke P, Van Ongeval C, Verellen S, Marchal G, Wilms G, Plets C, Goffin J, Van Calenbergh F et al.: Localized 1H NMR spectroscopy

in fifty cases of newly diagnosed intracranial tumors. J Comput Assist Tomogr 15(1): 67–76, 1991

81. Kugel H, Heindel W, Ernestus RI, Bunke J, du Mesnil R, Friedmann G: Human brain tumors: spectral patterns detected with localized H-1 MR spectroscopy. Radiology 183(3): 701–709, 1992

82. Vigneron D, Bollen A, McDermott M, Wald L, Day M, Moyher-Noworolski S, Henry R, Chang S, Berger M, Dillon W, Nelson S: Three-dimensional magnetic resonance spectroscopic imaging of histologically confirmed brain tumors. Magn Reson Imaging 19(1): 89–101, 2001

83. Kurhanewicz J, Swanson MG, Wood PJ, Vigneron DB: Magnetic resonance imaging and spectroscopic imaging: Improved patient selection and potential for metabolic intermediate endpoints in prostate cancer chemoprevention trials. Urology 57(4 Suppl 1): 124–128, 2001

84. Wagenaar DJ, Weissleder R, Henegerer A. Glossary of molecular imaging technology. Acad Radiol 8: 409–420, 2001

85. Weissleder R, Mahmood U: Molecular imaging. Radiology 219(2): 316–333, 2001

86. Phelps ME: Inaugural article: positron emission tomography provides molecular imaging of biological processes. Proc Natl Acad Sci USA. 97(16): 9226–9233, 2000

87. Phelps ME: PET: the merging of biology and imaging into molecular imaging. J Nucl Med 41(4): 661–681, 2000

88. Bugaj JE, Achilefu S, Dorshow RB, Rajagopalan R: Novel fluorescent contrast agents for optical imaging of in vivo tumors based on a receptor-targeted dye-peptide conjugate platform. J Biomed Opt 6(2): 122–133, 2001

89. Mahmood U, Tung CH, Bogdanov A Jr, Weissleder R: Near-infrared optical imaging of protease activity for tumor detection. Radiology 213(3): 866–870, 1999

90. Jacobs RE, Ahrens ET, Meade TJ, Fraser SE: Looking deeper into vertebrate development. Trends Cell Biol 9(2): 73–76, 1999

91. Marten K, Bremer C, Khazaie K, Sameni M, Sloane B, Tung CH, Weissleder R: Detection of dysplastic intestinal adenomas using enzyme-sensing molecular beacons in mice. Gastroenterology 122(2): 406–414, 2002

92. Tung CH, Bredow S, Mahmood U, Weissleder R: Preparation of a cathepsin D sensitive near-infrared fluorescence probe for imaging. Bioconjug Chem 10(5): 892–896, 1999

93. Tung CH, Mahmood U, Bredow S, Weissleder R: in vivo imaging of proteolytic enzyme activity using a novel molecular reporter. Cancer Res 60(17): 4953–4958, 2000

94. Walter G, Barton ER, Sweeney HL: Noninvasive measurement of gene expression in skeletal muscle. Proc Natl Acad Sci USA 97: 5151–5155, 2000

95. Pozzilli P, Pozzilli C, Pantano P, Negri M, Andreani D, Cudworth AG: Tracking of indium-111-oxine labelled lymphocytes in autoimmune thyroid disease. Clin Endocrinol (Oxf) 19(1): 111–116, 1983

96. Melder RJ, Brownell AL, Shoup TM, Brownell GL, Jain RK: Imaging of activated natural killer cells in mice by positron emission tomography: preferential uptake in tumors. Cancer Res 53(24): 5867–5871, 1993

97. Melder RJ, Elmaleh D, Brownell AL, Brownell GL, Jain RK: A method for labeling cells for positron emission

tomography (PET) studies. J Immunol Methods 175(1): 79–87, 1994

98. Schoepf U, Marecos EM, Melder RJ, Jain RK, Weissleder R: Intracellular magnetic labeling of lymphocytes for in vivo trafficking studies. Biotechniques 24(4): 642–646, 648–651, 1998

99. Hardy J, Edinger M, Bachmann MH, Negrin RS, Fathman CG, Contag CH: Bioluminescence imaging of lymphocyte trafficking in vivo. Exp Hematol 29(12): 1353–1360, 2001

100. Koike C, Oku N, Watanabe M, Tsukada H, Kakiuchi T, Irimura T, Okada S: Real-time PET analysis of metastatic tumor cell trafficking in vivo and its relation to adhesion properties. Biochim Biophys Acta 1238(2): 99–106, 1995

101. Weissleder R, Cheng HC, Bogdanova A, Bogdanov A Jr: Magnetically labeled cells can be detected by MR imaging.J Magn Reson Imaging 7(1): 258–263, 1997

102. Kan Z, Liu TJ: Video microscopy of tumor metastasis: using the green fluorescent protein (GFP) gene as a cancer-cell-labeling system. Clin Exp Metastasis 17(1): 49–55, 1999

103. Yang M, Baranov E, Wang J-W, Jiang P, Wang X, Sun F-X, Bovet M, Moossa AR, Penman S, Hoffman RM: Direct external imaging of nascent cancer, tumor progression, angiogenesis, and metastatsis on internal organs in the fluorescent orthotopic model. Proc Natl Acad Sci USA 99: 3824–3829, 2002

104. Perrottii M, Han KR, Epstein RE et al.: Efficacy of endorectal magnetic resonance imaging to detect tumor foci in men with prior negative prostatic biopsy: a pilot study. J Urol 162: 1314–1317, 1999

105. Torricelli P, De Santis M, Pollastri CA: Magnetic resonance with endorectal coil in the local staging of prostatic carcinoma: comparison with histologic macrosections in 40 cases. Radiol Med (Torino) 97: 491–498, 1999

106. Perrotti M, Han KR, Epstein RE, Kennedy EC, Rabbani F, Badani K, Pantuck AJ, Weiss RE, Cummings KB: Prospective evaluation of endorectal magnetic resonance imaging to detect tumor foci in men with prior negative prostastic biopsy: a pilot study. J Urol 162(4): 1314–1317, 1999

107. Torricelli P, Lo Russo S, Pecchi A, Luppi G, Cesinaro AM, Romagnoli R: Endorectal coil MRI in local staging of rectal cancer. Radiol Med (Torino) 103(1–2): 74–83, 2002

108. Other atomic species can be used to produce a signal, notably Cl-Chlorine. However, the majority of machines deployed are configured for proton (^{1}H) spectra, and the detection of other substances using proton spectroscopy often entails nothing more than software changes. Thus, most of the improvements now heading toward clinical use tend to be based on hydrogen. There is a large body of literature on cellular energetics using phosphorus resonance, with a suggestion of clinical utility from the analysis of high energy stores such as phosphocreatine, ATP, ADP, AMP, adenosine, and the like

109. Scheidler J, Hricak H, Vigneron DB, Yu KK, Sokolov DL, Huang RL, Zaloudek CJ, Nelson SJ, Carroll PR, Kurhanewicz J: 3D ^{1}H-MR spectroscopic imaging in localizing prostate cancer: clinico-pathologic study. Radiology 213: 473–480, 1999

298

110. Kurhanewicz J, Vigneron DB, Hricak H, Narayan P, Carroll P, Nelson SJ: Three-dimensional H-1 MR spectroscopic imaging of the in situ human prostate with high (0.24–0.7 cm³) spatial resolution. Radiology 198: 795–805, 1996

111. Vigneron D, Bollen A, McDermott M, Wald L, Day M, Moyher-Norworolski S, Henry R, Chang S, Berger M, Dillon W, Nelson S: Three-dimensional magnetic resonance spectroscopic imaging of histologically confirmed brain tumors. Magn reson imaging 19: 89–101, 2001

112. Menard C, Smith IC, Somorjai RL, Leboldus L, Patel R, Littman C, Robertson SJ, Bezabeh T: Magnetic resonance spectroscopy of the malignant prostate gland after radiotherapy: a histopathologic study of diagnostic validity. Int J Radiat Oncol Biol Phys 50(2): 317–323, 2001

113. Hahn P, Smith IC, Leboldus L, Littman C, Somorjai RL, Bezabeh T: The classification of benign and malignant human prostate tissue by multivariate analysis of 1H magnetic resonance spectra. Cancer Res 57(16): 3398–3401, 1997

114. Arnold DL, Shoubridge EA, Villemure JG, Feindel W: Proton and phosphorus magnetic resonance spectroscopy of human astrocytomas in vivo. Preliminary observations on tumor grading. NMR Biomed 3(4): 184–189, 1990

115. Rutter A, Hugenholtz H, Saunders JK, Smith IC: Classification of brain tumors by ex vivo 1H NMR spectroscopy. J Neurochem 64(4): 1655–1661, 1995

116. Merchant TE, Kasimos JN, Vroom T, de Bree E, Iwata JL, de Graaf PW, Glonek T: Malignant breast tumor phospholipid profiles using (31)P magnetic resonance. Cancer Lett 176(2): 159–167, 2002

117. Gohagan JK, Spitznagel EL, Murphy WA, Vannier MW, Dixon WT, Gersell DJ, Rossnick SL, Totty WG, Destouet JM, Rickman DL et al.: Multispectral analysis of MR images of the breast. Radiology 163(3): 703–707, 1987

118. Swanson MG, Vigneron DB, Tran T-K, Sailasuta N, Hurd RE, Kurhanewicz J: Single-voxel oversampled J-resolved spectroscopy of in vivo human prostate tissue. Mag Reson Med 45: 973–980, 2001

119. Costello LC, Franklin RB: The intermediary metabolism of the prostate: a key to understanding the pathogenesis and progression of prostate malignancy. Oncology 59(4): 269–282, 2000

120. Costello LC, Franklin RB, Narayan P: Citrate in the diagnosis of prostate cancer. Prostate 38(3): 237–245, 1999

121. The word signal, rather than concentration, is used, as the resonance signal is a convolution of many effects, including concentration and environmental factors.

122. Simmons ML, Frondoza CG, Coyle JT: Immunochemical localization of N-acetyl-aspartate with monoclonal antibodies. Neuroscience 45: 37–45, 1991

123. Janus TJ, Kim EE, Tilbury R, Bruner JM, Yung WK: Use of [18F]fluorodeoxyglucose positron emission tomography in patients with primary malignant brain tumors. Ann Neurol 33(5): 540–548, 1993

124. Aronen HJ, Gazit E, Louis DN, Buchbinder BR, Pardo FS, Weisskoff RM, Harsh GR, Cosgrove CR, Halpern EF, Hochberg FH, Rosen BR: Cerebral blood volume maps of gliomas: comparison with tumor grade and histologic findings. Radiology 191: 41–51, 1994

125. Kurhanewicz J, Vigneron DB, Males RG, Swanson MG, Yu KK, Hricak H: The prostate: MR imaging and spectroscopy. Present and future. Radiol Clin North Am 38(1): 115–138, viii–ix, 2000

126. DiBiasi SJ, Hosseinzadeh K, Gullapalli RP, Jacobs SC, Naslund MJ, Sklar GN, Alexander RB, Yu C: Magnetic reasonance spectroscopic imaging-guided brachytherapy for localized prostate cancer. Int J Radiat Oncol Biol Phys 52(2): 429–438, 2002

127. Smith BR, Johnson GA, Groman EV, Linney E: magnetic resonance microscopy of mouse embryos. Proc Nat Acad Sci USA 91: 3530–3533, 1994

128. Bremer C, Weissleder R: Molecular Imaging: in vivo imaging of gene expression: MR and optical technologies. Acad Radiol 8: 15–23, 2001

129. Enochs WS, Hyslop WB, Bennett HF, Brown RDd, Koenig SH, Swartz HM: Sources of the increased longitudinal relaxation rates observed in melanotic melanoma: an in vitro study of synthetic melanins. Invest Radiol 24: 794–804, 1989

130. Okazzaki M, Kuwata K, Miki Y, Shiga S, Shiga T: Electron spin relaxation of synthetic melanin and melanin-containing human tissues as studied by electron spin echo and electron spin resonance. Arch Biochem Biphys 242: 197-205, 1985

131. Isiklar I, Leeds NE, Fuller GN, Kumar AJ: Intracranial metastatic melanoma: correlation between MR imaging characteristics and melanin content. AJR Am J Roentgenol 165: 1503–1512, 1995

132. Louie AY, Huber MM, Ahrens ET et al.: In vivo visulalization of gene expression using magnetic resonance imaging. Nat Biotechnol 18: 321–325, 2000

133. Weissleder R, Bogdanov A Jr, Tung CH, Weinmann HJ: Size optimization of synthetic graft copolymers for in vivo angiogenesis imaging. Bioconjug Chem 12(2): 213–219, 2001

134. Weissleder R, Simonova M, Bogdanova A, Bredow S, Enochs WS, Bogdanov A Jr: MR Imaging and scintigraphy of gene expression through melanin induction. Radiology 204: 425–429, 1997

135. Kayyem JF, Kumar RM, Fraser SE, Meade TJ: Receptor-targeted co-transport of DNA into eukaryotic cells. Methods Enzymol 217: 618–644, 1993

136. Koretsky A, Lin Y, Schorle H, Jaenisch R: Genetic control of MRI contrast by expression of the transferring receptor. Proceedings of the fourth meeting of the International Society for Magnetic Resonance in Medicine. International Society for Magnetic Resonance in Medicine, Berkeley, CA, 5471, 1996 (Abstract)

137. Folpe AL, Lyles RH, Sprouse JT, Conrad EU 3rd, Eary JF: (F-18) fluorodeoxyglucose positron emission tomography as a predictor of pathologic grade and other prognostic variables in bone and soft tissue sarcoma. Clin Cancer Res 6(4): 1279–1287, 2000

138. Kostakoglu L, Leonard JP, Kuji I, Coleman M, Vallabhajosula S, Goldsmith SJ: Comparison of fluorine-18 fluorodeoxyglucose positron emission tomography and

Ga-67 scintigraphy in evaluation of lymphoma. Cancer 94(4): 879–888, 2002

139. Kernstine KH, Mclaughlin KA, Menda Y, Rossi NP, Kahn DJ, Bushnell DL, Graham MM, Brown CK, Madsen MT: Can FDG-PET reduce the need for mediastinoscopy in potentially resectable nonsmall cell lung cancer? Ann Thorac Surg 73(2): 394–401; discussion 401–402, 2002

140. Mijnhout GS, Hoekstra OS, van Tulder MW, Teule GJ, Deville WL: Systematic review of the diagnostic accuracy of (18)F-fluorodeoxyglucose positron emission tomography in melanoma patients. Cancer 91(8): 1530–1542, 2001

141. Kato H, Kuwano H, Nakajima M, Miyazaki T, Yoshikawa M, Ojima H, Tsukada K, Oriuchi N, Inoue T, Endo K: Comparison between positron emission tomography and computed tomography in the use of the assessment of esophageal carcinoma. Cancer 94(4): 921–928, 2002

142. Arulampalam TH, Costa DC, Bomanji JB, Ell PJ: The clinical application of positron emission tomography to colorectal cancer management. Q J Nucl Med 45(3): 215–230, 2001

143. Glasspool RM, Evans TRJ: Clinical imaging of cancer metastasis. Eur J Cancer 36: 1661–1670, 2000

144. Dwamena BA, Sonnad SS, Angobaldo JO, Wahl RL: Metastases from non-small cell lung cancer: mediastinal staging in the 1990s – meta-analytic comparison of PET and CT. Radiology 213: 530–536, 1999

145. Lewis P, Griffin S, Marsden P, Gee T, Nunan T, Maisey M: Whole-body F-18 fluorodeoxyglucose positron emission tomography in preoperative evaluation of lung cancer. Lancet 344: 1265–1266, 1994

146. Bury T, Dowlati A, Paulus P, Hustinx R, Radermecker M, Rigo P: Staging of non-small-cell lung cancer by whole-body fluorine-18 deoxyglucose positron emission tomography. Eur J Nucl Med 23: 204–206, 1996

147. Valk PE, Pounds TR, Hopkins DM, Haseman MK, Hofer GA, Greiss HB: Staging non-small cell lung cancer by whole-body positron emission tomography imaging. Ann Thorac Surg 60: 1573–1581, 1995

148. Macfarlane DJ, Sondak V, Johnson T, Wahl RL: Prospective evaluation of 2-[F-18]-2-deoxy-D-glucose positron emission tomography in staging of regional lymph nodes in patients with cutaneous malignant melanoma. J Clin Oncol 16: 1770–1776, 1998

149. Wagner JD, Schauwecker D, Hutchins G, Coleman JJ: Initial assessment of positron emission tomography for detection of nonpalpable regional lymphatic metastases in melanoma. J Surg Oncol 64: 181–189, 1997

150. Moog F, Bangerter M, Diederichs CG, Gulhman A, Kotzerke J, Merkle E, Kolokythas O, Frickhofen N, Reske SN: Lymphoma: role of whole-body 2-deoxy-2-[F-18]fluoro-D-glucose (FDG) PET in nodal staging. Radiology 203: 795–800, 1997

151. Blankenberg FG, Naumovski L, Tait JF, Post AM, Strauss HW: Imaging cyclophosphamide-induced intramedullary apoptosis in rats using 99mTc-radiolabeled annexin V. J Nucl Med 42(2): 309–316, 2001

152. Blankenberg FG, Katsikis PD, Tait JF, Davis RE, Naumovski L, Ohtsuki K, Kopiwoda S, Abrams MJ, Darkes M, Robbins RC, Maecker HT, Strauss HW: in vivo detection and imaging of phosphatidylserine expression during programmed cell death. Proc Natl Acad Sci USA 95(11): 6349–6354, 1998

153. Ray P, Bauer E, Iyer M, Barrio JR, Satyamurthy N, Phelps ME, Herschman HR, Gambhir SS: Monitoring gene therapy with reporter gene imaging. Semin Nucl Med 31(4): 312–320, 2001

154. Heppeler A, Froidevaux S, Eberle AN, Maecke HR: Receptor targeting for tumor localisation and therapy with radiopeptides. Curr Med Chem 7(9): 971–994, 2000

155. Alauddin MM, Shahinian A, Gordon EM, Bading JR, Conti PS: Preclinical evaluation of the penciclovir analog 9-(4-[(18)F]fluoro-3-hydroxymethylbutyl)guanine for in vivo measurement of suicide gene expression with PET. J Nucl Med 42(11): 1682–1690, 2001

156. Berger F, Gambhir SS: Recent advances in imaging endogenous or transferred gene expression utilizing radionuclide technologies in living subjects: applications to breast cancer. Breast Cancer Res 3(1): 28–35, 2001

157. Liang Q, Satyamurthy N, Barrio JR, Toyokuni T, Phelps MP, Gambhir SS, Herschman HR: Noninvasive, quantitative imaging in living animals of a mutant dopamine D2 receptor reporter gene in which ligand binding is uncoupled from signal transduction. Gene Ther 8(19): 1490–1498, 2001

158. Henze M, Schuhmacher J, Hipp P, Kowalski J, Becker DW, Doll J, Macke HR, Hofmann M, Debus J, Haberkorn U: PET imaging of somatostatin receptors. J Nucl Med 42(7): 1053–1056, 2001

159. Nakamoto Y, Saga T, Misaki T, Kobayashi H, Sato N, Ishimori T, Kosugi S, Sakahara H, Konishi J: Establishment and characterization of a breast cancer cell line expressing Na+/I- symporters for radioiodide concentrator gene therapy. J Nucl Med 41(11): 1898–1904, 2000

160. Scearce-Levie K, Coward P, Redfern CH, Conklin BR: Engineering receptors activated solely by synthetic ligands (RASSLs). Trends Pharmacol Sci 22(8): 414–420, 2001

161. Moore A, Basilion JP, Chiocca EA, Weissleder R: Measuring transferrin receptor gene expression by NMR imaging. Biochim Biophys Acta 1402(3): 239–249, 1998

162. Tjuvajev JG, Stockhammer G, Desai R, Uehara H, Watanabe K, Gansbacher B, Blasberg RG: Imaging the expression of transfected genes in vivo. Cancer Res 55(24): 6126–6132, 1995

163. Hustinx R, Shiue CY, Alavi A, McDonald D, Shiue GG, Zhuang H, Lanuti M, Lambright E, Karp JS, Eck SL: Imaging in vivo herpes simplex virus thymidine kinase gene transfer to tumour-bearing rodents using positron emission tomography. Eur J Nucl Med 28(1): 5–12, 2001

164. Gambhir SS, Herschman HR, Cherry SR, Barrio JR, Satyamurthy N, Toyokuni T, Phelps ME, Larson SM, Balatoni J, Finn R, Sadelain M, Tjuvajev J, Blasberg R: Imaging transgene expression with radionuclide imaging technologies. Neoplasia 2(1–2): 118–138, 2000

165. Yaghoubi S, Barrio JR, Dahlbom M, Iyer M, Namavari M, Satyamurthy N, Goldman R, Herschman HR, Phelps ME,

300

Gambhir SS: Human pharmacokinetic and dosimetry studies of ^{18}F-FHBG: a reporter probe for imaging herpes simplex virus type-1 thymidine kinase reporter gene expression. J Nucl Med 42(8): 1225–1234, 2001

166. Doubrovin M, Ponomarev V, Beresten T, Balatoni J, Bornmann W, Finn R, Humm J, Larson S, Sadelain M, Blasberg R, Gelovani Tjuvajev J: Imaging transcriptional regulation of p53-dependent genes with positron emission tomography *in vivo*. Proc Natl Acad Sci USA 98(16): 9300–9305, 2001

167. Benaron DA, Stevenson DK: Optical time-of-flight and absorbance imaging of biologic media. Science 259(5100): 1463-1466, 1993

168. Light propagates through tissue much as a gas diffuses through air, in a random, scattered walk called photon diffusion. At wavelengths near the blue, the absorbance of tissue is high, such that photons travel a few hundred microns or less before being absorbed; in contrast in the red and infrared wavelengths, photons scatter but travel millimeters to centimeters before absorption, and this scattering dominates the transport of photons across tissue. Scattering of light redirects photons based upon local changes in index-of-refraction. These refraction changes come from objects with structures on the size order of the wavelength of light (typically nucleus and cell membranes, and to a lesser extent mitochondria). The physics of the imaging has been well studied, is complex, and continues to evolve, in part because unlike in the transport of high-energy photons from PET or X-ray, a linear photon path often cannot be assumed.

169. AntiCancer, Inc. Image from web site at www.anticancer.com.

170. Shah N, Cerussi A, Eker C, Espinoza J, Butler J, Fishkin J, Hornung R, Tromberg B: Noninvasive functional optical spectroscopy of human breast tissue. Proc Natl Acad Sci USA 98(8): 4420–4425, 2001

171. Cerussi AE, Jakubowski D, Shah N, Bevilacqua F, Lanning R, Berger AJ, Hsiang D, Butler J, Holcombe RF, Tromberg BJ: Spectroscopy enhances the information content of optical mammography. J Biomed Opt 7(1): 60–71, 2002

172. Fishkin JB, Coquoz O, Andersen ER, Brenner M, Tromberg BJ: Frequency-domain photon migration measurements of normal and malignant tissue optical properties in a human subject. Appl Optics 36: 141–153, 1997

173. De Blasi RA, Fantini RA, Franceschini MA, Ferrari MA, Gratton E: Cerebral and muscle oxygen saturation measurement by frequency-domain near-infrared spectrometer. Med Biol Eng Comp 33: 228–230, 1995.

174. Benaron DA, Rubinski B, Hintz SR, et al.: Automated Quantitation of tissue components using real-time spectroscopy. In Benapon DA, Chance B, Ferrori M, eds. Photon Propagation in Tissues II. SPIE 3194: 500–511, 1997

175. Time-resolved spectroscopy of hemoglobin and myoglobin in resting and ischemic muscle. Anal Biochem 174: 698–707, 1988

176. Quaresima V, Homma S, Azuma K, Shimizu S, Chiarotti F, Ferrari M, Kagaya A: Calf and shin muscle oxygenation patterns and femoral artery blood flow during dynamic plantar flexion exercise in humans. Eur J Appl Physiol 84(5): 387–394, 2001

177. De Blasi RA, Quaglia E, Gasparetto A, Ferrari M: Muscle oxygenation by fast near infrared spectrophotometry (NIRS) in ischemic forearm. Adv Exp Med Biol 316: 163–172, 1992

178. Chance B, Zhaung Z, UnAh C, Alter C, Lipton L: Cognition activated low-frequency modulation of light absorption in human brain. Proc Natl Acad Sci USA 90: 3770–3774, 1993

179. Benaron DA, Hintz SR, Villringer A, et al.: Noninvasive functional imaging of human brain using light. J Cereb Blood Flow Metab 20: 469–477, 2000

180. Hintz SR, Benaron DA, Siegel AM, Zourabian A, Stevenson DK, Boas DA: Bedside functional imaging of the premature infant brain during passive motor activation. J Perinat Med 29: 335–343, 2001

181. Chance B: Near-infrared (NIR) optical spectroscopy characterizes breast tissue hormonal and age status. Acad Radiol 8: 209–210, 2001

182. Under the name FireFly™ tissue oximeter. Unpublished data, under review. See www.spectros.com up to date information on FireFly™ trials and results

183. Schomacker KT, Frisoli JK, Compton CC, Flotte TJ, Richter JM, Nishioka NS, Deutsch TF: Ultraviolet laser-induced fluorescence of colonic tissue: basic biology and diagnostic potential. Lasers Surg Med 12(1): 63–78, 1992

184. Ramanujam N, Mitchell MF, Mahadevan A, Thomsen S, Malpica A, Wright T, Atkinson N, Richards-Kortum R: Spectroscopic diagnosis of cervical intraepithelial neoplasia (CIN) *in vivo* using laser-induced fluorescence spectra at multiple excitation wavelengths. Lasers Surg Med 19(1): 63–74, 1996

185. Drezek R, Sokolov K, Utzinger U, Boiko I, Malpica A, Follen M, Richards-Kortum R: Understanding the contributions of NADH and collagen to cervical tissue fluorescence spectra: modeling, measurements, and implications. J Biomed Opt 6(4): 385–396, 2001

186. Nordstrom RJ, Burke L, Niloff JM, Myrtle JF: Identification of cervical intraepithelial neoplasia (CIN) using UV-excited fluorescence and diffuse-reflectance tissue spectroscopy. Lasers Surg Med 29(2): 118–127, 2001

187. Schantz SP, Kolli V, Savage HE, Yu G, Shah JP, Harris DE, Katz A, Alfano RR, Huvos AG: *In vivo* native cellular fluorescence and histological characteristics of head and neck cancer. Clin Cancer Res 4(5): 1177–1182, 1998

188. Georgakoudi I, Jacobson BC, Muller MG, Sheets EE, Badizadegan K, Carr-Locke DL, Crum CP, Boone CW, Dasari RR, Van Dam J, Feld MS: NAD(P)H and collagen as *in vivo* quantitative fluorescent biomarkers of epithelial precancerous changes. Cancer Res 62(3): 682–687, 2002

189. Georgakoudi I, Sheets EE, Muller MG, Backman V, Crum CP, Badizadegan K, Dasari RR, Feld MS: Trimodal spectroscopy for the detection and characterization of cervical precancers *in vivo*. Am J Obstet Gynecol 186(3): 374–382, 2002

190. Herman P, Maliwal BP, Lin HJ, Lakowicz JR: Frequency-domain fluorescence microscopy with the LED as a light source. J Microsc 203(Pt 2): 176–181, 2001

191. Cubeddu R, Canti G, Pifferi A, Taroni P, Valentini G: Fluorescence lifetime imaging of experimental tumors in hematoporphyrin derivative-sensitized mice. Photochem Photobiol 66(2): 229–236, 1997

192. McGill N, Dieppe PA, Bowden M, Gardiner DJ, Hall M: Identification of pathological mineral deposits by Raman microscopy. Lancet 337(8733): 77–78, 1991

193. Baraga JJ, Feld MS, Rava RP: *In situ* optical histochemistry of human artery using near infrared Fourier transform Raman spectroscopy. Proc Natl Acad Sci USA 89(8): 3473–3477, 1992

194. Manoharan R, Baraga JJ, Feld MS, Rava RP: Quantitative histochemical analysis of human artery using Raman spectroscopy. J Photochem Photobiol B 16(2): 211–233, 1992

195. Stone N, Stavroulaki P, Kendall C, Birchall M, Barr H: Raman spectroscopy for early detection of laryngeal malignancy: preliminary results. Laryngoscope 110(10 Pt 1): 1756–1763, 2000

196. Bakker Schut TC, Witjes MJ, Sterenborg HJ, Speelman OC, Roodenburg JL, Marple ET, Bruining HA, Puppels GJ: *in vivo* detection of dysplastic tissue by Raman spectroscopy. Anal Chem 72(24): 6010–6018, 2000

197. Rollins AM, Yazdanfar S, Barton JK, Izatt JA: Real-time *in vivo* color Doppler optical coherence tomography. J Biomed Opt 7(1): 123–129, 2002

198. Benaron DA, Cheong WF, Stevenson DK: Tissue optics. Science 276(5321): 2002–2003, 1997

199. Stanga PE, Bird AC: Optical coherence tomography (OCT): principles of operation, technology, indications in vitreoretinal imaging and interpretation of results. Int Ophthalmol 23(4–6): 191–197, 2001

200. Jesser CA, Boppart SA, Pitris C, Stamper DL, Mielsen GP, Brezinski ME, Fujomoto JG: High resolution imaging of transitional cell carcinoma with optical coherence tomography: feasibility for the evaluation of bladder pathology. Br J Radiol 72: 1170–1176, 1999

201. Li XD, Boppart SA, Van Dam J, Mashimo H, Mutinga M, Drexler W, Klein M, Pitris C, Krinsky ML, Brezinski ME, Fujimoto JG: Optical coherence tomography: advanced technology for the endoscopic imaging of Barrett's esophagus. Endoscopy 32(12): 921–930, 2000

202. Poneros JM, Brand S, Bouma BE, Tearney GJ, Compton CC, Nishioka NS: Diagnosis of specialized intestinal metaplasia by optical coherence tomography. Gastroenterology 120(1): 7–12, 2001

203. Tearney GJ, Brezinski ME, Bouma BE, Boppart SA, Pitris C, Southern JF, Fujimoto JG: *in vivo* endoscopic optical biopsy with optical coherence tomography. Science 276(5321): 2037–2039, 1997

204. Jang IK, Bouma BE, Kang DH, Park SJ, Park SW, Seung KB, Choi KB, Shishkov M, Schlendorf K, Pomerantsev E, Houser SL, Aretz HT, Tearney GJ: Visualization of coronary atherosclerotic plaques in patients using optical coherence tomography: comparison with intravascular ultrasound. J Am Coll Cardiol 39(4): 604–609, 2002

205. Backman V: Polarized light scattering spectroscopy for quantitative measurement of epithelial structures *in situ*. IEEE J Sel Topics Quant Elec 5(4): 1019–1026, 1999

206. Mourant JR, Canpolat M, Brocker C, Esponda-Ramos O, Johnson TM, Matanock A, Stetter K, Freyer JP: Light scattering from cells: the contribution of the nucleus and the effects of proliferative status. J Biomed Opt 5(2): 131–137, 2000

207. Mourant JR, Hielscher AH, Eick AA, Johnson TM, Freyer JP: Evidence of intrinsic differences in the light scattering properties of tumorigenic and nontumorigenic cells. Cancer 84(6): 366–374, 1998

208. Jiang H, Pierce J, Sevick-Muraca E: Measurement of particle-size distribution and volume fraction in concentrated suspensions with photon migration techniques. Appl Optics 36(15): 3310–3318, 1997

209. Balgi G, Reynolds J, Mayer RH, Cooley RE, Sevick-Muraca EM: Measurements of multiply scattered light for on-line monitoring of changes in size distribution of cell debris suspension. Biotechnol Prog 15(6): 1106–1114, 1999

210. Beauvoit B, Evans SM, Jenkins TW, Miller EE, Chance B: Correlation between the light scattering and the mitochondrial content of normal tissues and transplantable rodent tumors. Anal Biochem 226(1): 167–174, 1995

211. Beuthan J, Minet O, Helfmann J, Herrig M, Muller G: The spatial variation of the refractive index in biological cells. Phys Med Biol 41(3): 369–382, 1996

212. Cotran RS, Kumar V, Collins T (eds) Robbins Pathological Basis of Disease, WB Saunders. Toronto, 1425 pp

213. Hawrysz DJ, Sevick-Muraca EM: Developments toward diagnostic breast cancer imaging using near-infrared optical measurements and fluorescent contrast agents. Neoplasia 2(5): 388–417, 2000

214. Achliefu S, Dorshow RB, Bugal JE, Rajagopalan R: Novel receptor-targeted fluorescent contrast agents for *in vivo* tumor imaging. J Inves Radiol 35: 479–485, 2000

215. Ballou B, Fisher GW, Waggoner AS, Farkas DL, Reiland JM, Jaffe R, Mujumdar RB, Mujumdar SR, Hakala TR: Tumor labeling *in vivo* using cyanine-conjugated monoclonal antibodies. Cancer Immnol Immunother 41: 257–263, 1995

216. Licha K, Riefke B, Ntziachristos V, Becker A, Chance B, Semmler W: Hydrophilic cyanine dyes as contrast agents for near-infrared tumor imaging: synthesis, photophysical properties and spectroscopic *in vivo* characterization. Photochem Photobiol 72(3): 392–398, 2000

217. Bornhop DJ, Hubbard DS, Houlne MP, Adair C, Kiefer GE, Pence BC, Morgan DL: Fluorescent tissue site-selective lanthanide chelate, Tb-PCTMB for enhanced imaging of cancer. Anal Chem 71(14): 2607–2615, 1999

218. Chen Y, Kalas RM, Faris GW: Spectroscopic properties of upconverting phosphor reporters. In: Bornhop, DJ, Contag CH, Sevick-Muraca EM (eds) Biomedical Imaging: Reporters, Dyes, and Instrumentation, Proceedings of SPIE Vol 3600, 1999, pp 151–157

219. Becker A, Riefke B, Ebert B, Sukowski U, Rinneberg H, Semmler W, Licha K: Macromolecular contrast agents for optical imaging of tumors: comparison of indotricarbocyanine-labeled human serum albumin and transferrin. Photochem Photobiol 72(2): 234–241, 2000

302

220. Hirsch JI, Tisnado J, Cho SR, Beachley MC: Use of iso-sulfan blue for identification of lymphatic vessels: experimental and clinical evaluation. AJR Am J Roentgenol 139(6): 1061–1064, 1982

221. Andersson-Engels S, Klinteberg C, Svanberg K, Svanberg S: in vivo fluorescence imaging for tissue diagnostics. Phys Med Biol 42(5): 815–824, 1997

222. Andersson-Engels S, Canti G, Cubeddu R, Eker C, af Klinteberg C, Pifferi A, Svanberg K, Svanberg S, Taroni P, Valentini G, Wang I: Preliminary evaluation of two fluorescence imaging methods for the detection and the delineation of basal cell carcinomas of the skin. Lasers Surg Med 26(1): 76–82, 2000

223. Svanberg K, Wang I, Colleen S, Idvall I, Ingvar C, Rydell R, Jocham D, Diddens H, Bown S, Gregory G, Montan S, Andersson-Engels S, Svanberg S: Clinical multi-colour fluorescence imaging of malignant tumours – initial experience. Acta Radiol 39(1): 2–9, 1998

224. Benaron DA, Contag PR, Contag CH: Imaging brain structure and function, infection and gene expression in the body using light. Philos Trans R Soc Lond B Biol Sci 352(1354): 755–761, 1997

225. Contag CH, Contag PR, Mullins JI, Spilman SD, Stevenson DK, Benaron DA: Photonic detection of bacterial pathogens in living hosts. Mol Microbiol 18(4): 593–603, 1995

226. Nicolas JC: Applications of low-light imaging to life sciences. J Biolumin Chemilumin 9(3): 139–144, 1994

227. Dirnagl U, Lindauer U, Them A, Schreiber S, Pfister HW, Koedel U, Reszka R, Freyer D, Villringer A: Global cerebral ischemia in the rat: online monitoring of oxygen free radical production using chemiluminescence in vivo. J Cereb Blood Flow Metab 15(6): 929–940, 1995

228. Cutrin JC, Boveris A, Zingaro B, Corvetti G, Poli G: In situ determination by surface chemiluminescence of temporal relationships between evolving warm ischemia-reperfusion injury in rat liver and phagocyte activation and recruitment. Hepatology 31(3): 622–632, 2000

229. Proposal to the Baxter Foundation, Stanford University School of Medicine, Benaron DA and Contag CH (DA Benaron, PI) 1994

230. Bhaumik S, Gambhir SS: Optical imaging of Renilla luciferase reporter gene expression in living mice. Proc Natl Acad Sci USA 99(1): 377–382, 2002

231. Image provided by Anticancer, Inc., San Diego, CA

232. Chalfie M, Tu Y, Euskirchen G, Ward WW, Prasher DC: Green fluorescent protein as a marker for gene expression. Science 263: 802–805, 1994

233. Girotti M, Banting G: TGN38-green fluorescent protein hybrid proteins expressed in stably transfected cells provide a tool for the real-time, in vivo study of membrane traffic pathways and suggest a possible role for ratTGN38. J Cell Sci 109: 2915–2926, 1996

234. Hoogenraad, JH, van der Mark MB, Colak SB, Hooft GW, van der Linden, ES: First results from the Philips optical mammoscope, In: Benaron DA, Chance B, Ferrari M (eds)

Photon Propagation in Tissues III Proceedings of SPIE, Vol 3194, 1997, pp 184–190

235. Gotz L, Heywang-Kobrunner SH, Schutz O, Siebold H: [Optical mammography in preoperative patients]. Aktuelle Radiol 8(1): 31–33, 1998 (German)

236. Karwinski B, Svendsen E, Hartveit F: Clinically undiagnosed malignant tumours found at autopsy. APMIS 98(6): 496–500, 1990

237. Yang CR, Ou YC, Ho HC, Kao YL, Cheng CL, Chen JT, Chen LP, Ho WL: Unsuspected prostate carcinoma and prostatic intraepithelial neoplasm in Taiwanese patients undergoing cystoprostatectomy. Mol Urol 3(1): 33–39, 1999

238. Brawn PN, Kuhl D, Speights VO, Johnson CF 3rd, Lind M: The incidence of unsuspected metastases from clinically benign prostate glands with latent prostate carcinoma. Arch Pathol Lab Med 119(8): 731–733, 1995

239. Redding WH, Coombes RC, Monaghan P: Detection of micrometastases in patients with primary breast cancer. Lancet 2: 1271–1273, 1983

240. Stahel RA, Mabry M, Sharkin AT, Speak J, Bernal SD: Detection of bone marrow metastases in small-cell lung cancer by monoclonal antibody. J Clin Oncol 3: 455–456, 1985

241. Edelstein RA, Zietman AL, de las Morenas A et al.: Implication of prostatic micrometastases to the pelvic lymph nodes: an archival tissue study. Urology 47: 370–375, 1996

242. Pan Y, Lavelle JP, Bastacky SI, Meyers S, Pirtskhalaishvili G, Zeidel ML, Farkas DL: Detection of tumorigenesis in rat bladders with optical coherence tomography. Med Phys 28(12): 2432–2440, 2001

243. Gurjar RS, Backman V, Perelman LT, Georgakoudi I, Badizadegan K, Itzkan I, Dasari RR, Feld MS: Imaging human epithelial properties with polarized light-scattering spectroscopy. Nat Med 7(11): 1245–1248, 2001

244. Weissleder R, Moore A, Mahmood U: In vivo magnetic resonance imaging of transgene expression. Nat Med 6: 351–355, 2000

245. Ghossein RA, Bhattacharya S: Molecular detection and characterization of circulating tumour cells and micrometastases in solid tumors. Eur J Cancer 36: 1681–1694, 2000

246. Benaron DA, Parchikon IH, Talmi YI, Scardino PT: Real-time optical imaging system for operating room use. Presented at 1st Annual Meeting of the Society for Molecular Imaging. Boston, MA, August 24–26 2002

247. Benaron DA: Optical Contrast Agents. Presented Joint Working Group on Quantitative in vivo Functional Imaging in Oncology. Washington DC, USA, January 6–8, 1999

248. Benaron DA, Cheong W-F, Duchworth JL: Automated classification of tissue by type using real-time spectroscopy. In Photon Propagation in Tissues III. Benaron DA, Chance B, Ferrari M, Kohl M, eds. SPIE 3194: 99–109, 1997

Antisense therapy: Current status in prostate cancer and other malignancies

Martin Gleave[1], Hideake Miyake[1], Uwe Zangemeister-Wittke[2] and Burkhard Jansen[1]
[1]*The Prostate Centre, Vancouver General Hospital, Division of Urology, University of British Columbia, Vancouver, BC, Canada;* [2]*Department of Internal Medicine, Division of Medical Oncology, University of Zurich, Zurich, Switzerland*

Key words: prostate cancer, antisense therapy, ASOs

Summary

Recent technological advances now allowing both large scale data generation and its in-depth analysis have opened new avenues to identify and target genes involved in neoplastic transformation and tumor progression. This accelerated identification and characterization of cancer-relevant molecular targets has sparked considerable interest in the development of new generations of anti-cancer agents. It is anticipated, that these agents will show enhanced specificity for malignant cells and a more favorable side-effect profile due to well-defined and tailored modes of action. Antisense oligonucleotides (ASOs) are short synthetic stretches of chemically modified DNA capable of specifically hybridizing to the mRNA of a chosen cancer-relevant target gene are close, after decades of challenges, close to fulfilling their promise in the clinical setting. Emerging clinical evidence supports the notion that ASOs stand a realistic chance of developing into one of the main players of rationally designed anti-cancer agents, although certainly not all of the challenges have been met to date. The status of antisense targeting of genes relevant to prostate cancer, including bcl-2, bcl-xL, clusterin, androgen receptor (AR) and IGFBPs, are reviewed.

Introduction

In the last few years cutting edge high throughput technological platforms have been developed and are now accessible to rapidly and cost effectively produce an entire 'transcriptome', 'genome'- or 'proteome'-wide view of tumor biology. Integrated gene and protein expression data gathered from these high throughput technologies and mined by advanced bioinformatics will dramatically transform our understanding and approach to human malignancies. These technologies, when harnessed to detailed phenotypic information and investigated in laboratory models have the power to explain complex biological phenomenon of tumor progression and direct the development of prognosticators and new therapeutic targets. From the foundation of tumor classification derived from molecular profiles, science is poised to make the next leap into individualized prognostication and treatment based on the unique genetic aspects of individual tumors. As therapeutics are developed to address specific genetic abnormalities, custom therapeutic protocols will become the standard of care. Already specific, aberrantly expressed genes in cancers have been directly targeted with such agents as antisense Bcl-2, Gleevec and Herceptin; these approaches are leading the way into specialized and customized strategies tailored to the tumor's aberrations, with low toxicity.

The focus of this review is to address the development and recent progress in the use of antisense oligonucleotides (ASOs) as potential therapeutics in oncology, with an emphasis on those of specific relevance to prostate cancer. Known nucleotide sequences of cancer-relevant genes offer the possibility to design tailored anti-cancer agents which lack many of the toxic side-effects displayed by conventional therapeutics. An ASO is designed to target the complementary sequence within a given RNA species, and once delivered into the target cell, hybridize with its RNA complement to inhibit translation of the disease-relevant protein. In contrast to the use of plasmid-derived endogenous expression of antisense RNA which has failed to overcome inefficient plasmid delivery, the oligonucleotide approach has overcome many of the hurdles on the way to successful clinical application. While the idea behind oligonucleotide-based antisense therapy is

M.L. Cher, K.V. Honn and A. Raz (eds.), Prostate Cancer: New Horizons in Research and Treatment, 303–316.
© 2002 *Kluwer Academic Publishers.*

304

appealing and dates back more than 30 years [1–3], recent advances in nucleic acid chemistry, along with the advent of automated DNA synthesis, has accelerated progress in the use of this technology for target validation and therapy.

Mechanisms of ASO-induced inhibition of protein expression

ASOs bind to a selected target mRNA by Watson–Crick base pairing, with subsequent inhibition of mRNA processing or translation by a variety of mechanisms including prevention of mRNA transport, splicing or translational arrest (Figure 1). The specificity of this approach is based on the estimate that any sequence of at least 13 bases in RNA and 17 bases in DNA is represented only once within the human genome. While small molecules designed for therapeutic use generally recognize a specific protein target based on its molecular domain structure, an ASO recognizes a specific mRNA based on its sequence.

Cleavage of target mRNA by RNase H, a ubiquitous endonuclease usually involved in DNA replication, that cleaves the RNA strand of a DNA–RNA heteroduplex, is presumably the most important mechanism of antisense action and underlies the activity of all oligonucleotides tested in clinical trials to date. While the exact recognition structure for RNase H is still unknown, oligonucleotides with DNA-like properties as short as

tetramers seem to be capable of activating this potent endonucleolytic activity [4]. High affinity oligonucleotides with a 5–7 base homology may provide sufficient overlap for RNase H competency [5]. Early last year, the first successful use of double-stranded 21-nucleotide small interfering RNAs (siRNAs) that specifically suppress the expression of homologous genes in mammalian cells has been described [6]. Although definitely promising as a strategy for the regulation of gene expression in theory, data available to date do not yet allow conclusions on the potential usefulness of this approach in animal models or in the clinic.

Designing an optimal antisense sequence

Tertiary structures blocking the accessibility of the target mRNA and shared sequence homologies with non-target genes are important issues that need to be considered in the design of ASOs. While ASOs hybridizing to the start codon have been used successfully for a number of target mRNAs, other sites, like 5′ untranslated regions for instance, may prove to be even more effective under certain conditions [7–9]. A variety of in vitro techniques have been employed to streamline the process of selecting target sites for antisense action, many of these are computational strategies or combinatorial approaches based on annealing reactions with arrays of antisense species

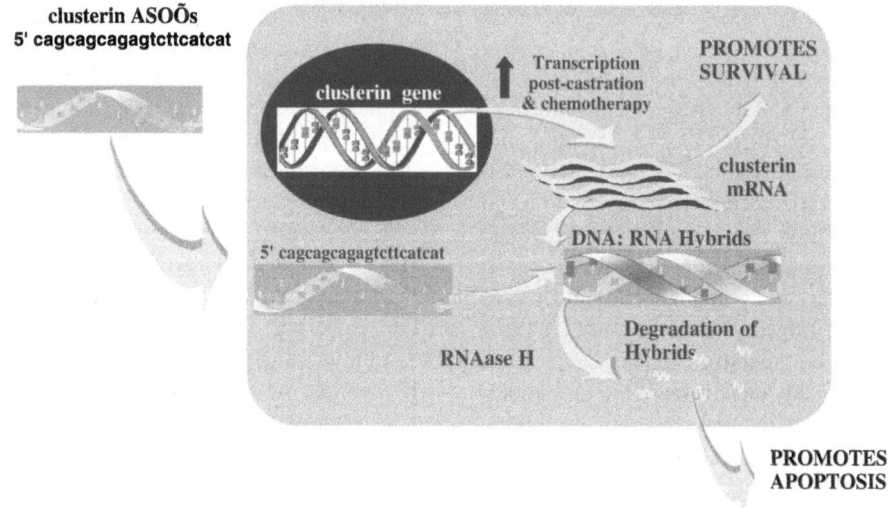

Figure 1. Schema illustrating mechanism of action of antisense oligonucleotide targeting the cell survival gene clusterin.

[10] and/or monitoring accessibility of target structures by RNase H mapping [11]. Although there are several shortcomings using these strategies they nevertheless significantly reduce cost by decreasing the number of oligonucleotides which have to be tested in high throughput screens.

Strategies to stabilize ASOs for *in vivo* application

Initially, the usefulness of ASOs under *in vivo* conditions was limited due to the susceptibility of the original phosphodiester backbone to degradation by cellular nucleases. A variety of backbone, sugar and base modifications have been investigated to reach stability characteristics required for clinical applications. Backbone modifications like the replacement of the oxygen atom of the PO moiety by sulfur (phosphorothioates, PS), a methyl group (methylphosphonates) or amines (phosphoramidates) led to significant improvements. Although these analogs largely overcome the stability problem, only the PS modification has resulted in antisense compounds combining serum stability with reasonably high RNA binding affinity and the ability to elicit RNase H cleavage of the target RNA [13]. Today, after more than a decade of intensive research, PS ASOs still represent the most widely used class of antisense compounds, and several of these analogs are currently being tested in clinical trials and have shown considerable promise. Nevertheless, the overall physico-chemical properties of PS oligonucleotides are sub-optimal, and primarily backbone-related issues, including complement activation, thrombocytopenia, inhibition of cell–matrix interaction or immune stimulation related to CpG motifs [14–16] warrant further study. The general observation that most effective drugs used to date in clinical oncology share the characteristic of having more than one distinct mode of action may also prove to be correct for antisense therapeutics, at least for the now most commonly used PS oligonucleotides.

To overcome the drawbacks associated with PS oligonucleotides, ongoing research has focused on backbone modifications that provide a more attractive pharmacological profile. The main goal of the modifications investigated so far was to further increase the metabolic stability and enhance the hybridization affinity of PS oligonucleotides for complementary mRNA. The affinity of ASOs to the target mRNA is a measure of stability of the nucleic acid hybrid, and higher affinity translates into higher gene repressing activity [5]. Among a number of different modifications at the 2′-sugar position, the 2′-O-(2-methoxy)ethyl (2′-MOE) incorporation was identified as enhancing both binding affinity and further resisting degradation by intracellular nucleases [18]. 2′-O,4′-C-methylene bridge (locked nucleic acid; LNA) [19] render ASOs in an RNA-like C3′-endo conformation also resulting in greatly enhanced affinity. The 2′-MOE modification resulted in decreased binding affinity to RNase H, the principal nuclease that cleaves ASO-bound mRNA. This problem was overcome by the use of 'gapped' ASO such that the 5′ and 3′ ends of the molecule contained 2′-MOE-modified sugar residues and the central portion of the ASO contained 2′-deoxy sugar residues that support RNaseH activity [5,19]. This chemical design is usually accompanied with a uniformly modified PS backbone. The incorporation of 2′-MOE modifications into 20-mer PS ASO showed a dramatic effect on the ability of the sequence to hybridize to a target mRNA as a result of the conformation of the sugar and the backbone. Furthermore, 2′-MOE gapmers exhibited substantially increased resistance to intracellular nucleases, compared to conventional PS ASO. Both increased hybridizing affinity toward the targeted mRNA and enhanced resistance toward both serum and intracellular nucleases resulted in a 20-fold increase in activity of 2′-MOE-modified ASO [20]. The enhanced potency of this new class of ASO did not lead to any decrease in specificity.

Antisense targets

The initial phase of the Human Genome Project left the field of nucleotide therapeutics with about 30,000–40,000 gene sequences and about 100,000 mRNAs as potential target structures. Although only a minority of these potential targets will prove to be suitable for therapeutic strategies, the potential for the development of tailored treatment approaches is certainly encouraging. The most attractive molecular candidates for antisense therapy are those that are engaged in cell proliferation [21], apoptosis [22], angiogenesis [23] and metastasis [24]. Antisense therapy that targets the apoptotic rheostat in cells or interferes with signaling pathways involved in cell proliferation and growth are particularly promising in combination with conventional anti-cancer treatments. An overview of key ASOs currently evaluated in clinical trials is

Table 1. Key antisense clinical trials in oncology

Phase of clinical trial	Target gene/ gene product	Antisense compound/ drug	Company or investigator	ASO size/ chemistry	Target malignancy	Combination treatment
I–III	PKC-α	ISIS 3521	ISIS	20-mer/PS	Solid tumors	+
I–II	c-raf	ISIS 5132	ISIS	20-mer/PS	Solid tumors	+
I–II	Ha-ras	ISIS 2503	ISIS	20-mer/PS	Solid tumors	−
III	bcl-2	Genasense™, G3139	Genta	18-mer/PS	Solid tumors, MM, CLL	+
I–II	Clusterin/TRPM-2	OGX-011	OncoGeneX	21-mer/SGO	Solid tumors	+
I–II	PKA-R1-α	GEM 231	Hybridon	18-mer/SGO	Solid tumors	−
I–II	c-myb	LR/INX-3001	Gewirtz et al.	24-mer/PS	CML	−
I–II	Ribonucleotide-reductase	GTI-2040	Lorus	21-mer/PS	Solid tumors	−
I–II	DNA methyltransferase	MG98	MethylGene	20-mer/SGO	Solid tumors	+

MM: Multiple myeloma, CLL: Chronic lymphatic leukemia, CML: Chronic myelogenous leukemia, AML: Acute myelogenous leukemia, MDS: Myelo-dysplastic syndrome, PS: Phosphorothioate oligonucleotide, SGO: Second generation oligonucleotide.

provided in Table 1. Biologic and clinical studies focusing on candidate genes with potential relevance to prostate cancer progression are discussed in greater detail.

For advanced or metastatic prostate cancer, androgen withdrawal is an effective form of systemic therapy. However, androgen-independent (AI) progression and death occurs within a few years in most cases. Progression to androgen-independence is a complex process involving variable combinations of clonal selection [25], adaptive up-regulation of anti-apoptotic survival genes [26–29], androgen receptor (AR) transactivation in the absence of androgen from mutations or increased levels of co-activators [30,31] and alternative growth factor pathways, including Her2/neu, EGFR and IGF-1 [31–33]. It is interesting and somewhat ironic to note that the very same agents used to kill or control cancer cells also trigger cascades of events that lead to a chemoresistant phenotype. Prostate cancer is highly chemoresistant, with objective response rates of 10% and no demonstrated survival benefit [34]. More recently phase II studies using taxane-based combination regimens are reporting objective responses in 20–30% and PSA responses in >50% of cases [35–37]. Hormone refractory prostate cancer (HRPC), is therefore, the main obstacle to improving the survival and quality of life in patients with advanced disease, and novel therapeutic strategies that target the molecular basis of androgen and chemo-resistance are required. A rational treatment strategy involves combinatorial therapies that target adaptive changes in gene expression precipitated by androgen withdrawal or chemotherapy in order to enhance apoptosis (e.g. Bcl-2, clusterin) and inhibit proliferation (IGF-1 or TK signaling).

Bcl-2 family

Bcl-2. Bcl-2 has emerged as a critical regulator of apoptosis in numerous tissues as part of a growing family of apoptosis regulatory gene products, which function as either death antagonists (e.g. Bcl-2, Bcl-xL) or death agonists (Bax, Bcl-Xs, Bad) [38–42]. The ratio of death antagonists to death agonists determines how a cell responds to an apoptotic signal. Alterations in this balance that favor cell survival may cause proliferative disorders such as cancer. In the prostate gland, Bcl-2 is expressed in the less differentiated basal cell layer of prostatic acini, but not in benign differentiated luminal cells or AD prostate cancer cells. In prostate cancer cells, Bcl-2 is up-regulated within months after androgen withdrawal [43] and remains increased in AI tumors [40,41]. Bcl-2 up-regulation after androgen withdrawal may be an adaptive mechanism that helps some prostate cancer cells survive castration-induced apoptosis and subsequently progress to androgen-independence [42]. Bcl-2 also blocks pro apoptotic signals by a variety of chemotherapy agents, and may contribute to the multi-drug resistant phenotype characteristic of HRPC and other cancers.

Induction of apoptotic cell death after androgen ablation or chemotherapy may be enhanced through functional inhibition of Bcl-2. Indeed, Bcl-2 ASOs induce apoptosis and enhance chemosensitivity in numerous cancers. Preclinical studies have shown that Bcl-2 ASOs decreased Bcl-2 protein and increased chemosensitivity in xenograft models of human melanoma [44] and prostate cancer [26,45,46]. In prostate cancer models, Bcl-2 ASO reduced the IC_{50} of paclitaxel, docetaxel and mitoxanthrone *in vitro* by a factor of 1 log. Adjuvant *in vivo*

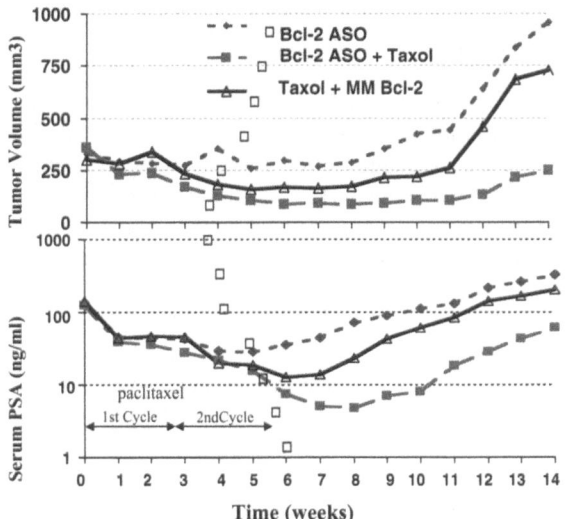

Figure 2. Human Bcl-2-specific antisense oligonucleotides (Genta, G3139) enhances the chemosensitiviy of human prostate LNCaP tumors to paclitaxel *in vivo*, delaying tumor progression and serum PSA increases compared to either paclitaxel alone or Bcl-2 ASO alone.

administration of Bcl-2 ASO plus paclitaxel following castration significantly delayed AI progression compared to administration of either agent alone. Furthermore, paclitaxel-induced regression of established AI Shionogi [45] or LNCaP [46] tumors was synergistically enhanced when combined with Bcl-2 ASO (Figure 2). Synergistic activity between Bcl-2 ASO and taxanes results from ASO-induced decreases in Bcl-2 mRNA and protein levels and taxol-induced Bcl-2 phosphorylation.

Initial data of a phase I clinical study evaluating single-agent bcl-2 ASO G3139 (Genasense, Table 1), a 18-mer PS oligonucleotide targeting the bcl-2 translation initiation site, was reported in 21 patients with non-Hodgkin's lymphoma (NHL) in 1997 [47,48]. The dose-limiting toxicity in this study was thrombocytopenia, and 1 complete response and 2 minor responses were seen. The disease stabilized in 9 patients, and 9 patients showed disease progression. However, reduction in Bcl-2 protein by ASO treatment was observed in only ~50% of evaluable patients. A second single agent phase I study in men with HRPC at Memorial Sloan–Kettering Cancer Center used a 14-day continuous intravenous infusion schedule of Genasense [49]. Dose escalations to 5.3 mg/kg/day for 14 days were well tolerated. Pharmacokinetic studies demonstrated dose levels of 2–4 mg/kg/day achieve

linear plasma concentrations between 1 and 4 μg/mL. Toxicity was mild in most patients, with a single patient experiencing Grade IV leukopenia which resolved in one day. Bcl-2 expression in peripheral blood lymphocytes was significantly decreased by day 7. An amendment to this protocol allows combination therapy with G3139 plus weekly paclitaxel starting with the second cycle of therapy.

In a phase I/II trial in patients with metastatic melanoma conducted in Vienna, Austria, Genasense was safely administered by continuous intravenous infusion in combination with full-dose DTIC [50]. This trial demonstrated that Genasense down-regulated Bcl-2 protein in serial melanoma biopsies, and that this biologic activity was associated with major clinical responses. Overall survival of the entire group of advanced-stage patients has exceeded 1 year. Transient thrombocytopenia at 12 mg/kg/d was dose-limiting in patients who also received full-dose DTIC treatment. An international, phase III, randomized trial is currently ongoing in patients with advanced melanoma using a 5-day pretreatment regimen of Genasense administered by continuous intravenous infusion at a dose of 7 mg/kg/day, followed by DTIC at 1000 mg/m².

A dose escalation study of combined Genasense plus mitoxantrone was recently completed in Vancouver [51]. Twenty-six patients with HRPC were treated, receiving Genasense and mitoxantrone at doses ranging from 0.6 to 5.0 mg/kg/day and 4 to 12 mg/m², respectively. Genasense was administered as a 14-day IV continuous infusion every 28 days with mitoxantrone given as an IV bolus on day 8. No dose-limiting toxicities were observed. Hematologic toxicities were transient and included neutropenia, thrombocytopenia and lymphopenia. Non-hematologic toxicities included cardiac dysfunction, fatigue, arthralgias and myalgias, none of which were severe. Two patients had >50% reductions in PSA. Of these, one had received Genasense at 1.2 mg/kg/day and a low dose (4 mg/m²) of mitoxantrone; he had symptomatic improvement in bone pain, and received a total of 6 cycles. The other had measurable disease with a documented partial response and received 8 cycles. Bcl-2 expression in peripheral blood lymphocytes decreased in all patients treated at the 5 mg/kg/day dose of Genasense. Results from this trial suggest that biologically active doses of Genasense are well tolerated in combination with mitoxantrone at without significant additional toxicity.

A phase II trial is now underway in San Antonio and Vancouver to determine activity of combination docetaxel plus G3139 Bcl-2 ASO in men with HRPC. Additional controlled multicenter trials in multiple myeloma, CLL, lung cancer and other indications (Table 1) with the goal to enhance the efficacy of available and experimental treatment strategies are ongoing.

Bcl-xL. Alternative splicing of the bcl-x pre-mRNA results in two distinct mRNAs, bcl-xL which codes for the anti-apoptotic protein and bcl-xS that codes for the pro-apoptotic variant [36]. Bcl-xL ASOs have been reported to induce apoptosis in various tumor cells and sensitize tumor cells to chemotherapy [52–54]. In the androgen-dependent Shionogi xenograft model, Bcl-xL expression increases 3-fold post-castration and remained elevated in recurrent AI tumors, and could be decreased by Bcl-xL ASO treatment [55]. Although treatment of Shionogi cells with Bcl-xL ASO marginally enhanced chemosensitivity and delayed AI progression, combined adjuvant treatment using Bcl-xL and/or Bcl-2 ASO plus paclitaxel acted synergistically to further enhance chemotherapy and delay time to AI progression beyond that of either agent alone. These findings illustrate that combinatorial regimens that inhibit two or more specific gene targets can produce additive effects and provide the basis for identifying additional anti-apoptotic genes that may serve as targets in a multi-agent approach to enhance the activity of existing chemotherapy and hormonal therapy.

Which of the anti-apoptotic bcl-2 family members may prove to be the most important survival factor in a given malignancy has sparked considerable interest since many tumor cells co-express the Bcl-2, Bcl-xL, as well as other bcl-2 family members. Although Bcl-2 and Bcl-xL are functionally similar, there is evidence in support of distinct biological roles of these proteins in protecting from apoptosis induced by different stimuli [56]. Together with the finding that the bcl-2 and the bcl-xL mRNA share homology regions with high sequence identity, it would be potentially advantageous to design an ASO which targets these two key inhibitors of apoptosis. The design and preclinical testing of a bcl-2/bcl-xL bispecific antisense oligonucleotide was reported recently [56,57]. This 20-mer MOE gapmer oligonucleotide efficiently down-regulated bcl-2 expression simultaneously with bcl-xL, and induced apoptosis in tumor cells of diverse histological origins *in vitro* and *in vivo*. Future plans for clinical trials using Bcl-xL or Bcl-2/Bcl-xL bispecific ASO are unknown.

Protein kinase C

Protein kinase C (PKC) belongs to a class of serine-threonine kinases that fine-tune numerous intracellular responses arising from G-protein coupled receptors, receptors with tyrosine kinase activity and non-receptor tyrosine kinases [58]. Increased PKC expression has been implicated in both oncogenesis and tumor progression [59]. A large number of ASOs that specifically target individual members of the PKC family have been screened systematically. Of these, a 20-mer PS ASO targeting human PKCα (ISIS 3521) inhibited the growth of glioblastoma xenografts and prolonged survival of tumor-bearing mice [59]. Based on the biologic evidence implicating PKC in the pathogenesis of solid tumors and on the activity of ISIS 3521 against human tumor xenografts in mice [60], clinical studies were initiated. While not well studied in prostate cancer, ISIS 3521 is, along with G3139, the only other ASO now in phase III trials and hence warrants mention in this review. The phase I dose escalation trials of ISIS 3521 in patients with treatment resistant solid tumors reported minimal toxicity and responses at several dose levels. Two patients with lymphoma experienced complete responses after 18 and 9 months of treatment with no recurrence of disease in either patient after 21 and 14 months, respectively [61]. In one of the phase I trials, a maximum tolerated dose was established at 2.0 mg/kg/day which corresponded well with doses showing anti-tumor activity in xenograft models [62]. There was evidence of tumor responses lasting up to 11 months in 3 of 4 patients with ovarian cancer. Continuous intravenous infusion of ISIS 3521 over a 3-week period has so far not shown objective clinical benefit in patients with recurrent high grade astrocytomas [63].

Based on extensive single-agent experience with ISIS 3521, a phase I/II study combining the PKC ASO with carboplatin and paclitaxel in patients with stage IIIB or IV non-small cell lung cancer (NSCLC) was initiated [64,65]. A recent update of 24 evaluable patients with NSCLC showed 1-year survival rates of 78% with a median survival of 18 months, more than twice that of comparable patient cohorts receiving chemotherapy alone. The combination of ISIS 3521, carboplatin and paclitaxel was well tolerated with manageable thrombocytopenia and neutropenia as the main side-effects. Based on acceptable toxicity and promising activity in NSCLC, a randomized phase III clinical trial of ISIS 3521 in combination with chemotherapy for NSCLC is underway.

Clusterin/TRPM-2

Testosterone-repressed prostate message-2 (*TRPM-2*), also known as *clusterin* or *sulfated glycoprotein-2*, was first isolated from ram rete testes fluid and has been implicated in tissue remodeling, lipid transport, reproduction, complement regulation and apoptotic cell death. Although clusterin was initially reported as an androgen-repressed gene in prostate tissue, the functional role of clusterin in apoptosis was poorly defined. Because clusterin binds to a wide variety of biological ligands [66], and the recent identification of a 14 bp element in its promoter that is recognized by transcription factor HSF1 (heat-shock factor 1) [67], an emerging view suggests that clusterin functions like small heat-shock proteins (Hsp) to chaperone and stabilize protein conformations at times of cell stress. Indeed, clusterin is substantially more potent than other Hsps at inhibiting stress-induced protein precipitation.

Clusterin levels increase following androgen ablation in androgen-dependent Shionogi tumors, and following chemotherapy and other cell death triggers in other cancer lines [27,68–70]. Immunostaining of prostate tissue arrays spotted with hormone naïve and post neoadjuvant hormone therapy (NHT)-treated specimens confirmed that clusterin is highly expressed in specimens after NHT, but low or absent in untreated specimens [68]. Increased clusterin levels have also been documented in renal cell, urothelial and ovarian cancers relative to benign tissues [70,71]. Forced over-expression of clusterin induces a chemoresistant and hormone resistant phenotype [27,72–74]. The up-regulation of clusterin after cell death signals like castration or chemotherapy, along with accumulating evidence implicating clusterin in protection of apoptosis, suggests that preventing this up-regulation of clusterin may enhance castration- or chemotherapy-induced apoptosis and delay tumor progression.

Clusterin ASOs were designed that reduced mRNA levels in a dose-dependent and sequence-specific manner (Figure 3A) [27,69,70,73,75]. Post-castration (adjuvant) treatment of mice bearing androgen-dependent Shionogi tumors decreased clusterin mRNA levels by 70% and resulted in earlier onset and more rapid apoptotic tumor regression, with significant delay in recurrence of AI tumors [27]. Clusterin ASOs also increased the cytotoxic effects of mitoxanthrone, docetaxel and paclitaxel *in vitro*, reducing the IC-50 by 75–90%. Although treatment with single-agent clusterin ASOs had no effect on the growth of established prostate, renal and urothelial tumors, clusterin ASOs synergistically enhanced paclitaxel-induced tumor regression in these cancers (Figure 3B) [69,70,73,75]. A second generation 2'-MOE ASO targeting the translation initiation site of the clusterin gene (OGX-011, Table 1), more potently suppressed clusterin mRNA compared to the PS ASO,

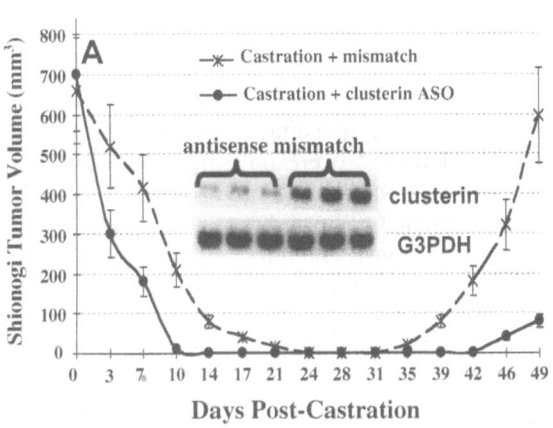
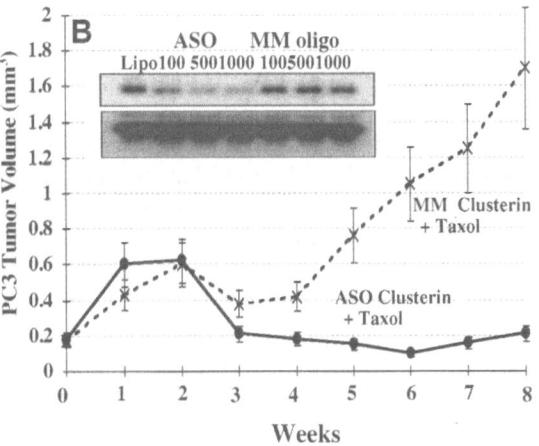

Figure 3. (A) Preclinical *in vivo* data illustrating inhibition of clusterin up-regulation (Northern analysis, insert) in murine androgen-dependent Shionogi tumors after castration using murine-specific clusterin ASO, with enhanced castration-induced apoptosis and delayed progression to androgen-independence. (B) Preclinical *in vivo* data illustrating paclitaxel chemosenstization in human androgen-independent PC3 tumors human-specific clusterin ASO, with enhanced taxol-induced apoptosis and delayed tumor progression. Insert shows dose-dependent and sequence-specific inhibition of clusterin levels in PC3 cells *in vitro*.

and had a significantly longer (5 days vs. 0.5 days) *in vivo* tissue half-life [76]. Weekly administration of OGX-011 was equivalent to daily PS clusterin ASO in enhancing paclitaxel efficacy *in vivo*, with no additional side-effects. These results support the use of 2'-MOE-modified ASO over conventional PS ASO by potentially increasing potency and allowing longer dosing intervals in clinical trials. A phase I/II clinical trial to determine the serum and tissue pharmacokinetics and biologic activity (i.e. the ability of clusterin ASOs to inhibit the up-regulation of clusterin after androgen ablation) of OGX-011 when combined with NHT prior to radical prostatectomy will begin in mid-2002.

Androgen receptor

Androgens act to regulate the expression of specific genes by binding to the AR, a ligand responsive transcription factor. Androgen ablation causes prostate cancer cell death through apoptosis, but despite high initial response rates, remissions are temporary because surviving tumor cells eventually recur. Failure of endocrine therapy and tumor progression is characterized by androgen-independent growth despite high levels of AR expression in recurrent disease. Furthermore, the AI phenotype is characterized by the up-regulation of genes that initially required androgens for expression, such as PSA, but become constitutively re-expressed in the absence of androgens [77]. Indeed, PSA may be a sentinel of other androgen-regulated genes that likewise become re-expressed in the absence of androgens during AI progression. Accumulating data implicates the AR as a key transcription factor activated in a ligand-independent fashion during AI progression. How androgen-regulated genes become dysregulated during AI progression remains incompletely understood, but potential mechanisms include aberrant phosphorylation of the AR via growth factor activated pathways, expression of co-activator, or mutations in the ligand-binding domain allowing activation by other steroids (reviewed in [78]). It is clear from clinical studies that anti-androgens are not able to prevent AI gene expression in prostate tumors *in vivo* [79], although these molecules can effectively block AR action in cultured prostate cell lines. This suggests that AI tumor progression is likely independent of the ligand-driven activity of AR.

Antisense inhibition of AR expression may offer one method to inhibit ligand-independent activation of the AR. Eder et al. [80] inhibited AR expression in LNCaP prostate tumor cells by using a 15-mer AR ASO targeting the CAG repeats encoding the poly-glutamine region of the AR (as750/15). Treatment of LNCaP cells with as750/15 appropriately reduced AR expression, and resulted in significant cell growth inhibition, strongly reduced secretion of the androgen-regulated prostate-specific antigen, and increased the number of apoptotic cells. Antisense inhibition was also very efficient in LNCaP-abl cells, a subline established after long-term androgen ablation of LNCaP cells, resulting in inhibition of AR expression and cell proliferation that was similar to that seen for parental LNCaP cells. This study suggests AR ASOs may be one method of inhibiting AI progression and warrants further study.

IGF-1 and IGF binding proteins

Accumulating evidence implicates insulin-like growth factor (IGF)-I in the pathophysiology of prostatic disease. The biological response of cells to IGFs, a potent mitogen for prostate cells, is regulated by various factors in the microenvironment, including the IGF-binding proteins (IGFBPs) [81]. After castration, the expression levels of certain IGFBPs change rapidly in the rat ventral prostate [82]. Differences in expression of various IGFBPs in benign and malignant prostatic epithelial cells have also been reported, with increases in IGFBP-2 and IGFBP-5, and decreases in IGFBP-3 in malignant vs. benign cells [83]. Increased IGFBP-5 levels after castration has been shown to be an adaptive cell survival response that helps potentiate the anti-apoptotic and mitogenic effects of IGF-I, thereby accelerating AI progression [29,84]. Forced overexpression of IGFBP-5 stimulated LNCaP cell proliferation, with corresponding increases in PI3K activity. *In vivo*, IGFBP-5-overexpressing LNCaP tumors progressed significantly faster to androgen-independence after castration compared to controls. PI3K inhibitor-induced apoptosis could be prevented by IGF-I treatment of IGFBP-5 transfectants, suggesting that high IGFBP5 levels can potentiate the anti-apoptotic effects of IGF-1. Systemic administration of IGFBP-5 ASOs in mice bearing Shionogi tumors after castration attenuated castration-induced increases in IGFBP-5 and significantly delayed time to AI progression. IGFBP-2 levels also increase in LNCaP and human prostate tumors after castration and during AI progression, and like IGFBP-5, appear to potentiate IGF-1 signaling [85]. IGFBP-2 ASOs decreased IGFBP-2 levels and reduced LNCaP cell growth rates *in vitro* and *in vivo*. Increased IGFBP-5 and -2 levels after androgen ablation may represent adaptive responses to potentiate IGF-I-mediated survival and mitogenesis. Use of ASOs to target IGFBP-modulation of IGF signaling is a potentially useful anti-proliferative therapy that warrants further study.

Inhibitors of apoptosis proteins

The inhibitors of apoptosis proteins (IAPs) regulate apoptosis signaling by directly binding to caspases, thereby blocking their processing and activity. Survivin is a human IAP family member that regulates apoptosis by directly binding and inhibiting a certain caspase-family cell death protease [86–88]. The IAPs have shown a remarkable ability to block apoptosis induced by a wide spectrum of non-related apoptotic triggers [89]. Survivin associates with the mitotic spindle, is involved in cytokinesis, and inhibits apoptosis induced by various apoptotic stimuli [90,91]. A possible oncogenic role for survivin is suggested by its cancer-specific expression and regulation by NF-kB transcription factor, the latter exerting its anti-apoptotic effect through up-regulation of various Bcl and IAP family members [89]. Survivin is detected in many human cancers but not in adjacent normal cells [89–95]. Survivin expression is prominent and developmentally regulated in embryonic and fetal tissue, is limited to the thymus in normal adult tissues, but has been detected in most lung, breast, colorectal, prostate, and pancreas tumor samples and many transformed cell lines.

Although the case for a role for survivin in drug resistance is correlative so far, survivin has been shown to protect against apoptosis induced by various diverse signals. Survivin lacks expression in terminally differentiated tissues but becomes re-expressed during neoplastic transformation, which identifies this IAP as a truly tumor-specific target for antisense therapy. Indeed, ASOs targeting different sites within the survivin mRNA in different cell systems induce apoptosis directly or sensitize cells to additional apoptotic stimuli [96,97]. IAP-mediated anti-apoptosis appears to be a highly trigger- and cell type-specific phenomenon, and what is observed in one system may not hold true for another. Hence it remains important to characterize the functional role of survivin in prostate cancer. The functional significance of survivin in *in vivo* prostate cancer models is unknown and is the subject of ongoing investigations.

Additional potential targets for antisense therapy in oncology

Many ASOs are being evaluated preclinically and in early clinical trials in numerous cancers and other diseases, and detailed discussion is beyond the scope of this review. Additional genes currently validated as targets for antisense therapy in preclinical studies include growth factor receptor tyrosine kinases such as HER-2/neu, the epidermal and vascular endothelial growth factor receptors, transcription factors involved in cell survival like NFκB, the myriad of protein kinases involved in cell cycle regulation, and thymidylate synthase. Examples include H-ras (ISIS 2503) [98], methyltransferase (MG98, MethylGene Inc) [99], BCR-ABL [100]. Hsp70 [101], c-myb [102], PKA (GEM 231) [103], c-raf (Isis 5132) [104], and p53 [105]. Despite of the preliminary nature of data available to date, there is hope that antisense strategies to some of these cancer-related targets will maintain their allure beyond the early stages of drug development.

The future of antisense therapy: Integrated combinatorial regimens

Contrary to critical notions voiced throughout the evolution of the field of antisense research, there is now increasing evidence that ASOs can work in a sequence-specific manner in patients and will hold their promise. While challenges remain, these are most likely easier to overcome in oncology than in any other field of large unmet medical needs. Recent clinical data strongly support the potential of combining ASOs with conventional anti-cancer treatment modalities. Antisense strategies designed to alter the apoptotic threshold of cancer cells, to hamper tumor micro-vasculature and to alter signal transduction pathways critical to the survival of cancer cells are certainly among the most promising and most obvious target choices. Since numerous genes and cellular pathways control the rate of tumor progression, inhibition of a single target gene will likely be insufficient to adequately suppress tumor progression. Exploration of additive or synergistic effects of combination antisense targeting in preclinical models will help guide further clinical protocols. Once target mechanisms and proof of principle for novel agents are established in preclinical model systems, significant methodological challenges confront clinicians, industry and regulatory agencies for

312

development in the clinical arena. Trial design for drug approval, which has traditionally required survival as an endpoint, is difficult and expensive in cancers with long natural history and inevitable contamination with crossover and uncontrolled additional treatments. The challenges inherent to successful translation of an integrated and combinatorial systemic therapy for prostate and other cancers will require close communication and collaboration amongst bench scientists, clinicians, industry and regulatory agencies.

References

1. Belikova AM ZVGN: Synthesis of ribonucleosides and diribonucleosides phosphates containing 2-chloroethylamine and nitrogen mustard residues. Tetrahedron Lett 37: 3357–3362, 1967
2. Paterson BM, Roberts BE, Kuff EL: Structural gene identification and mapping by DNA-mRNA hybrid-arrested cell-free translation. Proc Natl Acad Sci USA 74: 4370–4374, 1977
3. Zamecnik PC, Stephenson ML: Inhibition of Rous sarcoma virus replication and cell transformation by a specific oligodeoxynucleotide. Proc Natl Acad Sci USA 75: 280–284, 1978
4. Donis-Keller H: Site specific enzymatic cleavage of RNA 2. Nucleic Acids Res 7: 179–192, 1979
5. Monia BP, Lesnik EA, Gonzalez C, Lima WF, McGee D, Guinosso CJ, Kawasaki AM, Cook PD, Freier SM: Evaluation of 2'-modified oligonucleotides containing 2'-deoxy gaps as antisense inhibitors of gene expression. J Biol Chem 268: 14514–14522, 1993
6. Elbashir SM, Harborth J, Lendeckel W, Yalcin A, Weber K, Tuschl T: Duplexes of 21-nucleotide RNAs mediate RNA interference in cultured mammalian cells. Nature 411: 494–498, 2001
7. Bacon TA, Wickstrom E: Walking along human c-myc mRNA with antisense oligodeoxynucleotides: Maximum efficacy at the 5' cap region. Oncogene Res 6: 13–19, 1991
8. Monia BP, Johnston JF, Geiger T, Muller M, Fabbro D: Antitumor activity of a phosphorothioate antisense oligodeoxynucleotide targeted against C-raf kinase. Nat Med 2: 668–675, 1996
9. Ziegler A, Luedke GH, Fabbro D, Altmann KH, Zangemeister-Wittke U. Induction of apoptosis in small-cell lung cancer cells by an antisense oligodeoxynucleotide targeting the Bcl-2 coding sequence. J Nat Cancer Inst 89: 1027–1036, 1997
10. Milner N, Mir KU, Southern EM: Selecting effective antisense reagents on combinatorial oligonucleotide arrays. Nat Biotechnol 15: 537–541, 1997
11. Ho SP, Bao Y, Lesher T, Malhotra R, Ma LY, Fluharty SJ, Sakai RR: Mapping of RNA accessible sites for antisense experiments with oligonucleotide libraries. Nat Biotechnol 16: 59–63, 1998
12. Mathews DH, Sabina J, Zuker M, Turner DH: Expanded sequence dependence of thermodynamic parameters improves prediction of RNA secondary structure. J Mol Biol 288: 911–940, 1999
13. Crooke ST: Molecular mechanisms of antisense drugs: RNase H. Antisense Nucleic Acid Drug Development 8: 133–134, 1998
14. Galderisi U, Cascino A, Giordano A: Antisense oligonucleotides as therapeutic agents 4. J Cell Physiol 181: 251–257, 1999
15. Agrawal S: Importance of nucleotide sequence and chemical modifications of antisense oligonucleotides. Biochim Biophys Acta 1489: 53–68, 1999
16. Krieg AM, Yi AK, Hartmann G: Mechanisms and therapeutic applications of immune stimulatory cpG DNA. Pharmacol Ther 84: 113–120, 1999
17. Altmann KH, Dean NM, Fabbro D, Freier SM, Geiger T, Haener R, Huesken D, Martin P, Monia BP, Mueller M, Natt F, Nicklin P, Phillips J, Pieles U, Sasmor H, Moser HE: Second generation of antisense oligonucleotides: From nuclease resistance to biological efficacy in animals. Chimia 50: 168–176, 1996
18. Wahlestedt C, Salmi P, Good L, Kela J, Johnsson T, Hokfelt T, Broberger C, Porreca F, Lai J, Ren K, Ossipov M, Koshkin A, Jakobsen N, Skouv J, Oerum H, Jacobsen MH, Wengel J: Potent and nontoxic antisense oligonucleotides containing locked nucleic acids. Proc Natl Acad Sci USA 97: 5633–5638, 2000
19. Baker BF, Lot SS, Condon TP, Cheng-Flournoy S, Lesnik ES, Sasmor HM, Bennett CF: 2'-O-(2-methoxy)ethyl-modified anti-intercellular adhesion molecule 1 (ICAM-1) oligonucleotides selectively increase the ICAM-1 mRNA level and inhibit formation of the ICAM-1 translation initiation complex in human umbilical vein endothelial cells. J Biol Chem 272: 11994–12000, 1997
20. McKay RA, Miraglia LJ, Cummins LL, Owens RS, Sasmor H, Dean NM: Characterization of a potent and specific class of antisense oligonucleotide inhibitor of human protein kinase C-α expression. J Biol Chem 274: 1715–1722, 1999
21. Hanahan D, Weinberg RA: The hallmarks of cancer. Cell 100: 57–70, 2000
22. Adams JM, Cory S: The Bcl-2 protein family: Arbiters of cell survival. Science 281: 1322–1326, 1998
23. Folkman J: The role of angiogenesis in tumor growth. Semin Cancer Biol 3: 65–71, 1992
24. John A, Tuszynski G: The role of matrix metalloproteinases in tumor angiogenesis and tumor metastasis. Pathol Oncol Res 7: 14–23, 2001
25. Isaacs JT, Wake N, Coffey DS, Sandberg AA: Genetic instability coupled to clonal selection as a mechanism for progression in prostatic cancer. Cancer Res 42–48: 2353, 1982
26. Miyake H, Tolcher A, Gleave ME: Antisense Bcl-2 oligodeoxynucleotides delay progression to androgen-independence after castration in the androgen dependent Shionogi tumor model. Cancer Res 59: 4030–4034, 1999

27. Miyake H, Rennie P, Nelson C, Gleave ME, Miyake H, Rennie P, Nelson C, Gleave ME: Testosterone-repressed prostate message-2 (TRPM-2) is an antiapoptotic gene that confers resistance to androgen ablation in prostate cancer xenograft models. Cancer Res 60: 170–176, 2000

28. Bruchovsky N, Rennie PS, Coldman AJ, Goldenberg SL, To M, Lawson D: Effects of androgen withdrawal on the stem cell composition of the Shionogi carcinoma. Cancer Res 50: 2275–2282, 1990

29. Miyake H, Nelson C, Rennie P, Gleave ME: Overexpression of insulin-like growth factor binding protein-5 helps accelerate progression to androgen-independence in the human prostate LNCaP tumor model through activation of phosphatidylinositol 3′-kinase pathway. Endocrinology 141: 2257–2265, 2000

30. Sato N, Sadar MD, Bruchovsky N, Saatcioglu F, Rennie PS, Sato S, Lange PH, Gleave ME: Androgenic induction of prostate-specific antigen gene is repressed by protein–protein interaction between androgen receptor and AP-1c-Jun in the Human Prostate Cancer Cell Line LNCaP. J Bio Chem 272(28): 17485–17494, 1997

31. Craft N, Shostak Y, Carey M, Sawyers C: A mechanism for hormone-independent prostate cancer through modulation of androgen receptor signaling by the HER-2/neu tyrosine kinase. Nature Medicine 5: 280–285, 1999

32. Sherwood ER, Van Dongen JL, Wood CG, Liao S, Kozlowski JM, Lee C: Epidermal growth factor receptor activation in androgen-independent but not androgen-stimulated growth of human prostatic carcinoma cells. Br J Cancer 77(6): 855–861, 1998

33. Abreu-Martin MT, Chari A, Palladino AA, Craft NA, Sawyers CL: Mitogen-activated protein kinase kinase kinase 1 activates androgen receptor-dependent transcription and apoptosis in prostate cancer. Mol Cell Biol 19: 5143–5154, 1999

34. Oh WK, Kantoff PW: Management of hormone refractory prostate cancer: Current standards and future prospects. J Urol 60: 1220–1229, 1998

35. Hudes GR, Nathan F, Khater C, Haas N, Cornfield M, Giantonio B, Greenberg R, Gomella L, Litwin S, Ross E, Roethke S, McAleer C: Phase II trial of 96-hour paclitaxel plus oral estramustine phosphate in metastatic hormone-refractory prostate cancer. J Clin Oncol 15: 3156–3163, 1997

36. Petrylak DP, Macarthur R, O'Connor J, Shelton G, Weitzman A, Judge T, England-Owen C, Zuech N, Pfaff C, Newhouse J, Bagiella E, Hetjan D, Sawczuk I, Benson M, Olsson C: Phase I trial of docetaxel with estramustine in androgen-independent prostate cancer. J Clin Oncol 17: 958–967, 1999

37. Smith DC, Esper D, Strawderman M, Redman B, Pienta KJ: Phase II trial of oral estramustine, oral etoposide, and intravenous paclitaxel in hormone-refractory prostate cancer. J Clin Oncol 17: 1664–1671, 1999

38. Tsujimoto Y, Croce CM: Analysis of the structure, transcripts, and protein products of bcl-2, the gene involved in human follicular lymphoma. Proc Natl Acad Sci USA 83: 5214–5218, 1986

39. Sato T, Hanada M, Bodnig S, Ine S, Iwana N, Boise LH, Thompson C, Golemia E, Fong L, Wang H-G, Reed JC: Interactions among members of the bcl-2 protein family analysed with a yeast two-hybrid systems. Proc Nat Ass Sci USA 91: 9238–9242, 1994

40. McDonnell TJ, Troncoso P, Brisby SM, Logothetis CL, Chung LWK, Hsieh JT, Tu SM, Campbell ML: Expression of the protooncogene Bcl-2 in the prostate and its association with emergence of androgen-independent prostate cancer. Cancer Res 52: 6940–6944, 1992

41. Colombel M, Symmans F, Gil S, O'Toole KM, Chopin D, Benson M, Olsson CA, Korsmeyer S, Buttyan R: Detection of the apoptosis-suppressing oncoprotein Bcl-2 in hormone-refractory human prostate cancers. Am J Pathol 143: 390–400, 1993

42. Raffo AJ, Periman H, Chen MW, Streitman JS, Buttyan R: Overexpression of bcl-2 protects prostate cancer cells from apoptosis in vitro and confers resistance to androgen depletion in vivo. Cancer Res 55: 4438–4445.29, 1995

43. Patterson R, Gleave M, Jone E, Zubovits J, Goldenberg SL, Sullivan LD: Immunohistochemical analysis of radical prostatectomy specimens after 8 months of neoadjuvant hormone therapy. Mol Urol 3: 277–286, 1999

44. Jansen B, Schlagbauer-Wadl H, Brown BD, Bryan RN, van Elsas A, Muller M, Wolff K, Eichler HG, Pehamberger H: bcl-2 antisense therapy chemosensitizes human melanoma in SCID mice. Nature Med 4: 232–234, 1998

45. Miyake H, Tolcher A, Gleave ME: Antisense Bcl-2 oligodeoxynucleotides enhance taxol chemosensitivity and synergistically delays progression to androgen-independence after castration in the androgen dependent Shionogi tumor model. JNCI 92: 34–41, 2000

46. Gleave ME, Tolcher A, Miyake H, Beraldi E, Goldie J: Progression to androgen-independence is delayed by antisense Bcl-2 oligodeoxynucleotides after castration in the LNCaP prostate tumor model. Clinical Cancer Res 5: 2891–2898, 1999

47. Webb A, Cunningham D, Cotter F, Clarke PA, di Stefano F, Ross P, Corbo M, Dziewanowska Z: BCL-2 antisense therapy in patients with non-hodgkin-lymphoma. Lancet 349: 1137–1141, 1997

48. Waters JS, Webb A, Cunningham D, Clarke PA, Raynaud F, di Stefano F, Cotter FE: Phase I clinical and pharmacokinetic study of bcl-2 antisense oligonucleotide therapy in patients with non-Hodgkin's lymphoma. J Clin Oncol 18: 1812–1823, 1997

49. Morris MJ, Tong WP, Cordon-Cardo C, Drobnjak M, Kelly WK, Slovin SF, Terry KL, DiPaola RS, Rafi M, Rosen N, Scher HI: Intravenous BCL-2 antisense alone and in combination with paclitaxel in patients with advanced cancer. Clin Cancer Res 8(3): 679–683, 2002

50. Jansen B, Wacheck V, Heere-Ress E, Schlagbauer-Wadl H, Hoeller C, Lucas T, Hoermann M, Hollenstein U, Wolff K, Pehamberger H: Chemosensitisation of malignant melanoma by BCL2 antisense therapy. Lancet 356: 1728–1733, 2000

314

51. Chi KN, Gleave ME, Klasa R, Murray N, Bryce C, Lopes de Menezes DE, D'Aloisio S, Tolcher AW: A phase I dose-finding study of combined treatment with an antisense Bcl-2 oligonucleotide (Genasense) and mitoxantrone in patients with metastatic hormone-refractory prostate cancer. Clin Cancer Res 7(12): 3920–3927, 2001

52. Leech SH, Olie RA, Gautschi O, Simoes-Wust AP, Tschopp S, Haner R, Hall J, Stahel RA, Zangemeister-Wittke U: Induction of apoptosis in lung-cancer cells following bcl-xL anti-sense treatment. Int J Cancer 86: 570–576, 2000

53. Simoes-Wust AP, Olie RA, Gautschi O, Leech SH, Haner R, Hall J, Fabbro D, Stahel RA, Zangemeister-Wittke U: Bcl-xl antisense treatment induces apoptosis in breast carcinoma cells. Int J Cancer 87: 582–590, 2000

54. Lebedeva I, Rando R, Ojwang J, Cossum P, Stein CA: Bcl-xL in prostate cancer cells: Effects of overexpression and down-regulation on chemosensitivity 1. Cancer Res 60: 6052–6060.34, 2000

55. Miyaki H, Monia B, Gleave ME: Antisense Bcl-xL and Bcl-2 Oligodeoxynucleotides synergistically enhance taxol chemosensitivity and delay progression to androgen-independence after castration in the androgen dependent Shionogi tumor model. Int J Cancer 86: 855–862, 2000

56. Zangemeister-Wittke U, Leech SH, Olie RA, Simoes-Wust AP, Gautschi O, Luedke GH, Natt F, Haner R, Martin P, Hall J, Nalin CM, Stahel RA: A novel bispecific antisense oligonucleotide inhibiting both bcl-2 and bcl-xL expression efficiently induces apoptosis in tumor cells. Clin Cancer Res 6: 2547–2555, 2000

57. Gautschi O, Tschopp S, Olie RA, Leech SH, Simoes-Wust AP, Ziegler A, Baumann B, Odermatt B, Hall J, Stahel RA, Zangemeister-Wittke U: Activity of a novel bcl-2/bcl-xL-bispecific antisense oligonucleotide against tumors of diverse histologic origins. J Natl Cancer Inst 93: 463–471, 2001

58. Newton AC. Regulation of protein kinase C. Curr Opin Cell Biol 9: 161–167, 1997

59. Yazaki T, Ahmad S, Chahlavi A, Zylber-Katz E, Dean NM, Rabkin SD, Martuza RL, Glazer RI: Treatment of glioblastoma U-87 by systemic administration of an antisense protein kinase C-alpha phosphorothioate oligodeoxynucleotide. Mol Pharmacol 50: 236–242, 1996

60. Geiger T, Muller M, Dean NM, Fabbro D: Antitumor activity of a PKC-alpha antisense oligonucleotide in combination with standard chemotherapeutic agents against various human tumors transplanted into nude mice. Anticancer Drug Des 13: 35–45, 1998

61. Cotter FE: Antisense oligonucleotides for haematological malignancies. Haematologica 84: 19–22, 1999

62. Yuen AR, Halsey J, Fisher GA, Holmlund JT, Geary RS, Kwoh TJ, Dorr A, Sikic BI: Phase I study of an antisense oligonucleotide to protein kinase C-alpha (ISIS 3521/CGP 64128A) in patients with cancer. Clin Cancer Res 5: 3357–3363, 1999

63. Alavi JB, Grossman SA Supko J: Efficacy, toxicity, and pharmacology of an antisense oligonucleotide directed against protein kinase C-alpha (ISIS 3521) delivered as a 21 day continous intravenous infusion in patients with recurrent high grade astrocytomas (HGA). Proc Am Soc Clin Oncol 19: 167, 2000

64. Yuen A, Advani R, Fisher G: A phase I/II trial of ISIS 3521, an antisense inhibitor of protein kinase C alpha, combined with carboplatin and paclitaxel in patients with non-small cell lung cancer. Am Soc Clin Oncol 19: 459, 2000

65. Yuen A, Halsey J, Lum B: Phase I/II trial of ISIS 3521, an antisense inhibitor of PKC, with carboplatin and paclitaxel in non-small cell lung cancer. Clin Cancer Res 6(Suppl): 4572, 2000

66. Koch-Brandt C, Morgans C: Clusterin: A role in cell survival in the face of apoptosis? Prog Mol Subcell Biol 16: 130–149, 1996 (review)

67. Wilson MR, Easterbrook-Smith SB: Clusterin is a secreted mammalian chaperone. Trends Biochem Sci 25: 95–98, 2000

68. July LV, Akbari M, Zellweger T, Jones EC, Goldenberg SL, Gleave ME: Clusterin expression is significantly enhanced in prostate cancer cells following androgen withdrawal therapy. Prostate 50(3): 179–188, 2000

69. Miyake H, Chi KN, Gleave ME: Antisense TRPM-2 oligodeoxynucleotides chemosensitize human androgen-independent PC-3 prostate cancer cells both in vitro and in vivo. Clin Cancer Res 6: 1655–1663, 2000

70. Zellweger T, Miyake H, July LV, Akbari M, Kiyama S, Gleave ME: Chemosensitization of human renal cell cancer using antisense oligonucleotides targeting the antiapoptotic gene clusterin. Neoplasia 3: 360–367, 2001

71. Miyake H, Gleave M, Kamidono S, Hara I: Overexpression of clusterin in transitional cell carcinoma of the bladder is related to disease progression and recurrence. Urology 59(1): 150–154, 2000

72. Miyake H, Hara S, Zellweger T, Kamidono S, Gleave ME, Hara I: Acquisition of resistance to fas-mediated apoptosis by overexpression of clusterin in human renal-cell carcinoma cells. Mol Urol 5(3): 105–111, 2001

73. Miyake H, Rennie P, Nelson C, Gleave ME: Acquisition of chemoresistant phenotype by overexpression of the anti-apoptotic gene, testosterone-repressed prostate message-2 (TRPM-2), in prostate cancer xenograft models. Cancer Res 60: 2547–2554, 2000

74. Hara I, Miyake H, Gleave ME, Kamidono S: Introduction of clusterin gene into human renal cell carcinoma cells enhances their resistance to cytotoxic chemotherapy through inhibition of apoptosis both in vitro and in vivo. Jpn J Cancer Res 92(11): 1220–1224, 2001

75. Miyake H, Hara, I Kamidono S, Gleave ME: Synergistic chemsensitization and inhibition of tumor growth and metastasis by the antisense oligodeoxynucleotide targeting clusterin gene in a human bladder cancer model. Clin Cancer Res 7(12): 4245–4252, 2001

76. Zellweger T, Miyake H, Monia B, Cooper S, Gleave M: Efficacy of antisense clusterin oligonucleotides is improved *in vitro* and *in vivo* by incorporation of 2'-o-(2-methoxy) ethyl chemistry. J Pharmacol Exp Ther 298(3): 934–940, 2001

77. Gregory CW, Hamil KG, Kim D, Hall SH, Pretlow TG, Mohler JL, French FS: Androgen receptor expression in androgen-independent prostate cancer is associated with increased expression of androgen regulated genes. Cancer Res 58: 5718–5724, 1998

78. Feldman BJ, Feldman D: The development of androgen-independent prostate cancer. Nature Rev 1: 34–45, 2001

79. Denis L, Murphy GP: Overview of phase III trials on combined androgen treatment in patients with metastatic prostate cancer. Cancer 72: 3888–3895, 1993

80. Eder IE, Culig Z, Ramoner R, Thurnher M, Putz T, Nessler-Menardi C, Tiefenthaler M, Bartsch G, Klocker H: Inhibition of LncaP prostate cancer cells by means of androgen receptor antisense oligonucleotides. Cancer Gene Ther 7(7): 997–1007, 2000

81. Jones JI, Clemmons DR: Insulin-like growth factors and their binding proteins: Biological actions. Endocr Rev 16: 3–34, 1995

82. Nickerson T, Pollak M, Huynh H: Castration-induced apoptosis in rat ventral prostate is associated with increased expression of genes encoding insulin-like growth factor binding proteins 2, 3, 4 and 5. Endocrinology 139: 807–810, 1998

83. Figueroa JA, De Raad S, Tadlock L, Speights VO, Rinehart JJ: Differential expression of insulin-like growth factor binding proteins in high versus low Gleason score prostate cancer. J Urol 159: 1379–1383, 1998

84. Miyake H, Pollak M, Nelson C, Gleave ME: Antisense insulin-like growth factor binding protein-5 oligodeoxynucleotides inhibit progression to androgen-independence after castration in the Shionogi tumor model via negative modulation of insulin-like growth factor-I action. Cancer Res 60: 3058–3064, 2000

85. Kiyama S, Zellweger T, Akbari M, Cox M, Miyake H, Gleave M: Antisense oligonucleotides inhibit castration-induced increases in insulin-like growth factor-binding protein-2 and delay progression to androgen-independence in the human prostate LNCaP tumor model. Eur Urol 39: 94, 2001

86. Roy N, Deveraux Q, Takahashi R, Salvesen GS, Reed JC: The c-IAP and c-IAP-2 proteins are direct inhibitors of specific caspases. EMBO J 16: 6914–6925, 1997

87. Deveraux Q, Takahashi R, Salvesen GS, Reed JC: X-linked IAP is a direct inhibitor of cell-death proteases. Nature 17: 300–304, 1997

88. Deveraux Q, Leo E, Stennicke HR, Welsh K, Salvesen GS, Reed JC: Cleavage of human inhibitor of apoptosis protein XIAP results in fragments with distinct specificities for caspases. EMBO J 18: 5242–5251, 1999

89. Lacasse EC, Baird S, Korneluk RG, Mackenzie AE: The inhibitors of apoptosis (IAPs) and their emerging role in cancer. Oncogene 17: 3247–3259, 1998

90. Li F, Ambrosini G, Chu EY, Plescia J, Tognin S, Marchisio PC, Altieri DC: Control of apoptosis and mitotic spindle checkpoint by survivin. Nature 396: 580–583, 1998

91. Ambrosini G, Adida C, Altieri DC: A novel anti-apoptosis gene, survivin, expressed in cancer and lymphoma. Nature Med 3: 917–921, 1997

92. Tamm I, Wang Y, Sausville E, Scudiero DA, Vigna N, Oltersdorf T, Reed JC: IAP-family protein survivin inhibits caspase activity and apoptosis induced by Fas, Bax, and anticancer drugs. Cancer Res 58: 5315–5320, 1998

93. Lu CD, Altieri DC, Tanigawa N: Expression of a novel anti-apoptosis gene, survivin, corelated with tumor cell apoptosis and p53 acculmulation in gastric carcinomas. Cancer Res 58: 1808–1812, 1998

94. Kawasaki H, Altieri DC, Lu CD, Toyoda M, Tenjo T, Tanigawa N: Inhibition of apoptosis by survivin predicts shorter survival rates in colorectal carcinoma. Cancer Res 58: 5071–5074, 1998

95. Adida C, Berrebi D, Peuchmaur M, Reyes-Mugica M, Altieri DC: Anti-apoptosis gene, survivin, and prognosis of neuroblastoma. Lancet 351: 882–883, 1998

96. Olie RA, Simoes-Wust AP, Baumann B, Leech SH, Fabbro D, Stahel RA, Zangemeister-Wittke U: A novel antisense oligonucleotide targeting survivin expression induces apoptosis and sensitizes lung cancer cells to chemotherapy. Cancer Res 60: 2805–2809, 2000

97. Chen J, Wu W, Tahir SK, Kroeger PE, Rosenberg SH, Cowsert LM, Bennett F, Krajewski S, Krajewska M, Welsh K, Reed JC, Ng SC: Down-regulation of survivin by antisense oligonucleotides increases apoptosis, inhibits cytokinesis, and anchorage-independent growth. Neoplasia 235–241, 2000

98. Saleh M, Posey J, Pleasani L: A phase II trial of ISIS 2503, an antisense inhibitor of H-ras, as first line therapy for advanced colorectal carcinoma. Proc Am Soc Clin Oncol 19: 320, 2000

99. Siu LL, Gelmon KA, Moore MJ: A phase I and pharma-cokinetik (PK) study of the human DNA methyltransferase (Metase) antisense oligodeoxynucleotide MG98 given as a 21-day continous infusion every 4 weeks. Proc Am Soc Clin Oncol 19: 250, 2000

100. de Fabritiis P, Petti MC, Montefusco E, De Propris MS, Sala R, Bellucci R, Mancini M, Lisci A, Bonetto F, Geiser T, Calabretta B, Mandelli F: BCR-ABL antisense oligodeoxynucleotide *in vitro* purging and autologous bone marrow transplantation for patients with chronic myelogenous leukemia in advanced phase. Blood 91: 3156–3162, 1998

101. Nylandsted J, Rohde M, Brand K, Bastholm L, Elling F, Jaattela M: Selective depletion of heat shock protein 70 (Hsp70) activates a tumor-specific death program that is independent of caspases and bypasses Bcl-2. Proc Natl Acad Sci USA 97: 7871–7876, 2000

316

102. Ratajczak MZ, Hijiya N, Catani L, DeRiel K, Luger SM, McGlave P, Gewirtz AM: Acute- and chronic-phase chronic myelogenous leukemia colony-forming units are highly sensitive to the growth inhibitory effects of c-myb antisense oligodeoxynucleotides. Blood 79: 1956–1961, 1992

103. Tortora G, Bianco R, Damiano V, Fontanini G, De Placido S, Bianco AR, Ciardiello F: Oral antisense that targets protein kinase A cooperates with taxol and inhibits tumor growth, angiogenesis, and growth factor production. Clin Cancer Res 6: 2506–2512, 2000

104. Stevenson JP, Yao KS, Gallagher M, Friedland D, Mitchell EP, Cassella A, Monia B, Kwoh TJ, Yu R, Holmlund J, Dorr FA, O'Dwyer PJ: Phase I clinical/pharmacokinetic and pharmacodynamic trial of the c-raf-1 antisense oligonucleotide ISIS 5132 (CGP 69846A). J Clin Oncol 17: 2227–2236, 1999

105. Bishop MR, Iversen PL, Bayever E, Sharp JG, Greiner TC, Copple BL, Ruddon R, Zon G, Spinolo J, Arneson M, Armitage JO, Kessinger A: Phase I trial of an antisense oligonucleotide OL(1)p53 in hematologic malignancies. J Clin Oncol 14: 1320–1326, 1996

Address for offprints: Martin Gleave, The Prostate Centre, Vancouver General Hospital, Division of Urology, University of British Columbia, D9, 2733 Heather Street, Vancouver, BC, Canada V6H 3Z3; *Tel:* 604 875 5686; *Fax:* 604 875 5604; *e-mail:* gleave@interchange.ubc.ca

Antiangiogenesis therapeutic strategies in prostate cancer

Gordon R. Macpherson, Sylvia S.W. Ng, Nehal J. Lakhani, Douglas K. Price, Jurgen Venitz and William D. Figg
Molecular Pharmacology Section, Center for Cancer Research, National Cancer Institute, Bethesda, MD, USA

Key words: angiogenesis, prostate cancer, thalidomide, endostatin, carboxyamido-triazole, 2-methoxyestradiol

Summary

It is now well documented that tumor progression from its early stages to an advanced metastatic state requires the recruitment of new vasculature. The reliance on angiogenesis by tumors renders them susceptible to agents that can interfere with the angiogenic process. Recent interest in the therapeutic potential of using angiogenesis as a target mechanism for anticancer therapy has led to the identification of various antiangiogenic agents that interfere at various stages of the process. This review is a summary of recent progress in the identification and characterization of antiangiogenesis agents with a focus on their utility with respect to prostate cancer. Though we focus on prostate cancer, this knowledge is relevant to any cancer that involves angiogenesis.

Introduction

Prostate cancer has the highest incidence of any malignancy and is the second leading cause of cancer-related mortality in men in the US, accounting for an estimated 37,000 deaths in 1999 [1]. Since the 1940s when Huggins and Hodges demonstrated the antiproliferative effects of androgen ablation on prostate cancer, the established protocol for treatment of advanced disease has been surgical castration and/or chemotherapy to eliminate circulating androgens [2]. Androgen ablation therapy aims to down-regulate the expression of genes required for cell proliferation by precluding the formation of androgen–androgen receptor (AR) complexes required for their activation [3–6]. Although androgen ablation initially results in favorable response for most patients [7,8], androgen-independent disease ensues (likely influenced by *AR* gene amplification [9]), eventually progressing to a metastatic phenotype and ultimately causing patient death [10,11]. For some tumors it has been proposed that surgical excision of a primary tumor removes the source of endogenous angiogenesis inhibitors, allowing for subsequent growth of dormant micrometastases [12]. Limitations associated with the ubiquitous use of androgen ablation therapy for the treatment of advanced prostate cancer underscore the need for the development of alternative treatments that target mechanisms other than androgen-mediated regulation of cell proliferation and

differentiation. In this regard, angiogenesis represents a useful target mechanism.

Angiogenesis is the process by which new vasculature is recruited from pre-existing vessels [13,14], and it is particularly relevant to the pathology of most, if not all human tumors [15]. Recent data on the growth and metastasis of prostate cancer strongly suggest that angiogenesis is a crucial prerequisite for progression to advanced disease [16,17]. The angiogenic process in solid tumors is now known to be crucial for advanced tumor growth [18] and progression to a metastatic state [19]. Microvessel density is an indicator of biological agressiveness and metastatic potential in many primary tumors [20]. Developing tumors require new vasculature as they grow in order to ensure a constant supply of required nutrients and oxygen while allowing for the elimination of metabolic waste [15].

Interruption of this process would halt the progression of cancers that are dependent upon angiogenesis for advanced pathology by eliminating their potential for growth. Inhibition of angiogenesis is expected to augment the effects of other therapies such as chemotherapy and radiation by limiting the tumor to a dormant state of low metastatic potential [21]. To this end, interest in the potential of antiangiogenesis-related therapeutic strategies, including the development of new anticancer drugs has increased dramatically [22]. Concurrent advances in our understanding of the biology and biochemistry of the angiogenic process,

M.L. Cher, K.V. Honn and A. Raz (eds.), Prostate Cancer: New Horizons in Research and Treatment, 317–330.
© 2002 *Kluwer Academic Publishers.*

particularly the identification of biochemical end-points, have led to the identification of various small molecule and endogenous peptide inhibitors (Table 1) of neovascularization [23–30]. The upsurge in antiangiogenesis research continually generates new knowledge pertaining to biochemical determinants of the angiogenic process [24]. These experiments reveal a complex series of interconnected pathways operating synergistically to afford the genesis of new vasculature. In general, angiogenesis is initiated in quiescent endothelial cells following a shift in the balance between endogenous angiogenesis inhibitory factors and angiogenesis-promoting factors. Hanahan et al. [15] suggested that a shift in balance to a pro-angiogenic state occurs at an early to mid-stage in the development of cancers, leading to the activation of an 'angiogenic switch' or conversion to an angiogenic phenotype and consequently, the formation of new vasculature [31]. Cells thus activated synthesize matrix metalloproteinases required to degrade the extracellular matrix and allow for endothelial cell proliferation and organization into new vasculature [14,24]. Vessel formation is achieved by way of a biochemical cascade that results in parent vessel basement membrane degradation [13], migration of activated endothelial cells into the perivascular space and re-organization into new vasculature [24].

Although much remains to be discerned with respect to the molecular details of angiogenesis, several important biochemical determinants have been characterized. Angiogenesis requires (1) up-regulation of growth factors to induce cell proliferation, (2) degradation of the ECM both to provide space into which new vasculature can migrate and release of cytokines to modulate proliferation. Endogenous inhibitors of angiogenesis such as thrombospondin-1 [25], angiostatin [32] and endostatin [29] (Table 1) regulate this process and also have been identified as potentially useful therapeutic targets. Likewise, growth factors (Table 1) such as basic fibroblast growth factor (bFGF) [33] and vascular endothelial growth factor (VEGF) [34,35] that are up-regulated during angiogenesis have been identified and may also be important therapeutic targets and/or molecular indicators of disease stage. Thus, angiogenesis requires cooperating but distinct molecular pathways, each of which represents a potential therapeutic target (Figure 1).

Prostate cancer progression from primary neoplasia to advanced disease also requires the acquisition of microcirculation to support the developing neoplastic mass [36]. Molecular determinants of angiogenesis such as the growth factor VEGF are modulated in various prostate cancer models [37]. Significantly higher levels of VEGF are produced in malignant prostate tissues compared with benign prostatic hyperplasias [37]. Androgens are implicated in the induction of VEGF expression in human prostatic stroma, supporting the hypothesis that androgen ablation affects

Table 1. Endogenous angiogenesis promoting and inhibitory factors in prostate cancer

Angiogenesis promoters	Refs	Angiogenesis inhibitors	Refs
Vascular endothelial growth factor (VEGF)	[34,35]	Angiostatin	[32]
Basic fibroblast growth factor (bFGF)	[33]	Endostatin	[29]
Interleukin-8 (IL-8)	[39]	Thrombospondin	[25]
Tumor necrosis factor-α (TNF-α)	[59]	Maspin	[141]
Matrix metalloproteinases (MMPs)	[14]	Tissue inhibitor of metalloproteinase-1 (TIMP-1)	[142]
Transforming growth factor-β (TGF-β)	[142]	Prostate specific antigen (PSA)	[143]
Platelet-derived endothelial growth factor (PD-ECGF)	[144]	Interleukin-10 (IL-10)	[142]
Cyclooxygenase-2 (COX-2)	[85]	Interferon-β (IFN-β)	[145]

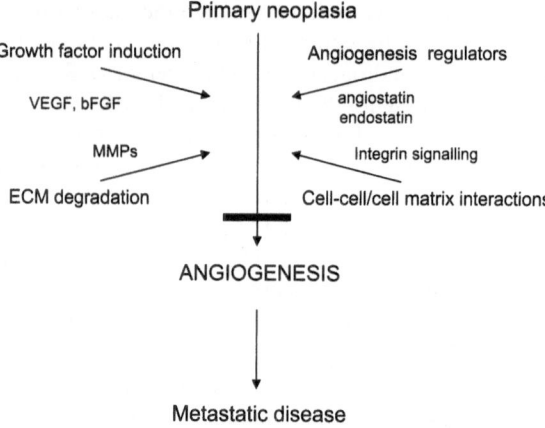

Figure 1. Molecular determinants of angiogenesis. Interruption of pathways required for angiogenesis would interrupt the progression to a metastaic phenotype. Abbreviations are as follows: VEGF; bFGF; MMPs; ECM.

prostate tumors at least in part through inhibition of angiogenesis [16]. The dependence of prostate tumors on androgens for growth factor induction of tumor growth and metastasis is unique to this cancer [16]. Aside from VEGF, highly metastatic prostate cancer cells have been shown to overproduce bFGF, interleukin-8 (IL-8) and matrix metalloproteinase-9 (MMP-9) mRNAs compared with a related but poorly metastatic cell line [38]. IL-8 and MMP-9 overexpression is correlated with a high level of angiogenesis in PC-3P cells [39], likely because IL-8 induces MMP expression [36] and subsequent ECM degradation required for angiogenesis. AG3340, an inhibitor of MMP-2 and MMP-9, was recently shown to inhibit tumor growth and increase survival of nude mice with PC-3 prostate tumors [40].

Recent data, therefore, demonstrate the requirement of angiogenesis for prostate tumor progression. Parallel observations with respect to molecular determinants of angiogenesis in prostate and other cancers suggest that antiangiogenic therapeutic strategies are relevant to prostate cancer. Antiangiogenic agents have demonstrated efficacy in the treatment of prostate cancer in various clinical trials [41–44]. Thus, future investigation into the development of antiangiogenic therapeutic strategies in prostate cancer is warranted. In this review, we summarize recent advances in knowledge pertaining to the molecular determinants of angiogenesis as they affect the identification of new drug targets and the development of new drug therapies with an emphasis on prostate cancer.

Thalidomide

No other drug currently under investigation for the treatment of vascular disorders has had such a colorful history as thalidomide, a glutamic acid-like synthetic racemate with a chiral center consisting of S(−)- and R(+) enantiomers which interconvert rapidly under physiological conditions [45] (Figure 2). Originally developed in the late 1950s as a sedative and tranquilizer, thalidomide was implicated a decade later in the incidence of severe congenital malformations in babies whose mothers were using the drug [46,47]. Tragically, thalidomide was an attractive alternative to barbituate sedatives due to its low acute toxicity, and was widely prescribed prior to the discovery of its teratogenicity with 14,580 kg sold in Germany in 1960 [45]. The resulting medical catastrophe led to the abolition of its use in most countries. Interest in the therapeutic value of thalidomide re-surfaced, however, when in 1965 it was shown to be effective in the treatment of erythema nodosum leprosum (EDL), a painful complication of lepromatous leprosy [48]. Thalidomide was subsequently re-introduced in clinical practice, albeit under strict regulations that require stringent control over access to the drug. Prescribing physicians, dispensing pharmacies and patients must now be registered and the quantity of the drug dispensed is now tightly controlled [49]. Unfortunately, such strict regulations for clinical use of the drug were not enforced in all countries. Brazil, tragically, did not impose restrictions on thalidomide use and even allowed for its sale over the counter without need of a doctor's prescription [45].

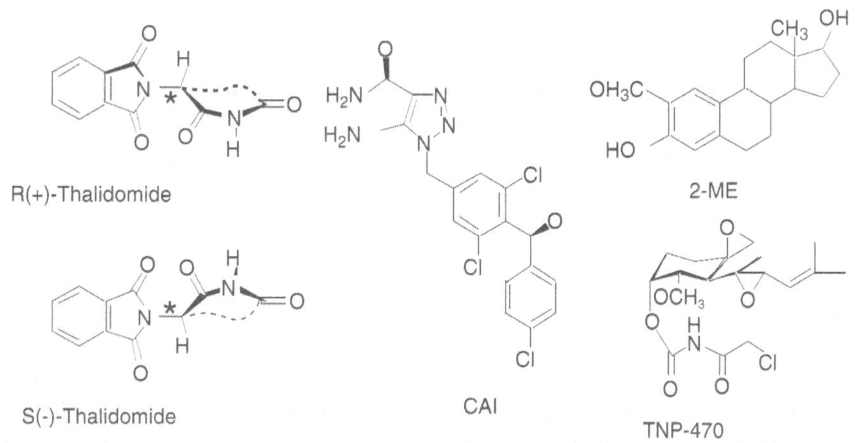

Figure 2. Structures of thalidomide (R(+) and S(−) enantiomers), CAI, 2-ME and TNP-470. The chiral center of thalidomide is indicated with an asterisk.

320

Although thalidomide is a potent and species-specific [50] teratogen, it has also proven to be a useful therapeutic agent for the treatment of various disorders other than ENL such as Behcet's disease [51] and graft versus host disease [52,53]. Thalidomide has also been shown to inhibit replication of HIV-1 [54] and is effective in the treatment of HIV-related aphthous stomatitis [55]. The observed bioactivity of thalidomide in ENL and other disorders inspired research into potential antiangiogenic activity [56]. D'Amato et al. [57] reported an inhibition of bFGF-induced angiogenesis following thalidomide treatment in a rabbit cornea micropocket assay. Kenyon et al. [58] demonstrated that thalidomide inhibited bFGF- and VEGF-induced corneal neovascularization in mice. Later, Bauer et al. [50] showed that thalidomide inhibits microvessel formation from rat aortas and slows human aortic endothelial cell proliferation. Observed antiangiogenic activity of thalidomide suggested that it might be useful in the treatment of cancer and other angiogenesis-dependent diseases [59], and it was eventually tested in various clinical trials [60]. The anticancer activity of thalidomide has been explored most intensely in myeloma where it is highly active, inducing clinically meaningful response in patients at various stages of the disease [60–62]. Other cancers are affected as well. Figg et al. [41] demonstrated a $\geq 40\%$ decline in prostate-specific antigen (PSA) in 27% of patients with androgen-independent prostate cancer who received thalidomide. PSA decline was often associated with improvement of clinical symptoms. A follow-up Phase II clinical trial conducted by the same group involved co-administration of thalidomide plus the cytotoxic taxane docetaxel. Fifty-three percent of patients who received both drugs had a PSA decline of at least 50% compared with 35% of patients who received docetaxel alone, suggesting that thalidomide may have increased efficacy in prostate cancer if administered in combination with other therapies [42]. Little et al. [63] demonstrated that thalidomide induced meaningful response in patients with Kaposi's sarcoma. Likewise, Fine et al. [64] reported partial response of high-grade glioma to thalidomide treatment while other groups recently noted significant responses in renal cancer [65,66], Crohn's disease [67] and glioblastoma multiforme [68]. As an immunomodulatory and antiangiogenic drug, thalidomide has re-surfaced and found a new niche, particularly in oncology where 90% of its current use resides [69]. Thalidomide clearly has therapeutic potential in prostate as well as various other cancers and should be considered in the setting of well-designed clinical trials alone or in combination with other therapies in patients whose therapeutic options are exhausted [60].

Thalidomide is a teratogenic, sedative, immunomodulatory and antiangiogenic agent but its mechanism of action is unknown [45]. Immunological experiments have identified potential molecular targets, however, that are intimately involved in oncogenesis. The most widely noted bioactivity of thalidomide is its inhibitory effect on tumor necrosis factor alpha (TNF-α), an angiogenic cytokine [70] that is overproduced in several malignancies [59,71,72]. Sampaio et al. [72] noted an inhibition of human monocyte TNF-α production in lipopolysaccharide-induced human monocytes. Inhibition of TNF-α production was later shown to correlate with thalidomide-induced TNF-α mRNA degradation rate [73]. This observation is consistent with later experiments conducted by Rowland et al. [74] in which thalidomide selectively inhibited the expression of TNF-α as assessed by RT-PCR. Thalidomide also inhibited the production of TNF-α in mouse macrophages in vitro and notably reduced (by 94%) the production of tumor-associated macrophages (TAMs) when administered to rats bearing MAT-Lu tumors. The inhibitory activity was associated with reduced tumor vessel density and tumor growth [75]. Ching et al. [76] likewise described an inhibition of TNF-α production upon co-administration of thalidomide structural analogs with the antitumor agent DMXAA (5,6-dimethylxanthenone-4-acetic acid) to mice bearing Colon 38 adenocarcinoma. Efficacy of thalidomide is directly related to its stereochemistry. The effect of S($-$)-thalidomide on TNF-α release from stimulated mononuclear blood cells in vitro was significantly higher than R($+$)-thalidomide at higher concentrations [77]. Likewise, the antiangiogenic properties of thalidomide in a bFGF- and VEGF-induced corneal neovascularization model are stereospecific, with the S($-$)- being more effective than the R($+$)-enantiomer [58]. Stereochemistry also determines the clinical profile of thalidomide with the sedative effects correlating with the R($+$)- but not the S($-$)-enantiomer [78,79].

Aside from its effects on TNF-α production, thalidomide has been shown to directly inhibit interleukin-6 (IL-6), a potent growth factor for malignant cells [60]. It was shown to cause a dose-dependent inhibition of IL-6, TNF-α and interferon-γ in mitogen-stimulated peripheral blood mononuclear cells (PBMC) [74] and it abolished the stimulating effects of insulin-like growth factor (IGF-1) on chondrogenesis and limb bud development [80]. Stephens and Fillmore [80] proposed a mechanism of action to explain the teratogenic activity of thalidomide that may also explain its activity in angiogenesis. This involves inhibition of growth factor-mediated activation of $\alpha_5\beta_3$-integrin genes, precluding their stimulation of angiogenesis in developing limb buds. This inhibition would be the direct result of thalidomide intercalation into GC promoter sites in the affected genes [81]. A similar effect of thalidomide on cancer cells may result in decreased production of integrins required for angiogenesis [45]. Thalidomide is also a co-stimulator of human T cells *in vitro*, increasing interleukin-2 (IL-2)-mediated T cell proliferation and γ-interferon production [82]. Taken in combination, research aimed at delineating thalidomide's mechanism of action appears to indicate a primary role for cytokine modulation. However, this is somewhat controversial. Neben et al. [83], for example, did not observe any decrease in TNF-α, VEGF or IL-6 levels in patients who responded to thalidomide treatment, raising questions as to whether the true mechanism of action is via inhibition of cytokine secretion. Nevertheless, the majority of reports implicating cytokine modulation as an antiangiogenic determinant warrant further investigation.

Interestingly, a potential new mechanism of action for thalidomide has emerged involving modulation of cyclooxygenase-2 (COX-2), a key enzyme in the synthesis of prostaglandins [84]. COX-2 is highly expressed in various human cancers including prostate cancer, and has been shown to be required for angiogenesis in a rat corneal model [85,86]. These results are consistent with the apoptotic and antiangiogenic response of human prostate cancer cells treated *in vitro* and *in vivo* with an inhibitor of COX-2 [87]. Fujita et al. [84] demonstrated that thalidomide inhibits lipopolysaccharride-mediated induction of COX-2 and subsequent prostaglandin-E_2 biosynthesis in a dose-dependent manner.

Whatever the mechanism(s) of action, thalidomide clearly has an important role to play in the treatment of prostate and other cancers. Future research should focus on the development and assay of thalidomide analogs with increased efficacy and/or reduced toxicity. Indeed, progress to this end has already been made with the development of analogs such as the so-called 'immunomodulatory drugs' (ImiDs), some of which are 1000 times more potent than thalidomide itself in blocking TNF-α production [69]. Thalidomide is susceptible to spontaneous hydrolytic cleavage under physiological conditions and has poor water solubility. To improve the pharmacokinetic profile of thalidomide,

Hess et al. [88] synthesized a series of analogs with greater water stability and solubility that retained the level of bioactivity observed with the parent compound. They noted a positive correlation between the stability of the thalidomide analogs and their bioactivity [88]. Clearly, development of new thalidomide analogs and further research into the bioactivity of thalidomide metabolites will shed new light on the affected molecular mechanism(s) as well as lead to the development of next-generation analogs with lower toxicity, improved efficacy and more favorable pharmacokinetic/pharmacodynamic profiles.

Endostatin

As noted above, angiogenesis is necessary for the growth of solid tumors and their metastatic foci. Tumors have the ability to up-regulate different angiogenic factors such as fibroblast growth factors (FGFs) both acidic and basic [89], and VEGF. Some tumors are also able to generate endogenous antiangiogenic [90] factors like thrombospondin [91], angiostatin [92], endostatin [93] and antithrombin III [94]. It has been proposed that the net balance of the positive and negative regulators of angiogenesis ultimately is responsible for the angiogenic phenotype [12,31].

In a 1997 report, O'Reilly et al. [93] described the discovery of endostatin, from the conditioned media of a murine hemangioendothelioma cell line (EOMA). When EOMA cell conditioned media was applied to bovine capillary endothelial cells stimulated with bFGF, a reversible inhibition of proliferation of the bovine cells as compared to controls was observed. It was also shown that the inhibition was not due to the previously discovered angiostatin. Upon isolation and subsequent microsequencing, the inhibitor was found to be a 20 kDa protein that was identical to the carboxy terminal end of collagen XVIII [93]. Using both baculovirus and *E. coli* expression systems, recombinant mouse endostatin was produced and used to show that inhibition of bovine capillary endothelial cells took place in a dose-dependent manner, inhibited angiogenesis in a chick chorioallantoic membrane assay, and inhibited the growth of Lewis lung carcinoma metastases. Metastases were maintained at a microscopic size while the primary tumor was reduced 150-fold. No re-growth of tumors, or evidence of drug resistance or toxicity was observed [93].

Murine recombinant endostatin specifically inhibits the proliferation [93] and migration of endothelial cells

[95–97]. In addition, several different xenograft mouse tumor models have been used to demonstrate murine endostatin's ability to suppress the growth of both primary and metastatic tumors. In the first set of experiments, Lewis lung carcinoma, T241 fibrosarcoma, EOMA hemangioendothelioma or B16F10 melanoma cells were all grown in syngeneic mice and treated with endostatin [93]. Purified nonrefolded endostatin was subcutaneously injected to form a pellet at the injection site, which resorbed over a 24–48-h period. The growth of Lewis lung primary tumors were severely suppressed by endostatin treatment, up to 97% at 10 mg/kg, and almost complete regression when that dose was doubled. Similar results were observed when the other tumor types were used, and in all cases, the tumors were held in a dormant state for as long as endostatin therapy was continued [93].

Acquired chemotherapy resistance is a major problem and is implicated in many of the cancer deaths described annually. To understand the drug resistance of endostatin Boehm et al. [98] repeated the xenograft experiments described above. Once the endostatin therapy regressed the tumors to the levels previously seen, treatment was discontinued and the tumor was permitted to re-grow. Treatment cycles of endostatin therapy, drug discontinuation followed by tumor re-growth, continued until no re-growth was observed. Six cycles of endostatin therapy were necessary to treat the mice with Lewis lung carcinoma, four cycles for T241 fibrosarcoma and two cycles for B16F10 melanoma with no evidence of drug resistance in the treated mice [98]. This was in contrast to control mice bearing Lewis lung carcinoma treated with cytotoxic chemotherapy (cyclophosphamide) that rapidly developed drug resistance. The tumor dormancy that resulted after endostatin therapy was not due to an immune response [98].

Endostatin therapy has been shown to be effective in other tumor types. Murine endostatin expressed in a yeast system, which has the advantages of its large-scale production of the protein and its ability to process post-translational modifications, was shown to inhibit the growth of renal cell carcinoma (RCC) [96]. In this report, the authors also showed that a mutant of endostatin protein was unable to inhibit RCC in their model. Human ovarian cells have been inhibited by endostatin, and a synergistic antiangiogenic effect was observed when endostatin was used in concert with angiostatin [99]. While all of the above mentioned studies were performed using tumors implanted in mice,

rat endostatin has also been demonstrated to inhibit primary mammary carcinomas in a rat model [100].

Human endostatin has been cloned after expression in a yeast system and purified to homogeneity in a soluble form. It inhibited the proliferation and migration of endothelial cells, caused G1 arrest and resulted in apoptosis of human derived endothelial cells [101]. A preclinical study using soluble human recombinant endostatin suppressed the growth of primary tumors and pulmonary metastases in a dose-dependent manner [102]. One drawback to the use of human endostatin is that it is produced in a large-scale yeast cell culture system and relatively large doses are required for the subcutaneous injections in the previous studies. Kisker et al. [103] in an effort to reduce the amount of endostatin needed, used continuous administration to accomplish this. Interestingly, the use of continuous administration via an i.p. implanted mini-osmotic pump showed that endostatin remained stable and active for at least 7 days, and 5-fold reduced doses resulted in more effective suppression of tumor burden. The authors suggest that this method of drug delivery results in sustained concentrations of the protein, and may more effectively inhibit angiogenesis within the vascular tumor bed [103].

To date, not much information is available on the potential role of endostatin in the treatment of prostate cancer. Prolonged survival time was noted in male C3(1)/Tag mice treated with endostatin. The male mice of this transgenic line are prone to develop prostate cancer and proliferative lesions in the genitourinary organs [104]. It has been noted that patients with Down's syndrome have a higher serum level of endostatin due to the three copies of the COL18A1 gene, and also have a decreased incidence of prostate cancer and other solid tumors [105]. It has been hypothesized that low levels or non-functioning endostatin might be associated with a higher risk of developing malignant solid tumors [106]. Recently a screen of polymorphic variants within the COL18A1 gene revealed a missense mutation located in the carboxy terminal endostatin encoding region. The mutation, an asparagine substituted for aspartic acid at position 104 (D104N), may lead to an impaired function of endostatin. Genotype analysis of the D104 SNP in 181 prostate cancer patients and 198 controls showed that individuals heterozygous for N104 have a 2.5 times greater chance of developing prostate cancer. Modeling methods suggest that the altered protein is stable, but might decrease the ability of endostatin to bind to other molecules, and thus, decrease its ability to be antiangiogenic [106]. Confirmation of the association of this polymorphism with prostate cancer in other populations is needed.

Carboxyamido-triazole

In the early 1990s, carboxyamido-triazole (CAI), initially developed as a coccidiostat, was first shown to have inhibitory effects on the proliferation, adhesion and motility of human melanoma, breast and ovarian cancer cells, and to prolonged survival of nude mice bearing ovarian cancer xenografts at a concentration ranging from 1 to $10 \mu M$ $(0.4–4 \mu g/ml)$ [107]. These findings were subsequently confirmed [108,109] and extended to other malignant cell lines including prostate [108,110], pancreas, colon, bladder, lymphoma [108] and glioblastoma [111], as well as xenografts [108,112]. Suppression of Ca^{2+}-sensitive pathways such as phospholipase A_2-induced generation of arachidonic acid, tyrosine phosphorylation of phospholipase C-γ, and regulation of *MMP-2* gene expression [113–115] has been indicated as one of the mechanisms contributing to the antiproliferative, antiinvasive and antimetastatic effects of CAI.

In addition to its activity against cancer cells, recent studies have unveiled the antiangiogenic effect of CAI. It was reported that CAI inhibits proliferation and spreading of human umbilical vein endothelial cells *in vitro* and angiogenesis in the chick chorioallantoic membrane assay [116,117]. Similar results were obtained in human aortic endothelial cells and in a rat aortic ring explant model with a concomitant decrease in nitric oxide synthase (NOS) expression as well as a decrease in VEGF production and secretion [22]. The antiangiogenic activity of CAI might be attributed in part to its inhibition of the Ca^{2+}-NOS-NO-VEGF pathway. Furthermore, CAI has been demonstrated to induce apoptosis in bovine aortic endothelial cells as well as human glioma and leukemia cells [118,119], indicating yet another mode of action of the drug.

Pharmacokinetic studies demonstrated that the steady concentrations, terminal half-life and volume of distribution of orally administered CAI are in the range of 2–5 $\mu g/ml$, 111 h and 100 to >400 liter, respectively [120]. Moreover, CAI is >99% protein-bound [120]. Ludden et al. [121] reported four metabolites

(M1, M2, M3, M4) of CAI *in vitro*. Phase I and Phase II enzymes appear to metabolize CAI, whereas CYP3A4 is responsible for the production of M3 and M4. Plasma samples from patients receiving CAI contained M1 and M2, and urine samples contained M3. M4 was not detectable in all samples [121].

Although no complete or partial response was evident, treatment with CAI in a liquid or a liquid gel cap preparation caused disease stabilization in 49% of a cohort of patients with RCC, pancreaticobiliary carcinoma, melanoma, ovarian, colorectal and non-small cell lung cancers lasting from 2 to 7 months [122]. Compliance-limiting gastrointestinal toxicities of these formulations prompted the development of a micronized powder capsule, which was found to be better tolerated [123]. Encapsulated micronized CAI also produced similar frequency of disease stabilization relative to the liquid formulation [123]. CAI was recently assessed in a Phase II clinical trial in patients with androgen-independent prostate cancer. Despite a 28% reduction of serum VEGF consequent to CAI monotherapy, clinical activity was not observed in patients with androgen-independent prostate cancer and soft tissue metastasis [44]. Thus, CAI may be more efficacious in the early stages of prostate cancer or in organ-confined disease [44]. In a Phase I trial, the sequential combination of CAI and paclitaxel was shown to be well tolerated, and yielded five partial and minor responses in melanoma, RCC, fallopian tube and ovarian cancer patients [124]. The therapeutic efficacy of CAI alone or in combination with cytotoxic agents in the treatment of various malignancies awaits further investigation.

2-Methoxyestradiol

2-Methoxyestradiol (2-ME) is an endogenous metabolite of estrogen, which is synthesized *in vivo* by hydroxylation at the 2-position of estradiol, and subsequent catechol-O-methyltransferase (COMT)-mediated O-methylation. Plasma 2-ME is in the picomolar range under normal physiological conditions; however, during late pregnancy the value reaches tens of nanomolar [125].

2-ME has been found to reduce tumor vasculature in mice injected subcutaneously with Meth A sarcoma and B16 melanoma cells and treated orally with 2-ME [126,127]. *In vivo* antiangiogenic activity of 2-ME has been demonstrated in the corneal micropocket [127]

324

and chick chorioallantoic model (CAM) systems [128]. In the corneal micropocket VEGF- and bFGF-induced neovascularization was reduced by 54% and 39% respectively. In the CAM model, 2 μM of 2-ME exposure for 3 days completely prevented bFGF-induced angiogenesis. *In vitro* 2-ME has been found to inhibit the neovascularization developing from the Rat Aortic ring assay [50,129]. 2-ME affects the angiogenesis cascade at various steps. In the rat aorta model 2-ME inhibited the proliferation, migration and tube formation [50,129]. It also blocks the tubule formation as well as the invasion through the collagen matrix [126]. In a human neuroblastoma xenograft model in mice, 2-ME resulted in a significant reduction in tumor growth after 14 days of treatment of tumors and showed a clear antiangiogenic and apoptotic effect [130].

The administration of 1 mg/day of 2-ME in female athymic mice having lung metastases induced by the injection of MIA PaCa-2 (Pancreatic Cancer) cells through the tail veins, did not show any significant difference in the number of blood vessels inside the colonies as examined by immunohistochemical staining for CD 31, a specific marker for endothelium [131]. Hence, ambiguity exists with respect to the exact mechanism of antiangiogenic properties of 2-ME. Although 2-ME has been labeled as antiangiogenic, endothelial cells are not necessarily more sensitive to its antiproliferative effects. And, the antiangiogenic and apoptotic activity of 2-ME vary with cell type and also with the regulatory microenvironment [132]. It has also been seen that administration of oral 2-ME in mice is associated with reducing the rate of tumor growth without signs of toxicity with a concomitant reduction in tumor vascularization [126], hence making it an ideal anticancer agent.

Thus, there is sufficient data to establish that 2-ME effectively inhibits angiogenesis but it is still difficult to pin point the exact mechanism through which it does so. Although clinical data on 2-ME is limited, animal and cell models have demonstrated that 2-ME is an effective antiangiogenic agent and the mechanism(s) of action are under investigation. In a Phase I clinical trial of 2-ME in patients with metastatic breast cancer conducted at the Indiana University Cancer Center, 67% of patients had stable disease after the first treatment period and continued therapy. Two patients had clinically significant improvement in bone pain and one patient with lymphangitic pulmonary metastases had a significant decrease in oxygen requirements. 2-ME was well tolerated and no grade IV toxicities occurred [133].

TNP-470

TNP-470 (*O*-(chloroacetyl carbamyl) fumagillol) is a semi-synthetic analog of the antibiotic fumagillin which has potent antiangiogenic, antitumor and antimetastatic properties [43,134–136]. The antitumor and antimetastatic properties are thought to be the result of the angiogenic inhibition of TNP-470 [136]. It is up to 50 times more potent and less toxic than the parent compound fumagillin, and plasma concentrations that achieve biological activity are transiently achievable in humans with moderate, reversible toxicity [43,134,137]. In addition, there is an active metabolite, AGM-1833. However, one of the biggest concerns in the development of TNP-470 is the short half-life. The terminal half-life has been estimated to be between 3 min and 0.8 h.

TNP-470 inhibits *in vitro* growth of endothelial cells more than other cells [135]. Fumagillin (the parent compound) inhibits methionine aminopeptidase-2, which is thought to play a role in the proliferation of endothelial cells [138]. A possible mechanism of antiangiogenesis is the inhibition of DNA synthesis in endothelial cells induced by growth factors (e.g. bFGF, VEGF) [136,139,140]. Prostate carcinomas that over express bcl-2 have a growth advantage that may be attributable to increased VEGF, this advantage reduced *in vitro* by TNP-470 [139].

TNP-470 has been shown, in both a clinical trial and *in vitro*, to increase PSA secretion [43,140]. This increase is through increase in transcription of the *PSA* gene, by both TNP-470 and AGM-1833 [140]. This clouds the interpretation of PSA as an indication of therapeutic response and disease progression in patients receiving TNP-470 therapy for prostate carcinoma. Additionally, attempts to quantify markers indicative of antiangiogenesis clinically (i.e. soluble E-selectin and thrombomodulin, urinary bFGF) did not show a correlation with trends in PSA levels, and require further investigation [43].

TNP-470 is one of the first antiangiogenic agents to enter clinical trials (entering human testing in 1992). The dose limiting toxicity of TNP-470 in dogs was cerebral bleeding [134]. There are seven Phase I trials using TNP-470 as a single agent in a variety of tumor types, as well as Phase II trials in renal cell, breast, cervical, pancreatic carcinomas and glioblastoma. In one Phase I trial, evidence of increased bleeding was not seen [43]. Dose-limiting toxicity in humans was neuropsychiatric symptoms, which resolved within 14 weeks of cessation of therapy, with a MTD in IV therapy of 70.88 mg/m^2 [43]. No evidence of GI toxicity or infectious complications was seen [43]. One diabetic patient was observed to have elevation in blood glucose levels during TNP-470 therapy, which normalized with cessation of therapy.

Logothetis and colleagues [43] completed a Phase I dose escalation trial of TNP-470 in 33 patients with metastatic prostate cancer. The drug was administered every other day. The patients were evaluated during therapy for evidence of neurological toxic effects. An assay of endothelial and vascular proliferation 'markers' and a sequential assay of serum PSA concentration were performed. The effects of TNP-470 could be evaluated in 32 of the 33 patients. The maximum tolerated dose was 70.88 mg/m^2 of body surface area. The dose-limiting toxic effect was a characteristic neuropsychiatric symptom complex (anesthesia, gait disturbance and agitation) that resolved upon cessation of therapy. The times to clinical recovery of neurological side effects were 6, 8 and 14 weeks. They concluded that no definite antitumor activity of TNP-470 was noted; however, transient stimulation of the serum PSA concentration occurred in some of the patients treated.

Conclusions

In prostate cancer, angiogenesis must function if progression from primary neoplasia to advanced metastatic disease is to occur. The angiogenic process is multistage, beginning with primary neoplasia and progressing to bone metastasis via the stimulatory effects of various metabolic determinants. Many of these molecular endpoints have been identified and their complex signaling pathways are continually being unraveled. The complex nature of the angiogenic process hinders the development of a complete understanding, but also provides an abundance of molecular target pathways against which therapeutic agents can be designed. Frequently, efficacious therapeutic agents have not been ascribed a detailed biochemical mode of action. In this paper, we have reviewed antiangiogenic agents with potential for clinical development in prostate cancer. Through the identification of agents with antiangiogenic activity in prostate cancer we can both increase our understanding of the role of angiogenesis in this disease and facilitate the development of related agents with lower toxicity and/or increased efficacy.

Key unanswered questions

Future research into therapeutic strategies to treat prostate cancer would benefit from improvement of our knowledge of the processes that determine the natural history and stages of prostate tumors. In particular, more work needs to be done to identify molecular endpoints required during the early stages of disease initiation, both to allow for the identification of potential molecular markers for diagnoses and to provide new drug targets. Known antiangiogenic drugs must be investigated further to determine their mechanisms of action. Also, molecular endpoints that govern the progression to late-stage hormone refractory prostate cancer must be characterized so that new drug therapies can be developed that are efficacious in late-stage disease.

References

1. Landis SH, Murray T, Bolden S, Wingo PA: Cancer statistics, 1999. CA Cancer J Clin 49: 8–31, 1, 1999
2. Huggins C, Hodges CV: Studies on prostatic cancer. I. The effect of castration, of estrogen and androgen injection on serum phosphatases in metastatic carcinoma of the prostate. CA Cancer J Clin 22: 232–240, 1941
3. Montgomery JS, Price DK, Figg WD: The androgen receptor gene and its influence on the development and progression of prostate cancer. J Pathol 195: 138–146, 2001
4. Stewart RJ, Panigrahy D, Flynn E, Folkman J: Vascular endothelial growth factor expression and tumor angiogenesis are regulated by androgens in hormone responsive human prostate carcinoma: Evidence for androgen dependent destabilization of vascular endothelial growth factor transcripts. J Urol 165: 688–693, 2001
5. Cude KJ, Dixon SC, Guo Y, Lisella J, Figg WD: The androgen receptor: Genetic considerations in the development and treatment of prostate cancer. J Mol Med 77: 419–426, 1999
6. Culig Z, Hobisch A, Hittmair A, Peterziel H, Cato AC, Bartsch G, Klocker H: Expression, structure, and function of androgen receptor in advanced prostatic carcinoma. Prostate 35: 63–70, 1998
7. The Veterans Administration Co-operative Urological Research Group: Treatment and survival of patients with cancer of the prostate. Surg Gynecol Obstet 124: 1011–1017, 1967
8. Scott WW, Menon M, Walsh PC: Hormonal therapy of prostatic cancer. Cancer 45: 1929–1936, 1980
9. Koivisto P, Visakorpi T, Kallioniemi OP: Androgen receptor gene amplification: A novel molecular mechanism for endocrine therapy resistance in human prostate cancer. Scand J Clin Lab Invest Suppl 226: 57–63, 1996
10. Crawford ED, Eisenberger MA, McLeod DG, Spaulding JT, Benson R, Dorr FA, Blumenstein BA,

326

Davis MA, Goodman PJ: A controlled trial of leuprolide with and without flutamide in prostatic carcinoma. N Engl J Med 321: 419–424, 1989

11. Group TCAS: A comparison of the treatment of metastatic prostate cancer by testicular ablation or total androgen blockade. Cancer Treat Res 59: 29–40, 1992

12. Folkman J: Angiogenesis in cancer, vascular, rheumatoid and other disease. Nat Med 1: 27–31, 1995

13. Nehls V, Schuchardt E, Drenckhahn D: The effect of fibroblasts, vascular smooth muscle cells, and pericytes on sprout formation of endothelial cells in a fibrin gel angiogenesis system. Microvasc Res 48: 349–363, 1994

14. Cockerill GW, Gamble JR, Vadas MA: Angiogenesis: Models and modulators. Int Rev Cytol 159: 113–160, 1995

15. Hanahan D, Weinberg RA: The hallmarks of cancer. Cell 100: 57–70, 2000

16. Choy M, Rafii S: Role of angiogenesis in the progression and treatment of prostate cancer. Cancer Invest 19: 181–191, 2001

17. Sokoloff MH, Chung LW: Targeting angiogenic pathways involving tumor-stromal interaction to treat advanced human prostate cancer. Cancer Metastasis Rev 17: 307–315, 1999

18. Kim KJ, Li B, Winer J, Armanini M, Gillett N, Phillips HS, Ferrara N: Inhibition of vascular endothelial growth factor-induced angiogenesis suppresses tumour growth in vivo. Nature 362: 841–844, 1993

19. Folkman J, Watson K, Ingber D, Hanahan D: Induction of angiogenesis during the transition from hyperplasia to neoplasia. Nature 339: 58–61, 1989

20. Weidner N, Carroll PR, Flax J, Blumenfeld W, Folkman J: Tumor angiogenesis correlates with metastasis in invasive prostate carcinoma. Am J Pathol 143: 401–409, 1993

21. McNamara DA, Harmey JH, Walsh TN, Redmond HP, Bouchier-Hayes DJ: Significance of angiogenesis in cancer therapy. Br J Surg 85: 1044–1055, 1998

22. Bauer KS, Cude KJ, Dixon SC, Kruger EA, Figg WD: Carboxyamido-triazole inhibits angiogenesis by blocking the calcium-mediated nitric-oxide synthase-vascular endothelial growth factor pathway. J Pharmacol Exp Ther 292: 31–37, 2000

23. Folkman J: Seminars in Medicine of the Beth Israel Hospital, Boston. Clinical applications of research on angiogenesis. N Engl J Med 333: 1757–1763, 1995

24. Suh DY: Understanding angiogenesis and its clinical applications. Ann Clin Lab Sci 30: 227–238, 2000

25. Dameron KM, Volpert OV, Tainsky MA, Bouck N: Control of angiogenesis in fibroblasts by p53 regulation of thrombospondin-1. Science 265: 1582–1584, 1994

26. Singh RK, Gutman M, Bucana CD, Sanchez R, Llansa N, Fidler IJ: Interferons alpha and beta down-regulate the expression of basic fibroblast growth factor in human carcinomas. Proc Natl Acad Sci USA 92: 4562–4566, 1995

27. Eriksson T, Bjorkman S, Hoglund P: Clinical pharmacology of thalidomide. European J Clin Pharmacol 57: 365–376, 2001

28. Kruger EA, Figg WD: TNP-470: An angiogenesis inhibitor in clinical development for cancer. Expert Opin Investig Drugs 9: 1383–1396, 2000

29. Kruger EA, Duray PH, Tsokos MG, Venzon DJ, Libutti SK, Dixon SC, Rudek MA, Pluda J, Allegra C, Figg WD: Endostatin inhibits microvessel formation in the ex vivo rat aortic ring angiogenesis assay. Biochem Biophys Res Commun 268: 183–191, 2000

30. Pribluda VS, Gubish ER, Lavallee TM, Treston A, Swartz GM, Green SJ: 2-Methoxyestradiol: An endogenous antiangiogenic and antiproliferative drug candidate. Cancer Metastasis Rev 19: 173–179, 2000

31. Hanahan D, Folkman J: Patterns and emerging mechanisms of the angiogenic switch during tumorigenesis. Cell 86: 353–364, 1996

32. Morikawa W, Yamamoto K, Ishikawa S, Takemoto S, Ono M, Fukushi JI, Naito S, Nozaki C, Iwanaga S, Kuwano M: Angiostatin generation by cathepsin D secreted by human prostate carcinoma cells. J Biol Chem 275: 38912–38920, 2000

33. Hori A, Sasada R, Matsutani E, Naito K, Sakura Y, Fujita T, Kozai Y: Suppression of solid tumor growth by immunoneutralizing monoclonal antibody against human basic fibroblast growth factor. Cancer Res 51: 6180–6184, 1991

34. Dvorak HF, Brown LF, Detmar M, Dvorak AM: Vascular permeability factor/vascular endothelial growth factor, microvascular hyperpermeability, and angiogenesis. Am J Pathol 146: 1029–1039, 1995

35. Neufeld G, Cohen T, Gengrinovitch S, Poltorak Z: Vascular endothelial growth factor (VEGF) and its receptors. FASEB J 13: 9–22, 1999

36. Izawa JI, Dinney CP: The role of angiogenesis in prostate and other urologic cancers: A review. CMAJ 164: 662–670, 2001.

37. Ferrer FA, Miller LJ, Andrawis RI, Kurtzman SH, Albertsen PC, Laudone VP, Kreutzer DL: Angiogenesis and prostate cancer: in vivo and in vitro expression of angiogenesis factors by prostate cancer cells. Urology 51: 161–167, 1998

38. Greene G, Kitadai Y, Pettaway C, von Eschenbach A, Bucana, C, Fidler I: Correlation of metastasis-related gene expression with metastatic potential in human prostate carcinoma cells implanted in nude mice using an in situ messenger RNA hybridization technique. Am J Pathol 150: 1571–1582, 1997

39. Inoue K, Slaton JW, Eve BY, Kim SJ, Perrotte P, Balbay MD, Yano S, Bar_Eli M, Radinsky, R, Pettaway CA, Dinney CP: Interleukin 8 expression regulates tumorigenicity and metastases in androgen-independent prostate cancer. Clin Cancer Res 6: 2104–2119, 2000

40. Shalinsky DR, Brekken J, Zou H, McDermott CD, Forsyth P, Edwards D, Margosiak S, Bender S, Truitt G, Wood A, Varki NM, Appelt K: Broad antitumor and antiangiogenic activities of AG3340, a potent and selective MMP inhibitor undergoing advanced oncology clinical trials. Ann NY Acad Sci 878: 236–270, 1999

41. Figg WD, Dahut W, Duray P, Hamilton, M, Tompkins A, Steinberg SM, Jones E, Premkumar A, Linehan WM, Floeter MK, Chen CC, Dixon S, Kohler DR, Kruger EA, Gubish E, Pluda JM, Reed E: A randomized phase II trial of thalidomide, an angiogenesis inhibitor, in patients with

androgen-independent prostate cancer. Clin Cancer Res 7: 1888–1893, 2001

42. Figg WD, Arlen P, Gulley J, Fernandez P, Noone M, Fedenko K, Hamilton M, Parker C, Kruger EA, Pluda J, Dahut W: A randomized phase II trial of docetaxel (taxotere) plus thalidomide in androgen-independent prostate cancer. Semin Oncol 28: 62–66, 2001

43. Logothetis CJ, Wu KK, Finn LD, Daliani D, Figg W, Ghaddar H, Gutterman JU: Phase I trial of the angiogenesis inhibitor TNP-470 for progressive androgen-independent prostate cancer. Clin Cancer Res 7: 1198–1203, 2001

44. Bauer KS, Figg WD, Hamilton JM, Jones EC, Premkumar A, Steinberg SM, Dyer V, Linehan WM, Pluda JM, Reed E: A pharmacokinetically guided Phase II study of carboxyamido-triazole in androgen-independent prostate cancer. Clin Cancer Res 5: 2324–2329, 1999

45. Diggle GE: Thalidomide: 40 years on. IJCP 55: 627–631, 2001

46. McBride W: Thalidomide and congenital abnormalities. Lancet 2: 1358, 1961

47. Lenz W: Thalidomide and congenital abnormalities. Lancet 1: 45, 1962

48. Sheskin J: Thalidomide in the treatment of lepra reactions. Clin Pharmacol Therapeut 6: 303–306, 1965

49. Calabrese L, Fleischer AB: Thalidomide: Current and potential clinical applications. Am J Med 108: 487–495, 2000

50. Bauer KS, Dixon SC, Figg WD: Inhibition of angiogenesis by thalidomide requires metabolic activation, which is species-dependent. Biochem Pharmacol 55: 1827–1834, 1998

51. Jorizzo JL, Schmalstieg FC, Solomon AR, Cavallo T, Taylor RS, Rudloff HB, Schmalstieg EJ, Daniels JC: Thalidomide effects in Behcet's syndrome and pustular vasculitis. Arch Intern Med 146: 878–881, 1986

52. Vogelsang GB, Farmer ER, Hess AD, Altamonte V, Beschorner WE, Jabs DA, Corio RL, Levin LS, Colvin OM, Wingard JR: Thalidomide for the treatment of chronic graft-versus-host disease. N Engl J Med 326: 1055–1058, 1992

53. Parker PM, Chao N, Nademanee A, O_Donnell MR, Schmidt GM, Snyder DS, Stein AS, Smith EP, Molina A, Stepan DE: Thalidomide as salvage therapy for chronic graft-versus-host disease. Blood 86: 3604–3609, 1995

54. Makonkawkeyoon S, Limson_Pobre RN, Moreira AL, Schauf V, Kaplan G: Thalidomide inhibits the replication of human immunodeficiency virus type 1. Proc Natl Acad Sci USA 90: 5974–5978, 1993

55. Revuz J, Guillaume JC, Janier M, Hans P, Marchand C, Souteyrand P, Bonnetblanc JM, Claudy A, Dallac S, Klene C: Crossover study of thalidomide vs placebo in severe recurrent aphthous stomatitis. Arch Dermatol 126: 923–927, 1990

56. Thomas DA, Kantarjian HM: Current role of thalidomide in cancer treatment. Curr Opin Oncol 12: 564–573, 2000

57. D' Amato RJ, Loughnan MS, Flynn E, Folkman J: Thalidomide is an inhibitor of angiogenesis. Proc Natl Acad Sci USA 91: 4082–4085, 1994

58. Kenyon BM, Browne F, D_Amato RJ: Effects of thalidomide and related metabolites in a mouse corneal model of neovascularization. Exp Eye Res 64: 971–978, 1997

59. Turk BE, Jiang H, Liu JO: Binding of thalidomide to alpha1-acid glycoprotein may be involved in its inhibition of tumor necrosis factor alpha production. Proc Natl Acad Sci USA 93: 7552–7556, 1996

60. Singhal S, Mehta J: Thalidomide in cancer: Potential uses and limitations. BioDrugs 15: 163–172, 2001

61. Barlogie B, Desikan R, Eddlemon P, Spencer T, Zeldis J, Munshi N, Badros A, Zangari M, Anaissie E, Epstein J, Shaughnessy J, Ayers D, Spoon D, Tricot G: Extended survival in advanced and refractory multiple myeloma after single-agent thalidomide: Identification of prognostic factors in a phase 2 study of 169 patients. Blood 98: 492–494, 2001

62. Rajkumar SV, Fonseca R, Dispenzieri A, Lacy MQ, Lust JA, Witzig TE, Kyle RA, Gertz MA, Greipp PR: Thalidomide in the treatment of relapsed multiple myeloma. Mayo Clin Proc 75: 897–901, 2000

63. Little RF, Wyvill KM, Pluda JM, Welles L, Marshall V, Figg WD, Newcomb FM, Tosato G, Feigal E, Steinberg SM, Whitby D, Goedert JJ, Yarchoan R: Activity of thalidomide in AIDS-related Kaposi's sarcoma. J Clin Oncol 18: 2593–2602, 2000

64. Fine HA, Figg WD, Jaeckle K, Wen PY, Kyritsis AP, Loeffler JS, Levin VA, Black PM, Kaplan R, Pluda JM, Yung WK: Phase II trial of the antiangiogenic agent thalidomide in patients with recurrent high-grade gliomas. J Clin Oncol 18: 708–715, 2000

65. Eisen T, Boshoff C, Mak I, Sapunar F, Vaughan MM, Pyle L, Johnston SR, Ahern R, Smith IE, Gore ME: Continuous low dose Thalidomide: A phase II study in advanced melanoma, renal cell, ovarian and breast cancer. Br J Cancer 82: 812–817, 2000

66. Stebbing J, Benson C, Eisen T, Pyle L, Smalley K, Bridle H, Mak I, Sapunar F, Ahern R, Gore ME: The treatment of advanced renal cell cancer with high-dose oral thalidomide. Br J Cancer 85: 953–958, 2001

67. Ginsburg PM, Dassopoulos T, Ehrenpreis ED: Thalidomide treatment for refractory Crohn's disease: a review of the history, pharmacological mechanisms and clinical literature. Ann Med 33: 516–525, 2001

68. Marx GM, Pavlakis N, McCowatt S, Boyle FM, Levi JA, Bell DR, Cook R, Biggs M, Little N, Wheeler HR: Phase II study of thalidomide in the treatment of recurrent glioblastoma multiforme. J Neuro-Oncology 54: 31–38, 2001

69. Stirling D: Thalidomide: A novel template for anticancer drugs. Semin Oncol 28: 602–606, 2001

70. Beckner ME: Factors promoting tumor angiogenesis. Cancer Invest 17: 594–623, 1999

71. Thomas DA, Kantarjian HM: The revitalization of thalidomide. Ann Oncol 12: 885–886, 2001

72. Sampaio EP, Sarno EN, Galilly R, Cohn ZA, Kaplan G: Thalidomide selectively inhibits tumor necrosis factor alpha production by stimulated human monocytes. J Exp Med 173: 699–703, 1991

73. Moreira AL, Sampaio EP, Zmuidzinas A, Frindt P, Smith KA, Kaplan G: Thalidomide exerts its inhibitory

action on tumor necrosis factor alpha by enhancing mRNA degradation. J Exp Med 177: 1675–1680, 1993

74. Rowland TL, McHugh SM, Deighton J, Dearman RJ, Ewan PW, Kimber I: Differential regulation by thalidomide and dexamethasone of cytokine expression in human peripheral blood mononuclear cells. Immunopharmacology 40: 11–20, 1998

75. Joseph IB, Isaacs JT: Macrophage role in the anti-prostate cancer response to one class of antiangiogenic agents. J Natl Cancer Inst 90: 1648–1653, 1998

76. Ching LM, Browne WL, Tchernegovski R, Gregory T, Baguley BC, Palmer BD: Interaction of thalidomide, phthalimide analogues of thalidomide and pentoxifylline with the anti-tumour agent 5,6-dimethylxanthenone-4-acetic acid: Concomitant reduction of serum tumour necrosis factor-alpha and enhancement of anti-tumour activity. Br J Cancer 78: 336–343, 1998

77. Wnendt S, Finkam M, Winter W, Ossig J, Raabe G, Zwingenberger K: Enantioselective inhibition of TNF-alpha release by thalidomide and thalidomide-analogues. Chirality 8: 390–396, 1996

78. Hoglund P, Eriksson T, Bjorkman S: A double-blind study of the sedative effects of the thalidomide enantiomers in humans. J Pharmacokinet Biopharm 26: 363–383, 1998

79. Eriksson T, Bjorkman S, Roth B, Hoglund P: Intravenous formulations of the enantiomers of thalidomide: Pharmacokinetic and initial pharmacodynamic characterization in man. J Pharm Pharmacol 52: 807–817, 2000

80. Stephens TD, Fillmore BJ: Hypothesis: Thalidomide embryopathy-proposed mechanism of action. Teratology 61: 189–195, 2000

81. Stephens TD, Bunde CJ, Fillmore BJ: Mechanism of action in thalidomide teratogenesis. Biochem Pharmacol 59: 1489–1499, 2000

82. Haslett PA, Corral LG, Albert M, Kaplan G: Thalidomide costimulates primary human T lymphocytes, preferentially inducing proliferation, cytokine production, and cytotoxic responses in the CD8+ subset. J Exp Med 187: 1885–1892, 1998

83. Neben K, Moehler T, Kraemer A, Benner A, Egerer G, Ho AD, Goldschmidt H: Response to thalidomide in progressive multiple myeloma is not mediated by inhibition of angiogenic cytokine secretion. Br J Haem 115: 605–608, 2001

84. Fujita J, Mestre JR, Zweldis JB, Subbaramaiah K, Dannenberg AJ: Thalidomide and its analogues inhibit lipopolysaccharide-mediated induction of cyclooxygenase-2. Clin Cancer Res 7: 3349–3355, 2001

85. Yamada M, Kawai M, Kawai Y, Mashima Y: The effect of selective cyclooxygenase-2 inhibitor on corneal angiogenesis in the rat. Curr Eye Res 19: 300–304, 1999

86. Daniel TO, Liu H, Morrow JD, Crews BC, Marnett LJ: Thromboxane A_2 is a mediator of cyclooxygenase-2-dependent endothelial migration and angiogenesis. Cancer Res 59: 4574–4577, 1999

87. Kirschenbaum A, Liu X, Yao S, Levine AC: The role of cyclooxygenase-2 in prostate cancer. Urology 58: 127–131, 2001

88. Hess S, Akermann MA, Wnendt S, Zwingenberger K, Eger K: Synthesis and immunological activity of water-soluble thalidomide prodrugs. Bioorg Med Chem 9: 1279–1291, 2001

89. Kandel J, Bossy-Wetzel E, Radvany F, Klagsburn M, Folkman J, Hanahan D: Neovascularization is associated with a switch to the export of bFGF in the multistep development of fibrosarcoma. Cell 66: 1095–1104, 1991

90. Chen C, Parangi S, Tolentino M, Folkman J: A strategy to discover circulating angiogenesis inhibitors generated by human tumors. Cancer Res 55: 4230–4233, 1995

91. Good D, Polverini P, Rastinejad F, LeBeau M, Lemons R, Frazier W, Bouck N: A tumor suppressor-dependent inhibitor of angiogenesis is immunologically and functionally indistinguishable from a fragment of thrombospondin. Proc Nat Acad Sci USA 87: 6624–6628, 1990

92. O'Reilly M, Holmgren L, Shing Y, Chen C, Rosenthal R, Moses M, Lane W, Cao Y, Sage E, Folkman J: Angiostatin: A novel angiogenesis inhibitor that mediates the suppression of metastases by a Lewis Lung carcinoma. Cell 79: 315–328, 1994

93. O'Reilly M, Boehm T, Shing Y, Fuakai N, Vasios G, Lane W, Flynn E, Birkhead J, Olsen B, Folkman J: Endostatin: An endogenous inhibitor of angiogenesis and tumor growth. Cell 88: 277–285, 1997

94. O'Reilly M, Pirie-Shepard S, Lane W, Folkman J: Antiangiogenic activity of a cleaved conformation of the serpin antithrombin. Science 285: 1926–1928, 1999

95. Yamiguchi N, Anand-Apte B, Lee M, Sasaki T, Fukai N, Shapiro R, Que I, Lowik C, Timpl R, Olsen B: Endostatin inhibits VEGF-induced endothelial cell migration and tumor growth independently of zinc binding. EMBO J 18: 4414–4423, 1999

96. Dhanabal M, Ramchandran R, Volk R, Stillman I, Lombardo M, Iruela-Arispe M, Simons M, VP S: Endostatin. Yeast production, mutants, and antitumor effect in renal cell carcinoma. Cancer Res 59: 189–197, 1999

97. Taddei L, Chiarugi P, Brogelli L, Cirri P, Magnelli L, Raugei G, Ziche M, Granger H, Chiarugi V, Ramponi G: Inhibitory effect of full-length human endostatin on in vitro angiogenesis. Biochem Biophys Res Commun 263: 340–345, 1999

98. Boehm T, Folkman J, Browder T, O'Reilly M: Antiangiogenic therapy of experimental cancer does not induce acquired drug reisistance. Nature 390: 404–407, 1997

99. Yokoyama Y, Dhanabal M, Griffioen A, Sukhatme V, Ramakrishnan S: Synergy between angiostatin and endostatin: inhibition of ovarian cancer growth. Cancer Res 60: 2190–2196, 2000

100. Perletti G, Concari P, Giardini R, Marras E, Piccinini F, Folkman J, Chen L: Antitumor activity of endostatin against carcinogen-induced rat primary mammary tumors. Cancer Res 60: 1793–1796, 2000

101. Dhanabal M, Volk R, Ramchandran R, Simons M, Sukhatme V: Cloning, expression, and in vitro activity of human endostatin. Biochem Biophys Res Commun 258: 345–352, 1999

102. Sim B, Fogler W, Zhou X, Liang H, Madsen J, Luu K, O'Reilly M, Tomaszewski J, Fortier A: Zinc

ligand-disrupted recombinant human endostatin: potent inhibition of tumor growth, safety and pharmacokinetic profile. Angiogenesis 3: 41–51, 1999

103. Kisker O, Becker C, Prox D, Fannon M, D'Amato R, Flynn E, Fogler W, Sim B, Allred E, Pirie-Shepard S, Folkman J: Continuous administration of endostatin by intraperitoneally implanted osmotic pump inproves the efficacy and potency of therapy in a mouse xenograft tumor model. Cancer Res 61: 7669–7674, 2001

104. Yokoyami Y, Green J, Sukhatme V, Ramakrishnan S: Effect of endostatin on spontaneous tumorigenesis of mammary adenocarcinomas in a transgenic mouse model. Cancer Res 60: 2000

105. Hasle H, Clemmensen I, Mikkelsen M: Risks of leukaemia and solid tumours in individuals with Down's syndrome. Lancet 355: 165–169, 2000

106. Iughetti P, Suzuki O, Godoi P, Alves V, Sertie A, Zorick T, Soares F, Camargo A, Moreira E, di Loreto C, Moreira-Filho A, Simpson A, Oliva G, Passos-Bueno M: A polymorphism in endostatin, an angiogenesis inhibitor, predisposes for the development of prostatic adenocarcinoma. Cancer Res 61: 2001

107. Kohn EC, Liotta LA: L651582: A novel antiproliferative and antimetastasis agent. J Natl Cancer Inst 82: 54–60, 1990

108. Kohn EC, Sandeen MA, Liotta LA: *In vivo* efficacy of a novel inhibitor of selected signal transduction pathways including calcium, arachidonate, and inositol phosphates. Cancer Res 52: 3208–3212, 1992

109. Lambert PA, Somers KD, Kohn EC, Perry RR: Antiproliferative and antiinvasive effects of carboxyamido-triazole on breast cancer cell lines. Surgery 122: 372–378; discussion 378–379, 1997

110. Wasilenko WJ, Palad AJ, Somers KD, Blackmore PF, Kohn EC, Rhim JS, Wright GL, Schellhammer PF: Effects of the calcium influx inhibitor carboxyamido-triazole on the proliferation and invasiveness of human prostate tumor cell lines. Int J Cancer 68: 259–264, 1996

111. Jacobs W, Mikkelsen T, Smith R, Nelson K, Rosenblum ML, Kohn EC: Inhibitory effects of CAI in glioblastoma growth and invasion. J Neuro-Oncology 32: 93–101, 1997

112. Qin LX, Tang ZY, Li XM, Bu W, Xia JL: Effect of antiangiogenic agents on experimental animal models of hepatocellular carcinoma. Ann Acad Med Singapore 28: 147–151, 1999

113. Gusovsky F, Lueders JE, Kohn EC, Felder CC: Muscarinic receptor-mediated tyrosine phosphorylation of phospholipase C-gamma. An alternative mechanism for cholinergic-induced phosphoinositide breakdown. J Biol Chem 268: 7768–7772, 1993

114. Felder CC, Ma AL, Liotta LA, Kohn EC: The antiproliferative and antimetastatic compound L651582 inhibits muscarinic acetylcholine receptor-stimulated calcium influx and arachidonic acid release. J Pharmacol Exp Ther 257: 967–971, 1991

115. Kohn EC, Jacobs W, Kim YS, Alessandro R, Stetler-Stevenson WG, Liotta LA: Calcium influx modulates expression of matrix metalloproteinase-2 (72-kDa type IV collagenase, gelatinase A). J Biol Chem 269: 21505–21511, 1994

116. Kohn EC, Alessandro R, Spoonster J, Wersto RP, Liotta LA: Angiogenesis: Role of calcium-mediated signal transduction. Proc Natl Acad Sci USA 92: 1307–1311, 1995

117. Alessandro R, Masiero L, Lapidos K, Spoonster J, Kohn EC: Endothelial cell spreading on type IV collagen and spreading-induced FAK phosphorylation is regulated by Ca2+ influx. Biochem Biophys Res Commun 248: 635–640, 1998

118. Ge S, Rempel SA, Divine G, Mikkelsen T: Carboxyamido-triazole induces apoptosis in bovine aortic endothelial and human glioma cells. Clin Cancer Res 6: 1248–1254, 2000

119. Waselenko J, Shinn C, Willis C, Flinn I, Grever M, Byrd J: Carboxyamido-triazole (CAI) – a novel 'static' signal transduction inhibitor induces apoptosis in human B-cell chronic lymphocytic leukemia cells. Leuk Lymph 42: 1049–1053, 2001

120. Figg WD, Cole KA, Reed E, Steinberg SM, Piscitelli SC Davis PA, Soltis MJ, Jacob J, Boudoulas S, Goldspiel B: Pharmacokinetics of orally administered carboxyamido-triazole, an inhibitor of calcium-mediated signal transduction. Clin Cancer Res 1: 797–803, 1995

121. Ludden L, Strong J, Kohn E, Collins J: Similarity of metabolism of CAI (NSC 609974) in human liver tissue *in vitro* and in humans *in vivo*. Clin Cancer Res 1: 399–405, 1995

122. Kohn EC, Reed E, Sarosy G, Christian M, Link CJ, Cole K, Figg WD, Davis PA, Jacob J, Goldspiel B, Liotta LA: Clinical investigation of a cytostatic calcium influx inhibitor in patients with refractory cancers. Cancer Res 56: 569–573, 1996

123. Kohn EC, Figg WD, Sarosy GA, Bauer KS, Davis PA, Soltis MJ, Thompkins A, Liotta LA, Reed, E: Phase I trial of micronized formulation carboxyamidotriazole in patients with refractory solid tumors: Pharmacokinetics, clinical outcome, and comparison of formulations. J Clin Oncol 15: 1985–1993, 1997

124. Kohn EC, Reed E, Sarosy GA, Minasian L, Bauer KS, Bostick-Bruton F, Kulpa V, Fuse E, Tompkins A, Noone M, Goldspiel B, Pluda J, Figg WD, Liotta LA: A phase I trial of carboxyamido-triazole and paclitaxel for relapsed solid tumors: Potential efficacy of the combination and demonstration of pharmacokinetic interaction. Clin Cancer Res 7: 1600–1609, 2001

125. Berg FD, Kuss E: Serum concentration and urinary excretion of 'classical' estrogens, catecholestrogens and 2-methoxyestrogens in normal human pregnancy. Arch Gynecol Obstet 251: 17–27, 1992

126. Fotsis T, Zhang Y, Pepper MS, Adlercreutz H, Montesano R, Nawroth PP, Schweigerer L: The endogenous oestrogen metabolite 2-methoxyoestradiol inhibits angiogenesis and suppresses tumour growth. Nature 368: 237–239, 1994

127. Klauber N, Parangi S, Flynn E, Hamel E, D-Amato RJ: Inhibition of angiogenesis and breast cancer in mice by the microtubule inhibitors 2-methoxyestradiol and taxol. Cancer Res 57: 81–86, 1997

330

128. Yue TL, Wang X, Louden CS, Gupta S, Pillarisetti K, Gu JL, Hart TK, Lysko PG, Feuerstein GZ: 2-Methoxyestradiol, an endogenous estrogen metabolite, induces apoptosis in endothelial cells and inhibits angiogenesis: Possible role for stress-activated protein kinase signaling pathway and Fas expression. Mol Pharmacol 51: 951–962, 1997

129. Nicosia RF, Ottinetti A: Growth of microvessels in serum-free matrix culture of rat aorta. A quantitative assay of angiogenesis *in vitro*. Lab Invest 63: 115–122, 1990

130. Wassberg E: Angiostatic treatment of neuroblastoma. Ups J Med Sci 104: 1–24, 1999

131. Schumacher G, Kataoka M, Roth JA, Mukhopadhyay T: Potent antitumor activity of 2-methoxyestradiol in human pancreatic cancer cell lines. Clin Cancer Res 5: 493–499, 1999

132. Shang W, Konidari I, Schomberg DW: 2-Methoxyestradiol, an endogenous estradiol metabolite, differentially inhibits granulosa and endothelial cell mitosis: A potential follicular antiangiogenic regulator. Biol Reprod 65: 622–627, 2001

133. Miller KD, Haney LG, Pribluda VS, Sledge GW: A phase I safety, pharmacokinetic and pharmacodynamic study of 2-methoxyestradiol (2ME2) in patients (Pts) with refractory metastatic breast cancer (MBC). American Society of Clinical Oncology (Abstract # 170), 2001

134. Figg WD, Pluda JM, Lush RM, Saville MW, Wyvill K, Reed E, Yarchoan R: The pharmacokinetics of TNP-470, a new angiogenesis inhibitor. Pharmacotherapy 17: 91–97, 1997

135. Miki T, Nonomura N, Nozawa M, Harada Y, Nishimura K, Kojima Y, Takahara S, Okuyama A: Angiogenesis inhibitor TNP-470 inhibits growth and metastasis of a hormone-independent rat prostatic carcinoma cell line. J Urol 160: 210–213, 1998

136. Yamaoka M, Yamamoto T, Ikeyama S, Sudo K, Fujita T: Angiogenesis inhibitor TNP-470 (AGM-1470) potently inhibits the tumor growth of hormone-independent human breast and prostate carcinoma cell lines. Cancer Res 53: 5233–5236, 1993

137. Kim J, Logothetis CJ: Serologic tumor markers, clinical biology, and therapy of prostatic carcinoma. Urol Clin North Am 26: 281–290, 1999

138. Gibaldi M: Regulating angiogenesis: a new therapeutic strategy. J Clin Pharmacol 38: 898–903, 1998

139. Fernandez A, Udagawa T, Schwesinger C, Beecken W, Achilles-Gerte E, McDonnell T, D-Amato R: Angiogenic potential of prostate carcinoma cells overexpressing bcl-2. J Natl Cancer Inst 93: 208–213, 2001

140. Horti J, Dixon SC, Logothetis CJ, Guo Y, Reed E, Figg WD: Increased transcriptional activity of prostate-specific antigen in the presence of TNP-470, an angiogenesis inhibitor. Br J Cancer 79: 1588–1593, 1999

141. Zhang M, Volpert O, Shi YH, Bouck N: Maspin is an angiogenesis inhibitor. Nat Me 6: 196–199, 2000

142. Stearns ME, Garcia FU, Fudge K, Rhim J, Wang M: Role of interleukin 10 and transforming growth factor beta1 in the angiogenesis and metastasis of human prostate primary tumor lines from orthotopic implants in severe combined immunodeficiency mice. Clin Cancer Res 5: 711–720, 1999

143. Papadopoulos I, Sivridis E, Giatromanolaki A, Koukourakis MI: Tumor angiogenesis is associated with MUC1 overexpression and loss of prostate-specific antigen expression in prostate cancer. Clin Cancer Res 7: 1533–1538, 2001

144. Miyadera K, Sumizawa T, Haraguchi M, Yoshida H, Konstanty W, Yamada Y, Akiyama S: Role of thymidine phosphorylase activity in the angiogenic effect of platelet derived endothelial cell growth factor/thymidine phosphorylase. Cancer Res 55: 1687–1690, 1995

145. Cao G, Su J, Lu W, Zhang F, Zhao G, Marteralli D, Dong Z: Adenovirus-mediated interferon-beta gene therapy suppresses growth and metastasis of human prostate cancer in nude mice. Cancer Gene Ther 8: 497–505, 2001

Address for offprints: W.D. Figg, Building 10, Room. 5A01, National Cancer Institute, National Institutes of Health, 9000 Rockville Pike, Bethesda, MD 20892, USA; *Tel:* 301 402 3622; *Fax:* 301 402 8606; *e-mail:* wdfigg@helix.nih.gov

Chemoprevention of prostate cancer

Omer Kucuk
Barbara Ann Karmanos Cancer Institute, Wayne State University, Detroit, Michigan, USA

Key words: prostate cancer, prevention, nutrition, chemoprevention, phytochemicals

Abstract

Chemoprevention is prevention of cancer by administering natural or synthetic chemicals. Anti-androgens are among the promising chemopreventive agents for prostate cancer because prostate epithelium is androgen dependent. A National Cancer Institute supported large, randomized, clinical prostate cancer chemoprevention trial has been conducted to test the efficacy of finasteride, an inhibitor of 5-α-reductase, which converts testosterone to 5-hydroxy-testosterone. Now the focus is on micronutrients and phytochemicals, which have potential preventive effects against prostate cancer. Lycopene, soy isoflavones, vitamin E and selenium are among the most promising nutritional chemopreventive agents. Another NCI supported large clinical chemoprevention trial was recently started to investigate the efficacy of selenium and vitamin E, alone or in combination in the prevention of prostate cancer. Inclusion of appropriate biomarkers in clinical trials will help elucidate the mechanisms by which genetic and epigenetic pathways of carcinogenesis are modulated by nutrients and phytochemicals.

Introduction

Prostate cancer is the second leading cause of cancer deaths in males in the US. It accounts for about 30% of all cancers that are diagnosed in men. In 2001, the American Cancer Society has predicted 198,100 new cases and 31,500 deaths from prostate cancer in the US [1]. The incidence of prostate cancer has increased dramatically in the last decade mainly due to the increase in screening using prostate-specific antigen (PSA). The prevalence of the precursor lesion, high grade prostatic intraepithelial neoplasia (HGPIN) and carcinoma of the prostate increase with aging starting in men in their early thirties [2]. Knowledge of the natural history of development, elucidation of critical genetic and epigenetic pathways and presence of risk factors for identifying target populations make prostate cancer a good target for prevention [3]. Thus, there is great interest in prostate cancer chemoprevention, which can be defined as the administration of natural and/or synthetic agents that inhibit one or more steps in prostate carcinogenesis [4].

Intermediate endpoints or surrogate endpoint biomarkers (SEBs) are used in small efficient phase I–II clinical chemoprevention trials to explore the efficacy and elucidate the mechanisms of action of potential chemopreventive compounds. Gap-junctional intercellular communication (GJIC) and Cx expression levels could be useful intermediate endpoints in prostate cancer chemoprevention clinical trials, because they are decreased in prostate cancer cells [5–7]. Therefore, chemopreventive agents modulating Cx expression and/or GJIC would be of great interest [8,9]. Retinoids and carotenoids are among the potent upregulators of Cx43 and GJIC [10–12]. In particular, lycopene increases GJIC by increasing the expression of the gap-junctional gene, connexin 43 [10,13,14]. This action correlates strongly with the ability of lycopene and other carotenoids to suppress neoplastic transformation in model cell culture systems [10]. This action of carotenoids has been proposed to have mechanistic significance by enabling the transfer of growth-regulatory signals between normal growth-inhibited cells and pre-neoplastic cells. Indeed, when neoplastic cells were forced into junctional communication with quiescent normal cells, the neoplastic cells became growth arrested in direct proportion to their extent of junctional communication [8]. Progressive decreases with disease severity in the expression of Cx43 have been reported in the human prostate [5], and there is evidence in prostatic carcinoma cell lines that some of this loss of junctional communication may result

M.L. Cher, K.V. Honn and A. Raz (eds.), Prostate Cancer: New Horizons in Research and Treatment, 331–344.
© 2002 *Kluwer Academic Publishers.*

from defects in the assembly of Cx43 protein into gap junctions [6]. When functional communication was restored in a human prostatic carcinoma cell line, cells had more normal differentiation, reduced proliferation and suppressed tumorigenicity [7]. Therefore, Cx43 and GJIC could be used as SEBs or intermediate endpoints in phase II clinical chemoprevention trials for prostate cancer.

It would be important to identify men at high risk for prostate cancer to enroll in chemoprevention trials. In addition to the presence of HGPIN in the prostate and elevated serum PSA levels, recent studies suggest high serum IGF-1 and/or low serum IGFBP-3 as good markers for high prostate cancer risk. Insulin-like growth factors have mitogenic and anti-apoptotic effects on normal and transformed prostate epithelial cells [15–17]. IGF-1 is an important mitogen for prostate cells. IGFBPs have opposing actions, in part by binding IGF-1, but also by direct inhibitory effects on target cells [15]. In recent epidemiologic studies, relatively high plasma IGF-1 and low IGFBP-3 levels have been independently associated with greater risk of prostate cancer [18–22]. Two- to four-fold elevated risk has been observed for prostate cancer in men in the top quartile of IGF-1 relative to those in the bottom quartile, and low levels of IGFBP-3 were associated with an approximate doubling of risk [18]. Recent data show that lycopene administration to humans with colon cancer for 1–5 weeks prior to surgery significantly reduces serum IGF-1 levels [23].

Since prostate carcinogenesis is a multistep process and takes many years to occur in humans, it is an ideal disease to conduct clinical chemoprevention trials. Currently, there are no chemopreventive agents approved by United States Food and Drug Administration for prostate cancer. Chemopreventive agents to be investigated should be non-toxic, inexpensive and available for use by mouth, because they are ultimately expected to be in used by healthy people in the general population. There are numerous natural and synthetic compounds with demonstrated activities against prostate cancer in cell culture and animal models (Table 1). Although potential chemopreventive agents are sometimes classified based on their structure or mechanism of action, many chemopreventive compounds have multiple mechanisms of action. For example, soy isoflavones have antioxidant, anti-inflammatory, anti-hormonal and anti-angiogenic effects. Chemopreventive agents can be found in vegetables and fruits, such as lycopene in tomatoes, lutein in spinach, quercetin in apples and onions.

Chemopreventive agents

Finasteride

Anti-androgens are among the first potential chemopreventive agents to be tested in large-scale clinical trials. Anti-androgens are expected to reduce cell proliferation in the prostate epithelium and thereby reduce

Table 1. Potential chemopreventive compounds for prostate cancer

Group	Compounds
Anti-androgens	Finasteride, bicalutamide, genistein
Carotenoids	Lycopene, phytoene, phytofluene, lutein, astaxanthin
Tocopherols, tocotrienols	Alpha-tocopherol, gamma-tocopherol, tocotrienols
Flavonoids, polyphenols	Genistein, quercetin, resveratrol, EGCG
Lipids	Omega-3 fatty acids
Vitamins	Vitamins D and E
Minerals	Selenium, zinc
Anti-inflammatory agents	
Cycloxygenase inhibitors	Celecoxib, rofecoxib
Lipoxygenase inhibitors	Zileuton, fish oil
Anti-proliferative agents	ODC inhibitors (DFMO)
PPAR-gamma agonists	Thiazolidinediones
Pro-apoptotic agents	Exisulind
Others	Curcumin

EGCG, epigallactocathecingallate; ODC, ornithine decarboxylase; DFMO, difluoromethylornithin.

the risk of developing cancer. Since prostate cancer is dependent on 5-hydroxytestosterone for growth, finasteride, a 5-α-reductase inhibitor, which prevents the conversion of testosterone to 5-hydroxytestosterone, was chosen for a large clinical trial for prostate cancer prevention [24]. Finasteride is being evaluated in a large prostate cancer prevention trial (PCPT) involving more than 18,800 healthy men at low to average risk [24]. This trial was designed to detect a 25% reduction in prostate cancer rate after 7 years of finasteride treatment. This drug does not induce histologic changes in prostate cancer or modulate the appearance of HGPIN but it is known to decrease serum PSA [25]. However, some nutritional agents and phytochemicals may have similar efficacy and may soon replace finasteride. For example, soy isoflavones also inhibit 5-α-reductase [26] and reduce serum PSA [27,28], in addition to their effects on prostate cancer growth in preclinical studies [29,30]. Therefore, they may be better than finasteride in the prevention of prostate cancer.

Selenium

Epidemiologic data suggest an association between selenium and prostate cancer risk. Health Professionals Follow-Up Study (HPFS) showed a significantly lower risk of advanced prostate cancer in men with toenail selenium levels in the highest quintile compared to those in the lowest quintile [31]. This suggests that selenium may not only prevent prostate cancer development but may also prevent its progression. A clinical trial that tested the effect of selenium supplementation on development of carcinomas of the skin showed a significant reduction in prostate cancer incidence but no reduction in skin cancer incidence [32,33]. In addition, compelling evidence that selenium might be a chemopreventive nutrient comes from preclinical studies in animals and cell cultures [34].

Vitamin E

In HPFS, supplemental vitamin E was inversely associated with the risk of metastatic or fatal prostate cancer among current smokers [35]. Furthermore, an inverse relationship between vitamin E and prostate cancer risk was supported by the ATBC Study, in which 32% fewer cases of prostate cancer and 16% fewer cases of colorectal cancer were diagnosed among men who received α-tocopherol supplements [36,37]. Preclinical studies suggest that several mechanisms may explain the ability of vitamin E to inhibit cancer.

These include quenching of free radicals, induction of cell differentiation, inhibition of cell growth, induction of apoptosis, and enhancement of the immune function [38].

Based on encouraging data from large clinical trials of vitamin E [36] and selenium [33], the Selenium and Vitamin E Cancer Prevention Trial (SELECT) has been started. This trial is investigating vitamin E, selenium, or the combination in more than 32,000 men (over age 55 for Caucasian and over age 50 for African-American) with normal PSA values. The study will have a minimum of 7 years of intervention [39].

Lycopene

Epidemiological studies have shown an inverse association between dietary intake of tomato products and lycopene and prostate cancer risk [40–43]. Lycopene, the major carotenoid in tomatoes, has been postulated to be a protective compound against prostate cancer [40–44]. Possible mechanisms by which lycopene may prevent prostate cancer include modulation of cell cycle regulatory proteins [45-49], IGF-1/IGFBP-3 system [49–59], gap-junctional tumor suppressor protein Cx43 [10,13,14,50,60–72,78], redox signalling [73], oxidative DNA damage [74,75,79] and carcinogen metabolizing enzymes [76].

IGF-1 has been identified as a risk factor for prostate cancer [18–22]. Lycopene, in cell culture, strongly inhibited IGF-1-mediated proliferation of human endometrial, mammary and lung cancer cells [49]. In contrast, normal human fibroblasts were less sensitive to lycopene, and the cells gradually escaped growth inhibition over time. In addition, lycopene suppressed IGF-1-stimulated growth of endometrial cancer cells. Lycopene treatment also resulted in a concentration-dependent reduction in HL-60 cell growth, which was accompanied by inhibition of cell cycle progression in the G0/G1 phase and induction of cell differentiation as measured by phorbol ester-dependent reduction of nitro blue tetrazolium and expression of the cell surface antigen CD14 [46]. Growth stimulation of MCF-7 mammary cancer cells by IGF-1 was also markedly reduced by physiological concentrations of lycopene [47]. Lycopene treatment markedly reduced the IGF-1 stimulation of tyrosine phosphorylation of insulin receptor substrate 1 and binding capacity of the AP-1 transcription complex [49]. Inhibitory effects of lycopene on MCF-7 cell growth were due to interference in IGF-1 receptor signaling and suppressed cell cycle progression. In another study, lycopene inhibited

334

proliferation and induced differentiation of mouse osteoblasts [48].

We conducted a pilot study to investigate the biological and clinical effects of lycopene supplementation on the prostate tissues and on serum levels of PSA, IGF-1 and IGFBP-3 in patients with localized prostate cancer [80]. We hypothesized that lycopene supplementation would decrease growth and induce apoptosis in premalignant and malignant prostate cells by up-regulating tissue Cx43 level, decreasing serum IGF-1 level and decreasing the ratio of bcl-2/bax in patients with localized prostate cancer. In a randomized clinical trial, we enrolled 35 men with clinical stages T1- or T2-localized prostate cancer, who were scheduled to undergo radical prostatectomy.

Data were collected from 26 subjects who were assigned to the lycopene arm ($n = 15$) or the control arm ($n = 11$) of the study. Nine patients were excluded because they had incorrect diagnosis (1 patient), or dropped out after randomization (2 patients) or had prior hormone therapy (6 patients). Detailed description of the methodology and the results of this trial have been published elsewhere [80].

Subjects were randomly assigned to receive either a tomato extract (Table 2) with 15 mg lycopene (Lyc-O-Mato® gel capsules, LycoRed Company, Beer Sheva, Israel) twice daily with meals or no supplement for 3 weeks prior to surgery. Biomarker studies were performed on blood samples collected at baseline and after 3 weeks of intervention prior to radical prostatectomy. At the time of surgery, entire prostate glands were resected and specimens were evaluated for pathologic stage, the volume of prostate cancer as well as the extent of HGPIN. Tissue levels of Cx43, bcl-2 and

Table 2. Contents of Lyc-O-Mato® capsules containing natural tomato extract

Contents	Percentage (w : w) in 250 mg tomato extract
Carotenoids	
Lycopene	5.8–6.2
Phytoene	0.5–0.7
Phytofluene	0.5–0.6
Beta-carotene	0.1–0.2
Total	6.9–7.7
Other components	
Tocopherols	1.5–2.5
Phospholipids	14–16
Phytosterols	0.5–0.7
Tomato oil	73–76

bax were assessed by Western analysis in benign and malignant areas of the tissue samples. Plasma and tissue levels of carotenoids were measured by HPLC. Plasma levels of IGF-1 and IGFBP-3 were measured by ELISA assay. Peripheral blood lymphocyte levels of 5-hydroxy-methyl-deoxyuridine (5-OHmdU) were measured by gas chromatography–mass spectrometry.

Changes in biological and clinical parameters after 3 weeks of Lyc-O-Mato® supplementation are shown in Table 3. Mean plasma PSA levels decreased by 18% in the intervention group, while it increased by 14% in the control group over the study period ($p = 0.22$). In the intervention group, 11 of 15 patients (73%) had tumor confined to the prostate, compared to 2 of 11 patients (18%) in the control group ($p = 0.02$). Twelve of fifteen patients (80%) in the lycopene group had tumors that measured 4 cc or less, compared to 5 of 11 (45%) in the control group ($p = 0.22$). Multifocal and/or diffuse involvement by HGPIN was observed in 10 of 15 subjects (67%) in the lycopene group, compared to all 11 subjects (100%) in the control group ($p = 0.05$).

Prostate cancer tissue was available for analysis in 4 subjects from the lycopene group and in 4 subjects from the control group. The level of Cx43 protein was 0.63 ± 0.19 optical density (OD) units in the lycopene group compared to the 0.25 ± 0.08 OD units in the control group ($p = 0.13$). The expression of cell cycle regulatory proteins, bcl-2 and bax, were not significantly different between the two groups, although bax level of the lycopene group (1.05 ± 0.29) was higher than the control group (0.68 ± 0.18).

Benign tissue was available for biomarker analysis in 8 subjects in the intervention group and 6 subjects in the control group. Prostatic tissue lycopene levels were 47% higher in the intervention group (0.53 ± 0.03 ng/gm of prostate tissue) compared to control group (0.36 ± 0.06), which was a significant difference ($p = 0.02$) despite the small number of samples ($n = 8$). Cx43 level was 0.64 ± 0.12 in the lycopene group compared to 0.51 ± 0.10 in the control group. The expression of bcl-2 was 0.63 ± 0.04 in the intervention group and 0.58 ± 0.04 in the control group, and the expression of bax was 0.62 ± 0.10 in the intervention group and 0.79 ± 0.11 in the control group.

Plasma samples were available from 13 subjects in the intervention group and 10 subjects in the control group. Mean plasma levels of IGF-1 decreased from 233 ± 21 to 169 ± 23 ng/ml in the lycopene group ($p = 0.0002$) and from 199 ± 20 to 140 ± 16 ng/ml in the control group ($p = 0.0003$). Interestingly,

Table 3. Post-treatment clinical and biological endpoints in the Lyc-O-Mato®[a] ($n = 15$) and control ($n = 11$) groups

	Lyc-O-Mato®	Control	p
Serum PSA (mean $\pm$ SE[b], ng/ml)	5.6 ± 0.9	7.7 ± 1.8	0.25[c]
Prostate HGPIN[d] (n)			
Focal	5	0	
Multifocal/diffuse	10	11	0.05
Prostate tumor volume (cm^3)			
$4\leq$	12	5	
>4	3	6	0.22
Surgical stage (n)			
Confined to prostate	11	2	
Not confined to prostate[e]	4	9	0.02
Prostate lycopene level (ng/gm tissue)	0.53 ± 0.03 ($n = 4$)	0.36 ± 0.06 ($n = 4$)	0.02
Prostate Cx43 expression (absorbance[f])			
In tumor tissue	0.63 ± 0.19	0.25 ± 0.08	0.13
In benign tissue	0.64 ± 0.04 ($n = 4$)	0.51 ± 0.10 ($n = 4$)	0.44
Prostate bax expression			
In tumor tissue	1.05 ± 0.29	0.68 ± 0.18	0.33
In benign tissue	0.62 ± 0.10 ($n = 4$)	0.79 ± 0.11 ($n = 4$)	0.28
Prostate bcl-2 expression			
In tumor tissue	0.54 ± 0.01	0.51 ± 0.06	0.59
In benign tissue	0.63 ± 0.04 ($n = 4$)	0.58 ± 0.04 ($n = 4$)	0.31
Prostate bax/bcl-2 ratio			
In tumor tissue	1.94	1.33	
In benign tissue	0.98	1.36	

[a]Lyc-O-Mato® is a tomato extract. See Table 2 for its composition.

[b]SE denotes standard error.

[c]p value is for comparing the change from pre- to post-intervention PSA in the two groups.

[d]HGPIN denotes high grade prostatic intraepithelial neoplasia.

[e]Resection margins are positive and/or extra-prostatic invasion is present.

[f]Absorbance corrected for expression of β-actin.

IGFBP-3 levels also decreased in both intervention and control groups during the study period. Plasma IGFBP-3 levels of the intervention group decreased from 5230 to 3924 ng/ml and control group decreased from 5200 to 4070 ng/ml, which were statistically significant ($p = 0.0002$ and $p = 0.0001$, respectively). In the intervention group, plasma lycopene level increased in 5 of 11 patients, whereas only 1 of 6 subjects in the control group had an increase (Fisher's exact test, $p = 0.33$). The level of post-intervention plasma lycopene was 23.5 μg/dL in the intervention group and 17.5 μg/dL in the control group ($p = 0.15$). However, there was no significant difference between the two groups with regard to percent change of plasma lycopene level, due to great variability in plasma lycopene levels and small numbers of subjects in each group. Peripheral blood lymphocyte levels of 5-OHmdU were similar in both groups before and after intervention.

The lycopene preparation that was used in this study was a mixture of tomato carotenoids and other tomato phytochemicals (Table 2). Although lycopene was the predominant carotenoid in the capsules, there were significant amounts of phytoene and phytofluene and other bioactive compounds. It is possible that the combination of the phytochemicals present in the tomato extract was responsible for the observed clinical effects rather than lycopene alone. There are *in vitro* data suggesting synergistic effects of lycopene with phytoene, phytofluene and beta-carotene against prostate cancer cells [81].

The differences observed in the bioavailability and the response to Lyc-O-Mato® preparation in this study are not easily explained, because the preparation contains the natural tomato oleoresin present in tomato matrix in the Lyc-O-Mato® capsules used in this study. Previous studies have shown excellent bioavailability of lycopene from this preparation [82]. However, it is possible that the fat and other nutrients in the diet might have influenced the bioavailablity of lycopene in our study population. In addition, ingestion of foods with lycopene (such as tomato, watermelon, pink grapefruit, guava), other carotenoids (β-carotene, lutein) and micronutrients (tocopherol, zinc, selenium, ascorbic acid) vary widely between individuals and also seasonally, which may have important interactions and influence the outcome of the study.

Genistein

Genistein is a soy isoflavone, a phytoestrogen found in soybeans [83,84]. It has a high affinity for estrogen receptor (ER)-β and low affinity for ER-α. The beneficial effects of estrogen, such as lowering of cholesterol and prevention of osteoporosis, are mediated by ER-β. Both antagonistic [85] and synergistic [86] effects have been observed between genistein and selective estrogen receptor modulator (SERM) tamoxifen in cell culture studies. Soy isoflavones have been of particular interest because of their possible cancer preventive effects as well as other beneficial health effects [87,88]. Epidemiologic studies have shown an inverse association between soy consumption and prostate cancer risk [89–92]. In addition, in some Asian countries with high soy consumption, the incidence of latent and small prostate carcinomas is the same as in Western countries; however, the mortality from clinically diagnosed prostate cancer is lower [93], suggesting that soy isoflavones may also inhibit the progression of prostate cancer.

The major soy isoflavones, genistein and daidzein, have been detected in human plasma, urine, feces, saliva, breast aspirate or cyst fluid, and prostatic fluid, and their bioavailability from oral consumption was demonstrated in women [94–98]. Mechanisms that have been proposed for the possible anti-carcinogenic effects of soy isoflavones include estrogen-like effects [99], prevention of oxidative DNA damage [100,101],

reduction in cancer cell proliferation [102], inhibition of angiogenesis [103], and modulation of steroid-metabolizing enzymes [104], tyrosine kinase [105], topoisomerase II [106], and signal transduction molecules [107].

We have previously observed that soy isoflavone genistein inhibits prostate cancer cell growth in culture in a dose-dependent manner which is accompanied by a G2/M cell cycle arrest [108]. Cell growth inhibition was observed with concomitant down-regulation of cyclin B, up-regulation of the p21[WAF1] growth inhibitory protein, and induction of apoptosis. Our recent data also show that TNF-α or H_2O_2-induced (oxidative stress) activation in NF-κB can be abrogated by genistein in prostate cancer cell lines [109] and by soy isoflavone supplementation in normal human volunteers [110].

Results of a phase II clinical study suggest that soy isoflavones are well tolerated and have evidence of significant clinical activity in patients with androgen-sensitive as well as -insensitive prostate cancer [111]. Disease stabilization was observed in 80% of hormone-sensitive patients and 30% of hormone-refractory patients. Soy isoflavones' biological activities mediated by their binding to estrogen and androgen receptors may explain the higher disease stabilization rate in patients with androgen-sensitive disease. However, the remarkable efficacy of soy isoflavones in hormone-refractory patients suggest that other mechanisms are also very important in the biological effects of soy isoflavones against prostate cancer.

Studies from our institution and others have demonstrated the *in vitro* effect of genistein on PSA synthesis and secretion by prostate cancer cells [112]. When LNCaP cells were treated *in vitro* with genistein, there was a significant decrease in the amount of PSA secretion. Immunohistochemistry and Western blot analysis suggested that this reduction was due to decreased PSA synthesis. In contrast, genistein did not alter the protein expression levels of another tumor-associated antigen, prostate-specific membrane protein [113]. These results indicate that the reduction of PSA level is a specific effect of genistein on PSA protein synthesis and secretion. In addition, genistein had *in vitro* growth-inhibitory and pro-apoptotic effects on hormone-dependent and -independent prostate cancer cells [108,112].

Considering that the effects of soy isoflavone supplementation on serum PSA were not known in the clinical setting, we conducted a phase II clinical trial to define the effects of soy isoflavone supplementation on prostate cancer and on serum PSA [111]. We found significant activity of soy isoflavones in patients with advanced prostate cancer. In addition, possible mechanisms of action of soy isoflavones were investigated by measuring blood DNA oxidation products and serum levels of IGF-1 and IGFBP-3.

In recent epidemiologic studies, relatively high plasma IGF-1 and low IGFBP-3 levels have been independently associated with greater risk of prostate cancer [113]. Two- to four-fold elevated risks have been observed for prostate cancer in men in the top quartile of IGF-1 relative to those in the bottom quartile, and low levels of IGFBP-3 were associated with an approximate doubling of risk. Insulin-like growth factors have mitogenic and anti-apoptotic effects on normal and transformed prostate epithelial cells [114,115]. Most circulating IGF-1 originates in the liver, but IGF bioactivity in tissues is related not only to circulating IGF and IGFBP levels, but also to local production of IGFs, IGFBPs, and IGFBP proteases [116]. Person-to-person variability in the levels of plasma IGF-1 and IGFBP-3 is considerable [117,118], and plasma IGF-1 levels appear to reflect heterogeneity in tissue IGF-1 bioactivity [119–121]. IGF-1 is an important mitogen for prostate cells. IGFBPs have opposing actions, in part by binding IGF-1, but also by direct inhibitory effects on target cells. As mitogens and anti-apoptotic agents, IGFs may be important in the development and progression of prostate cancer. However, in our clinical study, no significant change was observed in serum IGF-1 level and a significant decrease was observed in serum IGFBP-3 level [111]. The decrease in IGFBP-3 level after soy isoflavone supplementation is of concern. These findings have to be confirmed in larger studies.

Genistein is a potent antioxidant inhibiting the oxidation of low-density lipoprotein (LDL), alteration in electrophoretic mobility, and lipid hydroperoxides [122]. Healthy humans fed soy bars containing 36 mg genistein daily for 2 weeks exhibited large increases in plasma levels of genistein and reduced the susceptibility of LDL to oxidation [123]. Among selected isoflavones/flavones, genistein was the most potent inhibitor of oxidative DNA damage as measured by the formation of 8-hydroxy-2'-deoxyguanosine (8-OHdG) in HL-60 cells induced by TPA and $FeCl_2$ [101]. Similarly, Ruiz-Larrea et al. [124] found that genistein was the most potent antioxidant among a range of isoflavones, both in the aqueous and in the lipophilic phases. Cai and Wei [125] observed significant increases in the activities of antioxidant enzymes, catalase, superoxide dismutase, glutathione-S-transferase and glutathione peroxidase, in various tissues of mice

fed genistein in their diet. They also observed that genistein inhibited DNA oxidation [100]. Studies from our laboratory also suggested the antioxidant effect of genistein both *in vitro* [109] and in human volunteers [126]. In order to further elucidate the molecular mechanism by which genistein elicits its apoptotic effect, we investigated the role of a transcription factor, NF-κB, in the androgen-sensitive cell line LNCaP, and the androgen-insensitive cell line PC3 [109]. We showed that genistein decreases NF-κB DNA binding and abrogates NF-κB activation by oxidative stress inducing agents, H_2O_2 and TNF-α, in prostate cancer cells regardless of androgen sensitivity. Genistein's ability to abrogate NF-κB activation by oxidative stress inducing agents, strongly supports genistein's role as a cancer preventive agent. By inhibiting NF-κB activation, soy isoflavones may decrease proliferation of prostate cancer cells and serum PSA level. However, no significant change was observed in oxidative stress marker 5-OHmdU in our clinical study [111].

Omega-3 fatty acids

Diets high in animal fat are associated with an increased risk of prostate cancer, although the molecular mechanisms linking dietary fat to prostate cancer biology remain obscure. Animal fats are typically rich sources of arachidonic acid (either directly or through linoleic acid) and this fatty acid is converted to a wide range of powerful, biologically active compounds including leukotrienes and prostaglandins. Arachidonic acid (5,8,11,14-eicosatetraenoic acid), a member of the $n − 6$ PUFA's common in Western diet, was found to be an effective stimulator of human prostate cancer cell growth *in vitro* at micromolar concentrations [127]. Selective blockade of the different metabolic pathways of arachidonic acid (e.g. ibuprofen for cyclooxygenase, SKF-525A for cytochrome P-450, baicalein and BHPP for 12-lipoxygenase, AA861 and MK886 for 5-lipoxygenase, etc.) revealed that the growth stimulatory effect of arachidonic acid is inhibited by the 5-lipoxygenase specific inhibitors, AA861 and MK886, but not by others [127]. Addition of the eicosatetraenoid products of 5-lipoxygenase (5-hydroxyeicosatetraenoic acids (5-HETEs)) showed stimulation of prostate cancer cell growth similar to that of arachidonic acid, whereas the leukotrienes were ineffective. Moreover, the 5-series of eicosatetraenoids could reverse the growth inhibitory effect of MK886. Finally, prostate cancer cells fed with arachidonic acid showed a dramatic increase in the production of

5-HETEs, which is effectively blocked by MK886. These experimental observations suggested that arachidonic acid needed to be metabolized through the 5-lipoxygenase pathway to produce 5-HETE series of eicosatetraenoids for its growth stimulatory effects on human prostate cancer cells [128].

In another study, Ghosh and Myers [129,130] have reported that arachidonic acid stimulates proliferation of prostate cancer cells through production of the 5-lipoxygenase metabolite, 5-HETE. They also showed that 5-HETE is also a potent survival factor for human prostate cancer cells. These cells constitutively produce 5-HETE in serum-free medium with no added stimulus. Exogenous arachidonate markedly increases the production of 5-HETE. Inhibition of 5-lipoxygenase by MK886 completely blocks 5-HETE production and induces massive apoptosis in both hormone-responsive (LNCaP) and -nonresponsive (PC3) human prostate cancer cells. This cell death is very rapid: cells treated with MK886 showed mitochondrial permeability transition between 30 and 60 min, externalization of phosphatidylserine within 2 h, and degradation of DNA to nucleosomal subunits beginning within 2–4 h post-treatment. Cell death was effectively blocked by the thiol antioxidant, N-acetyl-L-cysteine, but not by androgen, a powerful survival factor for prostate cancer cells. Apoptosis was specific for 5-lipoxygenase. Programmed cell death was not observed with inhibitors of 12-lipoxygenase, cyclooxygenase, or cytochrome P450 pathways of arachidonic acid metabolism. Exogenous 5-HETE protects these cells from apoptosis induced by 5-lipoxygenase inhibitors, confirming a critical role of 5-lipoxygenase activity in the survival of these cells. These findings provide a possible molecular mechanism by which dietary fat may influence the progression of prostate cancer.

While epidemiological studies suggest an association between high intake of animal fat and an increased risk of prostate cancer development/progression, intake of fish oil has been associated with a reduced risk. Possible explanations for these observations include: (a) increased animal fat intake is associated with increased oxidative stress, while fish oil intake is associated with decreased oxidative stress [131]; (b) increased intake of animal fat is associated with increased arachidonic acid and eicasonoid levels, while fish oil intake is associated with decreased arachidonate and eicasonoid levels.

Despite the reported benefits associated with $n - 3$ fatty acids for cardiovascular disease, there remains concern that increased intake may lead to increased lipid peroxidation. To date, however, the data, particularly in vivo, are inconclusive. In contrast to previous reports, Mori et al. [131] demonstrated that $n - 3$ fatty acids reduce in vivo oxidant stress in humans. They reported the results of two interventions, one providing daily fish meals and the other eicosapentaenoic acid (EPA, $20 : 5$ $n - 3$) or docosahexaenoic acid (DHA, $22 : 6$ $n - 3$), the two principal omega-3 fatty acids in marine oils, in which in vivo lipid peroxidation was assessed by measurement of urinary excretion of F2-isoprostanes. In both trials, urinary F2-isoprostanes were significantly reduced by 20–27%.

Experimental studies suggest that the risk of prostate cancer is reduced with the intake of long-chain $n - 3$ polyunsaturated fatty acids derived from marine foods, such as EPA and DHA. However, few human studies have been conducted due to difficulties in assessing the dietary intake of these fatty acids. Norrish et al. [132] examined the relationship between prostate cancer risk and EPA and DHA in erythrocyte biomarkers in a population-based case-control study in Auckland, New Zealand during 1996–1997 involving 317 prostate cancer cases and 480 age-matched community controls. Reduced prostate cancer risk was associated with high erythrocyte phosphatidylcholine levels of EPA (multivariate relative risk $= 0.59$; 95% confidence interval 0.37–0.95, upper vs. lowest quartile) and DHA (multivariate relative risk $= 0.62$; 95% confidence interval 0.39–0.98, upper vs. lowest quartile). These analyses support evidence from in vitro experiments for a reduced risk of prostate cancer associated with dietary fish oils, possibly acting via inhibition of arachidonic acid-derived eicosanoid biosynthesis.

Herbs, dietary supplements and functional foods

One strategy in prostate cancer prevention may be the use of herbs, plant extracts, nutritional supplements and 'functional' foods as potential chemopreventive agents. Recently, a mixture of herbal compounds, PC-SPES, was found to be effective against prostate cancer [133]. Functional foods such as soymilk, tomato paste or fish oil may have significant amounts of bioactive compounds that may result in a chemopreventive effect. For example, an 8 ounce glass of soymilk may contain 38 mg of soy isoflavones, a cup of tomato paste may contain 30 mg of lycopene and a can of salmon or sardines may contain a large amount of omega-3 fatty acids. Soy isoflavones, lycopene and omega-3 fatty acids are excellent candidates as chemopreventive compounds in food extracts or whole foods for clinical investigation. Clinical trials should be conducted with functional foods as well as micronutrient supplements to investigate their potential cancer preventive activities, because the chemopreventive strategies would have a higher success rate if they provide a wider range of choices for different segments of the public. Some individuals may prefer supplements because of their life style or other personal restrictions, while others may prefer whole foods to increase the intake of important cancer preventive components of the diet.

Future studies

Dose response to lycopene, α-tocopherol, selenium and genistein should be investigated in subjects with localized prostate cancer scheduled for surgery or radiation, as well as subjects with high risk of disease, such as those with HGPIN or those with elevated PSA and negative biopsy. Clinical trials should be conducted in patients with HGPIN or elevated PSA but without a diagnosis of prostate cancer as they are at a high risk of developing prostate cancer or having occult disease. Lycopene could be compared to other promising agents such as vitamin E, selenium or soy in future clinical trials. We are currently conducting clinical trials investigating the effects of lycopene alone or in combination with soy isoflavones in patients with advanced prostate cancer. Because of the observed *in vitro* synergistic effects of tomato carotenoids against prostate cancer cells [81], we plan to conduct a clinical trial comparing the effects of pure lycopene with a mixture of tomato carotenoids (Lyc-O-Mato®) in patients with localized prostate cancer prior to prostatectomy. Lycopene should also be combined with vitamin E [36] and selenium [134] in future clinical trials. To support this idea, synergistic effects have been observed between lycopene and α-tocopherol against prostate cancer cells [135].

Conclusions

Prostate cancer accounts for over 30% of all cancer in men. Although, curative treatments exist they are associated with significant morbidity and a significant number of men still succumb to this deadly disease every year. Preventing the development of prostate cancer through chemopreventive strategies may be possible. Therefore, investigating how micronutrients and phytochemicals can reduce prostate cancer risk

is an important step in the right direction. A modest future investment in this area of research should pay a high dividend by preventing millions of men from developing this disease. Although there are no proven chemopreventive agents approved for human use by FDA, two large clinical trials supported by the National Cancer Institute should produce much needed information regarding some of the most promising preventive agents such as finasteride, selenium and vitamin E.

References

1. Greenlee RT, Hill-Harmon MB, Murray T, Thun M: Cancer statistics. CA Cancer J Clin 51: 15–36, 2001
2. Sakr WA, Haas GP, Cassin BJ, Pontes JE, Crissman JD: The frequency of carcinoma and intraepithelial neoplasia of the prostate in young male patients. J Urol 150: 379–385, 1993
3. Greenwald P, Lieberman R: Chemoprevention trials for prostate cancer. In: Chung L, Isaacs W, Simons J (eds) Prostate Cancer in the Twenty-First Century, Humana Press Inc, Totowa, NJ 2001, pp 499–518
4. Kelloff GJ, Lieberman R, Brawer MK, Crawford ED, Miller G: Strategies for chemoprevention of prostate cancer. Prostate Cancer and Prostate Dis 2: 27–33, 1999
5. Tsai H, Werber J, Davia MO, Edelman M, Tanaka KE, Melman A, Christ GJ, Geliebter J: Reduced connexin 43 expression in high grade, human prostatic adenocarcinoma cells. Biochem Biophys Res Commun 22: 64–69, 1996
6. Mehta PP, Lokeshwar BL, Schiller PC, Bendix MV, Ostenson RC, Howard GA, Roos BA: Gap-junctional communication in normal and neoplastic prostate epithelial cells and its regulation by cAMP. Mol Carcinog 15: 18–32, 1996
7. Mehta P, Perez-Stable C, Nadji M, Mian M, Asotra K, Roos BA: Suppression of human prostate cancer cell growth by forced expression of connexin genes. Develop Gene 24: 91–110, 1999
8. Mehta PP, Bertram JS, Loewenstein WR: Growth inhibition of transformed cells correlates with their junctional communication with normal cells. Cell 44: 187–196, 1986
9. Hossain MZ, Wilkens LR, Mehta PP, Loewenstein W, Bertram JS: Enhancement of gap junctional communication by retinoids correlates with their ability to inhibit neoplastic transformation. Carcinogenesis 10: 1743–1748, 1989
10. Zhang L-X, Cooney RV, Bertram JS: Carotenoids up-regulate connexin 43 gene expression independent of their pro-vitamin A or antioxidant properties. Cancer Res 52: 5707–5712, 1992
11. Rogers M, Berestecky JM, Hossain MZ, Guo HM, Kadle R, Nicholson BJ, Bertram JS: Retinoid-enhanced gap junctional communication is achieved by increased levels of connexin 43 mRNA and protein. Mol Carcinog 3: 335–343, 1990

12. Goldberg GS, Bertram JS: Retinoids, gap junctional communication and suppression of epithelial tumors. In Vivo 8: 745–754, 1994

13. Zhang L-X, Cooney RV, Bertram JS: Carotenoids enhance gap junctional communication and inhibit lipid peroxidation in C3H/10T1/2 cells: Relationship to their cancer chemopreventive action. Carcinogenesis 12: 2109–2114, 1991

14. Bertram JS, Pung A, Churley M, Kappock TJ 4th, Wilkins LR, Cooney RV: Diverse carotenoids protect against chemically induced neoplastic transformation. Carcinogenesis 12: 671–678, 1991

15. Rajah R, Valentinis B, Cohen P: Insulin-like growth factor (IGF)-binding protein-3 induces apoptosis and mediates the effects of transforming growth factor-beta-1 on programmed cell death through a p53- and IGF-independent mechanism. J Biol Chem 272: 12181–12188, 1997

16. Cohen P, Peehl DM, Rosenfeld RG: The IGF axis in the prostate. Hormone Metab Res 26: 81–84, 1994

17. Cohen P, Peehl DM, Lamson G, Rosenfeld RG: Insulin-like growth factors (IGFs), IGF receptors, and IGF-binding proteins in primary cultures of prostate epithelial cells. J Clin Endocrinol Metab 73: 401–407, 1991

18. Chan JM, Stampfer MJ, Giovanucci E, Gann PH, Ma J, Wilkinson P, Hennekens CH, Pollak M: Plasma insulin-like growth factor-1 and prostate cancer risk: A prospective study. Science 279: 563–566, 1998

19. Giovannucci E: Insulin-like growth factor-I and binding protein-3 and risk of cancer. Horm Res 51(Suppl 3): 34–41, 1999

20. Mantzoros CS, Tzonou A, Signorello LB, Stampfer M, Trichopoulos D, Adami HO: Insulin-like growth factor-1 in relation to prostate cancer and benign prostatic hyperplasia. Br J Cancer 76: 1115–1118, 1997

21. Wolk A, Mantzoros CS, Andersson SO, Bergstrom R, Signorello LB, Lagiou P, Adami HO, Trichopoulos D: Insulin-like growth factor-1 and prostate cancer risk: A population-based, case-control study. J Natl Cancer Inst 90: 911–915, 1998

22. Pollak M, Beamer W, Zhang JC: Insulin-like growth factors and prostate cancer. Cancer Met Rev 17: 383–390, 1998–1999

23. Sharoni Y, Levy Y, et al. (Personal communication and unpublished observations)

24. Feigl P, Blumenstein B, Thompson I, Crowley J, Wolf M, Kramer BS, Coltman CA Jr, Brawley OW, Ford LG: Design of the prostate cancer prevention trial (PCPT). Control Clin Trials 16: 150–163, 1995

25. Cote RJ, Skinner EC, Salem CE, Mertes SJ, Stanczyk FZ, Henderson BE, Pike MC, Ross RK: The effect of finasteride on the prostate gland in men with elevated serum prostate specific antigen (PSA) levels. Brit J Cancer 78: 413–418, 1998

26. Evans BA, Griffiths K, Morton MS: Inhibition of 5 alpha-reductase in genital skin fibroblasts and prostate tissue by dietary lignans and isoflavonoids. J Endocrinol 147(2): 295–302, 1995

27. Hussain M, Sarkar F, Djuric Z, Pollak M, Banerjee M, Doerge D, Fontana J, Chinni S, Davis J, Forman J, Wood D, Kucuk O: Soy isoflavones in the treatment of prostate cancer. J Nutr 132(3): 575S–576S, 2002

28. Davis JN, Muqim N, Bhuiyan M, Kucuk O, Pienta KJ, Sarkar FH: Inhibition of prostate specific antigen expression by genistein in prostate cancer cells. Int J Oncol 16: 1091–1097, 2000

29. Davis JN, Singh B, Bhuiyan M, Sarkar FH: Genistein induced up-regulation of p21, down regulation of cyclin B and induction of apoptosis in prostate cancer cells. Nutr Cancer 32(3): 123–131, 1998

30. Mentor-Marcel R, Lamartiniere CA, Eltoum IE, Greenberg NM, Elgavish A: Genistein in the diet reduces the incidence of poorly differentiated prostatic adenocarcinoma in transgenic mice (TRAMP). Cancer Res 61(18): 6777–6782, 2001

31. Yoshizawa K, Willett WC, Morris SJ, Stampfer MJ, Spiegelman D, Rimm EB, Giovannucci E: Study of prediagnostic selenium level in toenails and the risk of advanced prostate cancer. J Natl Cancer Inst 90: 1219–1224, 1998

32. Clark LC, Combs GF Jr, Turnbull BW, Slate EH, Chalker DK, Chow J, Davis LS, Glover RA, Graham GF, Gross EG, Krongrad A, Lesher JL Jr, Park HK, Sanders BB Jr, Smith CL, Taylor JR: Effects of selenium supplementation for cancer prevention in patients with carcinoma of the skin. JAMA 276: 1957–1963, 1996

33. Clark LC, Dalkin B, Krongrad A, Combs GF Jr, Turnbull BW, Slate EH, Witherington R, Herlong JH, Janosko E, Carpenter D, Borosso C, Falk S, Rounder J: Decreased incidence of prostate cancer with selenium supplementation: Results of a double-blind cancer prevention trial. Br J Urol 81: 730–734, 1998

34. Cohen LA (ed): Selenium and cancer: Larry C. Clark memorial issue. Nutr Cancer 40: 1–78, 2001

35. Chan JM, Stampfer MJ, Ma J, Rimm EB, Willett WC, Giovannucci EL: Supplemental vitamin E intake and prostate cancer risk in a large cohort of men in the United States. Cancer Epidemiol Biomark Prev 8: 893–899, 1999

36. Heinonen OP, Albanes D, Virtamo J, Taylor PR, Huttunen JK, Hartman AM, Haapakoski J, Malila N, Rautalahti M, Ripatti S, Maenpaa H, Teerenhovi L, Koss L, Virolainen M, Edwards BK: Prostate cancer and supplementation with alpha-tocopherol and beta-carotene: Incidence and mortality in a controlled trial. J Natl Cancer Inst 90: 440–446, 1998

37. Alpha-Tocopherol Beta-Carotene Cancer Prevention Study Group, Heinonen OP, Huttunen JK, Albanes D: The effect of vitamin E and beta carotene on the incidence of lung cancer and other cancers in male smokers. N Engl J Med 330: 1029–1035, 1994

38. Kline K, Yu W, Sanders BG: Vitamin E: Mechanisms of action as tumor cell growth inhibitors. J Nutr 131: 161S–163S, 2001

39. Klein EA, Thompson IM, Lippman SM, Goodman PJ, Albanes D, Taylor PR, Coltman C: SELECT: The next prostate cancer prevention trial. Selenium and Vitamin E Cancer Prevention Trial. J Urol 166: 1311–1315, 2001

40. Giovannucci E, Clinton SK: Tomatoes, lycopene, and prostate cancer. Proc Soc Exp Biol Med 218: 129–139, 1998

41. Gann PH, Ma J, Giovannucci E, Willett W, Sacks FM, Hennekens CH, Stampfer MJ: Lower prostate cancer risk in men with elevated plasma lycopene levels: Results of a prospective analysis. Cancer Res 59: 1225–1230, 1999

42. Giovannucci E: Tomatoes, tomato-based products, lycopene, and cancer: Review of the epidemiologic literature. J Natl Cancer Inst 91: 317–331, 1999

43. Giovannucci E, Ascherio A, Rimm EB, Stampfer MJ, Colditz GA, Willett WC: Intake of carotenoids and retinol in relation to risk of prostate cancer. J Natl Cancer Inst 87: 1767–1776, 1995

44. Kelloff GJ, Lieberman R, Steele VE, Boone CW, Lubet RA, Kopelovitch L, Malone WA, Crowell JA, Sigman CC: Chemoprevention of prostate cancer: Concepts and strategies. Euro Urol 35: 342–350, 1999

45. Bertram JS: Carotenoids and gene regulation. Nutr Rev 57: 182–191, 1999

46. Amir H, Karas M, Giat J, Danilenko M, Levy R, Yermiahu T, Levy J, Sharoni Y: Lycopene and 1,25-dihydroxyvitamin D3 cooperate in the inhibition of cell cycle progression and induction of differentiation in HL-60 leukemic cells. Nutr Cancer 33: 105–112, 1999

47. Levy J, Bosin E, Feldman B, Giat Y, Miinster A, Danilenko M, Sharoni Y: Lycopene is a more potent inhibitor of human cancer cell proliferation than either alpha-carotene or beta-carotene. Nutr Cancer 24: 257–266, 1995

48. Park CK, Ishimi Y, Ohmura M, Yamaguchi M, Ikegami S: Vitamin A and carotenoids stimulate differentiation of mouse osteoblastic cells. J Nutr Sci Vitaminol 43: 281–296, 1997

49. Karas M, Amir H, Fishman D, Danilenko M, Segal S, Nahum A, Koifmann A, Giat Y, Levy J, Sharoni Y: Lycopene interferes with cell cycle progression and insulin-like growth factor I signaling in mammary cancer cells. Nutr Cancer 36: 101–111, 2000

50. Kucuk O, Sarkar F, Sakr W, Djuric Z, Khachik F, Pollak M, Bertram J, Grignon D, Banerjee M, Crissman J, Pontes E, Wood DP Jr: Lycopene supplementation in men with localized prostate cancer: Modulation of biomarkers and clinical endpoints. Cancer Epidemiol Biomarkers Prev 10: 861–868, 2001

51. Chan JM, Stampfer MJ, Giovannucci E, Gann PH, Ma J, Wilkinson P, Hennekens CH, Pollak M: Plasma insulin-like growth factor-1 and prostate cancer risk: A prospective study. Science 279: 563–566, 1998

52. Nickerson T, Pollak M, Huynh H: Castration-induced apoptosis in the rat ventral prostate is associated with increased expression of genes encoding insulin-like growth factor binding proteins 2,3,4 and 5. Endocrinology 139: 807–810, 1998

53. Miyake H, Pollak M, Gleave ME: Castration-induced up-regulation of insulin-like growth factor binding protein-5 potentiates insulin-like growth factor-I activity and accelerates progression to androgen independence in prostate cancer models. Cancer Res 60: 3058–3064, 2000

54. Giovannucci E: Insulin-like growth factor-I and binding protein-3 and risk of cancer. Horm Res 51(Suppl 3): 34–41, 1999

55. Rajah R, Khare A, Lee PD, Cohen P: Insulin-like growth factor-binding protein-3 is partially responsible for high-serum-induced apoptosis in PC-3 prostate cancer cells. J Endocrinol 163: 487–494, 1999

56. Mantzoros CS, Tzonou A, Signorello LB, Stampfer M, Trichopoulos D, Adami HO: Insulin-like growth factor-1 in relation to prostate cancer and benign prostatic hyperplasia. Br J Cancer 76: 1115–1118, 1997

57. Wolk A, Mantzoros CS, Andersson SO, Bergstrom R, Signorello LB, Lagiou P, Adami HO, Trichopoulos D: Insulin-like growth factor-1 and prostate cancer risk: A population-based, case-control study. J Natl Cancer Inst 90: 911–915, 1998

58. Pollak M, Beamer W, Zhang JC: Insulin-like growth factors and prostate cancer. Cancer Met Rev 17: 383–390, 1998–1999

59. Rajah R, Valentinis B, Cohen P: Insulin-like growth factor (IGF)-binding protein-3 induces apoptosis and mediates the effects of transforming growth factor-beta-1 on programmed cell death through a p53- and IGF-independent mechanism. J Biol Chem 272: 12181–12188, 1997

60. Matsushima-Nishiwaki R, Shidoji Y, Nishiwaki S, Yamada T, Moriwaki H, Muto Y: Suppression by carotenoids of microcystin-induced morphological changes in mouse hepatocytes. Lipids 30: 1029–1034, 1995

61. Zhang L-X, Cooney RV, Bertram JS: Carotenoids enhance gap junctional communication and inhibit lipid peroxidation in C3H/10T1/2 cells: Relationship to their cancer chemopreventive action. Carcinogenesis 12: 2109–2114, 1991

62. Bertram JS, Pung A, Churley M, Kappock TJ 4th, Wilkins LR, Cooney RV: Diverse carotenoids protect against chemically induced neoplastic transformation. Carcinogenesis 12: 671–678, 1991

63. Zhang L-X, Cooney RV, Bertram JS: Carotenoids up-regulate connexin43 gene expression independent of their pro-vitamin A or antioxidant properties. Cancer Res 52: 5707–5712, 1992

64. Hotz-Wagenblatt A, Shalloway D: Gap junctional communication and neoplastic transformation. Crit Rev Oncogenesis 4: 541–558, 1993

65. Bertram JS, Bortkiewicz H: Dietary carotenoids inhibit neoplastic transformation and modulate gene expression in mouse and human cells. Am J Clin Nutr 62(Suppl 6): 1327S–1336S, 1995

66. Hossain MZ, Wilkens LR, Mehta PP, Loewenstein W, Bertram JS: Enhancement of gap junctional communication by retinoids correlates with their ability to inhibit neoplastic transformation. Carcinogenesis 10: 1743–1748, 1989

67. Mehta PP, Bertram JS, Loewenstein WR: The actions of retinoids on cellular growth correlate with their actions on gap junctional communication. Cell Biol 108: 1053–1065, 1989

68. Beyer EC, Paul DL, Goodenough DA: Connexin43: A protein from rat heart homologous to a gap junction protein from liver. J Cell Biol 105: 2621–2629, 1987

69. Mehta PP, Bertram JS, Loewenstein WR: Growth inhibition of transformed cells correlates with their junctional communication with normal cells. Cell 44: 187–196, 1986

70. Loewenstein WR: Junctional intercellular communication and the control of growth. Biochem Biophys Acta 560: 1–65, 1979

71. Yamasaki H: Gap junctional intercellular communication and carcinogenesis. Carcinogenesis 11: 1051–1058, 1990

72. Chen S-C, Pelletier DB, Peng A, Boynton AL: Connexin43 reverses the phenotype of transformed cells and alters their expression of cyclin/cyclin-dependent kinases. Cell Growth Diff 6: 681–690, 1995

73. Gius D, Botero A, Shah S, Curry HA: Intracellular oxidation/reduction status in the regulation of transcription factors NF-kappaB and AP-1. Toxicol Lett 106: 93–106, 1999

74. Riso P, Pinder A, Santangelo A, Porrini M: Does tomato consumption effectively increase the resistance of lymphocyte DNA to oxidative damage? Am J Clin Nutr 69: 712–718, 1999

75. Rao AV, Fleshner N, Agarwal S: Serum and tissue lycopene and biomarkers of oxidation in prostate cancer patients: A case-control study. Nutr Cancer 33: 159–164, 1999

76. Jewell C, O'Brien NM: Effect of dietary supplementation with carotenoids on xenobiotic metabolizing enzymes in the liver, lung, kidney and small intestine of the rat. Br J Nutr 81: 235–242, 1999

77. Giovannucci E, Rimm EB, Liu Y, Stampfer MJ, Willett WC: A prospective study of tomato products, lycopene, and prostate cancer risk. J Natl Cancer Inst 94: 391–398, 2002

78. Hotz-Wagenblatt A, Shalloway D: Gap junctional communication and neoplastic transformation. Crit Rev Oncogenesis 4: 541–558, 1993

79. Chen L, Stacewicz-Sapuntzakis M, Duncan C, Sharifi R, Ghosh L, van Breemen R, Ashton D, Bowen PE: Oxidative DNA damage in prostate cancer patients consuming tomato sauce-based entrees as a whole-food intervention. J Natl Cancer Inst 93: 1872–1879, 2001

80. Kucuk O, Sarkar F, Sakr W, Djuric Z, Khachik F, Pollak M, Khachik F, Li YW, Banerjee M, Grignon D, Bertram JS, Crissman JD, Pontes EJ, Wood DP Jr: Phase II randomized clinical trial of lycopene supplementation before radical prostatectomy. Cancer Epidemiol Biomarkers Prev 10: 861–868, 2001

81. Sharoni Y, Levy Y, et al. (Personal communication and unpublished observations)

82. Rao AV, Agarwal S: Bioavailability and in vivo antioxidant properties of lycopene from tomato products and their possible role in the prevention of cancer. Nutr Cancer 31(3): 199–203, 1998

83. Wang TT, Sathyamoorthy N, Phang JM: Molecular effects of genistein on estrogen receptor mediated pathways. Carcinogenesis 17: 271–275, 1996

84. Cassidy A, Bingham S, Setchell KD: Biological effects of a diet of soy protein rich in isoflavones on the menstrual cycle of premenopausal women. Am J Clin Nutr 60: 333–340, 1994

85. Schwartz JA, Liu G, Brooks SC: Genistein-mediated attenuation of tamoxifen-induced antagonism from estrogen receptor-regulated genes. Biochem Biophys Res Commun 253: 38–43, 1998

86. Shen F, Xue X, Weber G: Tamoxifen and genistein synergistically down-regulate signal transduction and proliferation in estrogen receptor-negative human breast carcinoma MDA-MB-435 cells. Anticancer Res 19: 1657–1662, 1999

87. Tham DM, Gardner CD, Haskell WL: Clinical review 97: Potential health benefits of dietary phytoestrogens: A review of the clinical, epidemiological, and mechanistic evidence. J Clin Endocrinol Metab 83(7): 2223–2235, 1998

88. Anderson JJ, Anthony MS, Cline JM, Washburn SA, Garner SC: Health potential of soy isoflavones for menopausal women. Public Health Nutr 2(4): 489–504, 1999

89. Giovanucci E: Epidemiological characteristics of prostate cancer. Cancer 75(Suppl): 1766–1777, 1995

90. Shimizu H, Ross RK, Bernstein L, Yatani R, Henderson BE, Mack TM: Cancers of the prostate and breast among Japanese and white immigrants in Los Angeles County. Br J Cancer 63: 963–966, 1991

91. Mills PK, Beeson WL, Phillips RL, Fraser GE: Cohort study of diet, lifestyle, and prostate cancer in Adventist men. Cancer 64: 598–604, 1989

92. Rose DP, Boyar AP, Wynder EL: International comparison of mortality rates for cancer of the breast, ovary, prostate and colon, and per capita food consumption. Cancer 58: 2363–2371, 1986

93. Adlercreutz H: Phytoestrogens: Epidemiology and a possible role in cancer prevention. Environ Health Perspect 103(Suppl 7): 103–112, 1995

94. Adlercreutz H, Fotsis T, Lampe J, Wahala K, Makela T, Brunow G, Hase T: Quantitative determination of lignans and isoflavonoids in plasma of omnivorous and vegetarian women by isotope dilution gas chromatography-mass spectrometry. Scand J Clin Lab Invest 53(Suppl 215): 5–18, 1993

95. Adlercreutz H, Fotsis T, Bannwart C, Wahala K, Brunow G, Hase T: Isotope dilution gas chromatographic-mass spectrometric identification of genistein. Clinica Chimica Acta 199: 263–278, 1991

96. Adlercreutz H, Fotsis T, Kurzer MS, Wahala K, Makela T, Hase T: Isotope dilution gas chromatographic-mass spectrometric method for the determination of unconjugated lignans and isoflavonoids in human feces with preliminary results in omnivorous and vegetarian women. Anal Biochem 225: 101–108, 1995

97. Finlay EMH, Wilson DW, Adlercreutz H, Griffiths K: The identification and measurement of phyto-estrogens in human saliva, plasma, breast aspirate or cyst fluid, and prostatic fluid using gas chromatography-mass spectrometry. J Endocrinol 129(Suppl): 49, 1991

98. Setchell KDR, Brown NM, Desai P, Zimmer-Nechemias L, Wolfe BE, Brashear WT, et al.: Bioavailability of pure isoflavones in healthy adults and analysis of commercial soy isoflavone supplements. J Nutr 131(Suppl): 1362S–1375S, 2001

99. Knight DC, Eden JA: A review of the clinical effects of phytoestrogens. Obstet Gynecol 87(5): 897–904, 1996

100. Wei H, Cai Q, Rahn RO: Inhibition of UV light- and Fenton reaction-induced oxidative DNA damage by the soybean isoflavone genistein. Carcinogenesis 17: 73–77, 1996

343

101. Giles D, Wei H: Effect of structurally related flavones/isoflavones on hydrogen peroxide production and oxidative DNA damage in phorbol ester-stimulated HL-60 cells. Nutr Cancer 29: 77–82, 1997

102. Shao Z, Alpaugh M, Fontana J, Barsky S: Genistein inhibits proliferation similarly in estrogen receptor-positive and negative breast carcinoma cell lines characterized by p21^{WAF1} induction, G2/M arrest and apoptosis. J Cell Biochem 69: 44–54, 1998

103. Fotsis T, Pepper M, Adlercreutz H, Fleischmann G, Hase T, Montesano R, Schweigerer L: Genistein, a dietary-derived inhibitor of in vitro angiogenesis. Proc Natl Acad Sci USA 90: 2690–2694, 1993

104. Wong CK, Keung WM: Bovine adrenal 3beta-hydroxy-steroid dehydrogenase (E.C. 1.1.1. 145)/5-ene-4-ene isomerase (E.C. 5.3.3.1): characterization and its inhibition by isoflavones. J Steroid Biochem Mol Biol 71(5–6): 191–202, 1999

105. Akiyama T, Ishida J, Nakagawa S, Ogawara H, Watanabe S, Itoh N, et al.: Genistein, a specific inhibitor of tyrosine-specific protein kinase. J Biol Chem 262: 5592–5595, 1987

106. Okura A, Arakawa H, Oka H, Yoshinari T, Monden Y: Effect of genistein on topoisomerase activity and on the growth of [val 12] Ha-ras transformed NIH 3T3 cells. Biochem Biophys Res Comm 57: 183–189, 1998

107. Axelsson L, Hellberg C, Melander F, Smith D, Zheng L, Andersson T: Clustering of beta(2)-integrins on human neutrophils activates dual signaling pathways to PtdIns 3-kinase. Exp Cell Res 256(1): 257–263, 2000

108. Davis JN, Singh B, Bhuiyan M, Sarkar FH: Genistein-induced upregulation of p21WAF1, downregulation of cyclin B, and induction of apoptosis in prostate cancer cells. Nutr Cancer 32: 123–131, 1998

109. Davis JN, Kucuk O, Sarkar FH: Genistein inhibits NF-kappaB activation in prostate cancer cells. Nutr Cancer 35: 167–174, 1999

110. Davis JN, Kucuk O, Djuric Z, Sarkar FH: Soy isoflavone supplementation in healthy men prevents NF-kappaB activation by TNF-alpha in blood lymphocytes. Free Rad Biol Med 30(11): 1293–1302, 2001

111. Hussain M, Sarkar F, Djuric Z, Pollak M, Banerjee M, Doerge D, Fontana J, Chinni S, Davis J, Forman J, Wood D, Kucuk O: Soy isoflavones in the treatment of prostate cancer. J Nutr 132(3): 575S–576S, 2002

112. Davis JN, Muqim N, Bhuiyan M, Kucuk O, Pienta KJ, Sarkar FH: Inhibition of prostate specific antigen expression by genistein in prostate cancer cells. Int J Oncol 16: 1091–1097, 2000

113. Chan JM, Stampfer MJ, Giovanucci E, Gann PH, Ma J, Wilkinson P, et al.: Plasma insulin-like growth factor-1 and prostate cancer risk: A prospective study. Science 279: 563–566, 1998

114. Cohen P, Peehl DM, Rosenfeld RG: The IGF axis in the prostate. Hormone Metab Res 26: 81–84, 1994

115. Cohen P, Peehl DM, Lamson G, Rosenfeld RG: Insulin-like growth factors (IGFs), IGF receptors, and IGF-binding proteins in primary cultures of prostate epithelial cells. J Clin Endocrinol Metab 73: 401–407, 1991

116. Jones JI, Clemmons DR: Insulin-like growth factors and their binding proteins: Biological actions. Endocr Rev 16: 3–34, 1995

117. Juul A, Bang P, Hertel NT, Main K, Dalgaard P, Jorgensen K, et al.: Serum insulin-like growth factor-I in 1030 healthy children, adolescents, and adults: Relation to age, sex, stage of puberty, testicular size, and body mass index. J Clin Endocrinol Metab 78: 744–752, 1994

118. Juul A, Dalgaard P, Blum WF, Bang P, Hall K, Michaelsen KF, et al.: Serum levels of insulin-like growth factor (IGF)-binding protein-3 (IGFBP-3) in healthy infants, children, and adolescents: The relation to IGF-I, IGF-II, IGFBP-1, IGFBP-2, age, sex, body mass index, and pubertal maturation. J Clin Endocrinol Metab 80: 2534–2542, 1995

119. Pollak M, Costantino J, Polychronakos C, Blauer SA, Guyda H, Redmond C, et al.: Effect of tamoxifen on serum insulin-like growth factor I levels in stage I breast cancer patients. J Natl Cancer Inst 82: 1693–1697, 1990

120. Huynh H, Yang X, Pollak M: Estradiol and antiestrogens regulate a growth inhibitory insulin-like growth factor binding protein 3 autocrine loop in human breast cancer cells. J Biol Chem 271: 1016–1021, 1996

121. Huynh H, Yang X, Pollak M: A role for insulin-like growth factor binding protein 5 in the antiproliferative action of the antiestrogen ICI 182780. Cell Growth Differ 7: 1501–1506, 1996

122. Kapiotis S, Hermann M, Held I, Seelos C, Ehringer H, Gmeiner BM: Genistein, the dietary-derived angiogenesis inhibitor, prevents LDL oxidation and protects endothelial cells from damage by atherogenic LDL. Arteriosclerosis, Thrombosis Vascular Biol 17: 2868–2874, 1997

123. Tikkanen MJ, Wahala K, Ojala S, Vihma V, Adlercreutz H: Effect of soybean phytoestrogen intake on low density lipoprotein oxidation resistance. Proc Natl Acad Sci USA 95: 3106–3110, 1998

124. Ruiz-Larrea MB, Mohan AR, Paganga G, Miller NJ, Bolwell GP, Rice-Evans CA: Antioxidant activity of phytoestrogenic isoflavones. Free Radical Research 26: 63–70, 1997

125. Cai Q, Wei H: Effect of dietary genistein on antioxidant enzyme activities in SENCAR mice. Nutr Cancer 25: 1–7, 1996

126. Djuric Z, Chen G, Doerge D, Heilbrun L, Kucuk O: Effect of soy isoflavone supplementation on oxidative stress in men and women. Cancer Lett 172: 1–6, 2001

127. Ghosh J, Myers CE: Arachidonic acid stimulates prostate cancer cell growth: Critical role of 5-lipoxygenase. Biochem Biophys Res Commun 235: 418–423, 1997

128. Hayes RB, Ziegler RG, Gridley G, Swanson C, Greenberg RS, Swanson GM, Schoenberg JB, Silverman DT, Brown LM, Pottern LM, Liff J, Schwartz AG, Fraumeni JF Jr, Hoover RN: Dietary factors and risks for prostate cancer among blacks and whites in the United States. Cancer Epidemiol Biomarkers Prev 8: 25–34, 1999

129. Ghosh J, Myers CE: Inhibition of arachidonate 5-lipoxy-genase triggers massive apoptosis in human prostate cancer cells. Proc Natl Acad Sci USA 95: 13182–13187, 1998

344

130. Myers CE, Ghosh J: Lipoxygenase inhibition in prostate cancer. Eur Urol 35: 395–398, 1999

131. Mori TA, Puddey IB, Burke V, Croft KD, Dunstan DW, Rivera JH, Beilin LJ: Effect of Omega-3 fatty acids on oxidative stress in humans: GC-MS measurement of urinary F2-isoprostane excretion. Redox Rep 5: 45–46, 2000

132. Norrish AE, Skeaff CM, Arribas GL, Sharpe SJ, Jackson RT: Prostate cancer risk and consumption of fish oils: A dietary biomarker-based case-control study. Br J Cancer 81: 1238–1242, 1999

133. DiPaola RS, Zhang H, Lambert GH, Meeker R, Licitra E, Rafi MM, Zhu BT, Spaulding H, Goodin S, Toledano MB, Hait WN, Gallo MA: Clinical and biologic activity of an estrogenic herbal combination (PC-SPES) in prostate cancer. N Engl J Med 339: 785–791, 1998

134. Clark LC, Dalkin B, Krongrad A, Combs GF Jr, Turnbull BW, Slate EH, Witherington R, Herlong JH, Janosko E, Carpenter D, Borosso C, Falk S, Rounder J: Decreased incidence of prostate cancer with selenium supplementation: Results of a double-blind cancer prevention trial. Br J Urol 81(5): 730–734, 1998

135. Pastori M, Pfander H, Boscoboinik D, Azzi A: Lycopene in association with alpha-tocopherol inhibits at physiological concentration proliferation of prostate carcinoma cells. Biochem Biophys Res Commun 250(3): 582–585, 1998

Address for offprints: Omer Kucuk, Professor of Medicine and Oncology, Barbara Ann Karmanos Cancer Institute, Wayne State University, 3990 John R, 5 Hudson, Detroit, MI 48201, USA; *Tel*: (313) 745-2748; *Fax*: (313) 993-0559; *e-mail*: kucuko@karmanos.org

Prostate brachytherapy

William J. Ellis
Department of Urology, University of Washington, Seattle, Washington, USA

Key words: prostatic neoplasms, radiotherapy, brachytherapy, adenocarcinoma, patient selection

Summary

Prostate brachytherapy has been practiced for nearly 100 years in various forms. However, technological advances over the past 20 years in imaging, computing, and devices have propelled this technique into the mainstream of prostate cancer treatments. A discussion of radiobiology principles is important to the understanding of modern brachytherapy technique. For low risk tumors, brachytherapy may be administered as monotherapy. For high risk tumors combination therapy with external beam therapy is indicated. Androgen ablation therapy is used for hormonal downsizing or for select high risk tumors. Diseases free survival appears similar to that seen with other definitive therapies for clinically localized prostate cancer. The short term morbidity of the procedure includes significant obstructive and irritative voiding symptoms. Future brachytherapy goals are discussed.

Introduction

Prostate brachytherapy, popularly known as prostate seed implantation, is a technique whereby small radiation implants are distributed within the prostate itself. While the basic technique has been practiced for decades, the procedure has enjoyed a resurgence in popularity in the past decade due to advances in imaging, computing, and medical devices.

History

Local application of radiation sources was first introduced by Pasteau in 1911, who used radium sources. Early techniques generally involved insertion of needles transperineally under digital guidance. Alternative applications, including insertion of urethral or rectal sources were also introduced. In 1950s, Flocks reported his experience with colloidal gold [1]. However, with the development of modern linear accelerators, external beam radiation became the primary modality of prostate irradiation.

In 1972, Whitmore reported his landmark procedure of retropubic I 125 implantation into the prostate [2]. This technique became the standard of prostate brachytherapy for the next 20 years. Through a lower abdominal incision the prostate was exposed in the retropubic space. The total dose of radiation, and by extension the number of seeds, was calculated from an estimation of the prostate volume. The seeds were then implanted into the prostate through needles passed parallel to one another at 0.5–1.0-cm intervals. Placement of the needles was confirmed by palpation of the needle tips through the rectum. In initial studies, the technique appeared very promising. Carleton adopted a similar approach to implantation of Au 198 seeds. However, the long-term results with this free-hand approach were disappointing. Follow-up of Whitmore's patients showed a biochemical diseased free rate of only 13% at 15 years [3]. In retrospect, the failure of this technique stemmed from the imprecise placement of the seeds within the prostate.

The problem of accurate seed placement was addressed by Holm in the early 1980s. Holm applied the new imaging modality of transrectal ultrasound to prostate brachytherapy and developed a technique of implanting the seeds under real-time guidance to pre-determined three-dimensional coordinates [4]. The basic technique developed by Holm is the most commonly used technique today. Ultrasound was used to obtain treatment planning images at 5 mm intervals through the prostate. These images allowed for much more accurate dosimetric calculations than the previous

M.L. Cher, K.V. Honn and A. Raz (eds.), Prostate Cancer: New Horizons in Research and Treatment, 345–349.
© 2002 *Kluwer Academic Publishers.*

nomograms based on prostate volume. Accurate needle placement was facilitated by the use of a template system with a coordinated system of holes drilled at 5 mm intervals. These techniques led to the precise minimally invasive technique of modern brachytherapy.

Technological advances have been responsible for most of the refinements of prostate brachytherapy. Transrectal ultrasound has been continually improved over the past two decades, allowing accurate real-time imaging as the seeds are placed. Equipment ranging from needles to stepping units has been developed and improved to support the procedure. Modern computers and software programs now allow sophisticated dosimetry to be calculated on personal computers so treatment plans can be individualized in a relatively short time frame. The software can be purchased from vendors specializing in this application. CT based imaging is able to accurately determine the final resting position of seeds with great accuracy. Based on these post-treatment images the actual dosimetry can be recalculated as a means of quality control.

Radiation principles

At the most simplistic level, radiation therapy is a form of electromagnetic energy applied to tumors. The putative target is DNA, which may be damaged either by direct effect or indirectly through the generation of free radicals. Rarely a cell will be damaged to the extent that it is killed within a short time. More typically, the cell suffers a loss of reproductive integrity. The cells then may die when attempting to divide, or produce daughter cells which will die upon attempted division. Thus, in the absence of cell division, the cell may live for quite some time before it ultimately dies. This can cause some difficulty in interpreting post-radiation biopsies.

Several factors regulate the efficacy of radiation therapy. The percentage of cells killed is related to radiation dose. Increasing the radiation dose increases the probability of all cells receiving a lethal dose. The radiation effect is cell cycle dependent. Cells are most sensitive to radiation in M and G2, and least sensitive in S phase. Many cells have the ability to repair even lethal DNA damage. Since cell death may not occur until mitosis, cells with slower doubling times (including normal cells) often are less radiosensitive, as they have more time for repair. Dose fractionation or continuous low radiation such as that used in permanent prostate dose rate decreases brachytherapy, improves cell kill in cells with better DNA repair mechanisms.

The therapeutic window attempts to exploit the differential radio-sensitivity of tumor and normal cells. The ultimate goal of radiotherapy is to lethally damage all cancer cells with minimal permanent damage to normal tissues.

Isotopes

Two isotopes, I 125 and Pd 103, are typically used for prostate brachytherapy. The key differences between the isotopes is their half-life which is 60 days for I 125 and 17 days for Pd 103. If one considers that the effective dose of radiation is largely delivered in the first three half-lives, then the duration of treatment can be estimated at 180 days for I 125 and 51 days for Pd 103. In order to achieve therapeutic doses, Pd 103 is administered at a much higher dose rate. The dose rate for an I 125 implant is approximately 10 cGy/h versus 24 cGy/h for Pd 103. Both are relatively low energy, 28 and 21 keV, respectively. Since tissue penetration is related to energy, I 125 has somewhat more penetration than Pd 103.

Two factors, seed strength and number determine the radiation dose to the target gland. With relatively few seeds, the dosimetry is dependent on precise placement of the point sources. Increasing the number of seeds decreases the contribution of each seed to the overall dose proportionately. With 75–100 seeds the array behaves more like a radiation 'cloud'. Implants of this many seeds are much more robust, as errors in the placement of an individual seed due to technical error or seed migration become relatively insignificant compared to the array as a whole.

In addition to using a large number of seeds, most modern implants employ a peripheral loading pattern. If implants are distributed homogeneously throughout the prostate, the radiation dose decreases radially from the center of the gland, as the center of the gland receives a contribution from many seeds compared to the periphery. The result is excessive urethral toxicity. A peripherally loaded implant will keep the central dose to within tolerable limits.

Technique

What will be described here is the permanent low dose brachytherapy approach. In order to adequately treat the prostate, the prostate volume must be captured in three dimensions so that the dosimetry may be calculated. Any form of cross-sectional imaging such as transrectal ultrasound, CT, or MRI may be used to capture these images. Normally transrectal ultrasound is used as this allows the images to be used in the operating room to align the prostate in the exact position relative to the grid coordinates that it was in for the treatment planning studies. Images of the prostate are captured at 5-mm increments from base to apex. The cross section of the prostate is identified at each level. Around the prostate a target is drawn with a margin around the actual prostate. These images are then transferred to the physicist for treatment planning.

The images are digitized into a computer and with treatment planning software a three-dimensional prostate is reconstructed. The physicist then determines the number of seeds and the three-dimensional coordinates of each seed. There are several seed distribution patterns, which will provide adequate dosimetry. The radiation oncologist works with the physicist to select the plan that optimizes the technical ease of the implants.

The treatment planning may also take place in the operating room immediately prior to the implant. Because there is a time constraint on planning the implant in this setting, pre-determined templates based on prostate volume are usually utilized. This results in less customization of the implant than with pre-planned implants. However dosimetry with both forms of planning is usually adequate.

The actual implant is accomplished under ultrasonic guidance. The prostate is aligned with the ultrasound equipment exactly as called for in the treatment plan. The needles are advanced to their proper three-dimensional coordinate within the prostate under real-time ultrasonic guidance. The seeds are then deposited at their assigned position within the prostate.

After the implant, the position of the seeds is confirmed. CT scanning is usually used for imaging the prostate. The seed coordinates are transferred into the treatment planning software, and the dosimetry is recalculated. If an implant is found to have under-treated a small area of the prostate, additional seeds may be implanted to correct the implant. Alternatively, if a large area of the prostate is undertreated, a supplemental course of external beam radiation may be appropriate.

Indications

Prostate brachytherapy is indicated for T1, T2 and select T3 tumors without evidence of metastatic dis-

ease. In certain cases as described below, brachytherapy may be combined with EBRT or hormonal therapy. The indications are similar to those of radical prostatectomy and external beam radiation. Prostate cancer has a long natural history. For older men with a life expectancy of less than 10 years, brachytherapy may not be indicated.

Combination therapy

Prostate brachytherapy may be combined with external beam radiation in select cases. Generally this combined therapy is used for higher risk disease with the intent of extending the treatment field and subjecting the prostate to a higher dose of radiation. Doses of the interstitial and external beam radiation must be modified with this approach, as combining full doses of each therapy would result in excessive toxicity. As a general rule, the implant and EBRT would be prescribed for approximately 75% and 60% of the typical monotherapy doses. There are two schools of thought regarding the sequence of treatment. Most physicians will initially treat with the external beam radiation and follow up with the permanent implant. With this schedule, the radiation is administered over a longer period of time, producing less toxicity. Alternatively, the EBRT may be administered after the implant. With this schedule the EBRT and brachytherapy are essentially administered simultaneously, potentially resulting in greater toxicity. However, the external beam schedule could be modified if the local toxicity is excessive.

Biologically, there is some controversy as to the value of combining treatment. Radical prostatectomy studies have suggested that microscopically visible extracapsular disease is confined to a radial distance of 4 mm from the prostate over 90% of the time [5]. Furthermore, relatively few patients fail monotherapy implants locally. Most fail with systemic disease. In this scenario the dose to the pelvic lymph nodes in the range of 45 cGy is relatively ineffective dose for prostate cancer.

A great value of the combination therapy is increasing the margin of safety in an implant. Certainly combination therapy results in greater dose homogeneity and can compensate for minor technical variations in seed placement. For this reason, we recommend that physicians be more liberal with combination therapy early in their experience with prostate brachytherapy. The prostate base and bladder neck is an area particularly vulnerable to under dosing with brachytherapy. In other areas of the prostate, seeds placed just outside the prostate will contribute to the dose applied to the prostate margin. However, at the prostate base, seeds placed just outside the prostate end up in the bladder. The margin for error for implants in this area is therefore much lower. Thus, combination therapy is often recommend for patients with extensive tumor at the base of the prostate.

Hormone therapy is used in three settings: (1) to downsize a large prostate in order to make the implant technically easier; (2) to reduce the severity or postoperative urinary symptoms; and (3) to combine the treatment effects of hormonal therapy and radiation therapy. A large prostate can be technically difficult to implant if some of the prostate tissue is inaccessible due to its location behind the bones of the pubic arch. Because the needles are directed into the prostate under the pubic arch, a large prostate may be partially 'covered' anterolaterally. Angulation of the needles will allow implantation in cases with minor arch interference. However, more severe arch interference may result in a technically inadequate implant. Hormonal downsizing will reduce pubic arch interference significantly.

Results and quality of life

As described earlier, long-term cancer control rates from the open implant technique of the 1970s were disappointing. The cancer control with modern prostate brachytherapy appears to be similar to radical prostatectomy for at least 10 years. Many studies suggest that 10-year disease free survival should be in the 85% range for tumors encountered with PSA levels of less than 10 ng/ml [6,7]. Most failures are distant.

Based on large published series, the overall cancer control rates and complication rates appear similar to that of radical prostatectomy. However, there are many variables in patient selection and follow-up, which make direct comparisons between radical prostatectomy and brachytherapy difficult. To that end, the American College of Surgeons Oncology Group has recently initiated a trial comparing radical prostatectomy with brachytherapy in the US and Canada. This is a randomized multi-center prospective trial comparing the two modalities in men with clinically localized tumors stages T1c and T2a with a PSA of less than 10 and a combined Gleason score of 6 or less.

Quality of life is an important consideration in prostate brachytherapy. The major complications are rectal, urinary, and sexual in nature. Most patients will experience transient rectal irritation manifested by more frequent looser stools and possibly painless bleeding. The symptoms are generally self-limited, but may be more severe in those receiving combined external beam radiation and brachytherapy. Long-term proctitis develops in 5% of men receiving brachytherapy as monotherapy and 15% of men receiving combination therapy.

Obstructive and irritative urinary symptoms are the most common side effect of prostate brachytherapy. The initial trauma of seed insertion causes prostatic swelling which can result in urinary obstruction or retention. Over a period of several weeks, the radiation causes irritation of the prostatic urethra to develop. This irritation presents as frequency, urgency, and dysuria. These irritative symptoms generally peak at 3–4 weeks post implant and the most bothersome symptoms resolve within 2–4 months. Complete urinary symptom resolution may take a year.

The cavernosal nerves which regulate erectile function course along the postero-lateral aspect of the prostate. These nerves, which can also be damaged by radical prostatectomy, receive a significant dose of radiation. This radiation induces a neurofibrosis, which is progressive over several years. With any prostate therapy, impotence rates are lower in younger men with better pre-treatment erectile function. Initial reports suggested that prostate brachytherapy produced significantly less impotence than surgery or external beam radiation. However, with longer follow-up, the rate of impotence appears similar to that of external beam radiation.

Future

The future of prostate brachytherapy is bright. This is a highly technical procedure, which was brought into the mainstream by technical advances in imaging, devices, and computing. All these disciplines will continue to advance the field. Probably the largest area of research is in the field of dosimetry. Intra-operative real-time pre- and post-operative dosimetry calculation, which could be accomplished in a reasonable time period, would be a major advance in prostate brachytherapy. Not only would patients be virtually guaranteed a high quality implant, but also the procedure would be much more convenient for the patient. Several techniques are under investigation. Intra-operative planning is much further advanced than post-operative dosimetry. Most intra-operative planning is based on activity per volume nomograms. Stock et al. [8] have described a technique whereby needle placement is captured by computer software to estimate dosimetry in real time. The Harvard group has devised a system of monitoring needle placement under MRI guidance [9]. However, like the pre-planned technique, these techniques still have inherent variability because prostates can be distorted by needle placement, and needle placement does not correlate perfectly with seed placement. Thus, what is truly needed is a system by which actual seed placement can be monitored in real time.

Intra-operative post-implant dosimetric calculation is a technical challenge. Since the goal of such dosimetry is to immediately correct any flaws in the implant, the process must be accurate and fast. The cost of operating suite time is on the order of $1000/h, and the anesthetic must be maintained until the calculations are performed. Trans-rectal ultrasound has many limitations in post-operative imaging. Seeds that have rotated from a perpendicular orientation to the ultrasound transducer may not be visualized, as they will not reflect the ultrasonic waves back to the transducer. Anterior seeds may also be poorly visualized due to acoustical interference from posterior seeds lying between anterior seeds and the rectal transducer. Foci of hemorrhage may produce echo patterns that mimic seeds. Finally, the prostate contour itself may be difficult to visualize due to seeds and hematoma formation. Technical advances in ultrasound may be able to accurately localize seeds in the post-operative setting. This could be through advances in either hardware or software. Increasing seed echogenicity has also been studied. This in theory will allow for better seed visualization.

CT and MRI are better imaging techniques for determining seed placement precisely. Portable units are now being developed which can be used in and operating room suite.

Investigations are ongoing relating dosimetry to brachytherapy complications. Decreasing the doses of radiation to these structures can minimize both impotence and urethral symptoms. With improved understanding of tissue responses to radiation and the amount of radiation necessary for tumor kill, dosimetry modifications may reduce complication rates without reducing cure rates.

Finally, devices for brachytherapy will undoubtedly improve in the future. These advances will lead to more rapid and more accurate distribution of radiation within the prostate. Ultimately, some type of robotic seed placement will become the implant technique of choice.

Conclusion

Prostate brachytherapy is a modern high technology method of prostate cancer control. The results obtained are competitive with other treatments of prostate cancer. As technology evolves, the field of prostate brachytherapy will continue to advance.

References

1. Flocks RH: Present status of interstitial irradiation in managing prostatic cancer. JAMA 210: 328–330, 1969
2. Whitmore WF Jr., Hilaris B, Grabstald H: Retropubic implantation to iodine 125 in the treatment of prostatic cancer. J Urol 108: 918–920, 1972
3. Zelefsky MJ, Whitmore WF Jr.: Long-term results of retropubic permanent 125iodine implantation of the prostate for clinically localized prostatic cancer. J Urol 158: 23–29, 1997
4. Holm HH, Juul N, Pedersen JF, Hansen H, Stroyer I: Transperineal 125iodine seed implantation in prostatic cancer guided by transrectal ultrasonography. J Urol 130: 283–286, 1983
5. Sohayda C, Kupelian PA, Levin HS, Klein EA: Extent of extracapsular extension in localized prostate cancer. Urology 55: 382–386, 2000
6. Critz FA, Levinson AK, Williams WH, Holladay DA, Holladay CT: The PSA nadir that indicates potential cure after radiotherapy for prostate cancer. Urology 49: 322–326, 1997
7. Grimm PD, Blasko JC, Sylvester JE, Meier RM, Cavanagh W: 10-year biochemical (prostate-specific antigen) control of prostate cancer with (125)I brachytherapy. Int J Radiat Oncol Biol Phys 51: 31–40, 2001
8. Stock RG, Stone NN, Lo YC: Intraoperative dosimetric representation of the real-time ultrasound-guided prostate implant. Tech Urol 6: 95–98, 2000
9. Cormack RA, Tempany CM, D'Amico AV: Optimizing target coverage by dosimetric feedback during prostate brachytherapy. Int J Radiat Oncol Biol Phys 48: 1245–1249, 2000

Address for offprints: William J. Ellis, Department of Urology, Box 356510, University of Washington, Seattle, Washington 98195, USA; *Tel:* (206) 543-3640; *Fax:* (206) 543-3272; *e-mail:* wjellis@u.washington.edu

Fast neutron irradiation for prostate cancer

Jeffrey D. Forman[1], Mark Yudelev[1], Susan Bolton[1], Sam Tekyi-Mensah[1] and Richard Maughan[2]
[1]Department of Radiation Oncology, Wayne State University, Detroit, MI; [2]Department of Radiation Oncology, University of Pennsylvania, Philadelphia, PA, USA

Key words: neutron radiation, prostate cancer, three-dimensional conformal radiation, high LED radiation

Abstract

The purpose of this study was to summarize the progress made using fast neutron irradiation in the treatment of prostate cancer at Wayne State University between 1991 and the year 2001. The results of three Phase II studies and one Phase III study involving nearly 700 patients is summarized in this paper. The Phase II studies were dose finding studies looking at doses of 15, 9, 10, and 11 nGy, respectively. The randomized protocol was a study of sequence looking at the results of treating patients with neutron first *versus* neutron radiation last. The results demonstrated that the best combination of tumor control probabilities and normal tissue complications was found in a mix of approximately 50% neutrons and 50% photons. Thus, the standard doses become 10 nGy and 40 Gy of photons. The randomized trial demonstrated that the sequence has significant importance and the disease-free survival was 93% for patients treated with neutrons first *versus* 73% for patients treated with neutrons last. There was no difference in the rate of acute or chronic complications. Finally, an analysis was performed demonstrating which patients may best benefit from the use of neutron irradiation. It was shown that patients with one, two, or three adverse risk factors had a significant improvement in disease-free survival when part of the treatment included neutron radiation *versus* standard photon radiation alone. Neutron radiation can be delivered safely with effort to see that it is superior to that which can be achieved by conformal photon irradiation by itself. Future work will be done to expand the role of neutron radiation in other clinical disease sites.

Introduction: The history of neutrons

The neutron was discovered by James Chadwick in 1932. Within 6 years neutrons had already been used to treat cancer patients. Although tumor responses were identified, the high normal tissue complication rates led investigators to consider neutrons to be unsuitable for clinical cancer treatment. Following this work there was a fallow period in the use of neutron irradiation until the 1960s. At that time Mary Catterall took advantage of what was known about the biological rationale for neutrons, i.e., that they were especially useful in large and slow growing cancers, and developed a clinical experience in which previously incurable patients were treated with neutrons with dramatic and often long lasting responses.

As a result of this pioneering work, many centers initiated trials including neutron irradiation therapy. However, there were serious limitations in machine design and availability. Most of the cyclotrons used during the 1970s were machines that were designed for either isotope production or physics research and were not designed specifically for patient care.

However, despite the equipment limitations, a number of randomized studies were initiated by the National Cancer Institute. Many patients with different types of tumors, were treated with mixtures of neutron and photon irradiation because of the limited access to the neutron machines on a daily basis. One study involved patients with locally advanced prostate cancer (stage T3N0/N1) and randomized them to a mixture of neutron and photon irradiation felt to be the normal tissue equivalent of 70 Gy in 7 weeks. This was compared to patients receiving the standard of photon irradiation of 70 Gy in 7 weeks. The 10-year overall survival of 49% for patients treated with mixed neutron and photon irradiation compared to 29% for the patients receiving photon irradiation alone. In addition,

M.L. Cher, K.V. Honn and A. Raz (eds.), Prostate Cancer: New Horizons in Research and Treatment, 351–355.
© 2002 *Kluwer Academic Publishers.*

352

there was no increase in normal tissue complication rates [1].

In response to this study, the National Cancer Institute sponsored a program in which $60 million was used to build four new neutron facilities. A new series of clinical trials was sponsored testing these new neutron facilities. Patients with locally advanced prostate cancer were randomized to either 70 Gy as the standard arm *versus* the experimental arm of 100% neutrons using a dose of 20.4 nGy in twelve fractions delivered in 4 weeks. This study demonstrated that the use of 100% neutron irradiation was associated with a significant increase in the overall complication rate. Patients treated with neutron irradiation alone had a 25% grade 3–4 complication rate compared to only 6% in the patients treated with photons alone [2]. Although there was a significant improvement in disease-free survival, biochemical disease-free survival and histologic control, there was no improvement in the overall survival. As a result of this, further trials involving neutron irradiation in this country were discontinued.

The Wayne State University experience

In 1991, a 10-year long project to develop a superconducting cyclotron to deliver fast neutrons was completed at Wayne State University in Detroit (Figure 1). The approach of this program involved the use of a state-of-the-art machine that allowed for the isocentric delivery of conformal neutron irradiation shaped with a unique multi-rod collimator combined with the benefits of three-dimensional treatment planning to optimize the delivery of neutron irradiation [3,4]. The cyclotron at Wayne State University relies on super-conducting technology which allows for a magnet which weighs only 25 tons. In this way, the entire cyclotron is able to rotate around the patient with a precision of rotation at the isocenter of 1 mm. This allows for fully conformal delivery of neutron irradiation [5].

A series of Phase II trials was initiated to determine the optimal dose and method of delivery of neutron irradiation. The initial dose used in the first Phase II study at Wayne State University was a dose of approximately 75% neutrons. In this study 15 nGy were combined with 18 photon Gy for an equivalent dose of 78 Gy to the prostate. The 58 patients entered on this study all had locally advanced disease. The 5 year rate of grade 3 GU and GI complications were 10% and 18%, respectively. In addition, 11% of patients had soft tissue injuries in and around the hips including fibrosis of the muscles characterized by hip stiffness.

Following this initial experience and high complication rate, the neutron doses were reduced. The doses

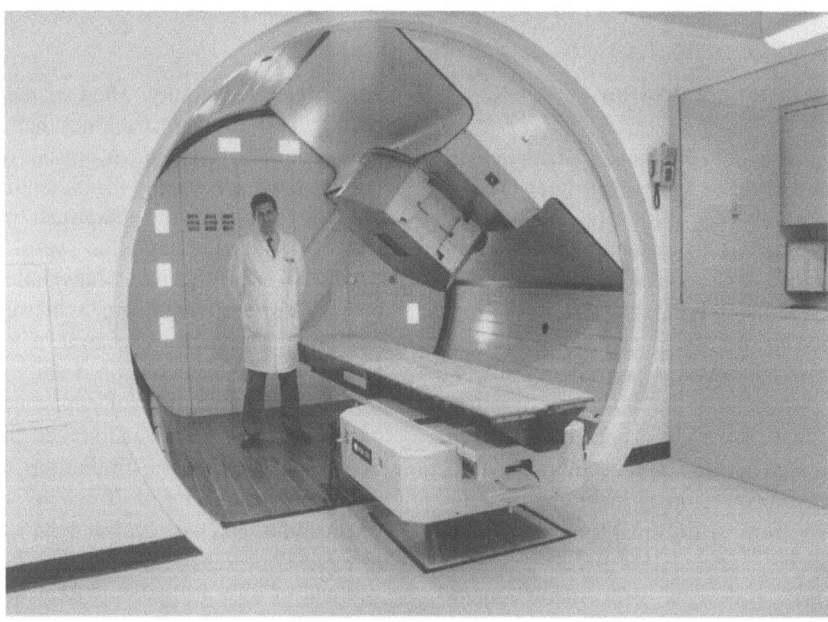

Figure 1. This is the gantry collimator and couch for the isocentric super-conducting cyclotron.

Table 1. 5-year grade 3 or higher actuarial complication rate

Neutron dose (nGy)	Photon dose (Gy)	Patient number	Gastro-intestinal (%)	Genitourinary (%)	Soft-tissue/hip stiffness (%)
15	18	58	10	18	11
9	38	75	0	0	0
10	38	150	2	5	2
11	40	100	7	5	0

that were subsequently looked at were 9 nGy plus 38 Gy of photons, 10 nGy plus 40 Gy of photons and 11 nGy plus 40 Gy of photons. Seventy-five patients were treated to a total dose of 9 nGy and there were no grade 3 complications seen at 5 years. At 10 nGy, 150 patients were treated on Phase II studies and the GI, GU and soft tissue complications rates were 2%, 5%, and 2%, respectively. By increasing the dose to 11 nGy in 100 patients, the complication rates again rose to 7% and 5% for GI and GU complications (Table 1). Thus, it appeared based on the experience of nearly 400 patients entered on Phase II studies, that the optimal mixture of neutron and photon irradiation was 10 nGy plus 40 Gy photons [6–8].

When the results were analyzed based on dose and compared to the RTOG experience, the rates of significant complications were dramatically lower. However, a patient self-assessment evaluation was undertaken to be certain that the initial patients treated with neutron irradiation were not suffering higher than anticipated complications. Our data with conformal neutron and photon radiation was compared to patients treated with conformal photon irradiation. As could be seen from the perspective of urinary function, bowel function and potency, there was no difference in the rates of complications in patients treated with neutron or photon irradiation suggesting that this mixture of 10 nGy plus 38–40 Gy of photons when delivered with three-dimensional conformal treatment techniques could be delivered as safely as conformal photons at standard doses (Table 2) [9].

Once the Phase II studies had been completed and the safe doses of neutron irradiation in combination with photon irradiation had been established, a study was conducted to determine if the sequence of neutron and photon irradiation would affect the therapeutic ratio. The rationale behind this study was based on pre-clinical data published by Joiner et al. [10], suggesting that *in vivo* and *in vitro* experiments, the sequence of neutron irradiation did make a difference in tumor control. In tumor models in which tumors were treated with neutron irradiation first, the tumor control probabilities

Table 2. Patient reported quality of life

	Neutron radiation (%)	Photon radiation (%)
Urinary function		
Pad use	8	11
Stricture	9	5
Drips with full bladder	23	36
Gastro-intestinal function		
Any symptoms	60	49
Severe diarrhea	11	10
Severe bleeding	2	5

were greater than when neutron irradiation was used second. The suggestion by Joiner was that this had to do with the presence of intracellular oxygen. However, if this was true and the sequence did make a difference, it would have significant impact in the clinical situation, thus this randomized study was designed.

Between June 1994 and October 1998, 300 patients were entered onto a Phase III randomized study. All patients had organ confined prostate cancer, clinically staged T1 or T2 disease. The maximum Gleason Score was seven or less and the median follow-up in time is 49 months (range of 30–80 months).

All patients were treated to a volume encompassing the prostate and seminal vesicles only. The patients received 10 nGy in 10 fractions and 40 Gy of photons delivered in 20 fractions. The field arrangements used for the neutron irradiation evolved from a four-field box, to a four-field non-axial technique and ultimately to a six-field technique. The photon irradiation was delivered either through a four-field and a four-field non-axial technique. The patients were well randomized and there was no difference in the two arms with respect to age, stage, Gleason Score, pre-treatment PSA level, race or the use of pre-treatment hormonal therapy (Table 3). At 5 years, the overall disease-free survival for the patients treated with neutrons first was 93% compared to 73% for the patients treated with photons first ($p = 0.008$) (Figure 2). There was no difference in the rate of grade 2 or 3 complications. In patients treated with neutrons first the rate of grade 3 or higher

Table 3. Randomized prospective trial

Randomization	Neutron first	Neutron last	*p* value
Age	69	67	0.2
Race AAM	36%	40%	0.3
Cancer	64%	60%	0.3
Stage T2	54%	61%	0.3
Gleason Score $= 7$	42%	44%	0.7
Pre-RT hormones	30%	26%	0.4
Median pre-RT PSA (ng/m)	8.3	7.4	0.4
Median follow-up (months)	49	49	0.9

Table 4. 5-year relapse survival – neutron *versus* photon

Risk factors	Neutron (%)	Photon (%)	*p* value
0	88	89	0.8
1	78	53	0.01
2	59	47	0.06
3	36	7	0.0004

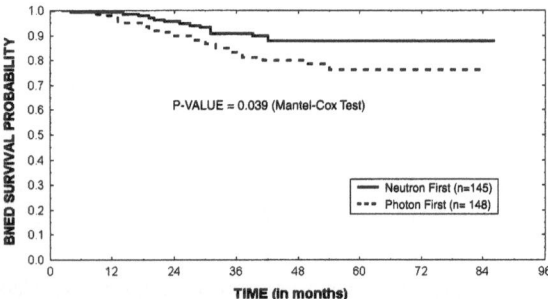

Figure 2. Disease-free survival for patients treated in randomized trial of neutrons/photon *versus* photon/neutron.

GI complications was 1% *versus* 4% in patients treated with photons first. In patients treated with neutrons first, the rate of grade 3 of higher GU complications was 3% as it was in patients treated with photon irradiation first. As a result of this study, using neutron irradiation first has become our standard approach.

Having determined the optimal dose mixture of neutron and photon irradiation, the optimal sequence of neutron and photon irradiation, and the optimal field arrangements, the next question to answer was what was the ideal patient population to be targeted with the use of neutron irradiation. The next study that was developed was designed to identify patients who had a post-radiotherapy follow-up period of greater than 5 years to allow for adequate assessment of failure, and to evaluate patients who had been treated with curative intent in order to compare the outcome of the mixed neutron and photon irradiation with photon irradiation by itself. The purpose of this was to identify if there were patient groups who would most benefit by the use of neutron irradiation as compared to photon irradiation alone and also to identify patient groups in need of additional treatment despite the use of neutron irradiation.

In total, 350 patients receiving irradiation in 1994 and 1995 in the Department of Radiation Oncology at Wayne State University were compared. They were matched for T-stage, Gleason Score and pre-treatment PSA level and the outcome was the 5-year relapse free survival. For every disease category analyzed, the use of neutron irradiation *versus* photon irradiation resulted in an improvement in outcome. For the patients with early stage disease, locally advanced disease, African-American patients, Caucasian patients, those with a low Gleason Score or high Gleason Score or a low PSA or high PSA, all had a numerical benefit through the use of neutron irradiation. These factors reached statistical significance for early stage disease for patients with a Gleason Score greater than 7 and for patients with a PSA level less than 10. When all patients were combined, four risk groups were identified. These were patients who had either no adverse risk factors, 1, 2, or 3 risk factors. An adverse risk factor was categorized as stage T3 or higher disease, a Gleason Score of 7 or higher and a PSA level greater than 10 ng/ml. For patients with no adverse risk factors, the 5-year relapse free survival was 88%. For patients with 1, 2, or 3 adverse risk factors, the disease-free survival at 5 years were 62%, 51%, and 24%, respectively ($p = 0.0001$).

However, when the data was analyzed for patients who did or did not receive neutron irradiation for patients with no adverse risk factors the disease-free survival with or without neutron irradiation was 88% *versus* 89%, respectively ($p = 0.8$). For patients with one adverse risk factor, the disease-free survival was 78% *versus* 53% for neutron *versus* photon irradiation ($p = 0.01$). For patients with two risk factors, the numbers were 59% *versus* 47% and 36% *versus* 7% for patients with three adverse risk factors (Table 4).

The impact of pre-radiation hormone therapy and neutron irradiation was analyzed. Patients who did receive neutron irradiation and hormones had a 74% 5-year disease-free survival *versus* 53% in patients who received photon irradiation and hormonal therapy ($p = 0.01$). As a result of these studies, we no longer use neutron irradiation on a routine basis in the low risk patients with no adverse risk factors. In those patients, we either use conformal photon irradiation or may recommend a radioactive seed implant. In patients with one or two adverse risk factors, we do recommend the use of mixed neutron or photon irradiation. However, for patients with two adverse risk factors we are currently analyzing the benefit of neoadjuvant hormonal therapy. For patients with three adverse risk factors we do use the mixed neutron/photon combination and recommend 2–3 years of adjuvant hormonal therapy based on the recent published data from the RTOG and EROTC. In addition, we are investigating the use of chemotherapy and hormonal therapy in this group of patients.

Conclusions

After 10 years of research involving clinical studies with nearly 900 patients, it has been demonstrated that neutron radiation can be delivered safely. Neutron radiation has an efficacy that is superior to that which has been seen with conformal photon irradiation by itself. Obviously utilization is limited by machine availability. Thus, the primary future goals of the program lie in understanding the cellular and molecular mechanisms and targets of action through which neutron radiation exerts its beneficial effect.

In the future we plan to increase the capacity of the current machine by adding a computer driven multi-leaf collimator in the summer of 2002. We also plan to expand this clinical data to other disease sites based on the observations that neutron irradiation has a demonstrable and proven superiority in patients with chemotherapy resistant large cell lymphomas and squamous cell carcinomas of the head and neck.

References

1. Laramore GE, Krall JM, Thomas FJ, Griffin TW, Maor MH, Hendrickson FR: Fast neutron radiotherapy for locally advanced prostate cancer: Results of an RTOG randomized study. Int J Radiat Oncol Biol Phys 11: 1621–1627, 1985

2. Russell KJ, Caplan RJ, Laramore GE, Burnison CM, Maor MH, Taylor ME, Zink S, Davis LW, Griffin TW: Photon *versus* fast neutron external beam radiotherapy in the treatment of locally advanced prostate cancer: Results of a randomized prospective trial. Int J Radiat Oncol Biol Phys 28: 47–54, 1994

3. Forman JD, Kocheril PG, Hart KB, Chuba PJ, Washington TA, Orton CG, Porter AT: Estimating the RBE for pelvic neutron irradiation in patients treated for carcinoma of the prostate. J Brachythera Int 13: 29–34, 1997

4. Forman JD, Duclos M, Sharma R, Chuba PJ, Hart KB, Yudelev M, Devi S, Court W, Shamsa F, Littrip P, Grignon D, Porter AT, Maughn RL: Conformal mixed neutron and photon irradiation in localized and locally advanced prostate cancer: Preliminary estimates of the therapeutic ratio. Int J Radiat Oncol Biol Phys 35: 259–266, 1996

5. Maughan RL, Blosser HG, Blosser EB, Yudelev M, Forman JD, Blosser H, Powers W: A multi-rod collimator for neutron therapy. Int J Rad Oncol Biol Phys 34(2): 411–420, 1996

6. Forman JD, Duclos M, Sharma R, Chuba P, Hart K, Yudelev M, Devi S, Court W, Shamsa F, Littrup P, Grignon D, Porter A, Maughan RL: Conformal mixed neutron and photon irradiation in localized and locally advance prostate cancer: Preliminary estimates of the therapeutic ratio. Int J Radiat Oncol Biol Phys 35(2): 259–266, 1996

7. Hart K, Duclos M, Shamsa F, Forman JD: Potency following conformal neutron/photon irradiation for localized prostate cancer. Int J Radiat Oncol Biol Phys 35(5): 881–884, 1996

8. Chuba PJ, Sharma R, Uudelev M, Duclos M, Shamsa F, Giacalone S, Orton CG, Maughan RL, Forman JD: Hip stiffness following mixed conformal neutron and photon radiotherapy: A dose–volume relationship. Int J Radiat Oncol Biol Phys 35(4): 693–699, 1996

9. Reddy S, Ruby J, Wallace M, Forman JD: Patient self-assessment of complications and quality of life after conformal neutron and photon irradiation for localized prostate cancer. Radiat Oncol Invest 5: 252–256, 1997

10. Carl UM, McNally NJ, Joiner MC: The effect of mixed fractionation with x-rays and neutrons on tumour growth delay and skin reactions in mice. Brit Jour Radiol 60: 583–588, 1987

Address for offprints: Jeffrey D. Forman, Gershenson Radiation Oncology Center, 3990 John R, Detroit, MI 48201, USA

Prostate cancer gene therapy: Past experiences and future promise

Thomas A. Gardner[1], James Sloan[2], Sudhanshu P. Raikwar[2] and Chinghai Kao[1]
[1]Department of Urology, Microbiology and Immunology and Walther Oncology Center, [2]Department of Urology, Indiana University Medical Center, Indianapolis, IN, USA

Key words: gene therapy, tumor-specific promoters, transcriptional targeting, metastatic, prostate cancer trials

Abstract

Gene therapy has been used to target prostate cancer with excellent pre-clinical efficacy but limited clinical efficacy. The concept of delivering genetic material to prostate cancer cells to alter their phenotype and ultimately their behavior has been demonstrated in the laboratory over the last decade. Translating those pre-clinical findings into novel therapies for prostate cancer has been difficult. The stigma of gene therapy and the aggressive regulation of clinical trials involving transfer of genetic material to patients are two major impediments to clinical successes in gene therapy. This review hopes to provide a snapshot of prior gene transfer protocol findings and forecast the exciting future directions investigators are heading.

1. Introduction – why gene therapy for prostate cancer

In 2002 it is estimated the prostate cancer will account for the most new cancer diagnoses at 189,000 men and will be second only to lung cancer for number of cancer related deaths at 30,200 men. The steady decline of the annual age-adjusted death rates in males according to the SEER data base over the past five years would suggest improvements in detection and treatment of clinically organ confined prostate cancer. The 1998 annual age-adjusted death rate now approximates that of the 1940 death rate of 20 per 100,000 person years [1]. The elucidation of prostate cancer's innate hormone dependency 60 years ago was the last big breakthrough in the treatment of the lethal form of prostate cancer that metastasizes to osseous sites. The greater understanding of the molecular events underlying the development of metastatic disease allows gene therapy approaches to be developed that specifically target these molecular events. For this reason, our group has focused on developing tumor-specific promoters, such as the osteocalcin (OC) promoter, based gene therapy that specifically targets osseous metastases, the most lethal form of the disease [2–4].

2. Basics of gene therapy for prostate cancer

Gene therapy can be defined as the transfer of genetic material with therapeutic intent. This raises several major questions: (1) Who to target with gene therapy? (2) How to transfer genetic material? (3) Which genetic material to transfer? and (4) What route to administer?

Starting with the first question of 'who' to target with prostate cancer gene therapy. Several stages of prostate cancer are both amenable and appropriate for current gene therapy approaches. Most of the stages in the progression from localized disease to metastatic disease have been targeted, as well as several others that could be targeted as improvements in the molecular understanding of prostate cancer and developments of vectors occur. Men with locally advanced, locally recurrent or metastatic prostate cancer are natural groups to target due to the lack of conventional therapeutics. Additionally, those men at high risk for local or distant failure have been targeted for neoadjuvant and adjuvant approaches. As with most therapies the ability to treat men with low volume disease should enhance the success of the therapy. This is probably a critical point for both the immune-based and cytoreductive

M.L. Cher, K.V. Honn and A. Raz (eds.), Prostate Cancer: New Horizons in Research and Treatment, 357–365.

approaches discussed below. For example, a patient with a detectable PSA recurrence after definitive conventional therapy may be the perfect patient for either an immune-based strategy or systemically administered and targeted cytoreductive approach.

In the future, a corrective approach could be used for men with high grade PIN if a genetic determinant of prostate cancer progression could be identified. A gene therapist with the knowledge of continually improved vectors, with enhanced targeting and greater killing ability, can easily envision the realization of a 'molecular prostatectomy' for the treatment of localized disease or even better a 'prophylactic molecular prostatectomy' to prevent morbidity and mortality associated with both benign prostatic hypertrophy and prostate cancer.

The currently available methods of 'how' to transfer genetic material are listed in Table 1. Each vector has been used in prostate cancer clinical gene transfer protocols. Each of the vector has advantages and disadvantages as couriers of genetic information. For example, the 'common cold virus' or adenovirus can transfer a large amount of genetic information with high efficiency, regardless of cell cycle considerations and without toxicity to the cellular genome (genotoxicity). Unfortunately, this virus results in only transient expression of the genetic material and most individuals will have innate immunity due to prior exposure to the 'common cold' which limits multiple dosing or systemic administration. The 'gutless' adenovirus has less immunogenicity and can transfer three times the amount of DNA as the conventional one.

The answer to the 'what DNA' question depends on the objective of the therapy. Gene therapy for cancer has been either corrective, allowing for the replacement of a defective tumor suppressor gene (i.e. p53, p16, etc.) or cytoreductive, allowing for direct cell killing (i.e. suicide, oncolytic) or indirect cell killing by immunomodulation (i.e. IL-2, GM-CSF, IL-12). Table 2 lists some common paradigms used in prostate cancer gene transfer protocols.

For example, the genetic material from the herpes simplex virus encoding for the thymidine kinase (TK) enzyme has been utilized in a number of gene transfer protocols for prostate cancer listed in Table 3 [5]. The HSV-TK enzyme encoded by this viral DNA segment remains the main pharmaceutical target for treating herpes viral infections. The viral form of the TK enzyme can convert a number of well-tolerated clinically approved pro-drugs (i.e. ganciclovir (GCV), acyclovir, valacyclovir, etc.) to a potent intracellular toxin, which interferes with DNA replication. Due to the activated pro-drugs effect on dividing DNA, this form of suicide gene therapy will effectively kill a cell when it attempts to proliferate or divide, but is limited to the cells infected by the virus and those immediately surrounding the infected cell ('bystander-effect').

The final question raised was by 'which' route to administer the gene therapy. This question can only be answered after answering the first three questions of whom, how and what. Currently, the vector being used generally dictates the route of administration. For instance, it would be illogical to treat locally recurrent prostate cancer after external beam radiotherapy using an intravenous delivery of adenoviral suicide approach. First, a majority of the dose of a currently available replication defective adenovirus will be filtered by the liver only leaving a small fraction of the dose to be delivered to the radiated prostate bed containing the recurrent disease. Second, the ability to visualize

Table 1. Comparison of vector systems in gene therapy. This table lists the important attributes of the currently used gene therapy vectors for prostate cancer. The bold items are felt to be the disadvantage of the particular vector

Attribute	Retrovirus/ lentivirus ('HIV')	Adenovirus/ 'gutless'	Adeno- associated virus	Vaccinia/fowl pox virus	Non-viral (liposome)
In vivo gene transfer rate	**Low**/high	High	High	High	Low
Gene transfer cell cycle independent	**Yes**/No	No	No	No	No
Size limit of DNA transfer	8 kb	10/35 kb	**<5 kb**	>30 kb	? Limit
Genome integration/genotoxicity	**Yes**	No	**Yes**	No	No
Period of DNA expression	Stable	Transient/ stable	Stable	Transient	Transient
Immunoreactive	No	**Yes**/No	No	Yes	No
Large scale production	Yes	Yes*/**No**	Yes*	Yes	Yes
Clinical safety profile	Yes/**No**	Yes/**No**	No	Yes	Yes

* Significant difficulties still persist in clinical grade large scale production.

Table 2. Current approaches for prostate cancer gene therapy

Strategy	Vector(s) used	DNA transferred
Immunotherapy	Retrovirus	GM-CSF
	Vaccina/	IL-2
	fowlpox	IL-12
	Liposome	PSA
	RNA	Tumor RNA
	AAV	
	Adenovirus	
Corrective/tumor	Retrovirus	P53
suppressor	Adenovirus	P16
		C-MYC
Suicide/toxic	Adenovirus	TK
pro-drug		CD
		TK/CD
Oncolytic	Adenovirus	OC promoter
		PB/PSA
		promoter
		PB/PSE
		promoter

the prostate and directly inject the prostate using ultrasound would be the obvious route for such a vector with limited abilities.

3. Past approaches

In the past seven years a variety of gene therapy paradigms have been used to target prostate cancer and can broadly be classified into immunotherapy, tumor suppressor therapy, suicide gene therapy and oncolytic therapy (Table 2). Each of these approaches has a strong foundation of pre-clinical data allowing for such clinical studies to be approved. Currently, 45 gene transfer protocols targeting prostate cancer can be found on the Office of Biologic Activities Protocol List (web page) out of 314 protocols targeted at cancer. Therefore, prostate cancer gene therapy trials account for 14% of all cancer gene therapy trials to date (Table 3) [5]. The details of each of the protocols listed in Table 3 can be found at the reference web address. Each investigator and all co-investigators involved in these protocols should be commended for their exhaustive efforts in getting a gene therapy protocol to the clinic. Prostate cancer remains a focus of the gene therapist because the prostate is accessible, and limited availability of treatments for locally advanced or metastatic disease states, represents a large enough population/market to obtain NIH/corporate dollars. Prostate cancer gene therapy protocols listed in Table 3 exemplify the translation

nature of trial development in the 21st century. Within the table there are several examples of trials that have come to the clinic based on pre-clinical findings which then lead to further refinement and improved therapeutic trials, demonstrating bi-directional flow from the clinic and the basic research labs [2–4].

3.1. Immune-mediated gene therapy

Multiple mechanisms allow tumors to go unrecognized by the host immune system. Immunomodulatory therapy can enhance the hosts' anti-tumor immune response. Fifty-six percent or 25 of the 45 clinical prostate cancer gene therapy protocols utilize an immune-based approach. Initially, after demonstrating that immunostimulatory molecules could transform cancer cells previously able to hide from the immune system to activate a tumor-directed immune response, the first gene therapy trial in prostate cancer demonstrated that autologous prostate cancer cells from patients could be amplified, retrovirally transduced to express GM-CSF, irradiated and given back to patients to elicit an immune response toward metastatic prostate cancer cells. Unfortunately, this required a number of *ex vivo* steps, which limited the successful vaccination rate to 73% [6].

This trial led to the development of a simple vaccine composed of irradiated prostate cancer cell line allografts expressing GM-CSF. This approach will allow for multiple dosing. Several centers have put forth protocols to evaluate this approach further as listed in Table 3.

More recently, *in vivo* immunomodulatory approaches are being used. These include the use of both vaccina or fowlpox viruses to illicit an immune response against prostate cancer-specific molecules PSA, PSMA, MUC-1 alone or in conjunction with immunumodulating molecules (i.e. B7) and the direct intralesional injections of adenovirus, adeno-associated virus expressing a multitude of cytokines, including IL-2, GM-CSF and IL-12. The goal of each approach is to achieve a systemic anti-tumor response. These more recent *in vivo* methods avoid the complexities associated with *ex vivo* gene transfer approaches. The *in vivo* approach has the potential of making the tumor increasingly immunogenic because the vector carrying a gene to produce a cytokine is directly placed into the patient's tumor cells allowing the patient's own tumor cell to trigger the immune response to itself and other prostate cancer cells. Several trials have been

Table 3. Prostate cancer gene therapy trials (OBA Protocol List 11/19/01) [5]

Principal investigator	Institution	Vector	Genetic material	Year reviewed	Ref.
1. Simons JW	Johns Hopkins, MD	Retro	GM-CSF	94	[6]
2. Steiner MS	Vanderbilt Univ., TN	Retro	c-myc	95	
3. Chen AP	Nat. Naval Med, MD	Vaccinia	PSA	95	
4. Paulson DF	Duke Univ., NC	Liposome	IL-2	95	
5. Scardino PT	MSKCC, NY	Adeno	HSV-TK	96	[17,18]
6. Eder JP	Dana-Farber, MD	Vaccinia	PSA	96	
7. Sanda MG	Univ. of Michigan, MI	Vaccinia	PSA	97	
8. Belldegrun AS	UCLA, CA	Liposome	IL-2	97	
9. Hall SJ	Mt. Sinai, NY	Adeno	HSV-TK	97	
10. Belldegrun AS	UCLA, CA	Adeno	P53	97	[19]
11. Simons JW	Johns Hopkins, MD	Retro	GM-CSF	97	
12. Logothetis CJ	MD Anderson, TX	Adeno	p53	97	
13. Kadmon D	Baylor, TX	Adeno	HSV-TK	98	
14. Simons JW	Johns Hopkins, MD	Adeno	PSA	98	[13]
15. Figlin RA	UCLA, CA	Vaccinia	MUC-1/IL-2	98	
16. Gardner TA	Univ. of Virginia, VA	Adeno	OC promoter-HSV-TK	98	[3]
17. Eder JP	Dana-Farber Cancer Inst., MD	Vaccinia/fowlpox	PSA	99	[20]
18. Small EJ	UCSF, CA	Retro	GM-CSF	99	
19. Kaufman HL	Albert Einstein, NY	Vaccinia/fowlpox	PSA	99	
20. Vieweg J	Duke Univ., NC	RNA	PSA	99	
21. Belldegrun AS	UCLA, CA	Liposome	IL-2	99	
22. Small EJ	UCSF, CA	Retro	GM-CSF	99	
23. Kim JH	Henry Ford Hosp, MI	Adeno	CD/TK	99	
24. Aguilar-Cordova E	Harvard Univ., MA	Adeno	TK	99	
25. Gingrich JR	Univ. of Tenn., TN	Adeno	p16	99	
26. Terris MK	Stanford Univ., CA	Adeno	PSA	99	
27. Wilding G	Univ. of Wisc., WI	Adeno	PSA	99	
28. Belldegrun AS	UCLA, CA	Liposome	IL-2	99	
29. Dahut WL	NIH/NCI	Vaccinia/fowlpox	PSA	99	
30. Arlen PM	NIH/NCI	Vaccinia/fowlpox	PSA	00	
31. Vieweg J	Duke Univ., NC	RNA	Total tumor RNA	00	
32. Pollack A	Univ. of Texas, TX	Adeno	p53	00	
33. Gardner TA	Indiana Univ., IN	Adeno	OC promoter	00	
34. Freytag SO	Henry Ford Hosp., MI	Adeno	CD/TK	00	
35. Lubaroff DM	Univ. of Iowa	Adeno	PSA	01	
36. Miles BJ	Baylor College, TX	Adeno	IL-12	01	
37. DeWeese TL	Johns Hopkins, MD	Adeno	PB/PSE promoter	01	
38. Small EJ	UCSF, CA	Adeno	PB/PSE promoter	01	
39. Dula E	West Coast Clinical Res.	AAV	GM-CSF	01	
40. Freytag SO	Henry Ford, MI	Adeno	CD/TK	01	
41. Scher H	MSKCC, NY	Liposome	PSMA	01	
42. Corman J	VA Puget Sound, WA	AAV	GM-CSF	01	
43. Pantuck AJ	UCLA, LA	Vaccinia	MUC-1/IL-2	01	
44. Vieweg J	Duke, NC	RNA	hTeRT	01	
45. Corman J	VA Puget Sound, WA	Adeno	PSE promoter	01	

initiated and limited published results are available for further comment.

3.2. Corrective gene therapy

Replacement of normal tumor suppressor genes (i.e. p53, p16) can reestablish the normal cell cycle progression and enhance apoptosis of abnormal cancer cells. Unfortunately, multiple genetic sites, as opposed to a single locus, have been implicated in the development and progression of prostate cancer. However, mutations in the p53 gene have been identified in multiple prostate cancer cell lines and clinical specimens. Replacement of wild type p53, or other tumor suppressor genes, *in vitro* and in animal models have resulted in inhibited tumor growth [7]. Clinical studies using replacement of p53 alone and also in combination with radiation therapy are being investigated (Table 3).

The over expression of particular oncogenes may be combated by the introduction of anti-sense mRNA to inhibit the translation of the oncogenic protein(s). The introduction of anti-sense c-myc mRNA into prostate cancer cell lines, such as LNCaP, result in decreased translation of the oncogenic protein. Mouse studies indicate that this approach results in tumor shrinkage. Clinical trials are also in progress.

3.3. Suicide gene therapy

The efficacy of suicide gene therapy relies on the conversion of a non-toxic pro-drug to a lethal metabolite by the enzymatic product of a previously delivered gene. Fortunately, the toxic effect is not limited to cells transfected by a suicide gene (i.e. TK, CD, etc.), but extends to nearby cells via the 'bystander effect'. The bystander effect is mediated primarily by intercellular communication (i.e. gap junctions) and phagocytosis of debris from dying cells by the neighboring cells.

The most well characterized suicide gene therapy utilizes the TK from the herpes simplex virus and one of several clinically available anti-herpetic medications (i.e. GCV, acyclovir, valacyclovir, etc.) to activate the suicide mechanism. Unlike its human counterpart, the viral DNA encodes for the TK enzyme, which can phosphorylate the un-phosphorylated nucleoside guanine or the guanine analogues (i.e. GCV, acyclovir, valacyclovir, etc.). Therefore, when a pro-drug such as GCV is administered it will be phosphorylated and incorporated into the DNA at the time of replication. This incorporation occurs at a guanine site and causes abnormal DNA replication, which in turn generates an apoptotic signal and kills the cell when it tries to divide.

The TK/pro-drug system is the most studied because it is a safe approach for cancer gene therapy for a number of reasons. First, suicide of the infected cell occurs only when they divide thus targeting cancer cells, which divide more rapidly then non-cancerous cells. Second, the toxic effect only occurs when the pro-drug is administered allowing the cessation of the pro-drug in the event of serious toxicities. Third, several anti-herpetic drugs used as pro-drugs are clinically available, therefore simplifying the approval process for the clinical trail. Finally, the bystander effect is limited to surrounding cells that can take up the toxin

produced by within the dying cell. All of these attributes allowed the pioneers of this form of gene therapy to apply and receive approval to conduct clinical trials in patients with advanced cancer.

Initially, TK was placed under the regulation of a universal promoter (i.e. retroviral LTR, RSV or CMV). The universal promoter is very active but it is activated in all cell types. This allows for the TK to be active in normal and cancer cells that are transduced by the vector. These vectors required direct injection or intralesional delivery due to the effect they would exert on normal cells trying to divide if administered systemically. The initial prostate cancer TK trial used a replication-defective adenovirus to transport RSV-TK followed by GCV in men with locally recurrent prostate cancer after definitive external beam radiotherapy. This trial realized the potential of this therapy by demonstrating anti-cancer activity as evidenced by sustained decreases in serum PSA and improved biopsies from these men with recurrent tumors. As a result of some of the adenovirus leaving the injection site and reaching the liver, several of the patients experienced a self-limiting toxicity and one patient experienced a grade III hepatic dysfunction and grade IV thrombocytopenia.

Our group tried to harness the abilities of TK and to allow for systemic therapy for men with metastatic disease by exchanging the universal promoter for a tumor-specific OC promoter and PSA promoter. After a series of pre-clinical studies demonstrating the specificity of the OC promoter, we performed a phase I trial by directly injecting post-surgical recurrences ($n = 2$) or metastatic prostate cancer lesions ($n = 9$) with a replication-defective adenovirus to transport the OC promoter driving TK expression followed by valacyclovir administration.

This trial demonstrated several novel principles upon which we are now building, first, an adenoviral vector that could be safely and repeatedly injected into either a prostate cancer osseous metastatic (Figure 1) or a post-surgical recurrence. Second, anti-tumor effect could be seen by transient declines in PSA or improved post-treatment biopsies in several patients. Third, despite transient detection of live viral particles in the serum of these men, valacyclovir administration did not lead to several hepatic toxicities, suggesting that the hepatocytes could not activate the OC promoter and did not produce TK even though exposed to the Ad–OC–TK virus and were unaffected by valacyclovir. Finally, TK gene expression could be detected in the biopsy specimens after treatment, demonstrating target tissue gene transfer and protein expression.

362

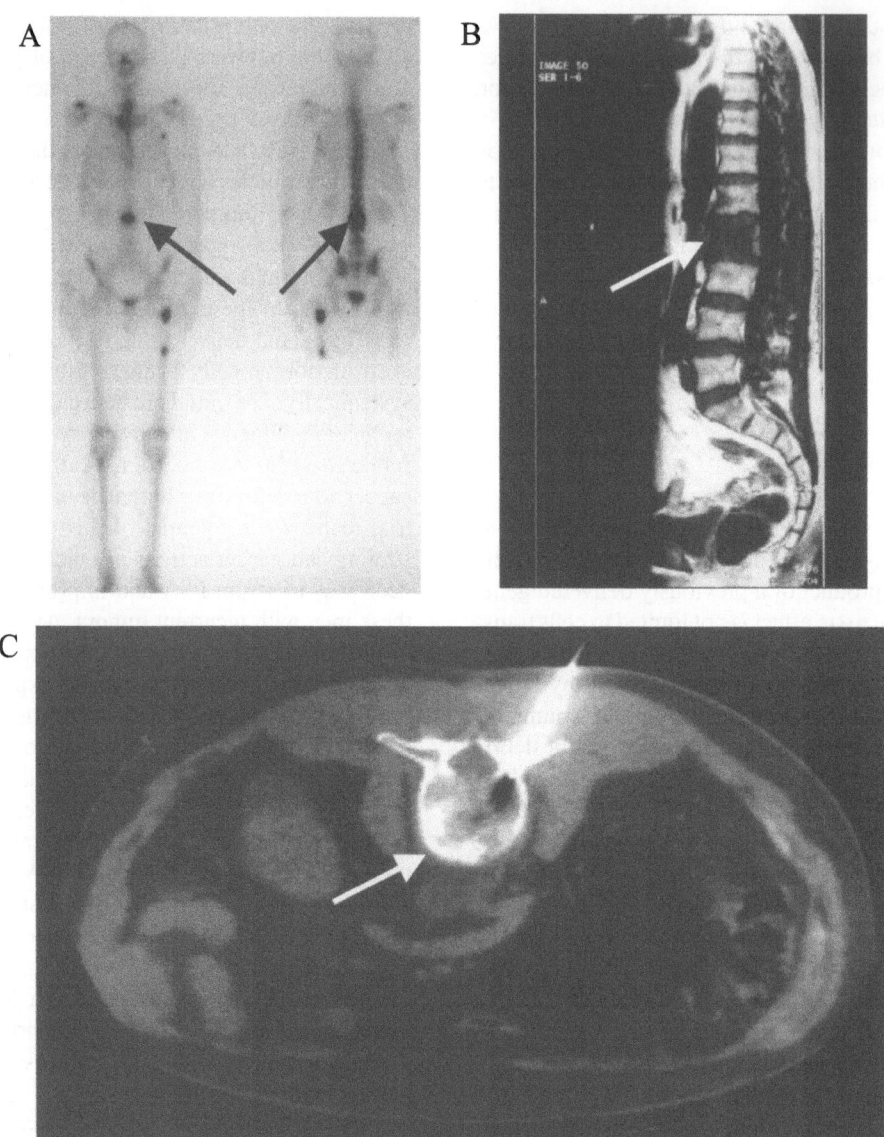

Figure 1. Intralesion administration of Ad–OC–TK to 2nd lumbar vertebral body osseous metastases delineated with an arrow by (A) Bone Scan, (B) MRI and (C) CT Scan during the actual injection.

It is important to note that as with many of these trials it took three years after demonstrating efficacy in pre-clinical models to produce and test cGMP grade Ad–OC–TK at a cost of $200,000 and perform GLP grade toxicology testing in mice at a cost of $100,000. The completion of this 11 patient trial including clinical monitoring, and personnel cost (PI and CRN) was $700,000 or about $91,000 per patient enrolled.

Fortunately, we received a gift from the Kluge Foundation to cover these costs or this trial may never have

been performed. It is also important to note that this trial was conducted prior to the unfortunate events at the University of Pennsylvania that have led to additional viral testing and toxicology requirements now being requested by the regulatory agencies.

This trail demonstrated that the prostate tumor-specific promoter OC could be used to target prostate cancer cells and protect normal surrounding cells. Phase II testing of this vector was proposed, but due to viral production delays and the development of an improved OC based oncolytic vector (see below) with more potential clinical efficacy based on pre-clinical studies, the phase II trial was appropriately shelved by the sponsor.

3.4. Oncolytic gene therapy

To overcome some of the limitations of replication-deficient viral vectors used in suicide gene approach, such as the incomplete delivery of virus to every tumor cell, viruses have been engineered that harness the natural lytic life cycle of the adenovirus under the regulation of tumor-specific promoter. Several oncolytic vectors have demonstrated strong and specific tumor killing in animal models of aggressive human prostate cancers and are currently being tested in the clinic.

Initially, our group [8] and others [9] demonstrated the prostate cancer-specific gene regulation of the PSA promoter in animal models of prostate cancer as has been demonstrated in other tumor models such as CEA promoter in colon cancer [10,11]. This finding combined with the advanced understanding of the adenoviral genes and their regulatory functions allowed for the creation of a series of conditionally replicative adenoviruses.

Rodriquez et al. demonstrated that a portion of the PSA promoter could provide prostate cancer-specific viral replication both *in vitro* and in animal models. Additionally, the element from the PSA promoter could be enhanced if androgens were applied [12]. This virus has been used in a clinical trial of men with recurrent prostate cancer after failed definitive external beam radiotherapy [13]. This trial demonstrated several important findings about tumor-specific oncolysis. Limited adverse events throughout the dose escalation in all 20 men, combined with 5 responders demonstrating a greater than 50% decline in serum PSA would suggest that the portion of the PSA promoter allowed conditional replication of the adenovirus only within prostate cancer cells (Table 3, #14). Additional modifications [14] to the above virus has demonstrated enhanced specificity and strength in pre-clinical models and is currently being tested in clinical trial at several centers (Table 3, #26, 27, 37, 38, 45).

Due to our groups continued interest in the OC promoter to provide gene expression in advanced prostate cancer cells and the supportive bone cells of osseous metastasis, we created an adenovirus that would replicate intracellularly and lyse them if the cell was able to activate the OC promoter (Figure 2). The Ad–OC–E1a

virus is a conditionally replicative adenovirus which has performed well in pre-clinical animal models of human prostate cancer [4]. A trial paralleling the design Ad–OC–TK trial with this virus has been proposed and is awaiting final approvals from regulatory agencies (Table 3, #33).

4. Future directions in prostate cancer gene therapy

The immediate future of gene therapy for prostate cancer appears to be found in four major paradigms as follows: (1) immune-based therapy (2) novel vectors (3) synthetic oncolytic viruses and (4) a combination of gene therapy with conventional therapies.

Immunotherapeutic approaches to prostate cancer still account for greater than 50% of the current gene transfer trials. The safety of these approaches has been demonstrated although the efficacy remains to be seen. The ability to target extremely low volume disease and the continual discovery of new prostate-specific targets permits continued optimism for this approach.

Several new vectors are being tested in pre-clinical models including oncolytic herpes viral vectors [15] and lenti viral vectors [16] containing prostate-specific regulatory elements (e.g. PSA promoter). Two adeno-associated virus trials are proposed and should provide great insight into stable gene transfer to prostate cancer cells (Table 3, #39, 42).

The third major focus will be to create synthetic or designer vectors that are genetically engineered to exert their DNA transfer to the target cell only. This will allow the gene therapist to keep the desired attributes of a vector while altering the undesired attributes. For example, the knob protein of the adenovirus binds to the Coxsackie-adenovirus receptor (CAR) on the surface of a cell and allows an infection of the cell to occur. The toxicity associated with systemic administration of adenoviral vectors is thought to be secondary to the presence of CAR on normal cells (e.g. hepatocytes). We are currently testing an oncolytic virus which has been modified at the knob protein to attach to a RGD sequence found on the surface of most cancer cells and less common on normal cells (e.g. hepatocytes). The combination of our ability to manipulate the viral genomes and the information about cancer cells is allowing us to design vectors that will specifically target and destroy prostate cancer cells with precision.

Finally, as demonstrated by several of the recent submission to the Office of Biologic Activities is the

364

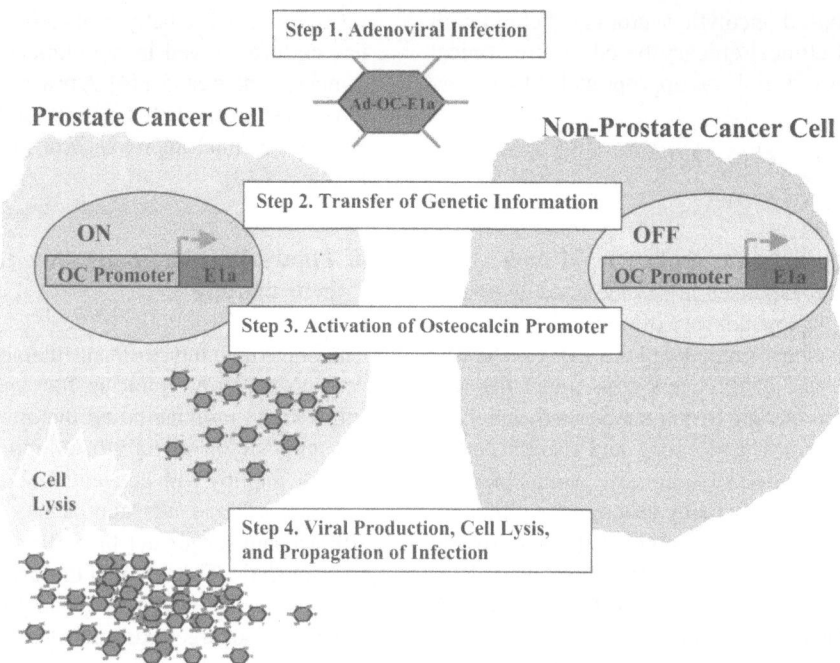

Figure 2. Steps of Ad–OC–E1a directed prostate cancer-specific oncolysis. The molecular steps required for all oncolytic viruses using conditionally replicating adenovirus employing the OC promoter to obtain prostate cancer specificity are illustrated. Step 1: the viral infection occurs in both the prostate cancer and non-prostate cancer cell. Step 2: the transfer of genetic material of cellular internalization of the DNA packaged in the virus occur in both cell type. Step 3: the activation of the OC promoter and subsequent initiation of new viral replication is specific to the prostate cancer due to the inability of the non-prostate cancer cell to activate the OC promoter. Step 4: the lytic cell death and the propagation of the adenoviral infection to neighboring cells can only occur in the prostate cancer cells therefore minimizing toxicities to the normal cells.

combination of a gene therapy strategy with more conventional therapy such as radiation or chemotherapy. There have been several elegant pre-clinical studies that demonstrate the ability of combining chemo-gene therapy and radio-gene therapy that have led to the proposed clinical trials (Table 3, #38) and (Table 3, #37, 40), respectively.

5. Conclusion

Gene therapy has been shown to be safe and effective in patients with prostate cancer. Principle investigators are currently using all available vectors and employing all available approaches as illustrated by Table 3. The paucity of gene therapy-related toxicities in the trials published to date would suggest that they could be added to conventional therapies with potentially additive or even synergistic improvements in efficacy without overlapping toxicity profiles. The main limitations to advances in this field are the time and expense producing and testing these biologics to meet the continually rising regulatory hurdles. The ability to target the delivery of vectors to prostate cancer cells as well as to limit the desired gene transfer to prostate cancer cells, currently exists in numerous labs throughout the world, but several years will pass before these non-traditional vectors will make it to patients in need of therapy.

Acknowledgements

Work referenced in this text has been financially supported by the American Foundation of Urologic Diseases, DOD – DAMD17-00-1-0027, NIH KO8 CA79544-01A2, New York Academy of Medicine-Edwin Beer Award, CaPCure Foundation, 5-T32-DK07642, Kluge Foundation. The authors would also like to acknowledge the past, present and future intellectual support of Leland W.K. Chung and his Molecular Urology and Therapuetic (MUT) Laboratory.

References

1. Jemal A, Thomas A, Murray T, Thun M: Cancer statistics. CA Cancer J Clin 52(1): 23, 2002

2. Gardner TA, Ko S-C, Kao C, Shirakawa T, Cheon J, Gotoh A, Wu T, Sikes RA, Zhau HE, Cui Q, Balian G, Chung LWK: Exploiting stromal–epithial interaction for model development and new strategies of gene therapy for prostate cancer and osteosarcoma metastases. Gene Therapy Mol Biol 2: 41, 1998

3. Koeneman KS, Kao C, Ko SC, Yang L, Wada Y, Kallmes DF, Gillenwater JY, Zhau HE, Chung LW, Gardner TA: Osteocalcin-directed gene therapy for prostate-cancer bone metastasis. World J Urol 18(2): 102, 2000

4. Matsubara S, Wada Y, Gardner TA, Egawa M, Park MS, Hsieh CL, Zhau HE, Kao C, Kamidono S, Gillenwater JY, Chung LW: A conditional replication-competent adenoviral vector, Ad–OC–E1a, to cotarget prostate cancer and bone stroma in an experimental model of androgen-independent prostate cancer bone metastasis. Cancer Res 61(16): 6012, 2001

5. Office of Biotechnology Activities' Recombinant DNA and Gene Transfer Web Page, http://www4.od.nih.gov/oba/Rdna.htm

6. Simons JW, Mikhak B, Chang JF, DeMarzo AM, Carducci MA, Lim M, Weber CE, Baccala AA, Goemann MA, Clift SM, Ando DG, Levitsky HI, Cohen LK, Sanda MG, Mulligan RC, Partin AW, Carter HB, Piantadosi S, Marshall FF, Nelson WG: Induction of immunity to prostate cancer antigens: Results of a clinical trial of vaccination with irradiated autologous prostate tumor cells engineered to secrete granulocyte-macrophage colony-stimulating factor using ex vivo gene transfer. Cancer Res 59(20): 5160, 1999

7. Ko SC, Gotoh A, Thalmann GN, Zhau HE, Johnston DA, Zhang WW, Kao C, Chung LW: Molecular therapy with recombinant p53 adenovirus in an androgen-independent, metastatic human prostate cancer model. Hum Gene Ther 7(14): 1683, 1996

8. Gotoh A, Ko SC, Shirakawa T, Cheon J, Kao C, Miyamoto T, Gardner TA, Ho LJ, Cleutjens CB, Trapman J, Graham FL, Chung LW: Development of prostate-specific antigen promoter-based gene therapy for androgen-independent human prostate cancer. J Urol 160(1): 220, 1998

9. Pang S, Taneja S, Dardashti K, Cohan P, Kaboo R, Sokoloff M, Tso CL, Dekernion JB, Belldegrun AS: Prostate tissue specificity of the prostate-specific antigen promoter isolated from a patient with prostate cancer. Hum Gene Ther 6(11): 1417, 1995

10. Richards CA, Wolberg AS, Huber BE: The transcriptional control region of the human carcinoembryonic antigen gene: DNA sequence and homology studies DNA Seq 4(3): 185, 1993

11. Huber BE, Richards CA, Austin EA: Virus-directed enzyme/prodrug therapy (VDEPT). Selectively engineering drug sensitivity into tumors. Ann N Y Acad Sci 716: 104, 1994

12. Rodriguez R, Schuur ER, Lim HY, Henderson GA, Simons JW, Henderson DR: Prostate attenuated replication competent adenovirus (ARCA) CN706: A selective cytotoxic for prostate-specific antigen-positive prostate cancer cells. Cancer Res 57(13): 2559, 1997

13. DeWeese TL, van der Poel H, Li S, Mikhak B, Drew R, Goemann M, Hamper U, DeJong R, Detorie N, Rodriguez R, Haulk T, DeMarzo AM, Piantadosi S, Yu DC, Chen Y, Henderson DR, Carducci MA, Nelson WG, Simons JW: A phase I trial of CV706, a replication-competent, PSA selective oncolytic adenovirus, for the treatment of locally recurrent prostate cancer following radiation therapy. Cancer Res 61(20): 7464, 2001

14. Yu DC, Chen Y, Seng M, Dilley J, Henderson DR: The addition of adenovirus type 5 region E3 enables calydon virus 787 to eliminate distant prostate tumor xenografts. Cancer Res 59(17): 4200, 1999

15. Varghese S, Newsome JT, Rabkin SD, McGeagh K, Mahoney D, Nielsen P, Todo T, Martuza RL: Preclinical safety evaluation of G207, a replication-competent herpes simplex virus type 1, inoculated intraprostatically in mice and nonhuman primates. Hum Gene Ther 12(8): 999, 2001

16. Yu D, Chen D, Chiu C, Razmazma B, Chow YH, Pang S: Prostate-specific targeting using PSA promoter-based lentiviral vectors. Cancer Gene Ther 8(9): 628, 2001

17. Herman JR, Adler HL, Aguilar-Cordova E, Rojas-Martinez A, Woo S, Timme TL, Wheeler TM, Thompson TC, Scardino PT: In situ gene therapy for adenocarcinoma of the prostate: A phase I clinical trial. Hum Gene Ther 10(7): 1239, 1999

18. Shalev M, Kadmon D, Teh BS, Butler EB, Aguilar-Cordova E, Thompson TC, Herman JR, Adler HL, Scardino PT, Miles BJ: Suicide gene therapy toxicity after multiple and repeat injections in patients with localized prostate cancer. J Urol 163(6): 1747, 2000

19. Pantuck AJ, Zisman A, Belldegrun AS: Gene therapy for prostate cancer at the University of California, Los Angeles: Preliminary results and future directions. World J Urol 18(2): 143, 2000

20. Eder JP, Kantoff PW, Roper K, Xu GX, Bubley GJ, Boyden J, Gritz L, Mazzara G, Oh WK, Arlen P, Tsang KY, Panicali D, Schlom J, Kufe DW: A phase I trial of a recombinant vaccinia virus expressing prostate-specific antigen in advanced prostate cancer. Clin Cancer Res 6(5): 1632, 2000

Address for offprints: Thomas A. Gardner, Assistant Professor of Urology, Microbiology and Immunology, Walther Oncology Center, Indiana University Medical Center, 535 N. Barnhill, RT 420, Indianapolis, IN 46202, USA; *Tel:* (317) 630-2636; *Fax:* (317) 630-6137; *e-mail:* thagardn@iupui.edu

Vitamin D-related therapies in prostate cancer*

Candace S. Johnson[2], Pamela A. Hershberger[3] and Donald L. Trump[1]
[1]*Department of Medicine*, [2]*Department of Pharmacology & Therapeutics, Roswell Park Cancer Institute, Buffalo, NY;* [3]*Department of Pharmacology, University of Pittsburgh, Pittsburgh, PA, USA*

Key words: calcitriol, vitamin D, VDR, vitamin D analogues, preclinical studies, animal models

Abstract

Calcitriol or 1,25-dihydroxycholecalciferol (vitamin D) is classically known for its effects on bone and mineral metabolism. Epidemiological data suggest that low vitamin D levels increase the risk and mortality from prostate cancer. Calcitriol is also a potent anti-proliferative agent in a wide variety of malignant cell types including prostate cancer cells. In prostate model systems (PC-3, LNCaP, DU145, MLL) calcitriol has significant anti-tumor activity *in vitro* and *in vivo*. Calcitriol's effects are associated with an increase in cell cycle arrest, apoptosis, differentiation and in the modulation of growth factor receptors. Calcitriol induces a significant G_0/G_1 arrest and modulates p21$^{Waf1/Cip1}$ and p27^{Kip1}, the cyclin dependent kinase inhibitors. Calcitriol induces PARP cleavage, increases the bax/bcl-2 ratio, reduces levels of phosphorylated mitogen-activated protein kinases (P-MAPKs, P-Erk-1/2) and phosphorylated Akt (P-Akt), induces caspase-dependent MEK cleavage and up-regulation of MEKK-1, all potential markers of the apoptotic pathway. Glucocorticoids potentiate the anti-tumor effect of calcitriol and decrease calcitriol-induced hypercalcemia. In combination with calcitriol, dexamethasone results in a significant time- and dose-dependent increase in VDR protein and an enhanced apoptotic response as compared to calcitriol alone. Calcitriol can also significantly increase cytotoxic drug-mediated anti-tumor efficacy. As a result, phase I and II trials of calcitriol either alone or in combination with the carboplatin, paclitaxel, or dexamethasone have been initiated in patients with androgen-dependent and -independent prostate cancer and advanced cancer. Patients were evaluated for toxicity, maximum tolerated dose (MTD), schedule effects, and PSA response. Data from these studies indicate that high-dose calcitriol is feasible on an intermittent schedule, the MTD is still being delineated and dexamethasone or paclitaxel appear to ameliorate toxicity. Studies continue to define the MTD of calcitriol which can be safely administered on this intermittent schedule either alone or with other agents and to evaluate the mechanisms of calcitriol effects in prostate cancer.

Vitamin D is a secosteroid hormone, which modulates calcium homeostasis through actions on kidney, bone, and the intestinal tract [1]. Vitamin D can be obtained from the diet or synthesized in the skin from 7-dehydrocholesterol in response to ultraviolet light. Vitamin D_3 is then transported to the liver by vitamin D binding protein (DBP) where it is 25-hydroxylated to 25-hydroxycholecalciferol. The level of 25-hydroxycholecalciferol reflects sunlight exposure and dietary intake and is often utilized as a marker of vitamin D stores. From the liver, it is transported to the kidney where it is 1-hydroxylated to the active form,

1,25-dihydroxycholecalciferol or calcitriol [1,2]. Concentrations of 25-hydroxycholecalciferol are often 1000-fold higher than the active metabolite calcitriol, whose concentrations are tightly regulated. Calcitriol is important in maintaining normal calcium homeostasis. When calcium is lowered, parathyroid hormone (PTH) is released and this stimulates production of calcitriol which thereby stimulates the small intestine to increase calcium absorption. Likewise, calcitriol can stimulate osteoclasts to mobilize calcium from bone.

VDR and calcitriol signaling

The effects of calcitriol are mediated primarily by the binding of 1,25-dihydroxycholecalciferol to a specific

*This work is supported by grants from the NCI (CA47904 and CA67267) and CaPCURE.

M.L. Cher, K.V. Honn and A. Raz (eds.), Prostate Cancer: New Horizons in Research and Treatment, 367–378.

368

intracellular receptor (VDR) a member of the steroid hormone receptor superfamily [3]. The VDR is a high-affinity, low-capacity receptor protein of 48–55 kDa primarily located in the nucleus, though evidence exists for the presence of cytoplasmic receptors [4–7]. In whole sections of prostate, VDR expression is localized primarily in the luminal epithelial cells, a potential site of cancer development [8,9]. The VDR acts as a ligand-dependent transcription factor and binds to the vitamin D response element(s) (VDRE) as a VDR: retinoid-X receptor (RXR) heterodimer. This interaction results in activation or repression of target genes. The identities and functions of all these genes, however, are unknown [5,6]. The VDR is a phosphoprotein and its function is regulated by phosphorylation on serine residues in the ligand/hinge domains [10,11]. The binding of calcitriol to the VDR induces receptor phosphorylation and the ligand-bound, phosphorylated receptor stimulates transcription [10]. While phosphorylation of the VDR is thought to play an important role in transcriptional activity, the details of this process are incompletely understood. Calcitriol may act independently of this genomic pathway [12]; and can activate protein kinase C [13], modulate phospholipid metabolism [14], stimulate formation of cyclic nucleotides [15], trigger calcium transport [16], and activate Raf and MAPK (Erk 1/2) activity [17], all in a manner which appears to be independent of VDR/DNA binding.

VDR polymorphisms

A number of polymorphisms have been identified in the VDR gene locus and include BsMI, TaqI, ApaI in intron 8 and exon 9 and a poly-A site in 3′UTR [18–22]. Studies demonstrated an association between VDR polymorphisms (TaqI and BsMI) and an increased risk of prostate cancer [18,19], however a study comparing men who died from prostate cancer with healthy controls showed no correlation [20]. Further, none of the polymorphisms are associated with changes in receptor sequence or function and may be related to VDR mRNA stability. A larger study in men over the age of 57, did not find a relationship with risk and BsMI polymorphisms, but found that the lowest risk of prostate cancer occurred in men with high 1,25-dihydroxycholecalciferol levels and low 25-hydroxycholecalciferol serum levels, and this was associated with older men with the BB genotype [22]. Although the functional role of these polymorphisms

is not clear, data suggest that polymorphisms within or near the VDR gene-encoding region may alter prostate cancer risk.

Epidemiology of prostate cancer and vitamin D

The major risk factors for prostate cancer are age, race, and geography [23]. Prostate cancer incidence increases with age; more than 80% of prostate cancer is found in men over the age of 65 [24]. African-Americans have a higher incidence and mortality of prostate cancer compared to Caucasians; in Japanese men, the incidence and mortality rates are substantially lower [25,26]. There is also a geographical risk for prostate cancer; higher mortality rates are seen in North America and Scandinavia and lower rates are evident in Africa and Central and South America [23]. Studies suggest that vitamin D may play a role in modifying the risk of prostate cancer in association with all of these risk factors. Serum vitamin D levels fall with increasing age. Individuals who reside in northern latitudes have a lower exposure to ultraviolet light and a higher rate of prostate cancer. Members of the African-American race are at an increased risk of prostate cancer and/or mortality from prostate cancer and have reduced serum levels of vitamin D due to skin pigments (melanin) which reduce vitamin D synthesis. In addition, higher serum vitamin D levels are associated with diets high in fish oil and increased exposure to ultraviolet light, and these represent factors that decrease risk or mortality from prostate cancer [24].

Vitamin D analogs

The dose-limiting toxicity of calcitriol is hypercalcemia [27]. To obviate this problem in the clinic, analogs have been developed to efficiently activate the VDR without inducing hypercalcemia. These analogs usually differ in their side chain and vary in their ability to bind to the VDR (Figure 1). A number of potent analogs have been developed. Several studies have demonstrated that a number of analogs can inhibit the growth of prostate tumor cells and other tumor types both *in vitro* and *in vivo* [28–31]. The analogs 16-dienes, 1-dienes, 19-nor, and fluorine derivatives all have demonstrated activity in prostate cells [32–34]. EB1089, an analog developed by Leo Pharmaceuticals, is more potent in binding to the VDR and has greater anti-proliferative activity against PC-3 and LNCaP compared to calcitriol [34]. A number of the analogs

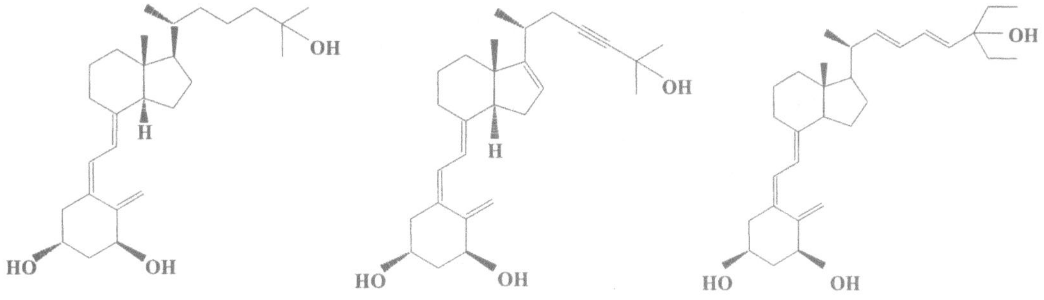

1,25-D$_3$ **Ro-23-7553**   **EB1089**

Figure 1. Structure of the parent compound vitamin D (1,25-dihydroxycholecalciferol or calcitriol) and the vitamin D analogs Ro-23-7553 (1,25-dihydroxy-16-ene-23-yne-cholecalciferol and EB 1089 [1 (s), 3 (R)-dihydroxy-20 (R)-(5′-ethyl-5′-hydroxy-hepta-1′ (E), 3′(E)-dien-1′-ye)-9,10-secopregna-5(2), 7(E), 10,19)-triene].

are not as calcemic as the parent and this may be related to a weaker affinity for the VDR, changes in the ability to bind to the DBP or differences in metabolic rate [35]. EB1089 is the analog that has been widely administered to patients in Europe where in a phase I trial, stabilization of disease was observed in patients with advanced breast and colorectal cancer [36]. Phase III trials in hepatoma are currently ongoing.

Anti-tumor activities

The VDR is found, not only in classical target organs (intestinal tract, kidney, and bone), but also in many other epithelial and mesenchymal cells as well as leukemic cells, osteosarcoma, breast and colon carcinoma, melanoma, glioma, lung and prostate carcinoma, and other malignant cell types [1,2]. Initial *in vivo* studies focused on the use of calcitriol in murine leukemia models where calcitriol has anti-proliferative and differentiating effects [37,38]. Calcitriol inhibits growth *in vitro* and *in vivo* in murine and human breast and colon cancer models [39–41]. Calcitriol has also been investigated in prostate cancer where anti-proliferative activity has been observed with established human prostate cell lines such as PC-3, DU145, and LNCaP [42–45]. PSA secretion and androgen receptor (AR) expression are enhanced in LNCaP cells in response to calcitriol, which also inhibits LNCaP proliferation, in a dose-dependent manner [43,44]. Calcitriol in combination with RXR ligands synergistically inhibits the growth of LNCaP cells [45]. Using *in vitro* assays, DU145 cells are highly invasive with significant inhibition by calcitriol [46].

Calcitriol can induce differentiation, cell cycle arrest, or apoptosis in leukemic and solid tumor cells [47–58]. Progression through the cell cycle is regulated by proteins known as cyclins and their associated cyclin dependent kinases (cdk). The cdk inhibitors p21$^{Waf1/Cip1}$ and p27^{Kip} are implicated in G$_1$ arrest [51,52]. In HL-60 cells, a human myelomonocytic leukemia cell line, calcitriol arrests cells in G$_1$; this effect is mediated through an increase in p27^{Kip} [49]. Calcitriol-mediated arrest in G$_0$/G$_1$ is also observed in human breast cancer lines [53]. In U937, a human myelomonocytic cell line, a functional VDRE has been identified in the p21 promoter region and transcriptional activation of p21 by the VDR induces differentiation in this cell line [50]. Apoptosis is mediated by biochemically diverse stimuli that activate caspases and bring about cellular destruction through specific cleavage of key cellular proteins [54]. The bcl-2 protein, which is overexpressed in many tumors, suppresses apoptosis and the bax protein promotes apoptotic cell death [55–57]. Calcitriol induces apoptosis associated with a decrease in bcl-2 expression in MCF-7 breast cancer cells [58]. In HL-60 leukemic cells apoptotic effects are varied, however, the expression of bcl-2 is consistently down-regulated by calcitriol in these cells [59,60].

In a murine syngeneic squamous cell carcinoma SCC VII/SF, metastatic Dunning rat prostate adenocarcinoma (MLL), and the human xenograft PC-3 prostate model systems, calcitriol has significant anti-proliferative effects *in vitro* and *in vivo* [61–63]. In the MLL model, calcitriol causes inhibition of tumor growth, but also a significant reduction in the number and size of lung metastases [62]. Calcitriol also causes arrest of tumor cells in G_0/G_1 and alters expression of cell cycle regulatory proteins [62,64]. In SCC *in vitro* calcitriol treatment results in decreased expression of p21 mRNA and protein, and increased expression of p27 mRNA and protein and Rb dephosphorylation [65]. *In vivo*, a decrease in SCC tumor volume induced by calcitriol correlates with a significant decrease in the intratumoral p21 expression.

Apoptotic cell death occurs through the activation of caspases, which results in specific cleavage of poly (ADP-ribose) polymerase or PARP [66–68]. We demonstrated by Western blot that calcitriol induced 90–100% PARP cleavage in MLL cells treated with 10 μM of calcitriol (half the IC50) [63]. Induction of apoptosis was confirmed using annexin binding as a measure of phosphatidylserine exposure. The caspase inhibitors, ZVAD-fmk and DEVD-fmk had no direct effect on cells but significantly inhibited calcitriol-mediated increase in annexin binding. In addition, bax was unchanged and bcl-2 was decreased at 24 h in MLL treated with calcitriol; this results in an increased bax/bcl-2 ratio, which favors death.

Effects of calcitriol on cell signaling

In vitro, exponentially growing tumor cells express significant levels of phosphorylated and hence activated mitogen-activated protein kinases (P-Erk1/2). Erk1/2 are known to transduce mitogenic and survival signals to the nucleus in response to a number of extra-cellular stimuli [69,70]. Treatment of SCC cells with calcitriol alone at 10 nM demonstrated no inhibition of P-Erk1/2 after 4 h, modest inhibition after 24 h, and strong inhibition after 48 h [71]. An increase in VDR expression accompanied the loss of P-Erk1/2 in calcitriol-treated cells. Similar effects were observed even at a lower dose of calcitriol (1 nM). Importantly, Erk-1 and Erk-2 protein levels were unchanged in any of the treatment groups. Upstream of Erk, the growth-promoting/pro-survival signaling molecule MEK is cleaved in a caspase-dependent manner in cells induced to undergo apoptosis with calcitriol. Cleavage results in nearly complete loss of full-length MEK and Erk1/2 phosphorylation. The phosphorylation and expression of Akt, a kinase regulating a second cell survival pathway, is also inhibited after treatment with calcitriol. The pro-apoptotic signaling molecule MEKK-1 is up-regulated in cells induced to undergo apoptosis after treatment with calcitriol. These results suggest that calcitriol exerts its growth inhibitory effects on tumor cells by inhibiting the mitogenic signaling pathway at a point upstream of Erk1/2 and by up-regulating the stress signaling kinase, MEKK-1.

Anti-angiogenic effects

Calcitriol has significant effects on vascular endothelium [72–76]. These studies have primarily utilized mature human/bovine vascular endothelial cells, isolated originally from umbilical veins or aorta and carried as established cell lines *in vitro*. Tumor and normal blood vessels differ in their permeability, composition of the basement membrane, or extra-cellular matrix and cellular composition [77–84]. Tumor microvessels are leaky with defective or limited extracellular matrix and are made up of immature neo-vascular cells with a higher proliferative capacity compared to more mature vessels which are found in normal tissues. We have developed a unique method, utilizing flow cytometry, to isolate fresh or early passage endothelial cells from tumors. Our procedures minimize the potential for phenotypic drift of the cells following removal from the *in vivo* tumor microenvironment [77,78]. Inherent in our approach is to characterize the response of endothelial cells freshly isolated from tumors that may be specific to these cells compared to normal.

Using these cells, we examined the ability of calcitriol to inhibit the growth of tumor-derived endothelial cells (TDECs) and normal endothelial cells and to modulate angiogenic signaling [79]. Calcitriol inhibited the growth of TDECs from two tumor models at nanomolar concentrations, but was less potent against normal aortic or yolk sac endothelial cells. The vitamin D analogs Ro-25-6760, EB1089, and Ro-23-7553 were also potent inhibitors of TDEC proliferation. Furthermore, the combination of calcitriol and dexamethasone had greater activity against TDECs than either agent alone. Calcitriol increased VDR and p27[kip1] protein levels in TDECs, while phospho-Erk1/2 and phospho-Akt levels were reduced. These changes were not observed in normal aortic endothelial cells. In SCC and RIF-1 tumor cells, calcitriol treatment caused a reduction in the angiogenic-signaling molecule, angiopoietin-2. Calcitriol and its analogs directly inhibit TDEC proliferation at concentrations comparable to those required to inhibit tumor cells. Further, calcitriol modulates cell cycle and survival signaling in TDECs and affects angiogenic signaling in cancer cells. This work suggests that angiogenesis inhibition may play a role in the anti-tumor effects of calcitriol.

Effect of calcitriol and dexamethasone on anti-tumor activity and VDR ligand binding

Treatment of cells with calcitriol, glucocorticoids, estrogens, retinoic acid, and PTH influences the cellular content of the VDR [85–89]. While glucocorticoids do not bind the VDR [90], they influence calcitriol–ligand binding to the VDR in normal cells and tissues [91–93]. Like vitamin D, glucocorticoids bind to the glucocorticoid receptor (GR) and then to the DNA recognition sequence or the glucocorticoid responsive element (GRE). Glucocorticoids can modulate calcitriol effects on Ca^{+2} transport and may alter the metabolism of calcitriol [94,95].

Dexamethasone significantly enhances calcitriol anti-tumor efficacy, *in vitro* and *in vivo* [96,97] (Figure 2). In PC-3, dexamethasone significantly enhances *in vitro* and *in vivo* clonogenic cell kill compared to either agent alone. This combination

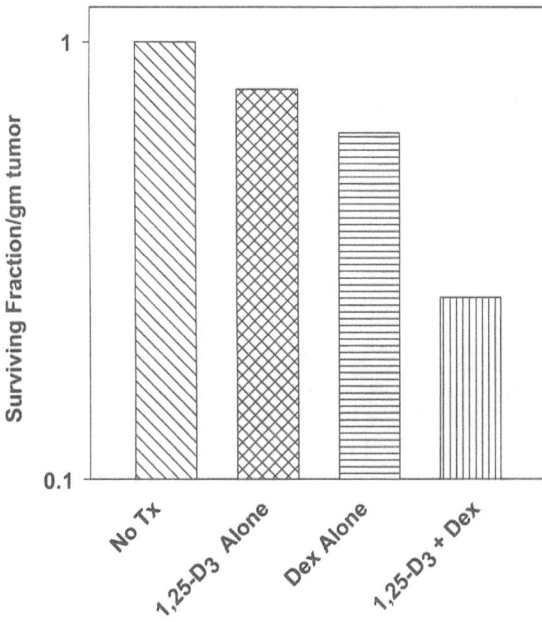

Figure 2. Dexamethasone enhancement of calcitriol-mediated clonogenic cell kill by *in vivo* excision assay. PC-3 tumor-bearing mice were treated with dexamethasone (9 μg/mouse, daily ×4, starting 24 h before calcitriol) and calcitriol (0.75 μg/mouse, daily ×3). 24 h after the last injection, tumors were harvested, plated, and enumerated in the clonogenic assay as described previously [96].

induces significant tumor regression in this model system. To further examine the effects of calcitriol and dexamethasone, we examined anti-proliferative cell cycle and apoptotic effects of this combination in SCC. In a crystal violet assay, the glucocorticoid antagonist, RU486 blocks the dexamethasone-induced enhancement of calcitriol anti-proliferative activity. As shown previously, calcitriol induces cell cycle arrest [62,64,97]. When cells were pretreated with dexamethasone, a significantly greater percentage of cells were in G_0/G_1 phase compared to either calcitriol or dexamethasone alone; RU486 significantly inhibits this enhancement. The combination of calcitriol/dexamethasone led to an increase in the cleaved, active form of caspase-3 and a further reduction in full length PARP compared to calcitriol alone; RU486 blocked this effect. In addition, the levels of phosphorylated, active Erk1/2 and Akt were reduced in cells treated with calcitriol and a further reduction was observed in combination with dexamethasone suggesting that dexamethasone enhances calcitriol pro-apoptotic signaling. RU486 inhibited the effects of dexamethasone on both Erk1/2 and Akt, suggesting that the GR may be required for these activities and that they may be important targets for anti-tumor activity.

Dexamethasone significantly increases VDR receptor content (number) without changing the affinity for calcitriol (Kd) [96]. To further examine the effects of steroids on calcitriol-mediated anti-tumor effects, treated cells were examined for changes in VDR protein by Western blot analysis. The combination of calcitriol and dexamethasone resulted in a significant increase in VDR protein as compared to calcitriol alone or dexamethasone alone. This increase was maximal at 48 h and correlated with an increase in VDR ligand binding. To determine whether dexamethasone mediates its effects through an increase in mRNA levels for the VDR, we isolated RNA from tumor cells treated *in vitro* with calcitriol with and without dexamethasone. By Northern blot analysis, no significant increase in mRNA levels was observed in any of the treatment groups. Treatment with calcitriol alone or other agents that enhance VDR protein do not significantly increase VDR mRNA expression in a number of cell types [98]. We also examined whether changes could be observed *in vivo* in animals treated with calcitriol. Tumor-bearing mice were treated for 3 days with calcitriol and tumors harvested 4 h later, homogenized, and whole cell extracts analyzed by Western blot. At 4 h after the last injection of calcitriol, VDR protein, especially the upper band of the doublet, was induced in the animals treated with calcitriol. Modulation of VDR demonstrates a biologic effect on the tumor; we also demonstrated that enhanced VDR in the tumor correlated with an increase in anti-tumor efficacy.

Calcitriol enhancement of chemotherapeutic activity

In vitro, pretreatment with calcitriol or the calcitriol analog, 1,25-dihydroxy-16-ene-23yne-cholecalciferol (Ro-23-7553) significantly enhanced cisplatin, carboplatin, or paclitaxel-mediated clonogenic cell kill compared to either agent alone [64] (Figure 3). In the *in vivo* excision clonogenic assay where tumors are removed 24 h after cytotoxic drug treatment and plated in a

7-day clonogenic assay, pretreatment with calcitriol markedly enhanced cytotoxic drug-mediated clonogenic tumor cell kill, even at low doses of drug as compared to drug alone. Similarly, a significant decrease in fractional tumor volume and an increase in regrowth delay are observed with calcitriol in combination with these drugs as compared to any agent alone. Schedule and timing are critical to optimal anti-tumor efficacy. Tumor-bearing animals were treated with calcitriol daily for 3 days and the cytotoxic agent was administered with calcitriol on day 3. Using this schedule, anti-tumor effects are maximized and less hypercalcemia was seen.

To explore how calcitriol enhances activity in combination with cytotoxics, we examined the molecular

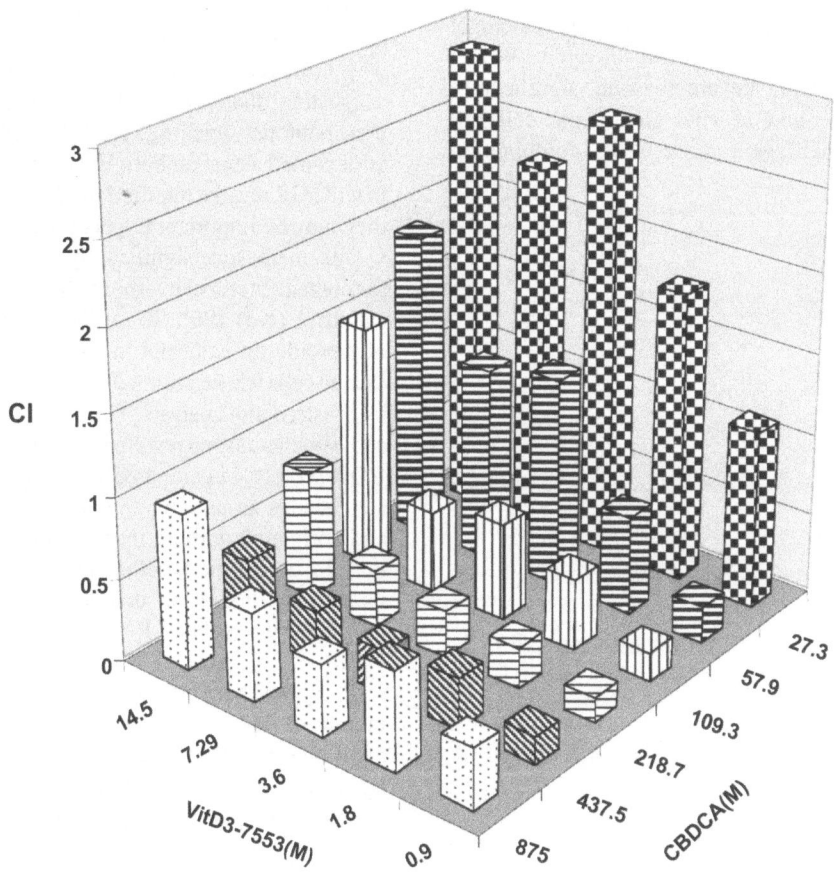

Figure 3. Assessment of the interaction between calcitriol and carboplatin in PC-3 cells. Cells were plated at 1.5×10^3 cells/well in 96-well tissue culture plates and then either untreated or pretreated for 24 h with the indicated doses of calcitriol. Cells were then treated with and without carboplatin (CBDCA) and after 24 h, plates were harvested by staining with MTT and the absorbance read at 460 nM. The dose-effect data obtained by each drug alone and in combination were used to calculate combination index (CI) values as described previously [99]. A combination index less than 1.0 is synergistic.

effects of paclitaxel cytotoxicity with and without calcitriol in PC-3 human prostatic adenocarcinoma cells [99]. The *in vitro* effects of calcitriol and paclitaxel on p21, bcl-2, caspase-3, and poly (ADP-ribose) polymerase (PARP) in PC-3 were evaluated by Western blot. Treatment *in vitro* with calcitriol resulted in a decrease in p21 expression in PC-3. Paclitaxel-induced apoptosis in PC-3 as evidenced by the time-dependent loss of procaspase-3 and full-length PARP. Paclitaxel caused increase of p21 and loss of bcl-2. An increase was observed in PARP cleavage in PC-3 treated with calcitriol/paclitaxel as compared to paclitaxel alone. Thus, calcitriol and paclitaxel have enhanced anti-tumor effects in PC-3 cells as compared to either agent alone and this is associated with a greater induction of apoptosis. Optimal activity for the combination is observed when cells are pre-treated with calcitriol followed by paclitaxel.

Clinical trials with calcitriol

Calcitriol supplement therapy is widely used for the treatment of osteoporosis and renal osteodystrophy in patients with chronic renal failure and hyperparathyroidism [100]. In cancer clinical trials, calcitriol has been utilized primarily in leukemia and myelodysplasia. Although some evidence of response was seen, the results were largely disappointing due to dose-limiting hypercalcemia [101,102].

We completed a study to evaluate the pharmacokinetics and MTD of calcitriol following subcutaneous (sc) QOD administration [103]. Thirty-six patients were entered at doses ranging from 2 to 10 μg QOD; dose-limiting toxicity (hypercalcemia) occurred in 3 of 3 patients entered at the 10 μg QOD dose. Hypercalciuria occurred at all dose levels examined. No other toxicity was seen. Assessment of serum calcitriol concentrations by a radioimmunoassay revealed a decrease in concentration–time curves on the seventh day compared to the first day of therapy. A dose-dependent increase in peak serum level and estimated area under the curve (AUC) were seen; the maximum serum levels occurred at the 10 μg QOD dose: 288±74 and 321 ± 36 pg/ml at days 1 and 7 respectively. The normal range of calcitriol serum concentrations using this assay is 16–56 pg/ml. Serum calcitriol levels were maintained at near peak concentrations for at least 8 h following sc injection. This study indicates that substantial doses of calcitriol can be administered via this route with tolerable toxicity.

In a recent phase I study by Beer et al. [104], patients with advanced cancer were treated once weekly for 4 weeks with calcitriol at a starting dose of 0.06 μg/kg. Dose escalation continued until 2.8 μg/kg without dose-limiting toxicity or hypercalcemia. Plasma calcitriol levels suggested a plateau in both serum levels and in AUC beyond 0.5 μg/kg and further dose escalation beyond 2.8 μg/kg was not attempted. Fifteen patients received 20 cycles of therapy with minimal toxicity and doses of 0.48 μg/kg produced mean calcitriol levels of 1625 pg/ml which is approximately 25 times the normal calcitriol serum levels and within the range utilized *in vitro* in tissue culture.

Calcitriol and glucocorticoids in prostate cancer

Earlier, we performed a small study to investigate the effect of calcitriol alone in prostate cancer [105]. In this study, 13 men with hormone independent prostate cancer received 1.5 μg daily and were monitored for effects of toxicity and effects on PSA. In this small group of patients, no responses were seen and 30% of the patients experienced dose-limiting hypercalcemia. Gross et al. [106] demonstrated that in 6 out of 7 patients with hormone refractory prostate cancer and a rising PSA, calcitriol significantly decreased the rate of rise of the PSA with an observed dose-limiting hypercalciuria.

Calcitriol causes hypercalcemia by increasing intestinal calcium absorption and mobilizing bone and calcium stores [1,2]. Glucocorticoids have been used to reverse the hypercalcemia of calcitriol intoxication [107]. Glucocorticoids have direct anti-tumor effects in many tumor systems. In prostate cancer, several large, randomized clinical trials have examined the efficacy of hydrocortisone or prednisone in hormone independent prostate cancer [108–110]. While clear palliative and PSA responses are seen, these occur in only 10–20% of cases. A recent report of high dose, short course dexamethasone alone indicates that dexamethasone did not result in a significant reduction in PSA [111].

As our preclinical data indicate, dexamethasone potentiates calcitriol anti-tumor effects and blocks hypercalcemia. As a result, we initiated a phase II study of calcitriol and dexamethasone in androgen-independent prostate cancer [112]. Calcitriol and dexamethasone are administered according to the following schedule: calcitriol 8 μg Monday, Tuesday, and Wednesday (MTW) weekly ×4, then if no toxicity was seen the dose was escalated to 10 μg MTW for one month. If no toxicity occurred the dose of calcitriol was increased to 12 μg MTW weekly for the duration of the study. Dexamethasone was administered orally 4 mg Sunday MTW each week. Forty-three patients were treated and 35 received 12 μg MTW ≥ 1 month; *no* patient has required dose reduction because of hypercalcemia. The only calcitriol related toxicity in this trial has been the development in 2 patients of urinary tract stones. All patients undergo pretreatment and Q3 month renal ultrasound to monitor for nephrolithiasis. Thirty-five patients are evaluable and 28% of the 35 evaluable patients experienced a 50% reduction in PSA; patients with bone pain at study entry have experienced pain relief. Eighty percent of patients have experienced a slowing in the rate of PSA rise. Our studies indicate that modification in the schedule and route of administration of calcitriol and dexamethasone permit dose escalation of this agent and that anti-tumor responses are seen in patients with androgen-independent disease treated with calcitriol and dexamethasone.

Clinical trials with calcitriol alone and in combination with cytotoxic agents

We are conducting two phase I trials of calcitriol + cytotoxics [113]: (1) carboplatin (AUC = 5) Q28 days + escalating doses of calcitriol QDX3 Q28 days. Calcitriol starting dose was 4 μg QDX3. Studies are designed such that in each patient, carboplatin is given on day 1 before calcitriol in one of the first two cycles of treatment and on day 3 after two days of high-dose calcitriol on the other. This permits comparison of AUC of carboplatin in the same patient before and after pretreatment with calcitriol. Dose-limiting toxicity has not been encountered in this trial; current doses of calcitriol are 13 μg po QDX3, Q4 week with carboplatin. AUC of carboplatin is higher in *each* patient following calcitriol than before calcitriol (mean AUC = 7.8 μg/ml · h ± 1.3, carboplatin day 3 vs. AUC = 6.7 μg/ml · h ± 1.5, carboplatin day 1). While no dose-limiting toxicity has been seen, myelosuppression (% change in platelet count) following the sequence carboplatin → calcitriol was less than that following calcitriol → carboplatin, consistent with the change in AUC. No clinically detectable renal impairment has been seen with either sequence. These data indicate that potentiation of carboplatin by calcitriol may in part be related to reduced carboplatin clearance. (2) paclitaxel

(80 mg/m^2 weekly ×6) + escalating doses of calcitriol, QDX3 weekly ×6. The starting dose of calcitriol was 4 μg po QDX3, weekly and we have entered patients through the 38 μg dose level where it appears that we have reached saturable concentrations at 16–20 μg. No limiting toxicity has been encountered. The study design calls for administration of paclitaxel on day 1 cycle 1 of therapy prior to any calcitriol therapy and on day 3 with the third dose of calcitriol week 2 and all subsequent weeks. This permits evaluation of the effect of calcitriol on paclitaxel pharmacokinetics – week 1 vs week 2. No changes in peak calcitriol concentration, AUC, or T 1/2 have been noted. To investigate the bioavailability of calcitriol, the studies continue where patients are entered at 14 μg using a liquid formulation of calcitriol with potentially greater bioavailability.

Conclusion

Epidemiology data suggest a role for vitamin D (calcitriol) in prostate cancer. Calcitriol induces antiproliferative effects in tumor cells characterized by induction of cell cycle arrest and apoptosis as well as perturbations of cell survival signals. Calcitriol induces a significant decrease in P-Erk1/2 and MEK, induces MEK cleavage and uniquely induces MEKK-1. These changes in the signaling pathway are associated with a significant anti-tumor activity both *in vitro* and *in vivo* in prostate tumor models. In addition, synergistic anti-tumor activity is observed when calcitriol is combined with glucocorticoids or chemotherapeutic agents, especially the taxanes. Clinical studies have demonstrated that calcitriol is safe and can be administered at high doses without toxicity. In addition, preliminary results suggest that clear anti-tumor responses as measured by a greater than 50% decrease in PSA are seen in men with androgen-independent prostate cancer with no observable or dose-limiting toxicities. Therefore, calcitriol has significant anti-tumor activities pre-clinically and clinically and results suggest that it could be an effective approach in combination with other agents (chemotherapeutic drugs, steroids, or antibodies) for the treatment of androgen-independent prostate cancer.

References

1. Bikle DD, Pillai S: Vitamin D, calcium, and epidermal differentiation. Endocrine Rev 14: 3–19, 1993

2. Reichel H, Koeffler HP, Norman AW: The role of the vitamin D endocrine system in health and disease. New Engl J Med 320: 980–991, 1989

3. Evans RM: The steroid and thyroid hormone receptor superfamily. Science 240: 889–895, 1998

4. Darwish HM, DeLuca HF: Recent advances in the molecular biology of vitamin D action. In: Progress in Nucleic Acid Research and Molecular Biology, Vol 53, Academic Press Inc, 1996, pp 321–344

5. Christakos S, Raval-Pandya M, Wernyj RP, Yang W: Genomic mechanisms involved in the pleiotropic actions of 1,25-dihydroxyvitamin D3. Biochem J 316: 361–371, 1996

6. Darwish H, DeLuca HF: Vitamin D-regulated gene expression. Critical Reviews in Eukaryotic Gene Expression 3(2): 89–116, 1993

7. Studzinski GP, McLane JA, Uskokovic MR: Signaling pathways for vitamin D-induced differentiation: Implications for therapy of proliferative and neoplastic diseases. Critical Reviews in Eukaryotic Gene Expression 3(4): 279–312, 1993

8. Kivineva M, Blauer M, Syvala H, Tammela T, Tuohimaa P: Localization of 1,25-dihydroxyvitamin D3 receptor (VDR) expression in human prostate. J Steroid Biochem Mol Biol 66: 121–127, 1998

9. Stevens A, Lowe JS: Male reproductive system. In: Stevens A, Lowe JS (eds) Histology, Gower Medical Publishing, London, 1992, pp 304–321

10. Weigel NL: Steroid hormone receptors and their regulation by phosphorylation. Biochem J 319: 657–667, 1996

11. Kuiper GGJM, Brinkmann AO: Steroid hormone receptor phosphorylation: Is there a physiological role? Mol Cell Endocrin 100: 103–107, 1994

12. Norman AW, Ilka N, Zhou LX, Bishop JE, Lowe KE, Maiyar AC, Collin ED, Taoka T, Sergeev I, Farach-Carson MC: 1,25(OH)$_2$-vitamin D3, a steroid hormone that produces biologic effects via both genomic and nongenomic pathways. J Steroid Biochem Mol Biol 41: 231–240, 1992

13. Slater SJ, Kelly MB, Taddeo, FJ, Larkin JD, Yeager MD, McLane JA, Ho C, Stubbs CD: Direct activation of protein kinase C by 1α,25-dihydroxyvitamin D3. J Biol Chem 270: 6639–6643, 1995

14. De Boland AR, Morelli S, Boland R: 1,25-(OH)$_2$-vitamin D3 signal transduction in chick myoblasts involves phosphatidylcholine hydrolysis. J Biol Chem 269: 8675–8679, 1993

15. Khare S, Tien XY, Wilson D, Wali RK, Bissonnette BM, Scaglione-Sewell B, Sitrin MD, Brasitus TA: The role of protein kinase-Cα in the activation of particulate guanylate cyclase by 1α,25-dihydroxyvitamin D$_3$ in CaCo-2 cells. Endocrinology 135: 277–283, 1994

16. De Boland AR, Norman AW: Evidence for involvement of protein kinase C and cyclic adenosine 3′,5′ monophosphate-dependent protein kinase in the 1,25-dihydroxyvitamin D3-mediated rapid stimulation of intestinal calcium transport (transcaltachia). Endocrinology 127: 39, 1990

17. Gniadecki R: Activation of Raf–mitogen-activated protein kinase signaling pathway by 1β25-dihydroxyvitamin D$_3$ in normal human keratinocytes. J Invest Derm 106: 1212–1217, 1996

18. Taylor JA, Hirvonen A, Watson M, Pittman G, Mohler JL, Bell DA: Association of prostate cancer with vitamin D receptor gene polymorphism. Cancer Res 56: 4108–4110, 1996

19. Ingles SA, Ross RK, Yu MC, Irvine RA, Lapera G, Haile RW, Coetzee GA: Association of prostate cancer risk with genetic polymorphisms in vitamin D receptor and androgen receptor. J Natl Cancer Inst 89: 166–170, 1997

20. Kibel AS, Isaacs SD, Isaacs WB, Bova GS: Vitamin D receptor polymorphisms and lethal prostate cancer. J Urol 160: 1405–1409, 1998

21. Morrison AN, Qi CJ, Tokita A: Prediction of bone density from vitamin D recptor alleles. Nature 67: 284–297, 1994

22. Ma J, Stampfer MJ, Gann PH, Hough HL, Giovannucci E, Kelsey KT, Hennekens CH, Hunter DJ: Vitamin D receptor polymorphisms circulating vitamin D metabolites and risk of prostate cancer in United States physicians. Cancer Epidemiol Biomarkers Prev 7: 385–390, 1998

23. Hanchette CL, Schwartz GG: Geographic patterns of prostate cancer mortality. Evidence for a protective effect of ultraviolet radiation. Cancer 70: 2861–2869, 1992

24. Schwartz GG, Hulka BS: Is vitamin D deficiency a risk factor for prostate cancer? (hypothesis). Anticancer Res 10: 1307–1312, 1990

25. Wu LY, Semenya KA, Hardy RE, Hargreaves MK, Robinson SB, Pederson L, Sung JF, Haynes MA: Cancer rate differentials between blacks and whites in three metropolitan areas: A 10-year comparison. J Natl Med Assoc 90: 410–416, 1998

26. Haenszel W, Jurihara M: Studies of Japanese migrants. I. Mortality from cancer and other diseases among Japanese in the United States. J Natl Cancer Inst 40: 43–68, 1968

27. Holick MF: The photobiology of vitamin D3 in man. In: Kumar R (ed) Vitamin D: Basic and Clinical Aspects, Martinus Nijhoff, Boston, 1984, pp 197–216

28. Campbell NJ, Elstner E, Holden S, Uskokovic M, Koeffler HP: Inhibition of proliferation of prostate cancer cells by a 19-nor hexafluoride vitamin D3 analogue involves the induction of p21[wafl], p27[kip1] and E-cadherin. J Mol Endocrinol 19: 15–27, 1997

29. Schwartz GG, Oeler TA, Uskokovic MR, Bahnson RR: Human prostate cancer cells: Inhibition of proliferation by vitamin D analogs. Anticancer Res 14: 1077–1081, 1994

30. Kubota T, Koshizuka K, Koike M, Uskokovic M, Miyoshi I, Koeffler HP: 19-nor-26,27-bishomo-vitamin D3 analogs: A unique class of potent inhibitors of proliferation of prostate, breast, and hematopoietic cancer cells. Cancer Res 58: 3370–3374, 1998

31. Hedlund TE, Moffatt KA, Uskokovic MR, Miller GJ: Three synthetic vitamin D analogues induce prostate-specific acid phosphatase and prostate-specific antigen while inhibiting the growth of human prostate cancer cells in a vitamin D receptor-dependent fashion. Clin Cancer Res 3: 1331–1338, 1997

376

32. Schwartz GG, Hill CC, Oeler TA, Becich MJ, Bahnson RR: 1,24-dihydroxy-16-ene-23-yne-vitamin D and prostate cancer cell proliferation *in vivo*. Urology 46: 365–369, 1995

33. Campbell MJ, Reddy GS, Koeffler HP: Vitamin D3 analogs and their 24-oxo metabolites equally inhibit clonal proliferation of a variety of cancer cells but have differing molecular effects. J Cell Biochem 66: 413–425, 1997

34. Hansen CM, Maenpaa PH: EB 1089, a novel vitamin D analog with strong antiproliferative and differentiation-inducing effects on target cells. Biochem Pharmacol 54: 1173–1179, 1997

35. Kissmeyer AM, Binderup E, Binderup L, Hansen M, Andersen NR, Makin HL, Schroeder NJ, Shankar VN, Jones G: Metabolism of the vitamin D analog EB1089: Identification of *in vivo* and *in vitro* liver metabolites and their biological activities. Biochem Pharmacol 53: 1087–1097, 1997

36. Gulliford T, English J, Colston KW, Menday P, Moller S, Coombes RC: A phase I study of vitamin D analogue EB1089 in patients with advanced breast and colorectoral cancer. Br J Cancer 78: 6–13, 1998

37. Mangelsdorf DJ, Koeffler HP, Donaldson CA, Pike JW, Haussler MR: 1,25-Dihydroxyvitamin D3 induced differentiation in a human promyelocytic leukemia cell line HL-60: Receptor mediated maturation to macrophage-like cells. J Cell Biol 98: 391–398, 1984

38. Zhou JY, Norman AW, Chen DL: 1,25-dihydroxy-16-ene-23-yne-vitamin D3 prolongs survival time of leukemic mice. Proc Natl Acad Sci USA 87: 3929–3932, 1990

39. Colston KW, Chander SK, Mackay AG, Coombes RC: Effects of synthetic vitamin D analogues on breast cancer cell proliferation *in vivo* and *in vitro*. Biochem Pharmacol 44: 693–702, 1993

40. Frappart L, Falette N, Lefebvre MF, Bremond A, Vauzelle JL, Saez S: *In vitro* study of effects of 1,25-dihydroxyvitamin D3 on the morphology of human breast cancer cell line BT.20. Differentiation 40: 63–69, 1989

41. Shabahang M, Buras RR, Davoodi F, Schmaker LM, Nauta RJ, Evans SR: 1,25-dihydroxyvitamin D3 receptors as a marker of human colon carcinoma cell line differentiation and growth inhibition. Cancer Res 53(16): 3712–3718, 1993

42. Peehl DM, Skowronski RJ, Leung GK, Wong ST, Stamey TA, Feldman D: Antiproliferative effects of 1,25-dihydroxyvitamin D_3 on primary cultures of human prostatic cells. Cancer Res 54: 805–810, 1994

43. Miller GJ, Stapleton GE, Ferrara JA, Lucia MS, Pfister S, Hedlund TE, Upadhya P: The human prostatic carcinoma cell line LNCaP expresses biologically active, specific receptors for 1,25-dihydroxyvitamin D3. Cancer Res 52: 515–520, 1992

44. Skowronski RJ, Peehl DM, Feldman D: Vitamin D and prostate cancer: 1,25-dihydroxyvitamin D3 receptors and actions in human prostate cancer cell lines. Endocr 132: 1952–1960, 1993

45. de Vos S, Holden S, Heber D, Elstner E, Binderup L, Uskokovic M, Rude B, Chen D, Le J, Cho SK,

Koeffler HP: Effects of potent vitamin D3 analogs on clonal proliferation of human prostate cancer cell lines. Prostate 31: 77–83, 1997

46. Schwartz GG, Wang MH, Zang M, Singh RK, Siegal GP: 1α,25-dihydroxyvitamin D (calcitriol) inhibits the invasiveness of human prostate cancer cells. Cancer Epidemiol Biomarkers Prev 6: 727–732, 1997

47. Godyn JJ, Xu H, Zhang F, Kolla SS, Studzinski GP: A dual block to cell cycle progression in HL-60 cells exposed to analogues of vitamin D3. Cell Proliferation 27: 37–46, 1994

48. Rigby WF, Noelle RJ, Krause K, Fanger MW: The effects of 1,25-dihydroxyvitamin D3 on human T lymphocyte activation and proliferation: A cell cycle analysis. J Immunol 135: 2279–2286, 1985

49. Wang QM, Jones JB, Studzinski GP: Cyclin-dependent kinase inhibitor p27 as a mediator of the G1-S phase block induced by 1,25-dihydroxyvitamin D3 in HL60 cells. Cancer Res 56: 264–267, 1996

50. Liu M, Lee M-H, Cohen M, Bommakanti M, Freedman LP: Transcriptional activation of the cdk inhibitor p21 by vitamin D3 leads to the induced differentiation of the myelomonocytic cell line U937. Genes & Devel 10: 142–153, 1996

51. Biggs JR, Kraft AS: Inhibitors of cyclin-dependent kinase and cancer. J Mol Med 73: 509–514, 1995

52. Sherr CJ, Roberts JM: Inhibitors of mammalian G^1 cyclin-dependent kinases. Genes & Devel 9: 1149–1163, 1995

53. Sheikh MS, Rochefort H, Garcia M: Overexpression of p21[WAF1/CIP1] induces growth arrest, giant cell formation and apoptosis in human breast carcinoma cell lines. Oncogene 11(9): 1899–1905, 1995

54. Henkart PA: ICE family proteases: Mediators of all apoptotic cell death? Immunity 4: 195–201, 1996

55. Hockenbery D, Nunez G, Milliman C, Schreiber RD, Korsmeyer SJ: Bcl-2 is an inner mitochondrial membrane protein that blocks programmed cell death. Nature (Lond) 348: 334–336, 1990

56. Hockenbery DM: The bcl-2 oncogene and apoptosis. Semin Immunol 4: 413–420, 1992

57. Oltvai Z, Milliman C, Korsmeyer SJ: Bcl-2 heterodimerizes *in vivo* with a conserved homolog, Bax, that accelerates programmed cell death. Cell 74: 609–619, 1993

58. Simboli-Campbell M, Narvaez CJ, Tenniswood M, Welsh J: 1,25-Dihydroxyvitamin D3 induces morphological and biochemical markers of apoptosis in MCF-7 breast cancer cells. J Steroid Biochem Mol Biol 58: 367–376, 1996

59. Elstner E, Linker-Israeli M, Umiel T, Le J, Grillier I, Said J, Shintaku IP, Krajewski S, Reed JC, Binderup L, Koeffler HP: Combination of a potent 20-epi-vitamin D3 analogue (KH 1060) with 9-cis-retinoic acid irreversibly inhibits clonal growth, decreases bcl-2 expression, and induces apoptosis in HL-60 leukemic cells. Cancer Res 56: 3570–3576, 1996

60. Xu H-M, Tepper CG, Jones JB, Fernandez C, Studzinski G: 1,25-Dihydroxyvitamin D3 protects HL60 cells against apoptosis but down-regulates the expression of the bcl-2 gene. Experimental Cell Res 209: 367–374, 1993

61. McElwain MC, Dettelbach MA, Modzelewski RA, Russell DM, Uskokovic MR, Smith DC, Trump DL, Johnson CS: Antiproliferative effects *in vitro* and *in vivo* of 1,25-dihydroxyvitamin D3 and a vitamin D3 analog in a squamous cell carcinoma model system. Mol Cell Diff 3(1): 31–50, 1995

62. Getzenberg RH, Light BW, Lapco PE, Konety BR, Nangia AK, Acierno JS, Shurin Z, Day RS, Trump DL, Johnson CS: Vitamin D inhibition of prostate adenocarcinoma growth and metastasis in the Dunning rat prostate model system. Urology 50: 999–1006, 1997

63. Modzelewski RA, Hershberger PA, Johnson CS, Trump DL: Apoptotic effects of paclitaxel and calcitriol in rat dunning MLL and human PC-3 prostate tumor cells *in vitro*. Proc Amer Assoc Cancer Res 40: 580a, 1999

64. Light BW, Yu W-D, McElwain MC, Russell DM, Trump DL, Johnson CS: Potentiation of cisplatin antitumor activity using a vitamin D analogue in a murine squamous cell carcinoma model system. Cancer Res 57: 3759–3764, 1997

65. Hershberger PA, Modzelewski RA, Shurin ZR, Rueger RM, Trump DL, Johnson CS: 1,25-dihydroxycholecalciferol (1,25-D$_3$) inhibits the growth of squamous cell carcinoma and down-modulates p21$^{Waf1/Cip1}$ *in vitro* and *in vivo*. Cancer Res 59: 2644–2649, 1999

66. Berger NA: Poly (ADP-ribose) in the cellular response to DNA damage. Radiat Res 101: 4–15, 1985

67. Wintersberger U, Wintersberger E: Poly ADP-ribosylation: A cellular emergency reaction? FEBS Lett 188: 189–191, 1985

68. Green DR, Reed JC: Mitochondria and apoptosis. Science 281: 1309–1312, 1998

69. Paul A, Wilson S, Belham CM, Robin CJM, Scott PH, Gould GW, Plevin R: Stress-activated protein kinases: Activation, regulation and function. Cell Signal 96: 403–410, 1997

70. Lewis TS, Shaprio PS, Ahn NG: Signal transduction through MAP kinase cascades. Advances in Cancer Res 74: 113–139, 1998

71. McGuire TF, Trump DL, Johnson CS: Vitamin D3-induced apoptosis of murine squamous cell carcinoma cells: Selective induction of caspase-dependent MEK cleavage and up-regulation of MEKK-1. J Biol Chem 276: 26365–26373, 2001

72. Koli K, Keski-Oja J: 1α,25-dihydroxyvitamin D3 and its analogues down-regulate cell invasion-associated proteases in cultured malignant cells. Cell Growth & Differentiation 11: 221–229, 2000

73. Iseki K, Tatsuta M, Uehara G, et al.: Inhibition of angiogenesis as a mechanism for inhibition by 1α-hydroxyvitamin D$_3$ and 1,25-dihydroxyvitamin D$_3$ of colon carcinogenesis induced by azoxymethane in Wistar rats. Int J Cancer 81: 730–733, 1999

74. Majewski S, Szmurlo A, Marczak M, Jablonska S, Bollag W: Inhibition of tumor cell-induced angiogenesis by retinoids, 1,25-dihydroxyvitamin D$_3$ and their combination. Cancer Lett 75: 35–39, 1993

75. Shokravi MT, Marcus DM, Alroy J, Egan K, Saornil MA, Albert DM: Vitamin D inhibits angiogenesis in transgenic murine retinoblastoma. Invest Opthalmol Vis Sci 36: 83–87, 1995

76. Oikawa T, Horotani K, Nakamura O, Hiragun A, Iwaguchi T: A highly potent antiangiogenic activity of retinoids. Cancer Lett 48: 157–162, 1989

77. Modzelewski RA, Davies P, Watkins SC, Auerbach R, Ming-Jei C, Johnson CS: Isolation and identification of fresh tumor-derived endothelial cells from a murine RIF-1 fibrosarcoma. Cancer Res 54: 336–339, 1994

78. Ming-Jei C, Modzelewski RA, Russell DM, Johnson CS: Interleukin 1alpha and gamma-interferon induction of nitric oxide production from murine tumor-derived endothelial cells. Cancer Res 56(4): 886–891, 1996

79. Bernardi RJ, Johnson CS, Modzelewski RA, Trump DL: Anti-proliferative effects of 1α,25-dihydroxyvitamin D3 and vitamin D analogs on tumor-derived endothelial cells (submitted)

80. Heuser LS, Miller FN: Differential macromolecular leakage from the vasculature of tumors. Cancer 57: 461–464, 1986

81. Gerlowski LE, Jain RK: Microvascular permeability of normal and neoplastic tissues. Microvasc Res 31: 288–305, 1986

82. Hori K, Suzuki M, Tanda S, Saito S: *In vivo* analysis of tumor vascularization in the rat. Jpn J Cancer Res 81: 279–288, 1990

83. Dvorak HF, Nagy JA, Dvorak JT, Dvorak AM: Identification and characterization of the blood vessels of solid tumors that are leaky to circulating macromolecules. Am J Pathol 133: 95–109, 1988

84. Blood CH, Zetter BR: Tumor interactions with the vasculature: Angiogenesis and tumor metastasis. Biochem Biophys Acta 1032: 89–118, 1990

85. Strom M, Sandgren ME, Brown TA, DeLuca HF: 1,25-Dihydroxyvitamin D3 up-regulates the 1,25-dihydroxyvitamin D3 receptor *in vivo*. Proc Natl Acad Sci USA 86: 9770–9773, 1989

86. Chen TL, Cone CM, Morey-Holton E, Feldman D: Glucocorticoid regulation of 1,25-(OH)2-vitamin D3 receptors in cultured mouse bone cells. J Biol Chem 257: 13564–13569, 1982

87. Levy J, Zuili I, Yankowitz N, Shany S: Induction of cytosolic receptors for 1,25-dihydroxyvitamin D3 in the immature rat uterus by estradiol. J Endocrinol 100: 265–269, 1984

88. Petkovich PM, Heersche JNM, Tinker DO, Jones G: Retinoic acid stimulates 1,25-dihydroxyvitamin D3 binding in rat osteosarcoma cells. J Biol Chem 259: 8274–8280, 1984

89. Reinhardt TA, Horst RL: Parathyroid hormone down-regulates 1,25-dihydroxyvitamin D receptors (VDR) and VDR messenger ribonucleic acid *in vitro* and blocks homologous up-regulation of VDR *in vivo*. Endocrin 127: 942–948, 1990

90. Bouillon R, Okamura WH, Norman AW: Structure–function relationships in the vitamin D endocrine system. Endocrine Reviews 16: 200–257, 1995

91. Hirst M, Feldman D: Glucocorticoid regulation of 1,25-(OH)$_2$-vitamin D3 receptors: Divergent effects on mouse and rat intestine. Endocrin 111: 1400–1402, 1982

92. Hirst M, Feldman D: Glucocorticoids down-regulate the number of 1,25-dihydroxyvitamin D3 receptors in mouse intestine. Biochem Biophys Res Comm 105: 1590–1596, 1982

93. Manolagas SC, Abare J, Deftos LJ: Glucocorticoids increase the 1,25-(OH)2 D3 receptor concentration in rat osteogenic sarcoma cells. Calcif Tissue Int 36: 153–157, 1982

94. Kimberg DV, Baerg RD, Gershon E, Graudusius RT: Effect of cortisone treatment on the active transport of calcium by the small intestine. J Clin Invest 50: 1309–1321, 1971

95. Haynes RC: Agents affecting calcification: Calcium, parathyroid hormone, calcitonin, vitamin D, and other compounds. In: Gilman AG, Rall TW, Nies AS, Taylor P (eds) The Pharmacological Basis of Therapeutics, Pergamon Press, New York, 1990, pp 1496–1522

96. Yu W-D, McElwain MC, Modzelewski RA, Russell DM, Smith DC, Trump DL, Johnson CS: Potentiation of 1,25-dihydroxyvitamin D3-mediated anti-tumor activity with dexamethasone. J Natl Cancer Inst 90: 134–141, 1998

97. Bernardi RJ, Trump DL, Yu WD, McGuire TF, Hershberger PA, Johnson CS: Combination of 1α,25-dihydroxyvitamin D3 with dexamethasone enhances cell cycle arrest and apoptosis: Role of nuclear receptor cross-talk and Erk/Akt signaling. Clin Cancer Res 7: 4164–4173, 2001

98. Norman AW: The mode of action of vitamin D. Biol Rev 243: 4055–4064, 1968

99. Hershberger PA, Yu W-D, Modzelewski RA, Rueger RM, Johnson CS, Trump DL: Enhancement of paclitaxel antitumor activity in squamous cell carcinoma and prostatic adenocarcinoma by 1,25-dihydroxycholecaciferol (1,25-D$_3$) Cancer Res 7: 1043–1051, 2001

100. Koeffler HP, Hirji K, Iltri L, the Southern California Leukemia Group: 1,25-Dihydroxyvitamin D3: *In vivo* and *in vitro* effects on human preleukemic and leukemic cells. Cancer Treat Rep 69: 1399–1407, 1985

101. French LE, Ramelet AA, Saurat J-H: Remission of cutaneous T-cell lymphoma with combined calcitriol and acitretin. Lancet 344: 686–687, 1994

102. Cunningham D, Gilchrist NL, Cowan RA, Forrest GJ, McArdle CS, Soukop M: Alfacalcidol as a modulator of growth of low grade non-Hodgkin's lymphomas. Brit Med J 291: 1153–1155, 1985

103. Smith DC, Johnson CS, Freeman CC, Muindi J, Wilson JW, Trump DL: A phase I trial of subcutaneous calcitriol (1,25-dihydroxycholecalciferol) in patients with advanced malignancy. Clin Cancer Res 5: 1339–1345, 1999

104. Beer TM, Munar M, Henner WD: A phase I trial of pulse calcitriol in patients with refractory malignancies. Cancer 91: 2431–2439, 2001

105. Osborne JL, Schwartz GG, Smith DC, Bahnson R, Day R, Trump DL: Phase II trial of oral 1,25-dihydroxyvitamin D (Calcitriol) in hormone refractory prostate cancer. Urol Oncol 1: 195–198, 1995

106. Gross C, Stamey T, Hancock S, Feldman D: Treatment of early recurrent prostate cancer with 1,25-dihydroxyvitamin D$_3$ (calcitriol). J Urol 159: 2035–2040, 1998

107. Davies M: High-dose vitamin D therapy: Indications, benefits and hazards. In: Walter P, Brubacher G, Stahelin H (eds) Elevated Dosages of Vitamins, Vol 81, Hans Huber, Lewistown, NY, 1989

108. Kantoff PW, Halabi S, Conaway M, Picus J, Kirshner J, Hars V, Trump DL, Winer EP, Vogelzang NJ: Hydrocortisone with or without mitoxantrone in men with hormone-refractory prostate cancer. J Clin Oncol 17: 2506–2513, 1999

109. Tannock I, Gospodarowicz M, Meakin W, Panzarella T, Stewart L, Rider W: Treatment of metastatic prostatic cancer with low-dose prednisone: Evaluation of pain and quality of life as pragmatic indices of response. J Clin Oncol 7: 590–597, 1989

110. Small EJ, Meyer M, Marshall, ME, Reyno LM, Meyers FJ, Natale RB, Lenchan PF, Chen L, Slichenmyer WJ, Eisenberger M: Suramin therapy for patients with symptomatic hormone-refractory prostate cancer: Results of a randomized phase III trial comparing suramin plus hydrocortisone to placebo plus hydrocortisone. J Clin Oncol 18(7): 1440–1450, 2000

111. Weitzman AL, Shelton G, Zuech N, Owen CE, Judge T, Benson M, Sawczuk I, Katz A, Olsson CA, Bagiella E, Pfaff C, Newhouse JH, Petrylak DP: Dexamethasone does not significantly contribute to the response rate of docetaxel and estramustine in androgen independent prostate cancer. J Urol 163(3): 834–837, 2000

112. Trump DL, Serafine S, Brufsky A, Potter D, Johnson CS: High dose calcitriol (1,25(OH)$_2$ vitamin D$_3$) + dexamethasone in androgen independent prostate cancer (AIPC). Proc Amer Soc Clin Oncol 19: 337a, 2000

113. Johnson CS, Egorin MJ, Zuhowski R, Parise R, Cappozolli M, Belani CP, Long GS, Muindi J, Trump DL: Effects of high dose calcitriol (1,25-dihydroxyvitamin D$_3$) on the pharmacokinetics of paclitaxel or carboplatin: Results of two phase I studies. Proc Amer Soc Oncol 19: 210a, 2000

Address for offprints: Candace S. Johnson, Department of Pharmacology and Therapeutics, Roswell Park Cancer Institute, Elm and Carlton Streets, Buffalo, NY 14263, USA; *Tel:* (716) 845-4443; *Fax:* (716) 845-8057; *e-mail:* candace.johnson@roswellpark.org

Osteoporosis and other adverse body composition changes during androgen deprivation therapy for prostate cancer

Matthew R. Smith

Massachusetts General Hospital, Boston, MA, USA

Key words: androgen deprivation therapy, bicalutamide, bone, estrogen, fat, fracture, gonadotropin-releasing hormone agonist, muscle, osteoporosis, prostate cancer

Abstract

Osteoporosis and other body composition changes are important complications of androgen deprivation therapy (ADT) for prostate cancer. Bilateral orchiectomy and gonadotropin-releasing hormone agonist treatment decrease bone mineral density and increase fracture risk. Other factors including diet and lifestyle may contribute to bone loss in men with prostate cancer. Estrogens play an important role in male bone metabolism. Androgen deprivation therapy with estrogens probably causes less bone loss than bilateral orchiectomy or gonadotropin-releasing hormone agonist treatment. Bicalutamide monotherapy increases serum estrogen levels and may also spare bone. Lifestyle modification including smoking cessation, moderation of alcohol use, and regular weight bearing exercise are recommended to decrease treatment-related bone loss. Supplemental calcium and vitamin D are also recommended. Pamidronate (Aredia®), an intravenous bisphosphonate, prevents bone loss during ADT. Other bisphosphonates are probably effective but have not been studied in hypogonadal men. Androgen deprivation therapy increases fat mass and decreases muscle mass. These body composition changes may contribute to treatment-related decreases in physical capacity and quality of life.

Introduction

Androgen deprivation therapy (ADT) by either bilateral orchiectomy or administration of a gonadotropin-releasing hormone agonist is the mainstay of treatment for advanced prostate cancer. The routine early use of ADT increases the importance of recognizing and preventing adverse effects of treatment. Adverse effects of ADT include loss of libido, vasomotor flushing, anemia, osteoporosis, weight gain, decreased muscle mass, and increased fat mass. This review focuses on the pathophysiology and management and osteoporosis and other body composition changes associated with ADT.

Male osteoporosis

In the United States, osteoporosis is prevalent in about 1.5 million men older than 65 years and another 3.5 million men are at risk [1]. One-third of hip fractures occur in men [2]. Male osteoporosis has not been adequately studied and most management decisions are based on research from postmenopausal osteoporosis.

Definition of osteoporosis

Low bone mineral density (BMD) correlates with fracture risk in men and women [3–6]. Every standard deviation decrease in BMD increases the relative risk of fracture in women by approximately two-fold [7]. A working group of the World Health Organization defines normal, osteopenia, and osteoporosis based on BMD compared to the mean value in young adults [8]. Normal is defined as BMD within 1 standard deviation of the young adult mean. Osteopenia is defined as BMD between 1.0 and 2.5 standard deviations below the young adult mean. Osteoporosis is defined as BMD 2.5 or more standard deviations below the young adult mean. Although these definitions are based primarily on the relationships between forearm BMD measurements by dual-energy X-ray absorptiometry and prevalent hip fractures in postmenopausal Caucasian

M.L. Cher, K.V. Honn and A. Raz (eds.), Prostate Cancer: New Horizons in Research and Treatment, 379–386.
© 2002 *Kluwer Academic Publishers.*

women, the World Health Organization definitions for osteopenia and osteoporosis have been widely applied to men, different skeletal sites, and different methods of BMD measurement. Because men have higher peak BMD and larger bones, additional studies are needed to develop appropriate definitions of osteopenia and osteoporosis in men [9].

Diagnosis of osteoporosis

Several noninvasive methods can be used to measure BMD [7]. Dual-energy X-ray absorptiometry is the method of choice for BMD measurement in most cases. Dual-energy X-ray absorptiometry easily and precisely measures BMD at multiple skeletal sites with minimal radiation exposure. Hip BMD is the most useful for predicting fractures whereas measurement of posterior–anterior lumbar spine BMD is most useful for assessing efficacy of treatment. Quantitative computed tomography can measure BMD of the spine, hip, or forearm. Quantitative computed tomography is more sensitive, less precise, and involves more radiation exposure than dual-energy X-ray absorptiometry. Ultrasound measurements of the heel, finger, tibia or patella are portable and inexpensive. Ultrasound measurements are less precise than other methods and evaluate skeletal sites that are unresponsive to treatment.

Quantitative computed tomography is more sensitive than dual-energy X-ray absorptiometry for detecting osteoporosis in men with prostate cancer [10]. Average BMD of the posterior–anterior lumbar spine increases in men after age 55 years due to the development of osteoarthritis in the posterior spinous elements [11–15]. Quantitative computed tomography restricts measurement of BMD to the central region of the vertebral bodies and eliminates the potential confounding effects of osteoarthritis [16]. Quantitative computed tomography discriminates between normal and osteoporotic bone significantly better than dual-energy X-ray absorptiometry [17].

Secondary causes of osteoporosis should be pursued in men with osteoporosis. A focused history, physical examination, and selected laboratory tests are sufficient in most patients. Measurement of serum concentrations of parathyroid hormone and 25-hydroxyvitamin D is recommended to exclude hypothyroidism and vitamin D deficiency. Serum thyroid-stimulating hormone levels can exclude hypothyroidism and routine serum chemistries can exclude renal or liver disease.

Serum concentrations of calcium, inorganic phosphate, and alkaline phosphatase are usually normal in men with osteoporosis. Serum alkaline phosphatase levels may be transiently elevated after fracture. In the absence of liver disease, persistent elevation of serum alkaline phosphatase levels suggests osteomalacia, Paget's disease, or bone metastases.

Measurement of biochemical markers of bone resorption and bone formation in the serum and urine complement measurement of BMD. High levels of bone turnover are associated with osteoporosis, increased rates of bone loss, and may independently predict fracture risk [18]. Changes in bone turnover also provide an early indication of treatment response. The clinical usefulness of bone turnover markers has not been established, however, and biochemical markers of bone turnover should not be used in place of BMD measurements.

Clinical manifestations of osteoporosis

Osteoporosis has no symptoms until it results in a fracture. Vertebral body compression fractures and fractures of the wrist, hip, ribs, pelvis, or humerus are the most common events. Vertebral body compression fractures may occur with minimal stress such as bending or lifting. The lumbar and thoracic vertebrae are the most frequently involved regions. Standing or sudden movements may exacerbate pain from collapse of the vertebra. Multiple vertebral fractures may cause loss of height, dorsal kyphosis, and cervical lordosis. Hip fractures are the most damaging complication of osteoporosis. Hip fractures are associated with falls. Thromboembolic events, infection, and other secondary complications of hip fracture result in mortality rates of approximately 20% in the elderly. About one-third of elderly hip fracture victims require long-term nursing home care.

Complications of osteoporosis may be mistaken for bone metastases in men with prostate cancer. Common symptoms from vertebral compression fractures, for example, are similar to typical clinical manifestations of bone metastases. Both bone metastases and vertebral body compression fractures from osteoporosis usually present with back pain and share radiographic features including increased uptake by bone scan [19]. Based on the prevalence of osteoporosis in this population, osteoporotic fractures should be considered when prostate cancer patients present with skeletal complaints.

Causes of osteoporosis in men

Adult bone mass reflects both peak bone mass achieved during development and the subsequent adult bone loss. Osteoporosis results from either deficient accumulation of bone during development, accelerated adult bone loss, or both. Accelerated adult bone loss accounts for most cases of osteoporosis. Smoking, excess alcohol intake, deficient dietary calcium intake, vitamin D deficiency, and sedentary lifestyle contribute to adult bone loss [20].

Alcohol abuse, chronic glucocorticoid therapy, and hypogonadism are the three major causes of osteoporosis in men and account for approximately one-half of all cases of male osteoporosis [9]. Primary hyperparathyroidism, hyperthyroidism, multiple myeloma, and other malignancies are less common causes of osteoporosis in men. Idiopathic osteoporosis refers to osteoporosis with no known cause.

ADT and osteoporosis

Four retrospective studies have evaluated the relationship between ADT and fractures in men with prostate cancer [21–24].

Daniell et al. [21] evaluated history of orchiectomy, other risk factors for osteoporosis, and incidence of fractures in 235 men with prostate cancer. Fourteen percent of men with a history of orchiectomy had at least one osteoporotic fracture compared to only 1% of men with no history of ADT. Thirty-eight percent of men surviving longer than five years after orchiectomy experienced an osteoporotic fracture. Osteoporotic fractures were more common than traumatic or pathological fractures.

Another retrospective review determined the incidence of fracture in men with prostate cancer receiving ADT with a GnRH agonist [22]. The median duration of ADT was 22 months. Twenty out of 224 (9%) men had at least one fracture. The median interval from start of ADT until fracture was 22 months. Seven of 22 fractures (32%) were attributed to osteoporosis. The remaining fractures were due to trauma (36%), the direct effect of bone metastases (9%), or multiple causes (23%).

In a Japanese study, osteoporotic fractures were observed in 14 out of 218 (6%) men during ADT for prostate cancer [23,24]. The mean interval from start of ADT to fracture was 28 months. Men with fractures

had lower BMD and higher biochemical markers of bone resorption than men without fractures.

In a recent study, fractures were evaluated in 181 consecutive men receiving ADT for prostate cancer [24]. Eighty percent of men survived for 10 years on ADT without a clinical fracture. Duration of ADT of was significantly associated with increased fracture risk. Black race and increased body mass index were significantly associated with decreased fracture risk.

Several studies have prospectively evaluated the effect of ADT on BMD [25–30]. ADT decreases BMD by 5–10% during the first year, a rate that exceeds bone loss associated with menopause [7]. Other factors including vitamin D deficiency and insufficient dietary intake of calcium may contribute to bone loss in men with prostate cancer [10].

Some but not all men develop osteoporosis during ADT. Baseline BMD varies between men due to individual differences in peak bone mass and adult bone loss prior to ADT. Accordingly, men begin ADT with different relative risks for developing osteoporosis. Although average bone loss is accelerated during ADT, there are also individual differences in rates of treatment-related bone loss. In the study of elderly men with benign prostatic hyperplasia, for example, treatment with a GnRH agonist decreased average BMD by approximately 10% although about one-third of men had little or no bone loss after one year [26].

Prevention and treatment of osteoporosis from ADT

Lifestyle modification including smoking cessation, moderation of alcohol consumption, and regular weight bearing exercise are recommended. Consistent with the National Institutes of Health and Food and Nutrition Board recommendations, dietary calcium intake should be maintained at 1200–1500 mg/day and supplemental vitamin D intake should be 400 IU/day [9]. Some men with prostate cancer are reluctant to take supplemental calcium based on the association between high dietary calcium intake (>2000 mg/day) and increased prostate cancer risk [31,32]. This association has been attributed to decreased conversion of 25-hydroxyvitamin D to the more active 1,25 dihydroxyvitamin D [33]. There is no established causal relationship between calcium intake and prostate cancer risk, however, and no evidence that dietary calcium intake at 1200–1500 mg/day is associated with prostate cancer progression. Moreover, concurrent treatment with supplemental calcium and

382

vitamin D during ADT increases serum concentrations of both 25-hydroxyvitamin D and 1,25 dihydroxy-vitamin D [34].

We recently reported the first randomized controlled study to prevent osteoporosis during ADT for non metastatic prostate cancer [34]. We evaluated pamidronate (Aredia®), an intravenous bisphosphonate known to prevent osteoporosis in other clinical settings. Forty-seven men with locally advanced or recurrent prostate cancer and no bone metastases were randomly assigned to ADT with leuprolide alone or ADT and pamidronate (60 mg intravenously every 12 weeks). Bone mineral densities of posterior–anterior lumbar spine and proximal femur were measured by dual-energy X-ray absorptiometry. Trabecular bone mineral density of lumbar spine was measured by quantitative computed tomography. In men receiving ADT alone, mean ($\pm$SE) bone mineral density decreased by 3.3% in posterior–anterior lumbar spine and 1.8% in total hip, and mean trabecular bone mineral density of lumbar spine decreased by 8.5% after 12 months. In contrast, mean bone mineral density did not change significantly at any skeletal site in men receiving both ADT and pamidronate. Mean changes in bone mineral density at 48 weeks differed significantly between groups in posterior–anterior lumbar spine ($P < 0.001$), trochanter ($P = 0.003$), and total hip ($P = 0.005$). Mean changes in trabecular bone mineral density of lumbar spine also differed significantly between groups ($P = 0.02$). These results indicate that pamidronate prevents bone loss in the hip and lumbar spine during ADT and provide the first demonstration of an effective therapy for prevention of osteoporosis in this setting.

Other bisphosphonates are probably effective but have not yet been evaluated in men during ADT. Alendronate (Fosamax®), an oral bisphosphonate, increases BMD and decreases vertebral fracture in men with osteoporosis and normal or near normal serum testosterone concentrations [35]. Zoledronate (Zometa®) is a third generation bisphosphonate indicated for the treatment of hypercalcemia of malignancy. In a randomized controlled study of men with androgen-independent prostate cancer and bone metastases, zoledronate decreased the incidence of skeletal related events, increased time to first skeletal related event, and increased time to first pathological fracture [36]. Another randomized controlled study will evaluate the effects of zoledronate on BMD and incident vertebral body fractures during ADT for nonmetastatic prostate cancer.

Estrogens and osteoporosis

Estrogens play an important role in male bone metabolism. Low serum estradiol concentrations are associated with decreased spinal BMD and increased vertebral fracture risk in older men [37–40]. Rare genetic defects that cause estrogen deficiency or estrogen resistance are characterized by osteoporosis. Skeletal maturation was delayed and BMD was decreased in a man with complete estrogen resistance due to a mutation in the estrogen receptor-alpha gene [41]. Severe osteoporosis and delayed skeletal maturation was also observed in a man with severe estrogen deficiency due to an inactivating mutation in the aromatase gene [42,43]. Estrogen treatment resulted in skeletal maturation and marked increase in bone density in the latter subject [43].

Medical castration with estrogens is not associated with bone loss in men with prostate cancer. In a nonrandomized study, changes in BMD were evaluated in men with nonmetastatic prostate cancer treated with either orchiectomy ($n = 11$) or estrogens ($n = 16$) [27]. Orchiectomy decreased femoral neck BMD by 10% after one year. In contrast estrogen treatment decreased femoral neck BMD by only 1%. The study should be interpreted cautiously, however, because of the small sample size and nonrandomized study design. Moreover, estrogens are no longer routinely used for ADT because of concerns about cardiovascular toxicity [44,45].

Bicalutamide monotherapy and osteoporosis

Bicalutamide is a nonsteroidal antiandrogen that competitively inhibits the action of androgens by binding to androgen receptors in the target tissue. Bicalutamide (50 mg by mouth daily) is indicated for use in combination with a GnRH agonist to treat metastatic prostate cancer. Monotherapy with bicalutamide (150 mg by mouth daily) has been compared to ADT in three randomized controlled clinical trials [46–48]. In men with locally advanced prostate cancer and no distant metastases, overall survival with bicalutamide monotherapy was similar to ADT. The most common adverse experiences with bicalutamide monotherapy are breast tenderness and enlargement. Men treated with bicalutamide monotherapy report less vasomotor flushing, less fatigue, and more sexual interest than men treated with GnRH agonists.

Bicalutamide monotherapy increases serum concentrations of testosterone and estradiol by 66% [49]. In contrast, ADT with a GnRH agonist decreases estradiol concentrations by 77% [34]. Because estrogens are important determinants of BMD and fracture risk in men, bicalutamide monotherapy may lack the adverse skeletal effects of ADT. Consistent with this hypothesis, preliminary evidence from a small cross-sectional study suggests that bicalutamide monotherapy maintains BMD in men with prostate cancer [50].

Changes in muscle and fat mass during ADT

Androgens are important determinants of body composition in men. Low serum testosterone concentrations are associated with decreased muscle mass and increased fat mass [51]. Testosterone replacement therapy increases lean body mass in men with hypogonadism due to aging, human immunodeficiency virus infection, and other chronic diseases [52–56]. Some but not all studies have reported that testosterone replacement therapy decreases fat mass in hypogonadal men [52,56,57].

Changes in body composition are generally recognized as adverse effects of ADT for prostate cancer although the effects of ADT on body composition are not well defined. Gonadotropin-releasing hormone agonist treatment increased weight and fat mass in ten men with locally advanced or metastatic prostate cancer [58]. Pretreatment weight loss and symptomatic metastatic disease, however, make it difficult to determine whether the reported body composition changes were due to hypogonadism or treatment-related improvements in cancer symptoms. In another study of 22 men with advanced prostate cancer, gonadotropin-releasing hormone agonist treatment increased fat mass and decreased lean body mass after 3 months [59].

We recently evaluated the effects of initial treatment with a GnRH agonist on body composition in asymptomatic men with nonmetastatic prostate cancer [60]. Forty men with locally advanced or recurrent prostate cancer, no radiographic evidence of metastases, and no prior ADT were treated with leuprolide 3-month depot intramuscularly every 12 weeks for 48 weeks. The main outcome measures were percentage changes in weight, percentage fat body mass, percentage lean body mass, fat distribution, and muscle size after 48 weeks. Body composition was measured by anthropometry, dual-energy X-ray absorptiometry, and quantitative computed tomography. Thirty-two subjects were evaluable. Serum testosterone concentrations decreased by 96% ($P < 0.001$). Weight increased by 2.4% ($P = 0.005$). Percentage fat body mass increased by 9.4% ($P < 0.001$) and percentage lean body mass decreased by 2.7% ($P < 0.001$). Cross-sectional areas of the abdomen and abdominal subcutaneous fat increased by 3.9% ($P = 0.003$) and 11.1% ($P = 0.003$), respectively. In contrast, cross-sectional area of intra-abdominal fat did not change significantly ($P = 0.94$). Cross-sectional paraspinal muscle area decreased by 3.2% ($P = 0.02$). These observations indicate that GnRH agonists increase weight and percentage fat body mass and decrease percentage lean body mass and muscle size in men with nonmetastatic prostate cancer. Increased fatness resulted primarily from accumulation of subcutaneous rather than intra-abdominal adipose tissue. Because these men had neither distant metastases nor disease-related symptoms, the marked changes in body composition changes represent an adverse effect of treatment rather than an improvement in disease-related symptoms.

Androgen deprivation therapy is associated with fatigue, loss of energy, emotional distress, and lower overall quality of life [61–63]. Treatment-related increases in fat mass and decreases in lean body mass may contribute to the adverse effects of ADT on physical function and quality of life. Additional studies are needed to determine whether diet, exercise, or alternative forms of hormonal therapy can diminish these adverse body composition changes.

Conclusions

Androgen deprivation therapy by bilateral orchiectomy or prolonged administration of a gonadotropin-releasing hormone agonist accelerates bone loss and increases fracture risk in men with prostate cancer. Other factors including diet and lifestyle may contribute to bone loss during ADT. Some but not all men develop osteoporosis and fractures during ADT. Lifestyle modification including smoking cessation, moderation of alcohol consumption, and regular weight bearing exercise are recommended. Supplemental calcium and vitamin D are also recommended. Pamidronate prevents bone loss during ADT. Other bisphosphonates are probably effective but have not been evaluated in this clinical setting. ADT increases

384

fat mass and decreases lean body mass and these body composition changes may contribute to decreases in quality of life. Additional research is needed to determine the best strategies to treat or prevent treatment-related osteoporosis and other adverse body composition changes in men with prostate cancer.

References

1. Siddiqui NA, Shetty KR, Duthie EH Jr: Osteoporosis in older men: Discovering when and how to treat it. Geriatrics 54: 20–22, 27–28, 30, 1999
2. Seeman E: The structural basis of bone fragility in men. Bone 25: 143–147, 1999
3. Cummings SR, Black DM, Nevitt MC, Browner WS, Cauley JA, Genant HK, Mascioli SR, Scott JC, Seeley DG, Steiger P: Appendicular bone density and age predict hip fracture in women. The study of osteoporotic fractures research group. JAMA 263: 665–668, 1990
4. Cummings SR, Black DM, Nevitt MC, Browner W, Cauley J, Ensrud K, Genant HK, Palermo L, Scott J, Vogt TM: Bone density at various sites for prediction of hip fractures. The study of osteoporotic fractures research group. Lan 341: 72–75, 1993
5. Gardsell P, Johnell O, Nilsson BE: The predictive value of forearm bone mineral content measurements in men. Bone 11: 229–232, 1990
6. Seeley DG, Browner WS, Nevitt MC, Genant HK, Scott JC, Cummings SR: Which fractures are associated with low appendicular bone mass in elderly women? The study of osteoporotic fractures research group. Ann Intern Med 115: 837–842, 1991
7. Eastell R: Treatment of postmenopausal osteoporosis. N Engl J Med 338: 736–746, 1998
8. Kanis JA, Melton LJ 3rd, Christiansen C, Johnston CC, Khaltaev N: The diagnosis of osteoporosis. J Bone Miner Res 9: 1137–1141, 1994
9. Bilezikian JP: Osteoporosis in men. J Clin Endocrinol Metab 84: 3431–3434, 1999
10. Smith MR, McGovern FJ, Fallon MA, Schoenfeld D, Kantoff PW, Finkelstein JS: Low bone mineral density in hormone-naive men with prostate carcinoma. Cancer 91: 2238–2245, 2001
11. Szulc P, Marchand F, Duboeuf F, Delmas PD: Cross-sectional assessment of age-related bone loss in men: The MINOS study. Bone 26: 123–129, 2000
12. Snyder PJ, Peachey H, Berlin JA, Hannoush P, Haddad G, Dlewati A, Santanna J, Loh L, Lenrow DA, Holmes JH, Kapoor SC, Atkinson LE, Strom BL: Effects of testosterone replacement in hypogonadal men. J Clin Endocrinol Metab 85: 2670–2677, 2000
13. Zojer N, Keck AV, Pecherstorfer M: Comparative tolerability of drug therapies for hypercalcaemia of malignancy. Drug Saf 21: 389–406, 1999
14. Zmuda JM, Cauley JA, Glynn NW, Finkelstein JS: Posterior–anterior and lateral dual-energy X-ray absorptiometry for the assessment of vertebral osteoporosis and bone loss among older men. J Bone Miner Res 15: 1417–1424, 2000
15. Finkelstein JS, Cleary RL, Butler JP, Antonelli R, Mitlak BH, Deraska DJ, Zamora-Quezada JC, Neer RM: A comparison of lateral versus anterior–posterior spine dual energy X-ray absorptiometry for the diagnosis of osteopenia. J Clin Endocrinol Metab 78: 724–730, 1994
16. Grampp S, Jergas M, Gluer CC, Lang P, Brastow P, Genant HK: Radiologic diagnosis of osteoporosis. Current methods and perspectives. Radiol Clin North Am 31: 1133–1145, 1993
17. Pacifici R, Rupich R, Griffin M, Chines A, Susman N, Avioli LV: Dual energy radiography versus quantitative computer tomography for the diagnosis of osteoporosis. J Clin Endocrinol Metab 70: 705–710, 1990
18. Delmas PD, Eastell R, Garnero P, Seibel MJ, Stepan J: The use of biochemical markers of bone turnover in osteoporosis. Committee of scientific advisors of the international osteoporosis foundation. Osteoporos Int 11: S2–S17, 2000
19. Schutte HE, Park WM: The diagnostic value of bone scintigraphy in patients with low back pain. Skeletal Radiol 10: 1–4, 1983
20. Orwoll ES: Osteoporosis in men. Endocrinol Metab Clin North Am 27: 349–367, 1998
21. Daniell HW: Osteoporosis after orchiectomy for prostate cancer. J Urol 157: 439–444, 1997
22. Townsend MF, Sanders WH, Northway RO, Graham SD Jr: Bone fractures associated with luteinizing hormone-releasing hormone agonists used in the treatment of prostate carcinoma. Cancer 79: 545–550, 1997
23. Hatano T, Oishi Y, Furuta A, Iwamuro S, Tashiro K: Incidence of bone fracture in patients receiving luteinizing hormone-releasing hormone agonists for prostate cancer. BJU Int 86: 449–552, 2000
24. Oefelein MG, Ricchuiti V, Conrad W, Seftel A, Bodner D, Goldman H, Resnick M: Skeletal fracture associated with androgen suppression induced osteoporosis: The clinical incidence and risk factors for patients with prostate cancer. J Urol 166: 1724–1728, 2001
25. Burton BT, Foster WR, Hirsch J, Van Itallie TB: Health implications of obesity: An NIH Consensus Development Conference. Int J Obes 9: 155–170, 1985
26. Goldray D, Weisman Y, Jaccard N, Merdler C, Chen J, Matzkin H: Decreased bone density in elderly men treated with the gonadotropin-releasing hormone agonist decapeptyl (D-Trp6-GnRH). J Clin Endocrinol Metab 76: 288–290, 1993
27. Eriksson S, Eriksson A, Stege R, Carlstrom K: Bone mineral density in patients with prostatic cancer treated with orchidectomy and with estrogens. Calcif Tissue Int 57: 97–99, 1995
28. Diamond T, Campbell J, Bryant C, Lynch W: The effect of combined androgen blockade on bone turnover and

bone mineral densities in men treated for prostate carcinoma: Longitudinal evaluation and response to intermittent cyclic etidronate therapy. Cancer 83: 1561–1566, 1998

29. Maillefert JF, Sibilia J, Michel F, Saussine C, Javier RM, Tavernier C: Bone mineral density in men treated with synthetic gonadotropin-releasing hormone agonists for prostatic carcinoma. J Urol 161: 1219–1222, 1999

30. Daniell HW, Dunn SR, Ferguson DW, Lomas G, Niazi Z, Stratte PT: Progressive osteoporosis during androgen deprivation therapy for prostate cancer. J Urol 163: 181–186, 2000

31. Giovannucci E, Rimm EB, Wolk A, et al.: Calcium and fructose intake in relation to risk of prostate cancer. Cancer Res 58: 442–447, 1998

32. Chan JM, Giovannucci E, Andersson SO, Yuen J, Adami HO, Wolk A: Dairy products, calcium, phosphorous, vitamin D, and risk of prostate cancer (Sweden). Cancer Causes Control 9: 559–566, 1998

33. Giovannucci E: Dietary influences of 1,25(OH)2 vitamin D in relation to prostate cancer: A hypothesis. Cancer Causes Control 9: 567–582, 1998

34. Smith MR, McGovern FJ, Zietman AL, et al.: Pamidronate to prevent bone loss in men receiving gonadotropin releasing hormone agonist therapy for prostate cancer. N Engl J Med 345: 948–955, 2001

35. Orwoll E, Ettinger M, Weiss S, Miller P, Kendler D, Graham J, Adami S, Weber K: Alendronate for the treatment of osteoporosis in men. N Engl J Med 343: 604–610, 2000

36. Novartis-Oncology. Data on file. 2001

37. Slemenda CW, Longcope C, Zhou L, Hui SL, Peacock M, Johnston CC: Sex steroids and bone mass in older men. Positive associations with serum estrogens and negative associations with androgens. J Clin Invest 100: 1755–1759, 1997

38. Khosla S, Melton LJ 3rd, Atkinson EJ, O'Fallon WM, Klee GG, Riggs BL: Relationship of serum sex steroid levels and bone turnover markers with bone mineral density in men and women: A key role for bioavailable estrogen. J Clin Endocrinol Metab 83: 2266–2274, 1998

39. Greendale GA, Edelstein S, Barrett-Connor E: Endogenous sex steroids and bone mineral density in older women and men: The Rancho Bernardo Study. J Bone Miner Res 12: 1833–1843, 1997

40. Barrett-Connor E, Mueller JE, von Muhlen DG, Laughlin GA, Schneider DL, Sartoris DJ: Low levels of estradiol are associated with vertebral fractures in older men, but not women: The Rancho Bernardo Study. J Clin Endocrinol Metab 85: 219–223, 2000

41. Smith EP, Boyd J, Frank GR, Takahashi H, Cohen RM: Estrogen resistance caused by a mutation in the estrogen-receptor gene in a man. N Engl J Med 331: 1056–1061, 1994

42. Morishima A, Grumbach MM, Simpson ER, Fisher C, Qin K: Aromatase deficiency in male and female siblings caused by a novel mutation and the physiological role of estrogens. J Clin Endocrinol Metab 80: 3689–3698, 1995

43. Bilezikian JP, Morishima A, Bell J, Grumbach MM: Increased bone mass as a result of estrogen therapy in a man

44. Robson M, Dawson N: How is androgen-dependent metastatic prostate cancer best treated? Hematol Oncol Clin North Am 10: 727–747, 1996

45. Moul JW: Hormonal therapy options for biochemical recurrence of prostate cancer after local therapy. Mol Urol 4: 267–272, 2000

46. Iversen P, Tyrrell CJ, Kaisary AV, Anderson JB, Baert L, Tammela T, Chamberlain M, Carroll K: Casodex (bicalutamide) 150-mg monotherapy compared with castration in patients with previously untreated nonmetastatic prostate cancer: Results from two multicenter randomized trials at a median follow-up of 4 years. Urology 51: 389–396, 1998

47. Tyrrell CJ, Kaisary AV, Iversen P, et al.: A randomised comparison of 'Casodex' (bicalutamide) 150 mg monotherapy versus castration in the treatment of metastatic and locally advanced prostate cancer. Eur Urol 33: 447–456, 1998

48. Boccardo F, Rubagotti A, Barichello M, et al.: Bicalutamide monotherapy versus flutamide plus goserelin in prostate cancer patients: Results of an Italian prostate cancer project study. J Clin Oncol 17: 2027–2038, 1999

49. Verhelst J, Denis L, Van Vliet P, et al.: Endocrine profiles during administration of the new non-steroidal anti-androgen Casodex in prostate cancer. Clin Endocrinol (Oxf) 41: 525–530, 1994

50. Abrahamsson PA: Treatment of locally advanced prostate cancer – a new role for antiandrogen monotherapy? Eur Urol 39: 22–28, 2001

51. Vermeulen A, Goemaere S, Kaufman JM: Testosterone, body composition and aging. J Endocrinol Invest 22: 110–116, 1999

52. Snyder PJ, Peachey H, Hannoush P, Berlin JA, Loh L, Lenrow DA, Holmes JH, Dlewati A: Effect of testosterone treatment on body composition and muscle strength in men over 65 years of age. J Clin Endocrinol Metab 84: 2647–2653, 1999

53. Bhasin S, Storer TW, Javanbakht M, et al.: Testosterone replacement and resistance exercise in HIV-infected men with weight loss and low testosterone levels. JAMA 283: 763–770, 2000

54. Grinspoon S, Corcoran C, Stanley T, Baaj A, Basgoz N, Klibanski A: Effects of hypogonadism and testosterone administration on depression indices in HIV-infected men. J Clin Endocrinol Metab 85: 60–65, 2000

55. Reid IR, Wattie DJ, Evans MC, Stapleton JP: Testosterone therapy in glucocorticoid-treated men. Arch Intern Med 156: 1173–1177, 1996

56. Katznelson L, Finkelstein JS, Schoenfeld DA, Rosenthal DI, Anderson EJ, Klibanski A: Increase in bone density and lean body mass during testosterone administration in men with acquired hypogonadism. J Clin Endocrinol Metab 81: 4358–4365, 1996

57. Bhasin S, Storer TW, Berman N, Yarasheski KE, Clevenger B: Testosterone replacement increases fat-free mass and muscle size in hypogonadal men. J Clin Endocrinol Metab 82: 407–413, 1997

with aromatase deficiency. N Engl J Med 339: 599–603, 1998

386

58. Tayek JA, Heber D, Byerley LO, Steiner B, Rajfer J, Swerdloff RS: Nutritional and metabolic effects of gonadotropin-releasing hormone agonist treatment for prostate cancer. Metabolism 39: 1314–1319, 1990

59. Smith JC, Bennett S, Evans LM, et al.: The effects of induced hypogonadism on arterial stiffness, body composition, and metabolic parameters in males with prostate cancer. J Clin Endocrinol Metab 86: 4261–4267, 2001

60. Smith MR, Finkelstein JS, McGovern FJ, et al.: Changes in body composition during androgen deprivation therapy for prostate cancer. J Clin Endocrinol Metab 87: 599–603, 2002

61. Stone P, Hardy J, Huddart R, A'Hern R, Richards M: Fatigue in patients with prostate cancer receiving hormone therapy. Eur J Cancer 36: 1134–1141, 2000

62. Herr HW, O'Sullivan M: Quality of life of asymptomatic men with nonmetastatic prostate cancer on androgen deprivation therapy. J Urol 163: 1743–1746, 2000

63. Potosky AL, Knopf K, Clegg LX, Albertsen PC, Stanford JL, Hamilton AS, Gilliland FD, Eley JW, Stephenson RA, Hoffman RM: Quality-of-life outcomes after primary androgen deprivation therapy: Results from the Prostate Cancer Outcomes Study. J Clin Oncol 19: 3750–3757, 2001

Address for offprints: Matthew R. Smith, Massachusetts General Hospital, Cox 640, 100 Blossom Street, Boston, MA 02114, USA; *Tel*: (617) 724 5257; *Fax*: (617) 726 4899; *e-mail*: smith.matthew@mgh.harvard.edu

Index

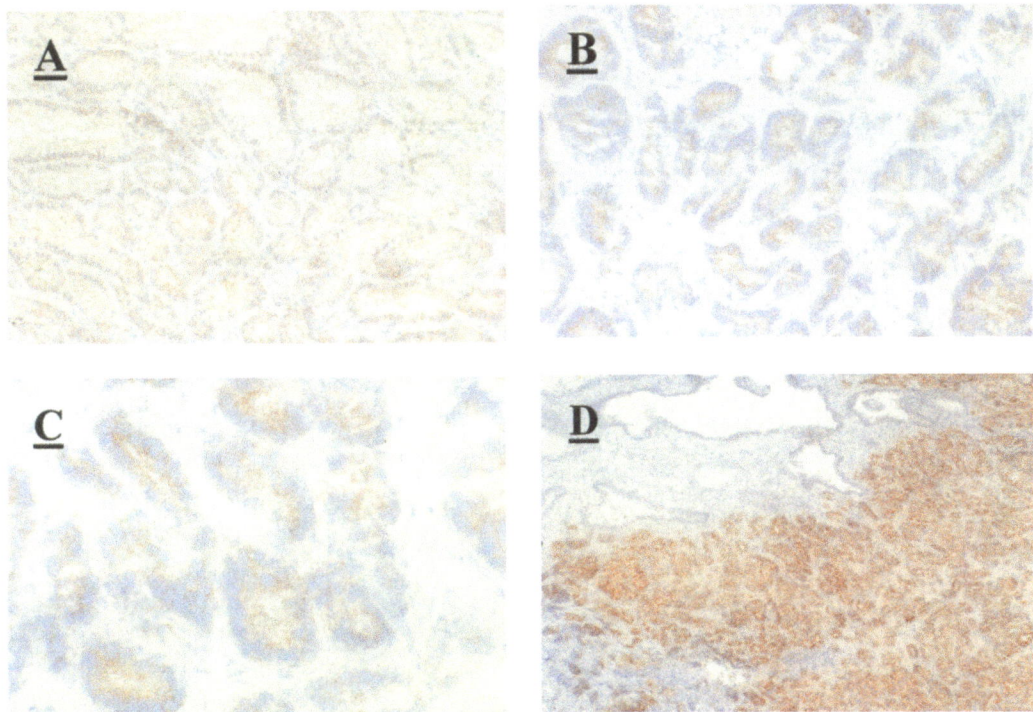

Figure 2. Immunohistochemical staining for 12-LOX in frozen prostate tumor tissues. Sections of frozen specimens were probed with a 12-LOX polyclonal antibody (Oxford Biomedical Research Inc, Oxford, MI). Positive immunoreactivity is indicated by staining with brownish color. A, A low-grade tumor; B,C, intermediate-grade tumor; D, a high-grade tumor.
This figure appears in black/white on page 65.

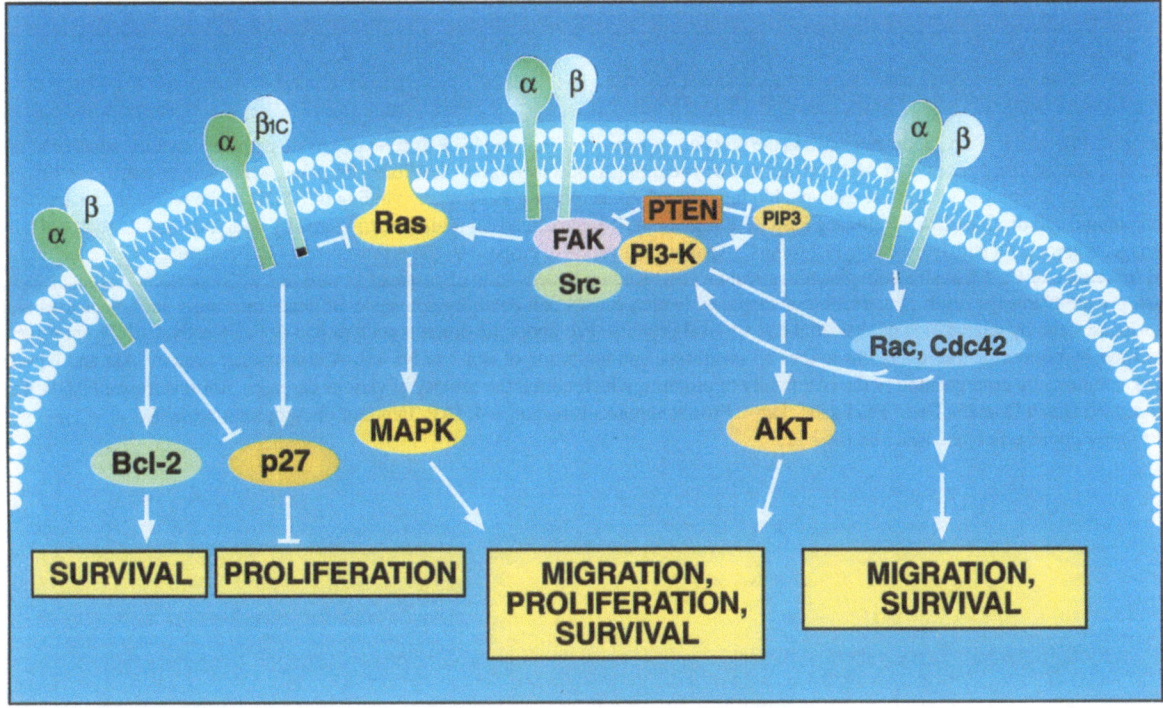

Figure 1. Signaling pathways activated by integrins and altered in prostate cancer. Schematic drawing showing the signal transduction pathways activated by integrins that control cell migration, survival and proliferation; these pathways are altered in prostate cancer. PIP3, phosphatidylinositol (3,4,5) triphosphate. *This figure appears in black/white on page 189.*

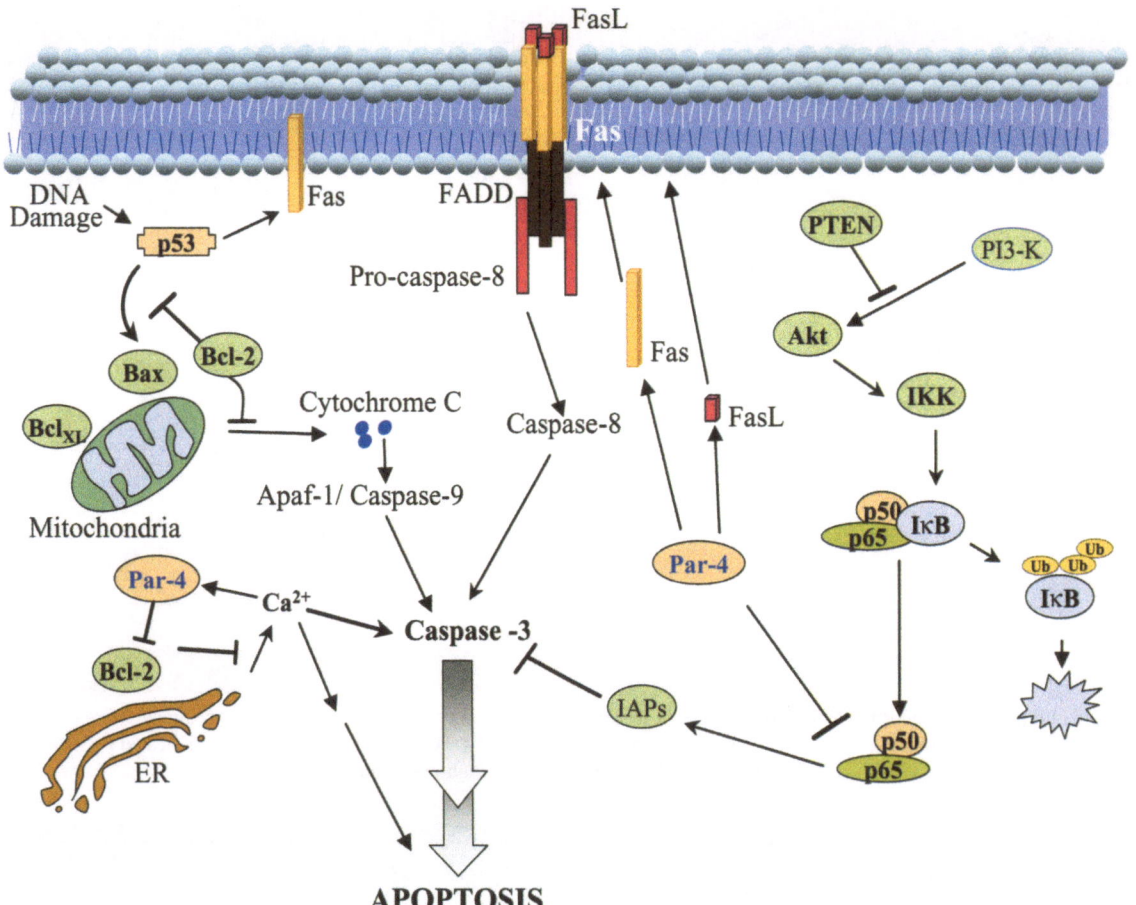

Figure 1. Pro- and anti-apoptotic pathways in the prostate. Apoptosis is initiated by activation of private pathways that are speci c to the type of apoptotic insult or activator. Most private pathways culminate in activation of the effector caspases, which induce cell death. Private pathways: (a) receptor-mediated, for example binding of FasL to its receptor Fas triggers binding of FADD to the receptor and activates the common cell death pathway following caspase-8 activation; (b) mitochondrial initiation, triggered by apoptotic insults such as DNA damage, is associated with release of cytochrome C, Apaf and activation of caspase-9, and is prevented by Bcl-2 members Bcl-2 and Bcl$_{XL}$ and (c) release of Ca^{2+} from the endoplasmic reticulum (ER) leading to activation of caspases as well as Ca^{2+} dependent endonucleases. Most private pathways result in activation of caspase-3 which causes cell death by activation of death mediators such nucleases and translocases and by degradation of structural and survival proteins. Pro-apoptotic proteins such as p53 or Par-4 activate different private pathways by promoting traf cking Fas to the cell membrane and inhibition of Bcl-2 or NF-κB. Anti-apoptotic proteins Akt and NF-κB block apoptosis by up-regulation of the IAP family of proteins, which inhibit the activity of various caspases. *Abbreviations*: FADD: Fas Associated Death Domain, FasL: Fas ligand, Par-4: Prostate apoptosis response-4, IAP: Inhibitor of Apoptosis proteins.
This figure appears in black/white on page 91.

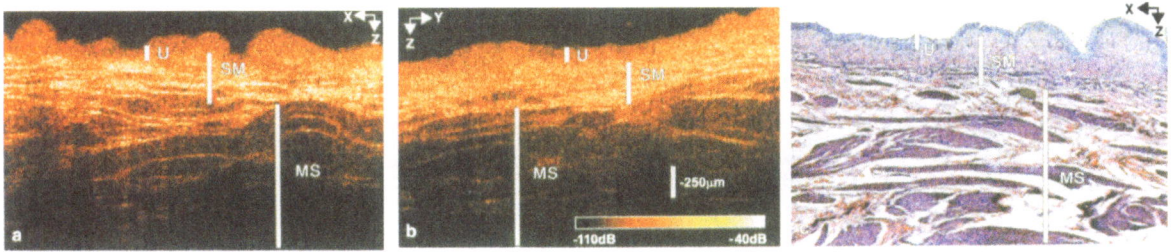

Figure 1. Ex vivo two-dimensional Optical Coherence Tomography (OCT) images of fresh porcine bladder. OCT images from the surface down, much like an ultrasound image, yielding a two-dimensional image of surface position and the tissue at depth. The structures seen in the OCT images (right) correspond to those seen in the H&E panel (left). Image size 4 mm × 4 mm. The urothelium (U), submucosa (SM) and muscularis (MS) layer of the urinary bladder wall are clearly seen, as indicated by white bars. Modified from Pan et al. [242].

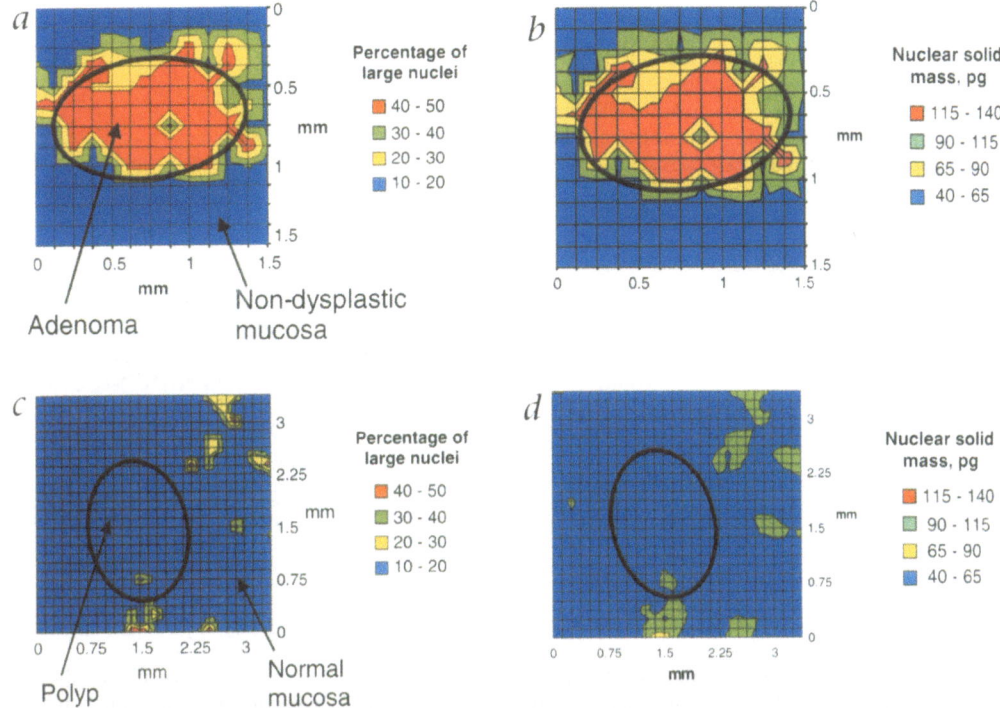

Figure 2. Optical Light Scattering Spectroscopy (LSS) images of nuclear size and density. In these images, (a and b) an adenoma shows as red, having a high percentage of large nuclei and high solid nuclear mass. In contrast, (c and d) a polyp is not visible by percent large nuclei, nor by high nuclear solid mass. These images required about 10 min to collect in a noninvasive, noncontact manner. From Gurjar et al. (2001) [243]. *These figures appear in black/white on page 275.*

394

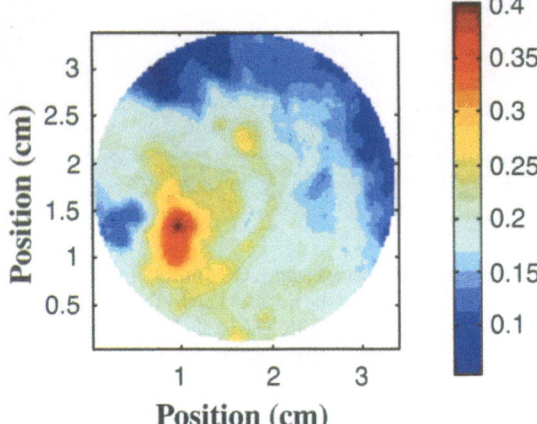

Figure 3. A optical canine breast image made after injection of a fluorescent optical contrast. The image was collected optically. A spontaneous canine mammary tumor shows up as red-dark red, due to retention of the contrast agent in the neovasculature and/or capillary leakage. Image provided by Sevick-Muraca et al. (1999).

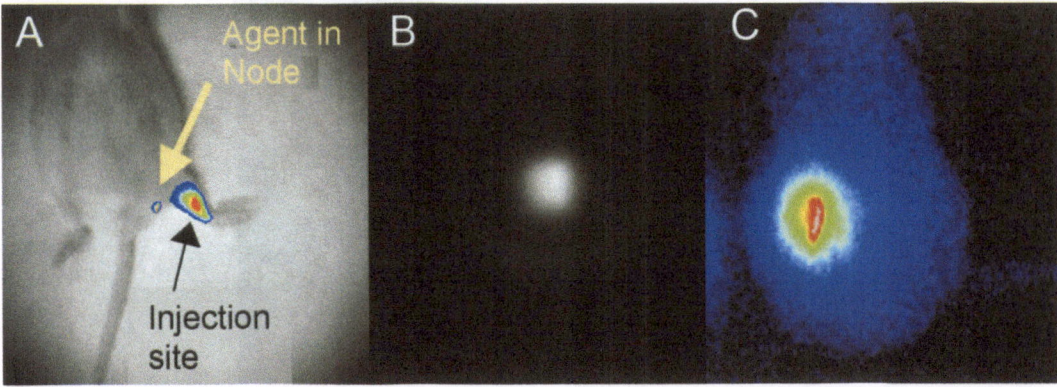

Figure 4. Optical contrast images collected in room light. (A) A subcutaneous injection of PEG conjugated to cyanine dyes for lymphatic tracking shows a lymph node in real time. (B) A 5 mm breast lymph node model at 2 cm depth is seen in real-time in this room light image. (C) One frame from a real-time optical fluorescence cine in which a 5 mm tumor model is imaged in real-time in a moving mouse. Importantly, these images were collected in room light, using a camera developed under National Cancer Institute support allowing trace fluorescence to be imaged in real-time during interventional surgical procedures. Images from Benaron et al. (2001) [65].

These figures appear in black/white on page 276.

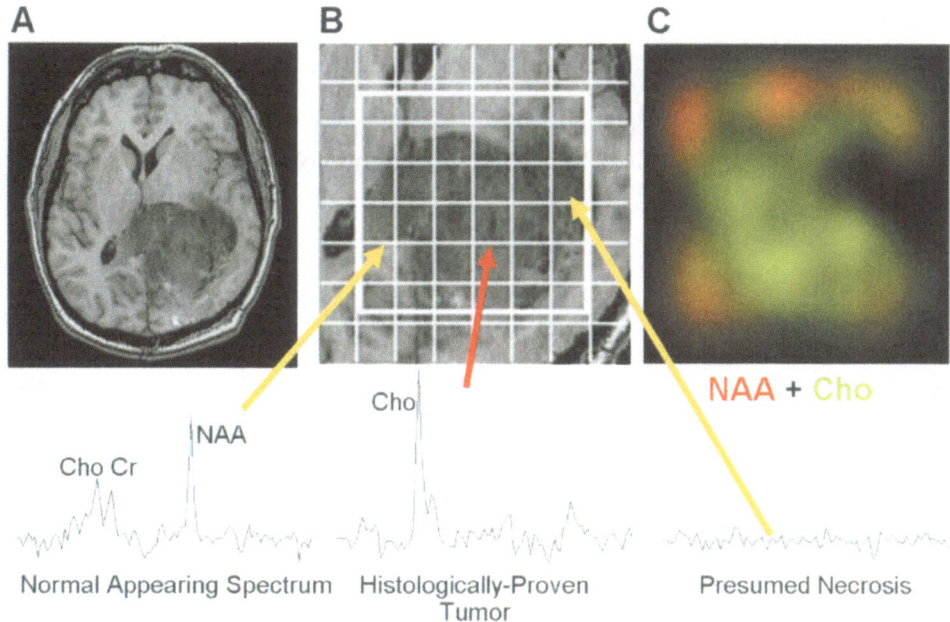

Figure 6. MRSI images from a brain tumor. (A) Conventional MRI image of a brain tumor before surgery. (B) A grid for spectroscopic analysis is overlayed on a region of the MRI scan in A, with MRSI spectra from three regions shown (arrows). (C) NAA is shown in red, choline in green. Regions of solid tumor appear green, normal brain tissue appears red-yellow, and necrotic tissue appears black. Modified from Vigneron et al. (2001) [82].

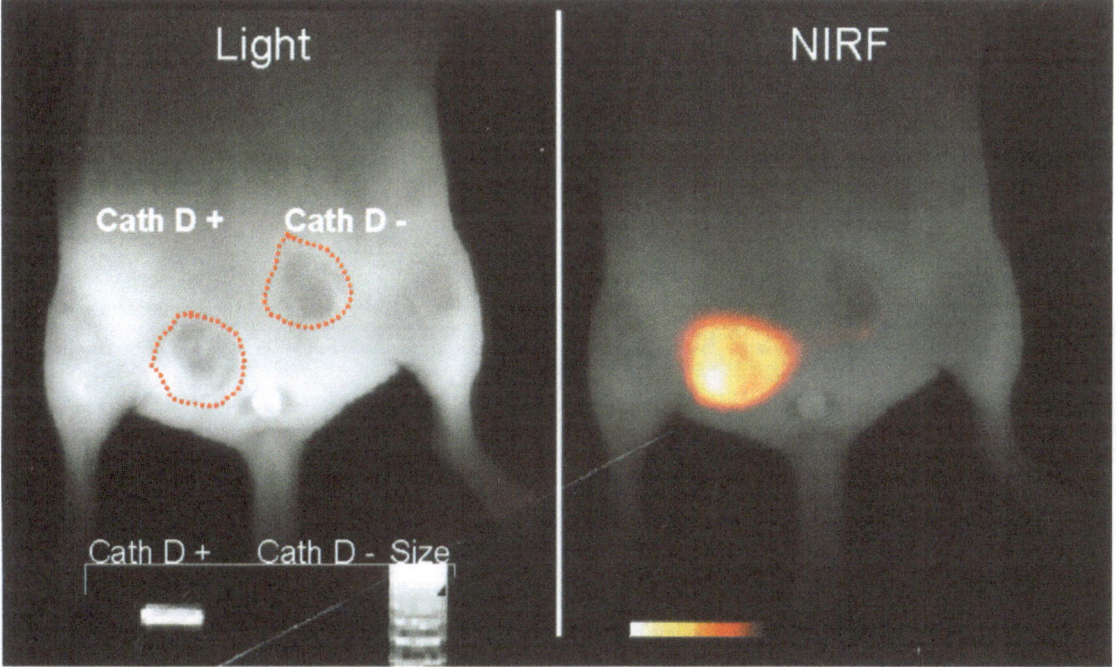

Figure 7. An activatable near-infrared fluorescent (NIRF) probe which is cleaved and activates in the presence of Cathepsin D. (Left) White light image showing the location of two tumors. (Right) Noninvasive NIRF image of dye activation *in vivo.* From Tung et al., *Cancer Research* (2001) [93]. *These figures appear in black/white on page 280.*

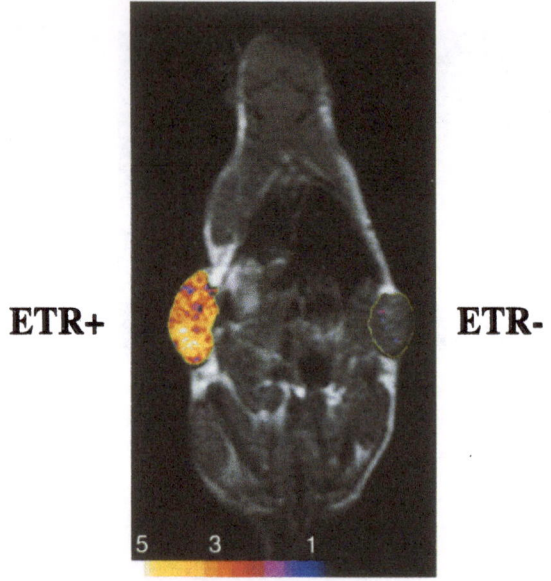

ETR+   **ETR-**

Figure 8. In vivo T1-weighted MR imaging of genetic expression. In this image, an engineered transferrin receptor (ETR) is transfected and expressed in a tumor cell line, which becomes detectable when a paramagnetic transferrin ligand probe is injected. (Left) With ETR expression, addition of the transferrin ligand produces a strong signal. (Right) In the absence of ETR expression, a control tumor does not enhance with ligand injection. From Weissleder et al. (2000) [244].

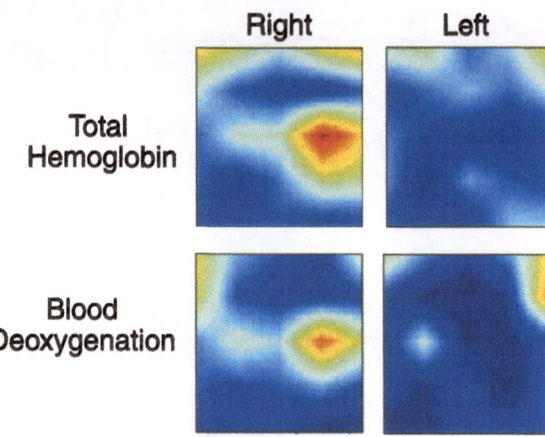

Figure 11. Breast model total hemoglobin and oxygenation imaged using a fast optical system developed by Chance et al. The right breast (with a suspicious lesion) shows a region of increased total hemoglobin and blood deoxygenation. The left breast (with no suspicious area) shows no comparable lesion. Image provided by Chance et al. (1999).
This figure appears in black/white on page 287.

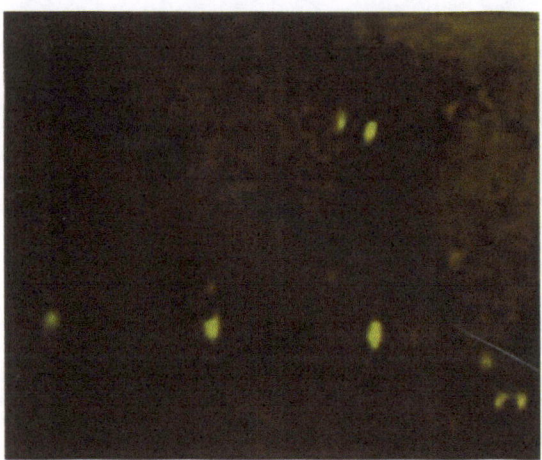

Figure 9. In vivo optical tracking and imaging of single glioma cells constitutively expressing GFP. The ability to externally image and identify single glioma cells labeled with GFP *in vivo* illustrates the power and sensitivity of optical techniques. From Yang et al. (2002) [103].
These figures appear in black/white on page 281.

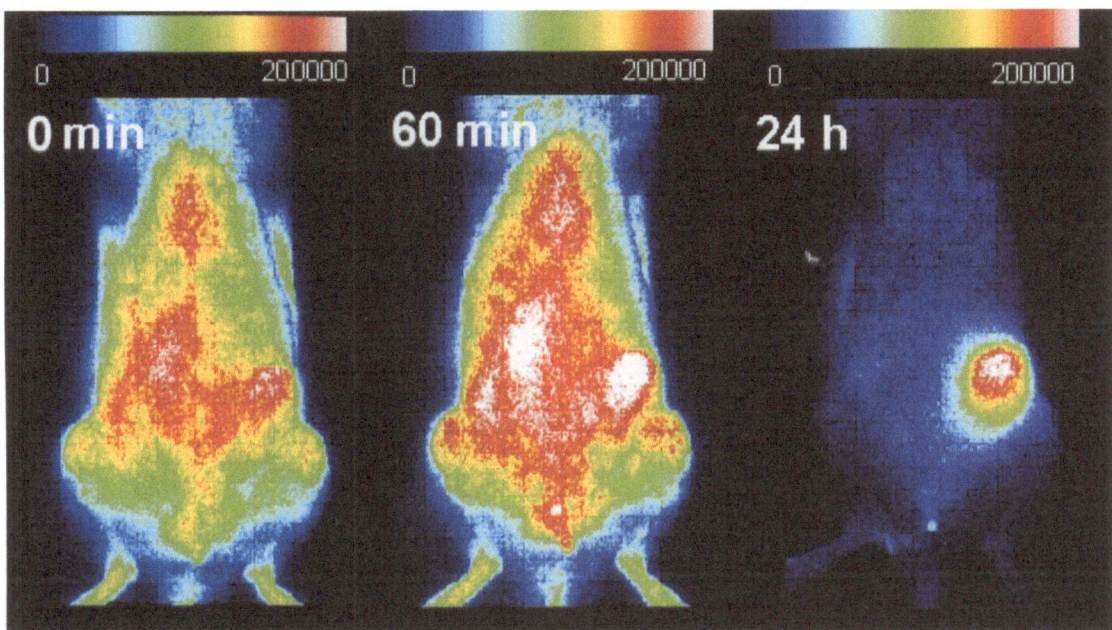

Figure 13. Optical image of a cyanine dye leaking from the vasculature in a mouse. Images obtained of MTLn-3 breast tumor in a rat, labeled by i.v. injection of optical contrast at 1 min, 60 min, and 24 h post-injection. Image provided by Licha et al. (2000).

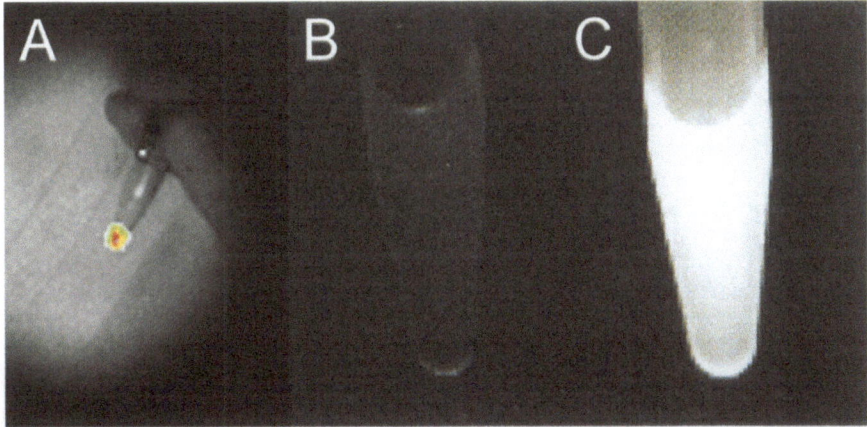

Figure 14. Two targeted optical dyes. (A) An antigenically targeted fluorescent dye, produced by our group for human use and targeted toward PSMA, as seen using a camera we developed for room light use. The concentration of dye in the tube is similar to that which can be achieved in tissue, or 1000 copies per cell. (B) A tube of enzymatically activatable optical dye, in which fluorescence is self-quenched prior to cleavage of a protein linkage by Caspase-3, after which the fluorescent substantially increases. (C) The dye is fluorescent in the presence of Caspase-3. In the presence of a Caspase-3 inhibitor, the activatable dye does not become fluorescent. (A) from Benaron et al. (2000) [67], (B) and (C) modified from Tung CH [93], in Weissleder et al. (2001) [85].

These figures appear in black/white on page 290.

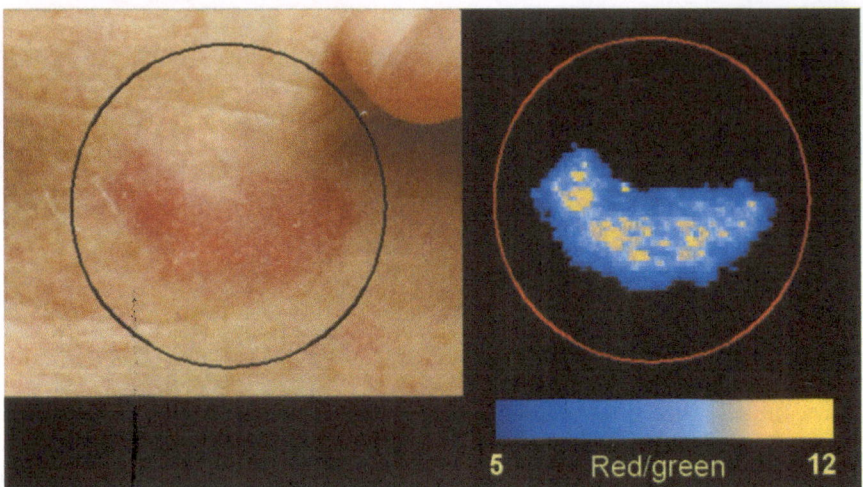

Figure 15. Photofrin® (porfimer sodium), a mixture of porphyrin derivatives used in photodynamic therapy, preferentially accumulates in metabolically active tissue, such as melanomas. (Left) A cutaneous human melanoma as seen by eye in room light after injection of Photofrin®, prior to photodynamic therapy treatment. (Right) A fluorescence red : green ratio image, demonstrating image contrast achieved based upon porphyrin trapping in the actively metabolic cutaneous melanoma. Using newer imaging techniques, this approach should be possible *in vivo* at depths of up to 4–6 cm. Image provided by Klinteberg and Svanberg, Lund (1999).

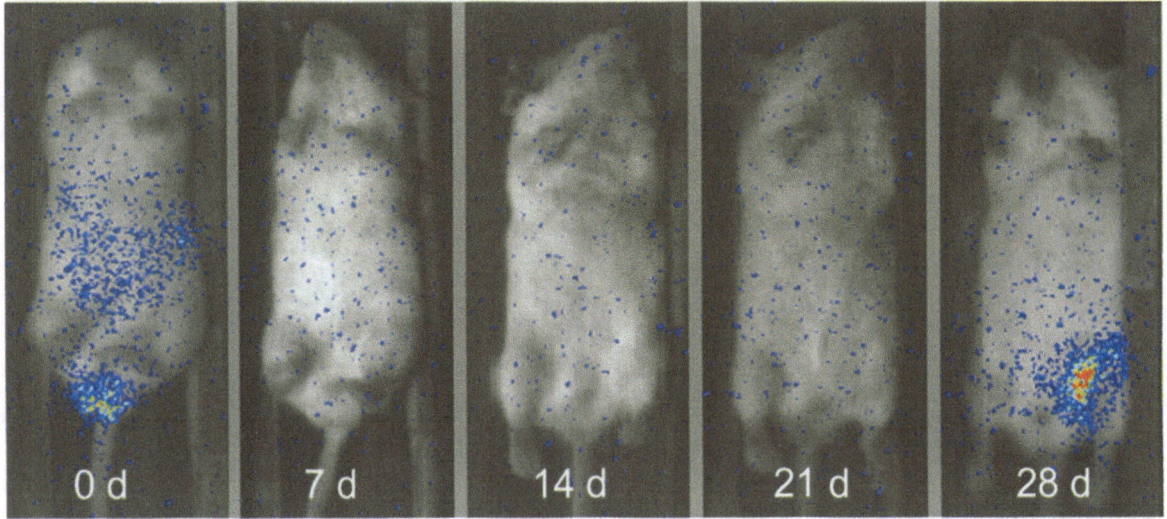

Figure 16. Quantitative imaging of tumor response using luciferase. An intraperitoneal tumor, labeled with luciferase, is injected by tail vein on day 0. During treatment with Cisplatin, the optical signal regresses, and then resurges on day 28, consistent with the development of resistance. Cell counts of under 1000 cells can be detected and imaged in 5 min. Image from Edinger et al. (2000) [9].
These figures appear in black/white on page 291.

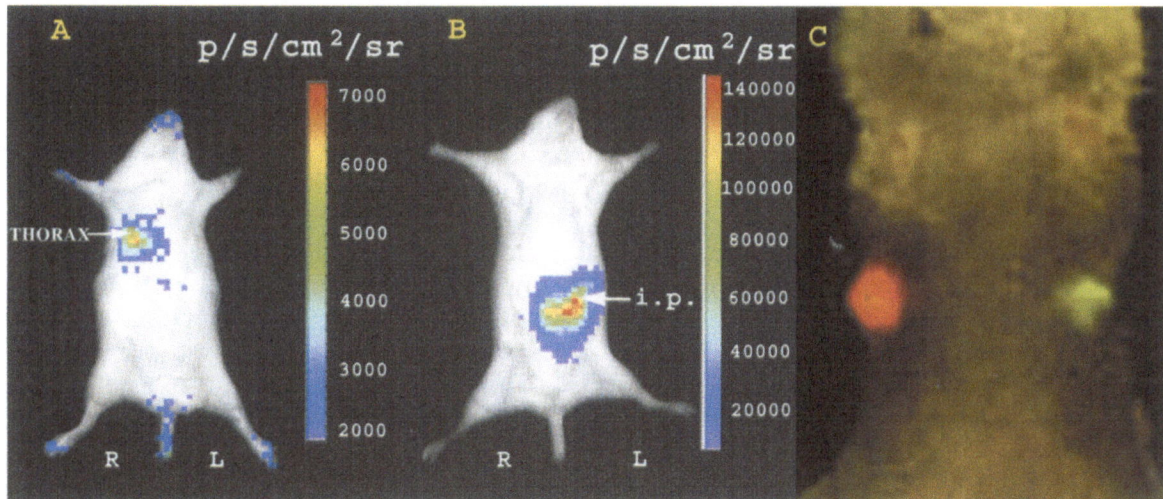

Figure 17. Dual optical reporter systems allow two molecular or genetic pathways to be simultaneously and independently monitoring using optical imaging. In this system, a dual reporter system in shown in which (A) a thoracic Renilla luciferase reporter and (B) an intraperitoneal firefly luciferase reporter can be independently switched on and off, with clear separation of the signals. From Bhaumik et al. (2002) [230]. (C) red and green fluorescent protein signals can be separated by wavelength, even when simultaneously produced. "From Anticancer [169]".

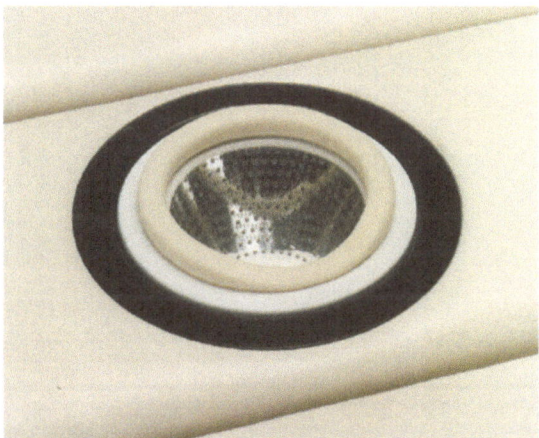

Figure 18. The breast imaging cup of a prototype commercial imaging device for the breast. The cup is filled with an index-matching solution, and the breast is suspended in the cup while the patient lies prone on the imaging table. Image provided by van der Mark, Philips Research (1997) [234].

These figures appear in black/white on page 292.